2nd edition

CHRONIC ILLNESS & DISABILITY

2nd edition

CHRONIC ILLNESS & DISABILITY

Principles for nursing practice

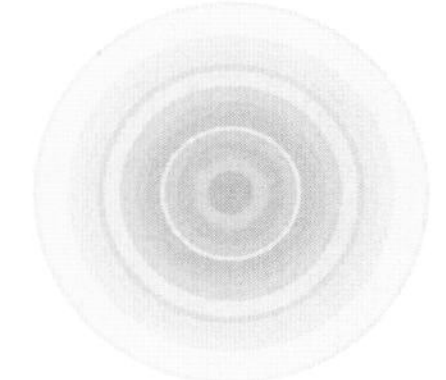

Edited by

Esther Chang

Amanda Johnson

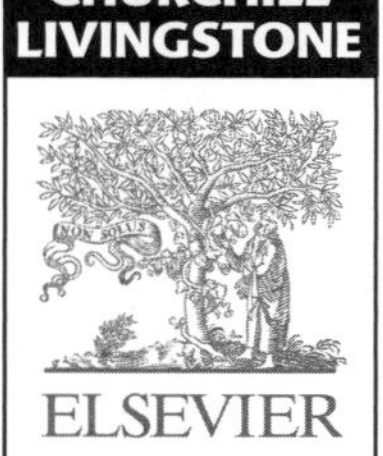

Sydney Edinburgh London New York Philadelphia St Louis Toronto

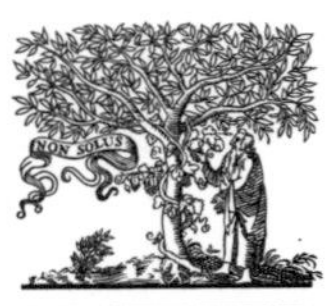

Churchill Livingstone
is an imprint of Elsevier

Elsevier Australia. ACN 001 002 357
(a division of Reed International Books Australia Pty Ltd)
Tower 1, 475 Victoria Avenue, Chatswood, NSW 2067

eISBN: 9780729581615

National Library of Australia Cataloguing-in-Publication Data

---

Chronic illness & disability: principles for nursing practice
/Esther Chang; Amanda Johnson.

2nd edition.
9780729541619 (paperback)
Includes index.

Nursing—Practice.
Chronically ill—Care.
People with disabilities—Care.
Palliative treatment.

Chang, Esther, editor.
Johnson, Amanda, editor.

610.73

Senior Content Strategist: Libby Houston
Content Development Specialists: Liz Coady and Vicky Spichopoulos
Senior Project Managers: Natalie Hamad and Nayagi Athmanathan
Edited by Forsyth Publishing Services
Proofread by Tim Learner
Permissions editor: Sarah Thomas
Cover and internal design by Lisa Petroff
Index by Robert Swanson
Typeset by Toppan Best-set Premedia Limited
Printed in China by China Translation & Printing Services Limited

CONTENTS

PREFACE

This book is developed for undergraduate nursing students, students in the TAFE sector, newly registered nurses and other health professionals who share our commitment to providing quality of care to people with chronic illness and disability. This book is based on principles for practice supported by evidence from Australian and international literature to enhance the understanding of some of the issues and challenges of caring for a person with chronic illness and disability. Across all chapters, the text illustrates a holistic approach highlighting quality of life in all aspects of care for chronic illnesses and disability. Concepts essential for underpinning best practice in self-management of chronic illness and disability are included, such as spirituality, individual education strategies, valuing the person's expertise, resources, culture, minimising socially stigmatising processes and social isolation. Issues affecting carers and family are also addressed. Attention to these concepts recognises the important shift nurses and other health professionals are making towards working in partnership with individuals, their family and carers. Through education and empowerment, individuals, their family and carers are supported in their adjustment and adaptation to chronic illness and disability to achieve optimal outcomes.

This second edition provides new case studies and reflective questions on chronic illness and disability for discussion. Where relevant, the text is supported by current statistics to illustrate key aspects of the discussion. Acquiring the knowledge and skills for people with a chronic illness and/or disability is vital in giving competent care. The reader will find viewpoints that are challenging but at the same time motivating and thought-provoking. The exercises and learning activities that are presented throughout the text offer the reader a range of helpful suggestions in understanding the context. This edition also includes one new chapter in models of management. In addition, each chapter has recommended readings for further exploration.

Nurses and other health professionals in clinical practice and academic roles have been involved in producing this text resource. We hope that readers will find the text scholarly, accessible, reality-based and practically useful. It is a resource intended for every student, practising nurse, educator and administrator in understanding the issues of caring for people with chronic illness and disability. By reading the text, reflecting on the issues and posing possible answers, the reader should be able to gain a comprehensive view of the issues, challenges and opportunities ahead of them in their practice.

We want to acknowledge a number of key people who contributed and assisted us in preparing this 2nd edition for publication. We wish to extend our sincere thanks and appreciation to the contributors for their shared interest and concern with the issues and challenges of caring for people and their families in nursing. This book would not be possible without them. We would like to extend our special appreciation to members of the Elsevier team: Libby Houston, Elizabeth Coady, Vicky Spichopoulos, Natalie Hamad and Nayagi Athmanathan. Elsevier Australia joins us in thanking all the reviewers who were involved in providing invaluable feedback during the development process (listed on page xiii). We would also like to thank our families for their endless support and encouragement through the years. Finally, we'd like to dedicate this important text to our past, present and future students.

Esther Chang
Amanda Johnson

CONTRIBUTORS

Prue Andrus, RN, BSc, MHMQL
Lecturer, Murdoch University, WA, Australia

Samar Aoun, BSc (Hons), MPH, PhD
Professor of Palliative Care, School of Nursing and Midwifery, Curtin University, WA, Australia

Susan Balandin, PhD, FSPAA
Professor of Education Research and Director of the Jessie Hetherington Centre for Educational Research, Victoria University of Wellington, New Zealand

Elizabeth Birchmore, BN, MNP, FACNP
Cardiac Nurse Practitioner, SA Heart Ashford, Tutor UNISA

Michelle Bissett, BAppSc (Hons) Occupational Therapy
Lecturer in Occupational Therapy, University of Western Sydney, NSW, Australia

Gilbert Blandin de Chalain, MPIA, BAppSci (EnvHth), MPlanning
Adjunct Fellow, University of Western Sydney, NSW, Australia

Ann Bonner, PhD, MA, BAppSc (Nurs), Renal Cert, RN, MACN
Professor of Nursing, School of Nursing, Queensland University of Technology, Qld, Australia
Visiting Research Fellow, Department of Renal Services, Royal Brisbane and Women's Hospital, Brisbane, Qld, Australia
Adjunct Professor of Nursing, School of Nursing, Midwifery & Indigenous Health, Charles Sturt University, NSW, Australia

Melissa Bonser, Dip App Sci (Nursing), Grad Cert (Neuroscience Nursing), Grad Cert (Rehabilitation Nursing)
Clinical Nurse Consultant, Brain Injury Unit, Royal Rehabilitation Centre, Sydney, NSW, Australia
Member of Australasian Rehabilitation Nurses Association, Member of Australian College of Nursing

Marina Boogaerts, RN, BHSci (Nursing)
Clinical Nurse Consultant Development and Research, ACT Health, Community Care Program, ACT, Australia

Keryln Carville, RN, STN (Cred), PhD
Professor Primary Health Care and Community Nursing, Silver Chain and Curtin University, Perth, WA, Australia

Esther Chang, RN, CM, DNE, BAppSc (Adv Nur), MEdAdmin, PhD (UNSW), FCN
Professor of Nursing, Director of Higher Degree Research Program, School of Nursing & Midwifery, University of Western Sydney, NSW, Australia

James Daley, Dip Nursing and Health Sciences, Grad Cert (Palliative Care), GradCert (Oncology), Palliative Care CNC, WNLHD
Clinical Nurse Consultant, Palliative Care, Greater Western Area Health Service, Sydney, NSW, Australia

Maree Daly, MClinPsy, MAPS
Education Coordinator, National Ageing Research Institute, Vic, Australia

Patricia M. Davidson, RN, BA, MEd, PhD, FACN, FAHA, FPCNA
Professor & Director, Centre for Cardiovascular and Chronic Care, Faculty of Health, University of Technology, Sydney, NSW, Australia
Professor of Cardiovascular Nursing Research, St Vincent's Hospital, Sydney, NSW, Australia

Bettina Douglas, RN, MMgt, MNPr, MN, Cert Nephrology Dialysis & Transplantation
Nurse Practitioner, Department of Nephrology, Princess Alexandra Hospital, Qld, Australia
Adjunct Senior Lecturer, School of Nursing & Midwifery, University of Queensland, Brisbane, Qld, Australia

Clint Douglas, RN, PhD
Lecturer, School of Nursing, Queensland University of Technology, Qld, Australia

Colleen Doyle, PhD, MAPS
Professor of Aged Care, Australian Catholic University and Catholic Homes, Vic, Australia
Principal Research Fellow, National Ageing Research Institute, Vic, Australia

Vicki Drury, PhD (Monash), MClNsg (CSU), PGCert Psych, Nsg (RMIT), Cert Men's Hlth (Curtin), BHlthSc (Nsg) (WACAE), BA (Ed) (Curtin), OND (Sydney Eye Hosp), RN, RMHN
Principal Consultant, Educare Consulting, Australia Visiting Scholar, The University of Leeds, United Kingdom
Visiting Senior Research Fellow, National University of Singapore

Tinashe Dune, BA (Hons), MPH, PhD
Lecturer in Interprofessional Health Sciences, University of Western Sydney, NSW, Australia

Isabelle Ellis, RN, RM, MPH&TM, PhD
Professor of Nursing, Rural and Regional Practice Development, University of Tasmania, Tas, Australia

Jennifer Evans, EdD, MNSt, BHSc (Nursing), AssocDipArts (VocRehab), RN
Lecturer, School of Nursing, Midwifery and Paramedicine
Australian Catholic University, North Sydney Campus, NSW, Australia

Scott Fanker, Dip Health Sc, BN, MN, MHSM
District Service Manager Mental Health, South Western Sydney Local Health District, NSW, Australia

Susan Gallagher, RN, BEd Nursing, MA (Ed), Cert Leadership in Health Care, MACMHN, MACN
Senior Lecturer, School of Nursing, Midwifery and Paramedicine, Faculty of Health Sciences, Australian Catholic University, NSW and ACT, Australia

Christophe von Garnier, MD
Senior Attending, Department of Pulmonology, Bern University Hospital, Switzerland

Gillian Garrett, RN, Cert Neurosciences, Grad Cert Change Management
Clinical Operations Manager, Spinal Injuries Unit, Royal Rehab Centre Sydney, NSW, Australia

Lynne S. Giddings, RN, RM, PhD
School of Health Care Practice, AUT University, Auckland, Aotearoa/New Zealand

Rhonda Griffiths, AM, RN, RM, BEd (Nursing), MSc (Hons), DrPH
Dean, School of Nursing & Midwifery, University of Western Sydney, NSW, Australia

Christine Haley, RN, CM, GCertWomensHlth, NSWCollNurs, BHSci (Nursing) CSturt MPHC Flinders
Lecturer, School of Nursing, Midwifery & Indigenous Health, Charles Sturt University, Bathurst, NSW, Australia

Karen Hancock, BSc (Psych) (Hons), PhD
Senior Research Psychologist, The Children's Hospital at Westmead, NSW, Australia

Mark Henrickson, PhD, RSW
Associate Professor, Massey University (Albany)

Mark Hughes, BSW (Hons), PhD
Associate Professor, Southern Cross University

Annette James, RN, DipT (secondary), GDAppSci (Nutritional Science)
Nutrition and Health Consultant, Sydney, NSW, Australia

Amanda Johnson, RN, DipT (Ng), MHScEd, PhD
Associate Professor, Director of Academic Programs (Undergraduate), UWS Inherent Requirements Strategy Leader, School of Nursing & Midwifery, University of Western Sydney, NSW, Australia

Anne Kavanagh, BAppSc (Speech Pathology) (Hons)
Senior Speech Pathologist, Cairns Outreach Home and Community Care Allied Health Service, Qld, Australia

Angela Marie Kucia, PhD, BN, MA, Grad Cert Ed
Senior Lecturer, School of Nursing and Midwifery, University of South Australia, SA, Australia
Chest Pain Assessment Nurse, Lyell McEwin Hospital, SA, Australia

Michelle Lincoln, B App Sci (Speech Path), PhD
Professor, Faculty of Health Sciences, The University of Sydney, NSW, Australia

Peter Simon Macdonald, MBBS, FRACP, PHD, MD
Senior Staff Cardiologist, St Vincent's Hospital, Sydney, Australia
Conjoint Professor of Medicine, University of New South Wales, Sydney, NSW, Australia
Head, Transplantation Research Laboratory, Victor Chang Cardiac Research Institute, NSW, Australia

Alan Merritt, RN, BN, MHSc (Education)
Accreditation Manager, Australian Nursing and Midwifery Accreditation Council, ACT, Australia

Geoffrey Mitchell, MBBS, PhD, FRACGP, FAChPM
Professor of General Practice and Palliative Care, University of Queensland, Brisbane, Qld, Australia

Phillip J. Newton, RN, PhD
Research Fellow, Centre for Cardiovascular & Chronic Care, University of Technology, Sydney, NSW, Australia

Stephen Neville, RN, PhD, FCNA (NZ)
Senior Lecturer & Director Postgraduate Programmes, School of Nursing, Massey University, Auckland, New Zealand

Tiffany Northall, Bachelor of Nursing (BN), Master of Nursing Research (MNR), Graduate Certificate Clinical Education
PhD candidate, Registered Nurse, Sydney & South Western Area Health Service, NSW, Australia
Associate Lecturer, University of Western Sydney, NSW, Australia

Louise O'Brien, RN, BA, PhD
Conjoint Professor of Nursing (Mental Health), University of Newcastle, NSW, Australia

Kate O'Reilly, BN, Grad Cert Community Nursing, MA Clinical Rehabilitation
Clinical Nurse Consultant, Royal Rehabilitation Centre Sydney, NSW, Australia

Julie Pryor, RN, RN, BA, GradCertRemoteHlth, MN, PhD
FACN Nursing Research and Development Leader, Royal Rehabilitation Centre Sydney, NSW, Australia
Associate Professor, Flinders University, Adelaide, SA, Australia

Robin Ray, RN, BEd, MHSc, PhD
Senior Lecturer, General Practice and Rural Medicine, James Cook University, Qld, Australia

John Xavier Rolley, RN, BN (Hons), PhD
Senior Lecturer of Nursing, School of Nursing and Midwifery, Deakin University, Vic, Australia

Dianne E. Roy, RN, PhD, FCNA (NZ)
Associate Professor, Department of Nursing, Unitec Institute of Technology, Auckland, New Zealand

Andrew Scanlon, DNP, MN (Nurse Practitioner), MNS, RN, NP, FACN
Lecturer, La Trobe University Clinical School of Nursing, Austin Health Heidelberg, Vic, Australia
Nurse Practitioner (Acute and Supportive care), Department of Neurosurgery, Austin Health Heidelberg, Vic, Australia

Sheree M. S. Smith, RN, BN, Cardiothoracic Cert, MSocPlan & Dev, PhD
Professor of Nursing and Director, Family and Community Health University Research Group, School of Nursing and Midwifery, University of Western Sydney, NSW, Australia
Visiting Professor Centre for Pharmacology and Therapeutics, Division of Experimental Medicine, Department of Medicine, Imperial College, London, UK

Philip A. Stumbles, BSc (Hons), PhD
Senior Lecturer in Pathology, Murdoch University, WA, Australia

Sandy Ward, RN Div 1, MEd, Grad Dip Women's Health, Adv Dip Business Studies
Manager, Templestowe Orchards Retirement Village, Vic, Australia
Joint Head, Transplantation Research Laboratory, Victor Chang Cardiac Research Institute, NSW, Australia

Michelle Woods, BSc-RN, Grad Cert Emergency Nursing, Grad Diploma Health Promotion and Education, MSN-NP, DNSc
Diabetes Nurse Practitioner/Senior Lecturer Tasmanian Department Health and Human Services (DHHS), University of Tasmania (UTAS), School of Nursing and Midwifery (SNM), Tas, Australia

Anthony Wright, BSc (Hons) (UU), GradCertEduc (Qld), MPhtySt (Qld), PhD (QUB)
Professor, School of Physiotherapy and Exercise Science, Curtin University, WA, Australia

Patsy Yates, PhD, RN, FACN
Professor, Queensland University of Technology, Qld, Australia

Lee Zakrzewski, DipOT (NSW), BAppSc (OT), MHlthScEd, HScD
Senior Lecturer in Occupational Therapy, University of Western Sydney, NSW, Australia

REVIEWERS

Jennifer Anastasi, RN, BHSci(N), MPH & TM, GD FET, MEd
Lecturer, School of Health, Charles Darwin University, Darwin, NT, Australia

Robyn Gallagher, RN, BA (Psych), MN, PhD
Associate Professor Chronic and Complex Care, Director, Research Students, Faculty of Health, UTS, NSW, Australia

Linda Goddard, RN BHltSci (Nursing), MEd (SpEd), PhD, MBBS, FRACGP
Senior Lecturer, School Nursing, Midwifery & Indigenous Health, Albury, NSW, Australia

Diana Guzys, RN, BPH, GradDipEd, GradDipAdolHlth&Welf, MN
Lecturer in Nursing, La Trobe Rural Health School, Bendigo, La Trobe University, Vic, Australia

Christine Hallinan, RN, DipAppSc, CertCritCare, MPH (Melb)
PhD Candidate, General Practice and Primary Health Care Academic Centre, Melbourne School of Medicine, The University of Melbourne, Vic, Australia

Sandy McLellan, Master Clinical Practice, Post Graduate Certificate Intensive Care
Lecturer in Nursing CQU, Central Queensland University, Qld, Australia

Karen Missen, RN, PhDstud, MHSc (NursEd), GradDip (ICU), BHSc (Nursing)
Lecturer, Monash University, Melbourne, Vic, Australia

Susan (Sue) Ronaldson, RN, DipNEd, BSc (Hons Class 1), PhD, FACN
Senior Lecturer, Sydney Nursing School, The University of Sydney, NSW, Australia

Natashia Scully, BA, BN, PGDipNSc, MPH, PhD (Candidate), MACN
Lecturer in Nursing, University of New England, NSW, Australia

Haakan Strand, MSocSci, MNP
Senior Lecturer, School of Nursing and Midwifery, The University of Queensland, Qld, Australia

Dean Whitehead, PhD, MSc, BEd, RN
Senior Lecturer, Massey University, Palmerston North, New Zealand

Tara Williams, RN, BPubHlth, GradDipHSM
Lecturer, Department of Rural Nursing & Midwifery, La Trobe University, Vic, Australia

Section 1

Frameworks for chronic illness and disability

CHAPTER 1

Amanda Johnson
Esther Chang

Chronic illness and disability: an overview

Learning objectives

When you have completed this chapter you will be able to:

- discuss chronic illness and disability within the global context
- describe and discuss the factors that contribute to chronic illness and disability in the Australian and New Zealand populations
- identify the challenges that a chronic illness and/or disability present for a person, their family, their caregiver and the wider community
- discuss the models of care and principles of holistic nursing as applied to caring for a person with a chronic illness and/or disability
- outline the role of healthcare professionals in the management of chronic illness and/or disability, with an emphasis on the nurse's role.

Key words

chronic condition, chronic disease, chronic illness, disability, models of care

INTRODUCTION

Nurses, now and into the future, will be exposed to caring for people with a chronic disease and/or disability across a wide range of care settings. This exposure requires nurses to have knowledge of, and the skills in, the principles of nursing practice required to provide optimal care to a person and their family. It is also important that they understand what it means for the person and their family to live with a chronic disease and/or disability. It is from this understanding that the needs of the person and their family can be best met by the nurse and other health professionals. It is the intent of this book, therefore, to give equal emphasis to what it means to live with a chronic disease and/or disability as to gaining specific practice knowledge and skills. The construction of the chapters reflect this emphasis through the case studies presented, highlighting that the person and their family are central to the nurse's understanding of their needs, as they commence on this life altering journey. What follows in Chapter 1 is an overview of the global context of chronic disease and disability followed by information specific to the Australian and New Zealand contexts.

THE GLOBAL PERSPECTIVE OF CHRONIC DISEASE AND DISABILITY

Chronic diseases remain the leading cause of deaths worldwide with projections that they will increase by a further 17% over the next 10 years (World Health Organization [WHO], 2008). These projections will most likely be attributed to: ageing populations; a rise in risk factors and increased survival of previous fatal diseases such as cancer (WHO, 2011a). In 2008, 63% (36 million) of the 57 million deaths that occurred in that year were directly attributed to chronic disease (WHO, 2011a). Nine million of these deaths were in people aged 60 years or younger. In middle to high income countries, chronic diseases were responsible for more deaths than all other causes of death combined (WHO, 2011a, p. 5). The four leading chronic diseases were: cardiovascular disease (48%); cancers (21%); chronic respiratory diseases (12%); and diabetes (3%) (WHO, 2011a, p. 5). In almost all deaths, preventable risk factors underlie the development of one or more chronic diseases and/or contribute to a disability burden (WHO, 2011a, p. 6). The following are the leading global risk factors and the percentage of deaths the factor directly contributes to:

- raised blood pressure (13%)
- tobacco use (9%)
- raised blood glucose (6%)
- physical inactivity (6%)
- overweight and obesity (5%).

(WHO, 2011a, p. 6)

To address these growing concerns about the health status of the world's population, nearly 90% of all countries have some government body responsible for determining targets, treatments and control, prevention and health promotion (WHO, 2011a, p. 8). Of these government departments, 92% have developed at least one policy, plan or strategy to address chronic disease and their risk factors in their country (WHO, 2011a, p. 9). The World Health Organization (WHO, 2008) continues to express that if preventive measures were instituted the number of premature deaths that countries currently experience could be significantly reduced. WHO believes this to be possible through the identification of risk factors, early detection and timely interventions (WHO, 2008). Many countries have tried to address the need for a systematic approach to managing and improving the quality of life for people with chronic disease and/or disability. With increasing numbers of people experiencing a chronic disease and associated mortality rapidly rising, WHO in 2008 released its 2008–2013 Action Plan.

The WHO Action Plan aims to reduce premature mortality and improve quality of life (WHO, 2008). Further, the plan is designed to illustrate the need for investment by countries in preventative strategies to ensure the sustainable socioeconomic development of the world's populations. For the most part, chronic diseases are largely preventable if the four key behavioural risk factors of tobacco use, unhealthy diet, physical inactivity and excess alcohol use (WHO, 2008) are effectively mitigated in an individual's lifestyle. The outcomes of these factors on an individual lead to: increased blood pressure; raised blood glucose levels; higher cholesterol levels; and excess body weight (WHO, 2011a). The basis for a large proportion of chronic disease is the presence of one or more of these outcomes. These outcomes represent a substantial burden on many levels for those individuals afflicted and the communities in which they live. In particular, costs to healthcare systems will continue to rise and many countries will be seriously impacted upon economically (WHO, 2008; 2011a). The Action Plan also requires an increased level of understanding by key stakeholders, of which nurses are one group, to prevent further development of chronic disease through education (WHO, 2005). It is also acknowledged that to best meet the needs of those who live with a chronic disease, evidence-based interventions are also required (Kralik, Paterson, & Coates, 2010; WHO, 2008).

With respect to disability, it is estimated worldwide that more than one billion people live with some form of disability (WHO, 2011b). This figure is expected to rise as a result of the world's ageing populations and the higher presence of disability in older people as well as the global rise of chronic diseases (WHO, 2011b, p. xi). The global impact of disability on communities has only been recently acknowledged by the first world report on disability (WHO, 2011b). This report demonstrates the attitudinal, physical and financial burden a person experiences every day with a disability. Further, this report shows the need for governments to remove the barriers to participation and to provide sufficient funds to allow people with disability access to health, rehabilitation, support, education and employment (WHO, 2011b, p. ix). Finally, the report concludes by illustrating the need for policymakers, researchers, practitioners, advocates and volunteers in disability to work together at local, national and international levels. This is necessary to bring about a reduction of the burden to society, to bring about changes to practice and to value more explicitly the contribution people with disability can make to the productivity of the community.

CHRONICITY AND DISABILITY IN THE AUSTRALIAN AND NEW ZEALAND CONTEXT

Understanding the term 'chronic disease'

Chronic disease is often difficult to define and frequently differing terms are used such as disease, illness, long-term conditions or non-communicable diseases (Australian Institute of Health and Welfare [AIHW], 2012a; Larsen, 2013; WHO, 2011a). However, in the context of chronicity, chronic disease and illness in particular have different meanings. Chronic disease refers to the pathophysiology that gives rise to an alteration in a person's body function and structure (Larsen, 2013). Chronic illness is 'the irreversible presence, accumulation or latency of disease states or impairments that involve the total human environment for supportive care and self-care, maintenance of function and prevention of further disability' (Curtin & Lubkin, 1995, pp. 6–7 as cited in Lubkin & Larsen, 2013, p. 6). While differing terms may be used to denote the same thing, all definitions are based on one or more of the following features (first outlined by the Commission on Chronic Illness) that have led to the impairment or deviation of normal function. These features include variations from normal that:

- are permanent
- leave a residual disability
- are caused by a non-pathological condition

- require special training of the patient for rehabilitation
- require a long period of supervision, observation or care (Mayo, 1956 cited in Lubkin & Larsen, 2013, p. 5).

New Zealand literature most commonly reports on chronic disease using the term 'chronic condition'. The varied use of terms signifies the difficulties health professionals face in determining the point along the illness trajectory line at which a disease becomes chronic (Larsen, 2013).

The term selected for use in this text is 'chronic illness'. This is the preferred term because, while it implies the irreversible presence of a disease state or impairment or disability, it emphasises the totality of the illness as experienced by the person. The term takes account of the resulting impact on all aspects of the person's life and the requirement by health professionals to address the person's needs holistically (Larsen, 2013). The implication therefore for nurses and other health professionals is the need to recognise that all dimensions of personhood are affected by the presence of a chronic disease and/or disability.

Understanding disability

People with disability, like people with chronic illness, have needs that require a range of supportive interventions to promote function and re-engagement with their life (Larsen, 2013). A revised definition of disability was endorsed by WHO to encompass impairments, activity limitations and participation restrictions (WHO, 2002). As a result of this expanded definition the term has moved away from being linked to specific biomedical causes and reoriented to focus on the impact disability has on the person's functioning capacity within their environment. The terms 'disability' and 'chronic disease' are sometimes used interchangeably, depending on the context and the implications for the person (Larsen, 2013, p. 5). Therefore, disability has the potential to be experienced either independently from chronic disease or as a consequence of chronic disease.

Disability in Australia is broadly defined and embraces a 'multidimensional concept relating to impairment in body structure or function, limitation in activities, restriction in participation and the affected persons' environment' (AIHW, 2006, p. 71). Persons are considered to have a disability 'if they have a limitation, restriction or impairment which has lasted, or is likely to last, for at least six months and restricts everyday activities' (Australian Bureau of Statistics [ABS], 2004, p. 20). One in five Australians or 20% of the total Australian population report a disability for both females and males (ABS, 2004, p. 3). Further, one in 17 people (5.9%) have a profound or severe level of core activity limitation, requiring help with self-care, mobility and communication activities (ABS, 2004, p. 3).

In Australia, physical conditions constitute the largest percentage of disability across the lifespan (84%), the remaining 16% consisting of mental or behavioural disorders (ABS, 2004, p. 4). The majority of people with disability report the origin of their disability to have stemmed from an accident or injury (15.2%) followed by disease, illness or hereditary (14%) and work-related conditions (11%) (ABS, 2004, p. 5). In 2003, 61% of people with a disability required assistance to manage their health condition or to cope with everyday activities (ABS, 2004, p. 4). Thirty-seven per cent of primary carers reported that they needed to provide care on an average of 40 hours or more a week and a further 18% indicated that they provided 20–39 hours of care per week, on average (ABS, 2004, p. 8).

The rate of disability increases with age. For example, in 2003 just over 51% of the Australian population reported disability (ABS, 2004, p. 2) while a further 22% reported a profound or severe limitation (AIHW, 2006, p. 215). The rate of increase is demonstrated in the following figures: of those aged 85 years or over, in Australia, 84% indicated the presence of a disability in their lives (ABS, 2004, p. 4) and by 90 years or over this percentage had risen to 92% (ABS, 2004, p. 3). Therefore, in the Australian population and similarly in New Zealand, more people over 65 years of age will have a disability (AIHW, 2006, p. 46) than in all other age groups (ABS, 2004). For this age group the following conditions were most commonly reported as posing a level of disability: arthritis (50%), hearing disorders (43%), hypertension (38%), heart disease (30%) and stroke (23%) (AIHW, 2006, p. 215).

In New Zealand, the term 'disability', as defined by the recent report *Living with Disability in New Zealand*, constitutes 'a long term limitation in the ability to carry out one or more activities' (Ministry of Health, 2005, p. 95). Similarly one in five New Zealanders has a disability, equating to nearly 750 000 people (Ministry of Health, 2012b, p. 1). Of this number 17% are Māori (Ministry of Health, 2012b, p. 1). In the latest report on disability in New Zealand, a new model has been developed focused on keeping people with a disability and their families in their own homes and within their communities (Ministry of Health, 2012b, p. 10). However, the prevalence is slightly lower (59%) for those aged 75 years or older (Ministry for Health, 2005, p. 15). In the New Zealand population 27% of those with disability are Māori and one in five Pacific peoples are children, illustrating the high prominence of Māori and Pacific ethnic groups in the disability population group (Ministry for Health, 2005, p. 8). This is in contrast to the Australian experience, where low levels of disability are found in the younger age groups: 4% of 0–4-year-olds, followed by a steady increase to 41% of 65–69-year-olds and 92% of those aged 90 years and over (ABS, 2004, p. 3). Disease or illness was the most common cause of disability (68% of adults) followed by ageing (37%) (Ministry for Health, 2005, p. 89). Mobility disability was the most commonly experienced disability in New Zealand adults followed by loss of agility and hearing (Ministry of Health, 2005, p. 11). Loss of mobility was identified as the greatest limitation on a person's everyday activity (Ministry of Health, 2005, p. 11). Lack of mobility affects 29% of those aged 65–74 years and 51% of those aged 75 years or over (Ministry of Health, 2005, p. 11).

AUSTRALIAN AND NEW ZEALAND PROFILES OF CHRONIC DISEASE

The populations of Australia and New Zealand both report chronic disease as a growing problem (AIHW, 2012a). The first WHO *Global Status Report on Noncommunicable Diseases* provides a profile for each country's chronic disease status on pages 23 and 136 respectively (WHO, 2011a). These profiles provide an indication of the country's capacity to respond to these diseases, the current mortality in each country and the prevalence of risk factors at the time of the data collection in 2008. With respect to the WHO Action Plan (2011a), the Australian and New Zealand governments have responded to the challenge of enacting the WHO action plan in their own countries by setting targets, developing strategies and formulating plans, some of which are specifically referred to throughout the course of this text.

In Australia chronic disease affects one in four Australians (AIHW, 2006) or, as reported in 2004–05, 77% of Australians had at least one long-term condition (AIHW, 2006, p. ix). In the total population these conditions were asthma (10%), osteoarthritis (7.9%), depression (5.3%) and diabetes (3.5%) (AIHW, 2006, p. ix). It is estimated that the mean number of chronic conditions is more than two for people in Australia aged 60 years and above (National Public Health Partnership [NPHP], 2001, p. 21). The top ten causes of disease burden in Australia consisted of chronic diseases (AIHW, 2005). This represented 43% of the total disease burden in Australia (AIHW, 2005). The Australian Chronic Disease Prevention Alliance estimate that this will increase to approximately 80% of the total disease burden in Australia by 2020 (2004, p. 5). In 2004, 50% of all Australian deaths were directly attributable to a chronic disease, the leading cause of death being coronary heart disease, followed by stroke (AIHW, 2006, p. ix). The profile of major chronic diseases in the Australian population constitutes heart disease, stroke, cancer, diabetes, asthma and osteoarthritis (AIHW, 2006, p. 60). Cardiovascular disease is the most prominent cause of death for 84-year-olds and older people (AIHW, 2012c).

Similarly, New Zealand reports that the most common chronic conditions facing their population include chronic neck or back problems (1 in 4 adults), mental illness (1 in 5 adults), asthma (1 in 5 adults aged 15–44 years), arthritis (1 in 6 adults) and heart disease (1 in 10 adults) (National Health Committee [NHC], 2007, p. 8). The explanation for the current growth of chronic conditions in New Zealand is linked to an increase in lifestyle factors especially tobacco use, low levels of physical activity and poor nutrition, ageing of the general population and social and economic determinants of health (NHC, 2007, p. 9). Chronic conditions in New Zealand are the leading cause of illness and account for more than 80% of deaths in the population (NHC, 2007, p. 8). The Australian and New Zealand patterns of chronic disease are both comparable to those outlined by WHO (2005).

The ageing population is a significant factor in the increasing prevalence of chronic illness and disability in both the Australian and the New Zealand populations. The number and proportion of people 65 years and over has been rapidly increasing in both Australia and New Zealand (AIHW, 2006; NHC, 2007). Correspondingly, the increase in the number and proportion of those aged 85 years and over is even more marked (AIHW, 2006; NHC, 2007). In 2005, more than 2.6 million Australians were aged 65 years and over and the proportion was similar to that of the USA and Canada but much lower than in Japan and Italy (AIHW, 2006, p. 17). The rising percentage of the population aged 65 years and over is a significant factor in the increasing prevalence of chronic illness (AIHW, 2006; NHC, 2007). Those 85 years and over represent 1.5% of the total Australian population while those between the ages of 65 and 84 years represent 13%. In 2005, there were 5178 centenarians and more than 110,000 persons aged over 90 years (AIHW, 2006, p. 17). By 2051, the proportion of the population aged 65 years and over will comprise 25.4% of the total population in New Zealand (NHC, 2007). The ageing process in itself increases the prevalence of co-morbidity and the complexity of chronic illness (NHC, 2007), which needs to be accounted for in the planning of resources and the modalities of care that are provided.

It is important to recognise that the prevalence of chronic disease increases with age (NPHP, 2001). For example, in Australia 80% of people aged 65 years or over have one or more long-term conditions (AIHW, 2006, p. ix). However, of greater concern is the high prevalence of chronic conditions now occurring in the 0–14 years age bracket, not previously seen in the numbers reported: 10% of all children are said to have three or more long-term conditions (AIHW, 2006, p. ix). Lifestyle risk factors are recognised worldwide as playing a significant role in the increasing prevalence of chronic disease over the last century and in the emergence of chronic disease in the child, early adult and middle adulthood age brackets. This is in stark contrast to previous generations (AIHW, 2006; NHC, 2007; WHO, 2005). Of equal concern to the mortality associated with chronic disease is the burden placed on the person, their family and the community by the consequences of their disease process and treatment regimens, and the resulting socioeconomic impact on all (WHO, 2005, p. 39).

Indigenous populations

Worldwide, there are vast disparities in the health of indigenous people and their subsequent experience of chronic illness and/or disability, as compared to non-indigenous

(WHO, 2008). This disparity is attributable to: a life expectancy which is reduced by 10–20 years less than the population; infant mortality 1.5 to 3 times greater than the national average; and a large proportion of indigenous people suffering from malnutrition and communicable diseases (WHO, 2008). Indigenous people's health is further exacerbated by damage to their habitat and resource base (WHO, 2008). In 2008 WHO, in its report *Primary Health Care: Now More Than Ever*, made explicit that health service providers take better account of the lack of services and the disadvantage remoteness plays in indigenous people accessing and achieving the same health status as non-indigenous people. The health disparity presented worldwide is also true for both the Australian and the New Zealand indigenous populations. They are more likely to have an increased presence of chronic disease; to be less healthy; to die at a much younger age; and to have a lower quality of life than non-indigenous people (AIHW, 2012a; Ministry of Health, 2012a). In 2008, Australian indigenous populations were more than twice as likely as non-indigenous people to have a disability (and to have a life expectancy less than 10 years) (Thomson et al., 2011). In New Zealand, the most recently reported figures (2006) show life expectancy for Pacific males were 6.7 years less than total males and for Pacific females it was 6.1 years less than total females (Ministry of Health, 2012a, p. 25). In New Zealand it is estimated that 18 700 Pacific adults had a disability with 43% ($n = 8100$) most likely attributed to chronic disease or illness as the most common cause of their disability (Ministry of Health, 2012a, p. 27).

By way of illustrating the disparity, Australian indigenous peoples are more likely to experience cardiovascular disease 12% more than non-indigenous Australians, were 3.4 times more likely to report some form of diabetes and had a 27% increase of having a respiratory disease (Thomson et al., 2011). In New Zealand the rate of diagnosed diabetes was significantly higher for Pacific men and women (45–64 years age group) than men and women in the total population by approximately 20% and 12% respectively (Ministry of Health, 2012a, p. 43). In terms of respiratory disease, the Ministry of Health (2012a) reports Pacific men are 3 times more likely to present for hospitalisations and Pacific women five times than the total population. The factors identified which contribute to indigenous health are: nutrition; physical activity; body weight; immunisation; breastfeeding; tobacco smoking; alcohol use; and illicit drug use (Thomson et al., 2011; Ministry of Health, 2012a). Indigenous peoples have and continue to experience substantial social disadvantage in relation to their: health through limited education; reduced employment opportunities; lower than national average income; higher levels of poverty; poorer housing; greater exposure to violence; limited access to services; underdeveloped social networks; connection with land; racism and incarceration; and impaired communication when English is a second language (Thomson et al., 2011; McMurray & Clendon, 2011; Ministry of Health, 2012a). It is important to recognise that for indigenous populations it is both the social determinants of health and the cultural concepts of indigenous health which strongly influence the health status of their communities (Thomson et al., 2011; McMurray & Clendon, 2011; Ministry of Health, 2012a). The presence of these risk factors either singly or in combination lead to a higher proportion of the indigenous population developing chronic disease and/or disability as compared to non-indigenous.

As a consequence, Indigenous Australians suffer much more ill health than non-Indigenous Australians (AIHW, 2012a). Indigenous Australians experience higher levels of disability when compared to the general population (36%): 8% experience a severe limitation of a core activity (AIHW, 2006, p. 56), which is twice that experienced by non-Indigenous Australians (AIHW, 2006, p. 56). In terms of chronic disease Indigenous Australians experience a higher mortality from diabetes (14 times higher than the general population), chronic kidney disease (8 times) and heart disease (5 times) (AIHW, 2006, p. ix). The resulting outcome for Indigenous Australians is that they are more likely to experience death four times more often as compared to non-Indigenous Australians (AIHW, 2006).

In New Zealand, 24% of Māori experience disability, followed by 18% of Europeans, and 17% of Pacific peoples (Ministry of Health, 2005, p. 8). The consequence of this is that Māori and Pacific peoples have a lessened life expectancy by 8.5 years compared with the European population, largely attributable to the increased incidence of chronic disease in these population groups (McMurray & Clendon, 2011; NHC, 2007, p. 10).

Risk factors in the development of chronic disease

Risk factors by definition are 'characteristics associated with an increased risk of developing a particular disease or condition' (AIHW, 2006, p. 13). They may be demographic, behavioural, biomedical, genetic, environmental, social or other factors acting independently or in combination (AIHW, 2006, p. 13; 2008). See Table 1.1 for a summary of potential risk factors for chronic disease.

The role risk factors play in the development of chronic disease is well understood (WHO, 2011a); however, available evidence now suggests that a person may have several risk factors coexisting or interacting with one another at any one time (AIHW, 2002) thereby creating the possibility of developing one or more chronic diseases. Recognition has also recently been afforded to the importance risk factors have on a person's life due to their interactive and cumulative effect at critical periods in the lifecycle (AIHW, 2002). While previously it was thought risk factors were exclusively adult behaviours, understanding of the role risk factors play now acknowledges the influence they pose from the period of gestation until death (AIHW, 2006; 2002). The global example of the increasing prevalence of young children being exposed to risk is demonstrated through the increased levels of tobacco usage, increased numbers of overweight and obese children and the increasing incidence of type 2 diabetes found in the younger generation (WHO, 2005, pp. 49–50), which manifests with younger children experiencing more chronic disease than ever before. Yet controlling body weight, eating nutritious foods, avoiding tobacco use, controlling alcohol consumption and increasing physical activity may lead to prevention or delay of many chronic diseases (AIHW, 2005, p. 1).

Controlling some risk factors and effectively managing others through initiatives such as screening and early intervention programs (AIHW, 2006; NPHP, 2006) can significantly reduce the presence of chronic disease within communities. In Australia, health promotion is acknowledged as the key to preventing chronic disease via prevention and management

TABLE 1.1

Risk factors and determinants for chronic diseases. Australian Institute of Health and Welfare (2006b) Chronic diseases and associated risk factors in Australia, 2006. Cat no PHE 81. Canberra: Australian Institute of Health and Welfare, page 13.

MODIFIABLE RISK FACTORS		BROAD INFLUENCES	
Behavioural	**Biomedical**	**May or may not be modifiable**	**Non-modifiable**
Tobacco smoking	Excess weight	Socio-environmental factors	Age
Excess alcohol use	High blood pressure	Psychosocial factors	Gender
Physical inactivity	High blood cholesterol	Early life factors	Indigenous status
Poor diet	Other	Political factors	Ethnic background
Other			Family history
			Genetic make-up

of risk factors (AIHW, 2006, p. 13). The most common, modifiable risk factors contributing to chronic disease are unhealthy diet, leading to raised glucose levels, increased body mass, abnormal blood lipids; physical inactivity, leading to increased body mass, increased blood pressure and increased blood lipids; and tobacco use, leading to raised blood pressure (AIHW, 2006, p. 13; WHO, 2011a). These risk factors are said to be modifiable because chronic disease can be prevented by the person changing their behaviour and/or medical intervention (AIHW, 2006, p. 13). The two key non-modifiable risk factors contributing to the development of chronic disease are age and heredity (WHO, 2005, p. 48). Identification of these factors within population groups allows for the development of prevention and management strategies that may be constructed to meet the cultural and linguistic needs of the group (AIHW, 2006, p. 13).

As you read over the chapters about specific chronic diseases, you will learn about the identification of risk factors in relation to disease and how these are best prevented and/or managed to prevent development of the chronic disease in the first instance.

Impact of chronic illness and disability

It is difficult to quantify the impact of chronic illness and disability experienced by the individual, family and community, as many of the costs are invisible. For example, in Australia 65% of people who experienced a severe or profound core activity limitation relied on informal carers for such activities as self-care, mobility and communication (AIHW, 2006, p. 49). The difficulty arises due to the nature of the chronic illness and/or disability and the resources available to manage the condition are highly variable, largely determined by each person's individual situation (Guillett, 2004).

Chronic disease is often thought of as a disease of the aged and yet, as we see the increasing evidence of lifestyle risk factors in younger generations, we will also see the outcomes of chronic disease (illness, disability, pain and death) being played out in other age groups (AIHW, 2006, p. 31). The implications of this are that individuals who acquire a chronic disease early on in life will need to live and adapt to their illness and sequelae for the rest of their life (AIHW, 2006, p. 31). Therefore, in order to prevent further extension of the disease and/or disability, the person needs to adopt a whole-of-life approach in the management of their condition (AIHW, 2006, p. 31).

People living with a chronic illness are more likely than the general population to experience periods of hospitalisation as a consequence of acute flare-ups of their underlying chronic disease. What is emerging is that due to the increasing prevalence of chronic disease, many admissions to hospital now constitute the underlying pathology of chronic disease. In 2003–04, for example, Australia reported that 21.6% of all hospital separations were directly attributable to one of the top chronic diseases in Australia (AIHW, 2006, p. 35). The single greatest reason for hospitalisation was from 'care involving dialysis', not because chronic kidney disease is the most prevalent disease but rather that it causes frequent, episodic admission for care (AIHW, 2006, p. 35). The consequences of this are lost productivity days, a reduction in the person's quality of life, cost to the community, burden on the family unit and disruption to 'normal' routine.

WHO (2005) has frequently warned of the need to take action to prevent chronic disease due to its economic impact and the community's inability to sustain large numbers of people accessing health services and their associated costs. AIHW (2004) estimates healthcare expenditure in Australia for chronic diseases to be 87.5% of the total recurrent health expenditure for 2000–01 (as cited in AIHW, 2006, p. 40). In 2005, the National Chronic Disease Strategy reported that 70% of the allocated health expenditure in 2000–01 went to a majority of diseases that are considered long-term conditions (as cited in AIHW, 2006, p. 40). This represents government and non-government funding for the costs incurred to prevent, diagnose, treat and manage disease (AIHW, 2006, p. 40). New Zealand's experience is that medical care for people with chronic conditions uses a giant proportion of health resources and accounts for a greater number of hospital admissions than for the general population (NHC, 2007, p. 9). Regardless of the underlying condition, the focus for a person living with a chronic illness is largely centred around the following three aspects: the demands created by the disease and/or treatments, for example medications; health professional visits; maintaining everyday life, for example chores, family responsibilities; and adjusting to an altered view of their future and managing their response, for example frustration, anger and/or depression (Lorig, 1996).

MODELS OF CARE

In the past our model of healthcare focused on infectious diseases and acute illness but now is required to be re-orientated to better manage longer term conditions (chronic disease and/or disability) (NHC, 2007, p. 14). Healthcare funding has also been traditionally centred on an acute care model. This model, however, is no longer sustainable in meeting the projected healthcare needs of individuals and their families in the 21st century and beyond. There are a number of chronic care models that aim to improve the practice and outcomes for patients and providers (Bodenheimer et al., 2002). Common to all models of chronic care are two key features:

1 system-wide integration of services based on the chronic care model
2 targeting of specific system components or populations at greatest risk of hospitalisation (Singh, 2005 cited in NHC, 2007).

What is required is the interface of both acute and chronic models of care to support the healthcare needs of people with chronic disease in an efficient and coordinated manner. Medical and nursing advances have resulted in the specialisation of health services, leading to fragmentation of care (NHC, 2007, p. 14). As a result, people with a chronic disease and/or disability often experience uncoordinated care, along with poor communication between different health service providers with an inflexible approach to the provision of care. It is well understood that people with chronic disease also experience times of acute illness (Larsen, 2013), requiring acute intervention and service provision. This requires different models of care to be implemented so that providers of healthcare promote continuity and sustainable relationships with people throughout their journey with a chronic illness and/or disability.

To understand the key differences between acute and chronic models of care, refer to Table 1.2.

The approach underpinning Australia's and New Zealand's models of chronic care in relation to the provision of health services is predicated on primary healthcare (NHC, 2007, p. 16). Three key aspects of primary healthcare incorporated into the models of chronic care include:

1 adopting a population health approach to address the prevention and management of chronic disease
2 recognising the integral role multidisciplinary teams play in achieving an effective population health approach
3 promoting a broad primary healthcare approach consisting of health promotion, early intervention and disease prevention (NHC, 2007, p. 16).

Guidelines to support the management of chronic disease in Australia and New Zealand have also been conceptualised and draw on the British National Health Service chronic

TABLE 1.2

Comparison between acute and chronic care models. National Health Committee (2007) Meeting the needs of people with chronic conditions. Hapai te whanau mo ake ake tonu. Wellington, New Zealand: National Advisory Committee on Health and Disability – table 1 'Acute and chronic care models – key differences' page 14

ACUTE MODEL	CHRONIC CARE MODEL
Disease-centred	Person-centred
Doctor-centred	Team-centred
Focus on individuals	Population health approach
Secondary care emphasis	Primary care emphasis
Reactive, symptom-driven	Proactive, planned intervention
Episodic care	Ongoing care
Cure focus	Prevention/management focus
Single setting: hospital, specialist centres, general practice	Community setting, collaboration across primary and secondary care
1 : 1 contact through visit by patient	1 : 1 or group contact through visit by patient or health professional, email, phone or Web contact
Diagnostic information provided	Support for self-management

care management, which has three levels: self-management, disease management and care management (NHC, 2007, p. 17). These levels refer to 'a group of interventions or activities, not a theoretical approach or model' (NHC, 2007, p. 17). In Australia this has been adapted by the Australian Government's National Health Priority Action Council as self-management, disease or care management and care coordination (NHC, 2007, p. 17). In New Zealand these three levels are referred to as self-management, care management and care coordination (NHC, 2007, p. 17). Combining these guidelines with models of care is considered to lead to greater effectiveness in the management of chronic disease (Renders et al., 2001, cited in NHC, 2007). A more detailed account of models of care is provided in Chapter 3.

ROLE OF THE INTERDISCIPLINARY TEAM

The person experiencing a chronic illness and/or disability requires access to a number of healthcare professionals and services such as counselling services, pharmacy, allied health and housing (AIHW, 2006, p. 31; NHC, 2007, p. 16; Neal, 2004, pp. 15–19). This access is far greater than for those individuals who experience an acute episode of ill health. Often the frequency and diversity of access required are due to the complexity of disease, or disability and/or treatment regimens that result in a myriad of needs.

The role of the nurse and other health professionals is therefore to support the person in managing their condition more effectively. The adoption of a team approach, often coordinated by the nurse, reduces fragmentation of services, enabling better integration of care and more effective support for the individual and their family (NHC, 2007, p. 16; Neal, 2004, p. 15). Chapter 2 discusses the specific roles other health professionals play in an inter/multi-disciplinary team in supporting individuals with a chronic disease and/or disability.

CHALLENGES PRESENTED BY CHRONIC ILLNESSES AND DISABILITIES

The challenges presented to health professionals by chronic illnesses and disabilities are vast. Consideration must be given to finding new ways of prevention to control the prevalence of chronic disease within our community. Controlling the prevalence of chronic disease is not the sole responsibility of government or health services but must emanate from individuals taking ownership of their health behaviours, working in collaboration with government and health services to eradicate the increasing presence of chronic disease in our communities (NHC, 2007, p. 12; WHO, 2005).

Some challenges that have been articulated are the rising costs of care, the number of people needing to access chronic disease care, inequities between the indigenous and general populations, the changing composition of the population experiencing chronic disease and/or disability, ethical issues, providing culturally competent care, caregiver issues (Remsburg & Carson, 2006, pp. 591–599), the mismatch between the needs of people with a chronic condition and what the health system offers (NHC, 2007, p. 13).

Part of the Australian Government's response to managing chronic disease has been to accord the most common and burdensome chronic diseases the status of National Health Priority Area (NHPA). This status was given on the 'basis of health impact; the potential to reduce their burden and community concern about them' (AIHW, 2006, p. 60). Nine national health priority areas now exist; the most recent, dementia, was added in 2012 (AIHW, 2012b). Of those nine priority areas, eight are explicitly linked to the pathophysiology of a chronic disease (AIHW, 2012b). The eight national health priority areas related to chronic disease are cancer, cardiovascular, mental illness, diabetes mellitus, asthma, arthritis and musculoskeletal conditions, obesity and dementia (AIHW, 2012b). The ninth area is related to injury prevention and in itself has the potential to contribute to the prevention of chronic disease and/or disability (AIHW, 2012b). Many of the chapters in this book are focused on NHPAs, recognising their importance to health professionals.

Other ways in which these challenges can be addressed include: improving the health experiences of various disadvantaged groups in Australia and New Zealand; providing public health programs in a more cohesive and non-fragmented manner; adopting a model of practice that recognises the importance of early life factors and their contribution to creating chronic disease in adulthood; using a multifaceted approach involving others outside the health area to reduce the prevalence of conditions such as obesity and depression to foster social norms of active living; acknowledging the contribution of psychosocial factors, for example resilience and family environment, to chronic disease and the need for multiple strategies to address these factors; and adopting a holistic approach in developing prevention and management strategies (NPHP, 2001, p. 2).

PRINCIPLES OF PRACTICE

To provide optimal care to a person and their family experiencing a chronic illness and/or disability which ensures all needs are met, a number of key principles of practice must be implemented by nurses in conjunction with other members of the inter/multi-disciplinary healthcare team. These principles are to:

1 recognise that chronic illness and/or disability affects all dimensions of personhood: physical, psychosocial, emotional, cognitive and spiritual (Guillett, 2004; Larsen, 2013)
2 recognise that cultural responses to illness are important when providing care (Larsen, 2013)

3 provide holistic care by incorporating a team approach to providing care that is relevant to the needs of the person experiencing the chronic illness and their family (Guillett, 2004, p. 19)
4 adopt a 'whole of life' approach, recognising that risk factors occur across the lifespan and play a significant role in the development of chronic disease (NPHP, 2001, p. 4)
5 provide care that is person-centred and inclusive of the family, however the person defines this for themselves (Morris & Edwards, 2006).

As you read through the following chapters you will see further expansion and application of these principles to assist you in your understanding of chronic illness and disability, as applied to the Australian and New Zealand context. The authors discuss critical components related to understanding the experience of chronic illness, such as: behaviours that contribute to the development of the condition; the relationship of chronic illness to activities of daily living; the impact of body image and identity on the person and their family or carers; issues concerning quality of life; a range of interventions to support restorative function and quality of life; the role of family and carers; and education of the person and family. Case studies are included to support your understanding and cover issues such as: culture; complementary and alternative therapies; rehabilitation/facilitation; financial considerations and their impact on the person's life; aspects of stigma; self-efficacy and social isolation; sexuality; the impact of psychosocial dimensions of disease, disability and treatments; spirituality; chronic pain; powerlessness; and the nurse's role in advocacy.

CONCLUSION

This chapter has provided an overview of the gravity of our health needs from global, Australian and New Zealand perspectives. The burden that chronic illness and/or disability currently places, and will continue to place, on our communities is significant. It is important to recognise that with the projected ageing population figures for both countries and the increasing prevalence of modifiable risk factors within our lifestyle and increased survival rates from potentially fatal diseases, chronic disease will emerge as the new epidemic of the twenty-first century. It is unlikely that our communities will be able to sustain health service provision to meet this growing demand. The resources (informal carers, equipment, qualified personnel and finance) required for the management of chronic illness and/or disability are not found in an endless supply. The challenge for nurses and other health professionals is to provide models of care aimed at preventing, reducing or eliminating modifiable risk factors from their communities' lifestyle in order to halt the growth of this cancer-like phenomenon and to promote sustainable healthy communities

Reflective questions

1 What challenges does the increasing prevalence of chronic disease and disability pose for you in terms of nursing practice?
2 What qualities, skills and knowledge do you think a nurse requires to practise effectively?
3 What practice models of care can you implement in your work environment?

Recommended reading

Australian Institute of Health and Welfare. (2012). *Australia's health 2012*. Cat. No. AUS 157. Canberra: AIHW.

Kralik, D., Paterson, B., & Coates, V. (Eds.). (2010). *Translating chronic illness research into practice*. United Kingdom: Blackwell publishing.

Ravenscroft, E. (2010). Navigating the health care system: insights from consumers with multi-morbidity. *Nursing and Healthcare of Chronic Illness*. doi: 10.1111/j.1752-9824.2010.01063.x

Thompson, N., MacRae, A., Brankovich, J., et al. (2011). Overview of Australian Indigenous health status. Retrieved from http://www.healthinfonet.ecu.au/overview_2012.pdf

World Health Organization. (2008). *2008–2013 Action plan for the global strategy for the prevention and control of noncommunicable diseases*. Geneva: Author.

References

Australian Bureau of Statistics. (2004). *Disability, ageing and carers, Australia: summary of findings 2003*. Canberra: Author.

Australian Chronic Disease Prevention Alliance. (2004). *Chronic illness: Australia's health challenge. The economic case for physical activity and nutrition in the prevention of chronic disease: full report*. Canberra: Australian Government Department of Health and Ageing.

Australian Institute of Health and Welfare. (2002). *Chronic diseases and associated risk factors in Australia*. Canberra: Author.

Australian Institute of Health and Welfare. (2005). Chronic disease and risk factor statistics. Retrieved June 7, 2007, from http://www.aihw.gov.au/cdarf/data_pages/index.cfm

Australian Institute of Health and Welfare. (2006). *Chronic diseases and associated risk factors in Australia, 2006*. Cat no PHE 81. Canberra: Author.

Australian Institute of Health and Welfare. (2008). Indicators for chronic diseases and their determinants, 2008. Retrieved March 12, 2008, from http://aihw.gov.au

Australian Institute of Health and Welfare. (2012a). *Australia's health 2012*. Cat. No. AUS 157. Canberra: Author.

Australian Institute of Health and Welfare. (2012b). National health priority areas. Retrieved February 20, 2013, from http;//www.aihw.gov.au/national-health-priorities

Australian Institute of Health and Welfare. (2012c). Deaths FAQ. Retrieved February 20, 2013, from http;//www.aihw.gov.au/deaths-faq/

Bodenheimer, T., Wagner, E., & Grumbach, K. (2002). Improving primary care for patients with chronic illness. *Journal of American Medical Association*, *288*(14), 1775–1779.

Guillett, S. (2004). Understanding chronic illness and disability. In L. J. Neal & S. E. Guillett (Eds.), *Care of the adult with a chronic illness or disability. A team approach*. St Louis: Elsevier.

Kralik, D., Paterson, B., & Coates, V. (Eds.), (2010). *Translating chronic illness research into practice*. Blackwell Publishing: United Kingdom.

Larsen, P. (2013). Chronicity. In I. M. Lubkin & P. D. Larsen (Eds.), *Chronic illness. Impact and interventions* (8th ed.). Sudbury, MA: Jones and Bartlett Learning.

Lorig, K. (1996). Chronic disease self-management: a model for tertiary prevention. *American Behavioural Scientist*, *39*(6), 676–678.

Lubkin, I. M., Larsen, P. D. (Eds.). (2013). *Chronic illness. impact and intervention* (8th ed.). Sudbury, MA: Jones and Bartlett Learning.

McMurray, A., & Clendon, J. (2011). *Community health and wellness. primary health care in practice* (4th ed.). Chatswood, N.S.W: Elsevier.

Ministry of Health. (2005). Living with disability in New Zealand: summary. Wellington, New Zealand: Ministry of Health. Retrieved August 29, 2012 from http://www.moh.govt.nz

Ministry of Health. (2012a). *Implementing the New Zealand health strategy 2011*. Wellington, NZ: Author. Retrieved July 30, 2012, from: www.health.govt.nz

Ministry of Health. (2012b). *Disability support services strategic plan 2010–2014*. Wellington, NZ: Author. Retrieved July 30, 2012, from www.health.govt.nz

Morris, T. L., & Edwards, L. D. (2006). Family caregivers. In I. M. Lubkin & P. D. Larsen (Eds.), *Chronic illness. Impact and interventions* (6th ed.). Sudbury, MA: Jones and Bartlett Learning.

National Health Committee. (2007). *Meeting the needs of people with chronic conditions. Hapai te whanau mo ake ake tonu*. Wellington, NZ: National Advisory Committee on Health and Disability.

National Health Priority Action Council. (2006). *National chronic disease strategy*. Canberra: Department of Health and Ageing.

National Public Health Partnership. (2001). *Preventing chronic disease: A strategic framework*. Background paper. Melbourne: Author.

National Public Health Partnership. (2006). *Blueprint for nation-wide surveillance of chronic diseases and associated determinant*. Melbourne: Author.

Neal, L. J. (2004). Settings of chronic care. In L. J. Neal & S. E. Guillett (Eds.), *Care of the adult with a chronic illness or disability. A team approach*. St Louis: Elsevier.

Remsburg, R. E., & Carson, B. (2006). Rehabilitation. In I. M. Lubkin & P. D. Larsen (Eds.), *Chronic illness. Impact and interventions* (6th ed.). Sudbury, MA: Jones and Bartlett Learning.

Thompson, N., MacRae, A., Brankovich, J., et al. (2011). Overview of Australian Indigenous health status, 2011. Retrieved July 30, 2012, from http://www.healthinfonet.ecu.au/overview_2012.pdf

World Health Organization. (2002). Towards a common language for functioning, disability and health. Retrieved March 12, 2008, from http://www3.who.int/icf/icftemplate.cfm?myurl=beginners.html&mytitle=Beginner%27s%20Guide

World Health Organization. (2005). Preparing a healthcare workforce for the 21st century. The challenge of chronic conditions. Retrieved July 30, 2012, from http://www.who.int/chp/chronic-disease-report/en/index.html

World Health Organization. (2008). 2008–2013 action plan for the global strategy for the prevention and control of noncommunicable diseases. Retrieved July 10, 2012, from http://www.who.int/chp/chronic_disease_report/en/index.html

World Health Organization. (2011a). The global status report on noncommunicable diseases 2010. Retrieved July 30, 2012, from http://whqlibdoc.who.int/publications/2011/9789240686458_eng.pdf

World Health Organization. (2011b). The world report on disability. Retrieved July 6, 2012, from http://www.who.int

CHAPTER 2

Sheree M. S. Smith
Annette James
Geoffrey Mitchell
Michelle Bissett
Lee Zakrzewski
Anthony Wright
Susan Balandin
Michelle Lincoln
Mark Hughes

Role of the interdisciplinary/ multidisciplinary team

Learning objectives

When you have completed this chapter you will be able to:

- discuss the concepts underpinning a interdisciplinary/multidisciplinary team approach
- recognise the importance of an interdisciplinary/multidisciplinary team approach in order to achieve optimal health outcomes
- understand the nature of an interdisciplinary/multidisciplinary team approach in the service provision of care for a person experiencing a chronic illness and/or disability
- appreciate the nurse's role in an interdisciplinary/multidisciplinary team in managing chronic illness and/or disability
- be aware of the roles and scope of practice offered by various members of the interdisciplinary/multidisciplinary team in the provision of care.

Key words

collaboration, goal setting, interdisciplinary, multidisciplinary, person-centred

INTRODUCTION

This chapter describes the contemporary roles of health professionals in caring for individuals with a chronic illness and/or disability. Every health professional plays an important role in the interdisciplinary/multidisciplinary team. The scope of practice implemented by these health professionals is also presented. The very nature of chronic illness and/or disability demands that health professionals from a diversity of disciplines work collaboratively to manage the complexity and variety of health issues that arise.

The terms 'interdisciplinary' and 'multidisciplinary' are often used interchangeably in the literature to denote the group of health professionals who comprise 'the team' responsible for the provision of care in chronic illness and/or disability. Neal (2004) does, however, distinguish between the two, essentially based on the approach to care employed by the team, which is worth noting. In a multidisciplinary team, it is most likely that the approach to care will be discipline focused (Neal, 2004). Here the health professionals largely work within their discipline base, independently of other health professionals, in determining goals in collaboration with the patient and family. Alternatively an interdisciplinary team comprises health professionals from several different disciplines who work collectively to identify and resolve issues through mutually agreed upon goals with the person and their family (Pierce & Lutz, 2013). Overall, regardless of the term applied, team meetings are used to share information and discuss possible solutions in achieving an optimal outcome for the person and their family (Pierce & Lutz, 2013).

In this chapter the terms 'interdisciplinary' and 'multidisciplinary' are used interchangeably by the various authors to enable both approaches to care to be illustrated and contextualised depending upon the needs of the person and their family. The approach in this chapter requires that health professionals and other allied disciplines work collaboratively in determining the priorities and the nature of the interventions to be implemented and in evaluating care provided in a more holistic and cohesive manner. This approach offers the flexibility needed to respond to the changing needs of a person with chronic illness and/or disability and their family. The partnerships created between the person and their family and among various members of the interdisciplinary team intersect with one another and make central the person and their health needs. The interdisciplinary team seeks to resolve issues for the person and their family by determining a shared goal of care, involving a number of strategies that are not discipline-specific but rather conceptualised from knowledge and experience to best suit the needs of the individual.

Effective communication is key to achieving the goals determined by the team in collaboration with the person. The nurse is equal to all other members of the interdisciplinary/multidisciplinary team and is most likely to be the primary carer in the majority of healthcare settings. As a result, the nurse will often assume a coordination role within the team to bring together the other health professionals. Having the primary carer assume this coordination role directly benefits the person and their family by bringing together the wealth of knowledge, experience and skills in the planning of a range of interventions to manage the issues arising for people with chronic illness and/or disability. This role is also pivotal in ensuring that the interventions and solutions implemented are evaluated on an ongoing basis and to recognise that as people's needs change so too does the plan of care.

This chapter begins therefore with a description of the nurse's role followed by the dietitian, general practitioner, occupational therapist, physiotherapist, speech pathologist and social worker.

References

Pierce, L. L., & Lutz, B. J. (2013). Family caregivers. In I. M. Lubkin & P. D. Larsen (Eds.), *Chronic illness. Impact and Interventions* (8th ed.). Burlington, Mass: Jones and Bartlett Learning.

Neal, L. J. (2004). Settings of chronic care. In L. J. Neal & S. E. Guillett (Eds.), *Care of the adult with chronic illness or disability: A team approach*. St Louis: Elsevier.

ROLE OF THE NURSE

Sheree Smith

As mentioned in the introduction to this chapter, the registered nurse often has a pivotal role in coordinating the multidisciplinary team. This role may encompass both ensuring the timely involvement of each discipline and being an advocate of quality assurance ensuring all patients have access to the most appropriate service or intervention within a reasonable timeframe. Whilst this role by registered nurses within a multidisciplinary team is well established in clinical practice, there have been concerns raised regarding the level of evidence to support the widespread implementation of this nurse coordination role in chronic disease management. Taylor and colleagues (2005) examined the literature associated with nurse-led multidisciplinary teams where registered nurses held the coordinating role and found the data were too sparse and the benefit and/or risk was unable to be ascertained. In contrast, nurse-led interventions for conditions such as COPD was significantly positive with nurse-led interventions being proven to be more effective in reducing the need for unscheduled primary care consultations and mortality. The differences between the review and Sridhar's clinical study (Sridhar et al., 2008) are primarily around the definition of the role, its implementation and outcome measures that are directly related to the role within a multidisciplinary team. Clear role description within the multidisciplinary teams enables others, including patients who are outside the team, to be able to discern what each member contributes to the overall functioning of the team. This view can be further established when we consider a study by Milisen et al. (2001) where they report on a nurse-led interdisciplinary intervention for reducing delirium in elderly hip-fracture patients. Milisen and colleagues were unable to demonstrate any effect on delirium as a discipline-based intervention a change in delirium health status had not been established that was discipline specific and therefore examining the nurse's role may not have been the most appropriate variable in measuring the outcome within a multidisciplinary team. Simply, Milisen had not established whether it was the discipline of the person who gave the intervention or the intervention itself that was under study.

The roles of registered nurses within multidisciplinary teams, models, programs and interventions can be varied and include coordination, patient assessment, being a meeting chairperson and/or an educator. Research into the effect of nurse-led multidisciplinary clinical rounds on patient outcomes is encouraging as Fakih et al. (2008) sought to address a known risk factor within the clinical setting of the unnecessary use of urinary catheters. Indwelling urinary catheters can increase the risk of patients developing urinary tract infections and systemic bacteraemia as well as increasing the patient's length of stay in hospital and thereby increasing health costs. Fakih et al.'s (2008) large study of 12 medical and surgical units found that a nurse-led multidisciplinary approach during clinical rounds reduced the use of indwelling urinary catheters and the morbidity in their patient population. In some chronic care models based in either primary or acute care settings nurses lead multidisciplinary teams and indeed share patient appointments. This shared-care multidisciplinary model has the medical officer and the nurse seeing the patient on alternate visits. Occurrence of this shared-care arrangement is increasing and the supporting evidence for this model is primarily financially based; however, with more research being undertaken in this area (Sabariego et al., 2010; Strand & Parker, 2012), significant benefit to patients is more likely to be established in the future (Watts et al., 2009). The clinical assessment by registered nurses who are leading a multidisciplinary program has been proven to have a significant clinical impact on patients with chronic illness (Zakrisson et al., 2012). Within multidisciplinary interventions, the role of the registered nurses is often to deliver the educational component of the intervention (Sabariego et al., 2010; Strand & Parker, 2012; Marsden et al., 2010) whilst other roles pertain to clinical assessment and tailoring of individual treatment plans (Melis et al., 2010; Filler & Lipshultz, 2012) and/or as a coordinator of an intervention (Wallasch, Angeli & Kropp, 2012).

CONCLUSION

As evidenced by the diversity of registered nurses' roles within a multidisciplinary team, program, intervention and/or service, the scope of the nursing discipline's unique contribution, flexibility and depth of knowledge and skill are demonstrated. With the development of new advanced practice roles in nursing and the need for fiscal restraint of health budgets, nurse-led multidisciplinary teams, programs and services will become more available for patients to access across all healthcare settings.

References

Fakih, M. G., Dueweke, C., Meisner, S., et al. (2008). Effect of Nurse-led multidisciplinary rounds in reducing the unnecessary use of urinary catheterization in hospitalized patients. *Infection Control and Hospital Epidemiology*, *29*(9), 815–819.

Filler, G., & Lipshultz, S. E. (2012). Why multidisicplinary clinics should be the standard for treating chronic kidney disease. *Pediatric Nephrology*, *27*(10), 1831–1834. doi: 10.1007/s00467-012-2236 -3. Epub 4 July 2012.

Marsden, D., Quinn, R., Pond, N., et al. (2010). A multidisciplinary group programme in rural settings for community-dwelling chronic stroke survivors and their carers: a pilot randomized controlled trial. *Clinical Rehabilitation*, *24*, 328–341.

Melis, R. J. F., Van Eijken, M. I. J., Boon, M. F., et al. (2010). Process evaluation of a trial evaluating a multidisciplinary nurse-led home visiting programme for vulnerable older people. *Disability and Rehabilitation*, *32*(11), 937–946.

Milisen, K., Foreman, M. D., Abraham, I. L., et al. (2001). A nurse-led interdisciplinary program for delirium in elderley hip-fracture patients. *Journal of American Geriatric Society*, *49*, 523–532.

Sabariego, C., Grill, E., Brach, M., et al. (2010). Incremental cost-effectiveness analysis of a multidiscilinary renal education program for patients with chronic renal disease. *Disability and Rehabilitation*, *32*(5), 392–401.

Sridhar, M., Taylor, R., Dawson, S., et al. (2008). A nurse led intermediate care package in patients who have been hospitalised with an acute exacerbation of chronic obstructive pulmonary disease. *Thorax*, *63*, 194–200.

Strand, H., & Parker, D. (2012). Effects of multidisciplinary models of care for adult pre-dialysis patients with chronic kidney disease: a systematic review. *International Journal of Evidence Based Healthcare*, *10*, 53–59.

Taylor, S. J. C., Candy, R., Bryar, R. M., et al. (2005). Effectiveness of innovations in nurse led chronic disease management for patients with chronic obstructive pulmonary disease: a systematic review of evidence. *British Medical. Journal*, *331*, 485.

Wallasch, T.-M., Angeli, A., & Kropp, P. (2012). Outcomes of a headache-specific cross-sectional multidisciplinary treatment program. *Headache*, *52*, 1094–1105.

Watts, S. A., Gee, J., O'Day, M. E., et al. (2009). Nurse practitioner-led multidisciplinary teams to improve chronic illness: The unique strengths of nurse practitioners applied to shared medical appointments/group visits. *Journal of the American Academy of Nurse Practitioners*, *21*, 167–172.

Zakrisson, A.-B., Engfeldt, P., Hagglund, D., et al. (2012). Nurse-led multidisciplinary programme for patients with COPD in primary health care: a controlled trial. *Primary Care Respiratory Journal*, *20*(4), 427–433.

ROLE OF THE DIETITIAN

Annette James

Learning objectives

- To appreciate the scope of professional dietetic practice.
- To value the importance of the dietitian in achieving positive health outcomes for clients as part of a professional interdisciplinary/multidisciplinary team.

Key words

dietitian, food and nutrition, nutritional assessment

In the hospital and in the community the dietitian is part of a professional interdisciplinary/multidisciplinary team that aims to prevent, treat, manage and improve individual and community health. Dietitians are specialists in human nutrition, the metabolic and physiological responses to food and the pathogenic impacts on health and wellbeing.

An Accredited Practising Dietitian (APD) is registered with the Dietitians Association of Australia (DAA) after qualifying from an accredited course in nutrition and dietetics. Such a course means at least 4 years of university training in the science and art of food and nutrition.

A dietitian's primary aim is to improve individual and community health and wellbeing through food. They assist people to understand the relationship of food to health and how to make healthy food choices. Nutritional advice is in strong demand, given the increase in the incidence of diet-related diseases, which often lead to chronic illness and disability (Wahlqvist, 2011). A dietitian uses a range of techniques to assess nutritional status, identify specific problems, counsel for better health outcomes and plan and evaluate for individual care.

Dietitians work in a range of public and private settings and with people of all ages. They may work in clinical nutrition, community and public health nutrition, nutrition and food service management, sports nutrition, education, nutrition research, government policy, the food industry or as private practitioners. The scope of dietetic practice will vary with each setting and often includes individual care, assessment, education and prevention. Dietitians have to deal with a range of scenarios from developmental anomalies to acute care, the ongoing management of chronic and debilitating conditions, through to peak athletic performance. Dietetic practice follows the DAA's best practice guidelines and National Competency Standards to support treatment and management protocols for individuals and specialised groups. With the rise in diet-related diseases dietitians are often engaged as public health nutritionists, working at the local community level or at a national level; to design and implement health improvement programs aimed at decreasing the risk factors associated with chronic and preventable diseases. Nutrition promotion has become an important aspect of a dietitian's role in any setting (DAA, 2012a).

A clinical dietitian works with people with particular medical conditions and is responsible for all aspects of nutritional care and nutritional intervention. This may include assessing needs for therapeutic or special diets. It may also include making recommendations to medical staff for biochemical tests, nutrition supplements and modes of feeding like tube feeding and total parenteral nutrition (TPN). Dietitians are great resources for other disciplines, patients and caregivers. They provide appropriate advice on nutrition for the interdisciplinary/multidisciplinary team, the patient and their family, and this may include enteral and parental as well as oral nutrition. Dietitians help translate technical information into practical advice on food and eating (DAA, 2012b).

Nutritional standards of reference

Dietitians use a range of nutritional standards of reference to analyse individual diets and promote healthy eating.

The *NUTTAB Australian Food Composition Table*

Food composition tables are used to convert information about food intake to nutrient intake (Wahlqvist, 2011). The *NUTTAB 2010 Australian Food Composition Table* contains nutrient data for 2668 foods available in Australia and up to 245 nutrients per food. NUTTAB is regularly updated by Food Standards Australia New Zealand (FSANZ) and is a useful summary of nutrient data for commonly consumed foods (FSANZ, 2010).

Nutrient reference value

In 2005 The National Health and Medical Research Council (NHMRC) endorsed a system of reference values that retains the concept of the recommended dietary intake (RDI) while attempting to identify the average requirements of essentials nutrients considered to be adequate to meet the known nutritional needs of practically all healthy people, based on available scientific knowledge. The NHMRC endorsed the nutrient reference value (NRV) as a more specific nutrient value to identify the average requirements needed by healthy individuals (NHMRC, 2005).

Dietitians use this information to develop and implement plans for the nutritional care of individuals during acute and chronic illness. In a food service setting the goals of a dietary department is to obtain, prepare and serve flavourful, attractive, safe and nutritious food (Wahlqvist, 2011).

In a consultation setting this information is used to advise and promote good health through proper eating. Dietitians help to develop and modify diets and educate individuals, family members, groups and healthcare providers on good nutritional habits (Wahlqvist, 2011).

Australian Dietary Guidelines

Dietitians also use the Australian Dietary Guidelines as a practical way of informing people about the general principles of healthy eating. These guidelines were first developed in 1981 to provide information about the types and amounts of foods, food groups and dietary patterns to promote health and wellbeing. The name has changed from *The Australian Guide to Healthy Eating* in 1998 to become *Food for Health; Dietary Guidelines for Australian Adults* and *Dietary Guidelines for Children and Adolescents in Australia* in 2003. These guidelines are currently under review by the NHMRC to ensure that they reflect the latest knowledge on nutrition, diet and health (NHMRC, 2003).

Nutritional anthropometric reference values

Height-for-age, weight-for-age, weight-for-height ratios and body mass index (BMI) are the most common anthropometric tools used to assess growth and the level of energy store. In children there is an expected range in variation, often referred to as a percentile. For example, the 50th percentile represents the median weight (or height) as the value below which the heights and weights of 50% of healthy children are expected to fall. For adults, BMI (weight in kg divided by the square of height in metres) is used as a measure of energy stores. It is the most common indicator to assess nutritional status (Wahlqvist, 2011).

Biochemical values

Serum biochemical assessments are important indicators of nutritional status and often signify the degree and severity of the disease process. It is used to help monitor management and progress in specific conditions.

CONCLUSION

A dietitian will make a nutritional assessment by:

- undertaking clinical assessment
- determining dietary intake
- using anthropometry
- interpreting biochemical indicators.

Integration of all this information will determine the individual's nutritional status. Once the assessment has been made a plan of management can be formulated. The client will receive personalised advice tailored to their specific health and food requirements. The dietitian will assist with meal and menu planning, recipe modification, reading food labels and communicating important health promotion messages to assist optimisation of individual and community health.

This process does not happen in isolation and the dietitian is an integral part of the interdisciplinary/multidisciplinary team that is working together to achieve the best possible health outcomes for every individual. All team members play an important role in observing and communicating with one another for signs of progress or signs of complications and this observation and communication between team members is an integral component to achieving maximised health outcomes for all.

Recommended reading

Wilson, T., & Temple, N. (2006). *Nutritional health — strategies for disease prevention* (2nd ed.). Totowa, NJ: Humana Press.

Mann, J., & Truswell, A. S. (2012). *Essentials of human nutrition* (4th ed.). UK: Oxford University Press.

References

Food Standards Australia New Zealand. (2010). NUTTAB. Retrieved May 7 2013, from http://www.foodstandards.gov.au/consumerinformation/nuttab2010/

Dietitians Association of Australia. (2012a). Dietetics in Australia. Retrieved May 7 2013, from http://daa.asn.au/universities-recognition/dietetics-in-australia/

Dietitians Association of Australia. (2012b). National competency standards. Retrieved May 7 2013, from http://daa.asn.au/universities-recognition/national-competency-standards/

National Health & Medical Research Council. (2005). Nutrient reference value. Retrieved May 7 2013, from http://www.nrv.gov.au/

National Health and Medical Research Council. (2003). Australian dietary guidelines. Retrieved May 7 2013, from http://www.nhmrc.gov.au/guidelines/publications/n29-n30-n31-n32-n33-n34

Wahlqvist, M. (Ed.), (2011). *Food and nutrition: food and health systems in Australia and New Zealand* (3rd ed.). Crows Nest, NSW: Allen & Unwin.

ROLE OF THE MEDICAL PRACTITIONER

Geoffrey Mitchell

The medical practitioner, with the other health professionals, assists the patient to achieve their goals in self-care. Clearly, the role of medical practitioners is to identify medical and other problems and, in concert with the patient, devise strategies to manage them. Problems identified may require a medical intervention such as a drug or an operation. However, many of the problems will require other assistance to manage the problem. This may involve health education, ventilation of anxieties, allied health support, the arrangement of aids of daily living or attendance to psychological or spiritual issues. This is a very complex role (Stewart et al., 2003). Full implementation of the development of a care plan requires coordination of care. In Australia, this role is evolving from a doctor-focused approach to a multidisciplinary one.

Community-based medical services are organised in different ways in different countries. The position of primary care in the health system varies. In the UK, Canada, Australia, the Netherlands and most Scandinavian countries, for example, the primary care practitioners are the patient's point of entry to the health system: referrals to specialist care take place via them. In other places, primary care doctors are but one of many medical specialties to whom a patient can present directly. Starfield and colleagues have shown conclusively that the health of a nation's population is directly proportional to the degree to which the primary care sector is valued and resourced (1991, 1994; Macinko, Starfield & Shi, 2003).

Primary care medicine is also funded in different ways. In Australia until 1999, the general practitioner (GP) was funded on a fee-for-service basis only, and no substitution of services by other health professionals on behalf of the GP was permitted. (These rules are identical to those related to consultation reimbursement currently in force (Medicare Australia, 2007).) That is, the GP had to see the patient and deliver the service personally in order to attract government-supported payments. Practice staff could not render the service for them. This is in sharp contrast to the UK model, where the general practice is the unit of care, and the GP heads a team of several health professionals who provide the care. The practice is paid a per capita fee to deliver primary care services to a defined group of patients, with the fee increasing if certain health targets (e.g. a percentage of patients immunised for influenza annually) are met. Teamwork in this setting is clearly encouraged (Weller & Maynard, 2004).

Since 1999, there has been a marked shift towards multidisciplinary care. Health planners have recognised that comprehensive care cannot be delivered by one health practitioner in isolation, and funding models have shifted to accommodate this. Health outcomes are better when patients are cared for in teams, with purposive planning of the care. For example, in the care of chronic obstructive pulmonary disease, patients have improved function, are more independent and have better quality of life when they are treated by multidisciplinary teams (Tieman et al., 2006). Similarly, diabetic patients who have comprehensive care by a general practice-based team have improved outcomes, to the point that their risk of an adverse vascular event such as a heart attack or stroke in the next 5 years actually falls by 25% over 2 years (Ackermann & Mitchell, 2006).

From the medical practitioner's perspective there are several models that can be used. All have the following requirements.

1 There has to be a structure both at the level of the system and at the practice to facilitate multidisciplinary care.
2 Patients have to be identified as requiring a multidisciplinary approach to care, preferably in a systematic way.

3 The team and the plan should be individualised according to the patient's healthcare needs.
4 There has to be a mechanism that allows the patient to receive the identified care from as many of the required medical and allied health professionals as possible (Tieman et al., 2006).

Such a system has evolved in Australia since 1999. This federal government initiative has facilitated multidisciplinary care, and funded GPs to take part in existing multidisciplinary care teams, such as those that exist in specialist palliative care services. In addition, the funding scheme allows certain patients (older people and intellectually disabled people) to be assessed for potential health problems that may not be readily detectable in a routine medical consultation. This allows appropriate multidisciplinary health interventions to be planned and delivered to prevent more serious and intractable problems from arising at a later date (Medicare Australia, 2007).

Once a multidisciplinary management plan has been devised, the funding mechanism supports limited allied health interventions. While an ideal multidisciplinary team would have equal input from all team members, in this case the practicalities of general practice and community-based private allied health provider service patterns means that the allied health team members generally sign off on a GP generated plan. The GP has to allocate a small number of allied health funding places among at least two providers, which creates dilemmas for the providers themselves if effective treatment requires a different level of service (Foster et al., 2009). Routine follow-up of patients is encouraged by the program. A similar but parallel scheme has been developed for the care of mental health problems in community patients, which provides more allied health access than that available in the Chronic Disease model.

Following are two examples of the way such programs can work. In Case Study 2.1 a multidisciplinary care program has been put in place within a rural general practice for diabetic patients. The features of this model are that every diabetic patient is offered the

CASE STUDY 2.1 Example of intra-practice multidisciplinary care (Ackermann & Mitchell, 2006)

Setting: Regional Australian town: district population 25 000.

Patients: All diabetic patients of the practice $n = 700$; 404 participated.

Multidisciplinary team members: GP, practice nurse, visiting diabetic educator, visiting dietitian.

Structure of multidisciplinary care: Patient reviewed by nurse, protocol of review developed by practice based on evidence-based best practice. GP reviews patient, being alerted to features required to manage. GP refers to other team members as required. Patients recalled for review every 3 months.

Outcomes: Population improvements in abdominal circumference, systolic and diastolic blood pressure, HDL and LDL cholesterol and 5 year risk of cardiovascular events, proportion of patients suffering severe hypoglycaemia in last 12 months, and proportion of foot lesions; proportion of patients at or below recommended blood pressure and cholesterol readings increased (all $p < 0.05$) over 2 years.

CASE STUDY 2.2 Example of interdisciplinary care planning between primary and secondary care — discharge after stroke (Indredavik et al., 2000)

Setting: Specialist stroke unit in a Norwegian city.

Patients: Patients to be discharged home after a completed strike.

Multidisciplinary team members: The mobile stroke team: physiotherapist, occupational therapist, nurse, consultant stroke specialist. Community caregivers—general practitioner, domiciliary nursing service; patient and caregivers.

Structure of multidisciplinary care: Home visit by the team before discharge. Planning meeting, then discharge meeting. Care by the mobile stroke team; outpatient review in 1 month, plan reviewed. Letter to GP with explicit issues to follow up. Responsibility for coordination was with the mobile team

Outcomes: 74% patients home (vs 55% for usual care) at 6 weeks post stroke. 23% (vs 40%) placed in institutions. Patients with moderate to severe stroke had the greatest benefit. 56% patients were independent (vs 45%) at 1 year post stroke.

service, and programmed recall is arranged every 3 months. The nurse works to a plan to review the patient, advising the doctor of findings to be reviewed. The doctor then arranges for individualised, ongoing care (Ackermann & Mitchell, 2006). In Case Study 2.2, case conferences and care planning take place between the team at a specialist inpatient stroke unit and all persons are involved in the early discharge of the patient to home. The participants all contribute to the care planning, the tasks are allocated clearly and there is a definite follow-up plan to ensure all planned treatments are carried out (Fjaertoft et al., 2004, 2005; Fjaertoft, Indredavik & Lydersen, 2003; Indredavik et al., 2000).

CONCLUSION

Multidisciplinary care is well placed in primary care. Primary medical practitioners such as GPs have the opportunity to care for patients over many years, and thus develop a deep understanding of the person as an individual, as well as a knowledge of the family and micro-environment in which that person operates (McWhinney, 1997). This enables healthcare planning to take into account local factors, making the plans more likely to be acceptable to the individual and thus more likely to be followed through.

Recommended reading

Tieman, J., Mitchell G., Shelby-James, T., et al. (2006). *Integration, coordination and multidisciplinary approaches in primary care: a systematic investigation of the literature.* Canberra: Australian Primary Health Care Research Institute.

Mitchell, G., Senior, H., Foster, M., et al. (2011). *The role of allied health in the management of complex conditions in primary care.* Canberra. Australian Primary Health Care Research Institute.

References

Ackermann, E. W., & Mitchell, G. K. (2006). An audit of structured diabetes care in a rural general practice. *The Medical Journal of Australia, 185*(2), 69–72.

Fjaertoft, H., Indredavik, B., Johnsen, R., et al. (2004). Acute stroke unit care combined with early supported discharge. Long-term effects on quality of life. A randomized controlled trial. *Clinical Rehabilitation, 18*(5), 580–586.

Fjaertoft, H., Indredavik, B., Lydersen, S. (2003). Stroke unit care combined with early supported discharge: long-term follow-up of a randomized controlled trial. *Stroke, 34*(11), 2687–2691.

Fjaertoft, H., Indredavik, B., Magnussen, J., et al. (2005). Early supported discharge for stroke patients improves clinical outcome. Does it also reduce use of health services and costs? One-year follow-up of a randomized controlled trial. *Cerebrovascular Diseases, 19*(6), 376–383.

Foster, M. M., Cornwell, P. L., Fleming, J. M., et al. (2009). Better than nothing? Restrictions and realities of enhanced primary care for allied health practitioners. *Australian Journal of Primary Health, 15*(4), 326–334.

Indredavik, B., Fjaertoft, H., Ekeberg, G., et al. (2000) Benefit of an extended stroke unit service with early supported discharge: A randomized, controlled trial. *Stroke, 31*(12), 2989–2994.

Macinko, J., Starfield, B., & Shi, L. (2003). The contribution of primary care systems to health outcomes within Organization for Economic Cooperation and Development (OECD) countries, 1970–1998. *Health Services Research*, June, *38*(3), 831–865.

McWhinney, I. R. (1997). Principles of family medicine. In I. R. McWhinney & T. Freeman (Eds.), *A textbook of family medicine*. New York: Oxford University Press.

Medicare Australia. (2007). Medicare Benefits Schedule. Retrieved 25 July 2007 from www.health.gov.au/mbsonline

Starfield, B. (1991). Primary care and health. A cross-national comparison. *The Journal of the American Medical Association, 266*(16), 2268–2271.

Starfield, B. (1994). Is primary care essential? *Lancet, 344*(8930), 1129–1133.

Stewart, M., Brown, J. B., Weston, W. W., et al. (2003). *Patient-centered medicine: transforming the clinical method*. Abingdon: Radcliffe Press.

Tieman, J., Mitchell, G., Shelby-James, T., et al. (2006). *Integration, coordination and multidisciplinary approaches in primary care: a systematic investigation of the literature*. Canberra: Australian Primary Health Care Research Institute.

Weller, D. P., & Maynard, A. (2004). How general practice is funded in the United Kingdom. *The Medical Journal of Australia, 181*(2), 109–110.

ROLE OF THE OCCUPATIONAL THERAPIST

Michelle Bissett
Lee Zakrzewski

Occupational therapists assert that daily life is comprised of participation in 'occupations' where occupations are the activities that people need to or want to do in day to day life. These occupations include tasks that people do to care for themselves (known as self-care), activities which are pleasurable (leisure) and activities that contribute to society (productivity). Participation in these occupations is known as 'occupational performance'. Occupational therapists believe that occupational performance is a result of the interaction of three main areas—the clients' personal skills, the nature of the occupations in which they engage and the influence of the environment on performance. Engagement in occupations, and people's abilities to self-select and perform meaningful tasks, are considered by occupational therapists to contribute to people's health, wellbeing and quality of life.

The ability to participate in and complete occupations can be reduced or eliminated when people experience illness or injury. Decreasing and/or fluctuating occupational performance is characteristic of people with chronic illness and correlates with deterioration of health status. Occupational therapists work with these clients to facilitate improvement or maintenance of their occupational performance within the limitations of their diagnosis.

Occupational therapists work across the healthcare continuum from acute care and rehabilitation to community care and health promotion. Clients with chronic conditions may be seen across any of these healthcare settings. Nursing staff can refer any patient who has identified difficulty completing day to day activities for occupational therapy assessment and intervention. Occupational therapy practice is commonly embedded within multidisciplinary or interdisciplinary teams. This has been documented as an effective approach for clients with chronic conditions (Engin & Pretorius, 2008; Firth, 2011; Oslund et al., 2009).

Some clients present to occupational therapists with chronic conditions that relate to a mental health issue. Others, with conditions that affect physical function, could have underlying issues of a psychosocial nature as a result of living with a chronic physical condition. Occupational therapists consider both the physical and the psychological aspects when considering the scope of the interventions with their clients.

With most clients, occupational therapists aim to improve occupational performance and subsequent ability in day to day tasks. The approach with clients with chronic health conditions is adapted in acknowledgment that their occupational performance will continue to decline as their condition progresses. The role of the occupational therapist with these clients can be to enhance function but frequently focuses on maintaining current levels of function.

Functional assessment of the client involves using a combination of both standardised and non-standardised assessments. A structured interview is used to identify individual asset and deficit areas. Assessments investigate how the client manages all aspects of self-care, productivity and leisure. This process also considers the personal characteristics of the client by assessing the areas of biomechanical, sensorimotor, cognitive, intrapersonal and interpersonal function. An environmental assessment considers the physical environment where clients need to perform tasks and the social and cultural environments in which clients function.

Occupational therapists employ a client-centred practice philosophy. When the assessment process is complete, therapists interact with clients, carers and family members to establish therapy goals (Shaw, Hill, & Robinson, 2011). The therapist identifies the client's strengths and weaknesses and the client participates by identifying the areas of deficit that they would like to work on. Therapy goals are typically centred on maintaining a balance in the areas of productivity, self-care and leisure in order to maintain the clients' quality of life (Klinger & Spaulding, 2001). This focus will vary between clients and within practice settings. For example, a patient on an acute medical ward may wish to be independent with showering whereas a client living in the community already independent in self-care tasks may wish to be able to independently complete household shopping and meal preparation.

Occupational therapy intervention focuses on self-management strategies to enable the client to achieve maximal occupational performance. While intervention focus is individualised, regularly used interventions are energy conservation, prescription of assistive devices and environmental modification. A detailed description of these interventions follows.

Energy conservation is particularly important for clients who experience decreased performance due to fatigue (Mathiowetz et al., 2005). Education about energy conservation is utilised to teach people to identify and modify their daily activity patterns (Finlayson, 2005). Energy conservation includes analysing and modifying tasks to reduce energy expenditure. The strategies implemented include planning ahead, delegation of tasks, balancing work and rest, using the body efficiently, modifying the task and using assistive technology (Finlayson, 2005; Mathiowetz et al., 2005). These principles enable clients to manage their energy use in order to have greater control and choice over activities in their day-to-day life. These strategies are also beneficial to clients who experience pain due to their condition.

Assistive devices can be described as equipment or systems that increase, maintain or improve the ability of clients to complete functional activities (Klinger & Spaulding, 2001). Devices can be utilised to prevent further impairment, to compensate for loss of function such as decreased strength or movement, to promote safety and to manage pain (Klinger & Spaulding, 2001). Assistive devices can be used in a range of tasks including dressing, feeding, grooming, communication, mobility and home management. The product prescribed can vary significantly depending on the client's functional problems. Popular products include shoe horns, modified cutlery, hand-held shower hoses, speaker phones, wheelchairs and easy-reachers. While in therapy clients are able to trial assistive devices to determine the effectiveness and impact on occupational performance.

Environmental modification—occupational performance occurs in a range of different environments; for example, the home, work or social environment. Occupational therapists are trained to assess these different environments in order to identify barriers for occupational performance and to recommend modifications that will enable ongoing participation. This requires assessment of the environmental layout and the client's performance within that environment (Sabata, Shamberg, & Williams, 2008). Modification of the home environment could include changing the design of taps for people with poor hand function or installation of external ramps for clients who, as the result of their diagnosis, require wheelchair access into and around their home. Other examples of environmental modifications include workplace redesign and vehicle adaptation.

In summary, occupational therapists are concerned with the client's ability to manage day to day activities. Therapists assist clients to maximise their performance in day-to-day activities through individualised treatment plans. Common strategies used with patients with chronic illness include education about energy conservation strategies, prescription of adaptive equipment and modification of their environments.

References

Engin, L., & Pretorius, C. (2008). Maintaining independence: A therapy pathway of a person with multiple sclerosis. *International Journal of Therapy and Rehabilitation, 15*(12), 580–585.

Finlayson, M. (2005). Pilot study of an energy conservation education program delivered by telephone conference call to people with Multiple Sclerosis. *NeuroRehabilitation, 20*(4), 267–277.

Firth, J. (2011). Rheumatoid arthritis: Diagnosis and multidisciplinary management. *British Journal of Nursing, 20*(18), 1179–1185.

Klinger, L., & Spaulding, S. J. (2001). Occupational therapy treatment of chronic pain and use of assistive devices in older adults. *Topics in Geriatric Rehabilitation, 16*(3), 34–44.

Mathiowetz, V. G., Finlayson, M. L., Matuska, K. M., et al. (2005). Randomized controlled trial of an energy conservation course for persons with Multiple Sclerosis. *Multiple Sclerosis, 11*, 592–601.

Oslund, S., Robinson, R. C., Clark, T. C., et al. (2009). Long-term effectiveness of a comprehensive pain management program: strengthening the case for interdisciplinary care. *Proceedings (Baylor University. Medical Center), 22*(3), 211–214.

Sabata, D. B., Shamberg, S., & Williams, M. (2008). Optimizing access to home, community and work environments. In M. V. Radomski & C. A. Trombly-Latham (Eds.), *Occupational therapy for physical dysfunction* (6th ed., pp. 951–973). Philadelphia: Lippincott Williams & Wilkins.

Shaw, N., Hill, S., & Robinson, P. (2011). *Goal setting for chronic illness rehabilitation: Experiences and views of patients and health professionals.* Paper presented at the Occupational Therapy Australia 24th National Conference and Exhibition, Gold Coast Australia.

ROLE OF THE PHYSIOTHERAPIST

Anthony Wright

Introduction

Physiotherapy is a healthcare profession with a therapeutic focus on healthy movement, enhancing mobility and maintaining physical activity and quality of life. Physiotherapists are experts in exercise and physical activity who assist people with movement-related problems and painful disorders, and help to improve and maintain movement, mobility and physical independence. They are key members of the interdisciplinary team in the management of a range of disabilities and chronic diseases and work collaboratively with nurses, medical practitioners and a range of allied health practitioners.

Physiotherapists practise in a wide variety of settings, including hospitals, private practices, primary care facilities, schools and universities, aged care facilities, sports facilities, workplaces, mental health services and public health services. They also work with people across the entire lifespan, from premature babies in neonatal intensive care to the very elderly. Physiotherapists work closely with nurses in many different settings including emergency departments, outpatient clinics, hospital wards and a range of community settings. Approximately half of all physiotherapists in Australia practise outside the public hospital system.

Physiotherapy profession

Physiotherapists are primary contact practitioners whose services can be directly accessed by members of the public without medical referral. They are registered by the Physiotherapy Board of Australia. The Australian Physiotherapy Association is the national peak body representing the interests of Australian physiotherapists and their patients. The organisation is active in a wide range of advocacy roles on behalf of physiotherapists and their clients.

Physiotherapists are eligible for registration upon completion of an accredited educational program. This may be a 4-year bachelor degree or a graduate-entry masters degree. Many physiotherapists complete postgraduate studies in areas such as manipulative therapy, sports physiotherapy, paediatrics and women's health. They may complete an examination process to become specialist physiotherapists and Fellows of the Australian College of Physiotherapists.

Physiotherapy practice

The physiotherapy profession places a strong emphasis on the provision of care based on evidence-based practice linked to sound clinical reasoning and clinical expertise. The physiotherapist establishes a clinical diagnosis based on a detailed assessment of the client, including a clinical history and detailed clinical examination. Specific movement-related impairments will be often identified and goals of treatment will be established in consultation with the client. The physiotherapist will then develop an individualised treatment plan and a broad approach to assisting the client to manage their particular disorder. Physiotherapists utilise a wide range of non-drug-based therapies to achieve their therapeutic goals and in most cases the treatment program will include an individualised exercise program and patient education related to prevention or management of the disorder. Commonly utilised treatments include joint mobilisation and other manual therapies, specific movement re-education, therapeutic exercise, gait re-education, electrophysical agents, hydrotherapy, assistive devices, behavioural therapy and education. For most people with a disability or a chronic disease or condition there is an emphasis on active interventions and empowering the individual and their carers to take an active role in self-management of their disorder and the promotion of health and activity.

Conditions treated

Physiotherapists treat clients with a wide range of conditions, including musculoskeletal disorders such as back pain, neck pain, headache and sports injuries. This includes assisting patients to manage a wide range of chronic pain problems. They are also actively involved in the management of patients with various forms of arthritis by providing specific treatments, encouraging preventive strategies and providing post-operative management and rehabilitation of individuals who receive joint replacements. At a community level physiotherapy places a strong emphasis on the importance of maintaining regular physical activity and exercise as a means of preventing or minimising the impact of arthritis.

Physiotherapists are also active in the management of a range of chronic cardiopulmonary disorders such as asthma, chronic obstructive pulmonary disease and cardiovascular disease. Interventions encourage exercise and physical activity, including specific exercises to retrain inspiratory muscle function and exercise programs to improve aerobic capacity. Physiotherapists have significant expertise in modifying exercise programs to ensure that they are safe for patients with significant pulmonary or cardiac pathology. The maintenance of optimal fitness is critical for many individuals living with significant pulmonary or cardiac disorders.

One of the most devastating outcomes of cardiovascular disease is stroke. Physiotherapists have a major role in the rehabilitation of patients after stroke. This includes movement re-education, re-education of gait and assisting patients to achieve the maximum possible level of functional independence. Physiotherapists often work closely with patients and their families for many months to ensure that they achieve the best possible outcomes and to assist them in adjusting to the major impact that stroke has on their lives.

Physiotherapy is also of benefit for patients with a variety of other neurological disorders such as Parkinson's disease and multiple sclerosis. Physiotherapists work closely with clients to assist them in managing the impacts of these chronic diseases over time. Physiotherapists can assist in maintaining movement and function and limiting disability associated with these conditions.

Physiotherapists are able to make an important contribution to the management of all chronic diseases for which exercise is known to be beneficial. This includes diseases such as diabetes mellitus and mental health problems such as depression. Physiotherapists have expertise in designing exercise programs for at-risk populations and addressing particular problems that clients may experience, such as foot disorders and balance problems in patients with diabetes.

As indicated previously, physiotherapists work actively with clients across the entire life span. Paediatric physiotherapists work with families and children who experience a variety of conditions that may affect normal motor development. This includes conditions such as cerebral palsy. Paediatric physiotherapy places a very strong emphasis on interdisciplinary practice and family-centred therapy. Physiotherapists work with parents to maintain and improve motor function in children with cerebral palsy and provide comprehensive rehabilitation programs after botulinum toxin injections and various surgical procedures. There are a number of other paediatric conditions for which physiotherapy interventions are beneficial.

Many developed countries are experiencing a rapid ageing of the population with a significant increase in the number of people living with chronic diseases. Physiotherapists work with older individuals to assist them in managing their disorders and maintaining healthy physical activity within the confines imposed by multiple chronic conditions. They can also provide specific interventions to address risk of falling and prevent the significant morbidity and mortality associated with falls.

Physiotherapists also provide significant assistance for women with continence problems related to pelvic floor disorders following childbirth.

CONCLUSION

Physiotherapy plays an important role in the management of a broad range of disabilities and chronic conditions that affect people throughout the lifespan. Physiotherapists work closely with many other members of the healthcare team including nurses across a range of settings to assist patients in managing their conditions. Physiotherapists place a strong emphasis on exercise and physical activity and are well equipped to tailor safe and effective exercise programs for people with a range of health conditions. They are also placing an increased emphasis on self-management and empowering and educating clients to take responsibility for the management of their own conditions. There is a strong emphasis on evidence-based interventions and an increased emphasis on primary and secondary prevention strategies.

ROLE OF THE SPEECH PATHOLOGIST

Susan Balandin
Michelle Lincoln

Speech pathologists specialise in the areas of speech, swallowing and memory (Speech Pathology Australia, 2003). Verbal communication is a distinguishing feature of humans and an essential component of adequate quality of life. Communication occurs in all situations across the hospital and community context. However, effective communication between nurses and people with communication disability and their carers and family is critical for achieving optimal healthcare. Successful communication between nurses and patients is an interaction in which both participants are satisfied that a message has been clearly conveyed and understood. Verbal communication fulfils four functions: communication of needs and wants, information transfer, social closeness and social etiquette (Light et al., 2003). Loss of or failure to develop normal verbal communication can have devastating effects on individuals and their families.

Nurses working in hospital and community contexts may encounter four broad types of conditions that result in communication impairments that require intervention and support from a speech pathologist.

1 Lifelong or developmental disability is disability that originated at birth or in childhood and is expected to continue throughout life. Lifelong disability includes intellectual disability and physical disability such as cerebral palsy. Patients with these conditions may routinely use a form of communication other than speech referred to as augmentative and alternative communication (AAC) (Beukelman, 2012). AAC includes signs, communication boards and computers with voice output. Training and advice from a speech pathologist may be necessary to ensure that these patients continue to be able to communicate effectively while in hospital and in the community.

2 Acquired disability such as sensory loss (especially hearing), cerebrovascular accident and traumatic brain injury or laryngectomy. These conditions may significantly impair an individual's ability to understand and produce speech and/or to use communication in a socially appropriate way.

3 Temporary disability, such as Guillain-Barré syndrome, intensive care unit admission and tracheostomy, which temporarily impair the person's ability to communicate verbally. Speech pathologists are able to provide patients with alternative means of communication during the period they are unable to speak.

4 Degenerative conditions such as motor neurone disease, Parkinson's disease and multiple sclerosis. Speech pathologists ensure that these patients continue to have a functional means of communication for as long as possible.

In addition, speech pathologists are actively involved in managing dysphagia (eating, drinking and swallowing disorders) with nurses on hospital wards or in residential aged care facilities (RACFs). The need to ensure communication and patient safety from the risks of choking or aspiration of food and drink means that it is important for speech pathologists and nurses to work collaboratively. This will help to ensure that not only patients' healthcare needs are met but all stakeholders feel confident that their swallowing and communication needs are being managed appropriately.

In hospital, patients with communication impairment may experience increased clinical and psychological risk if they cannot communicate effectively with nursing staff. Frequent outcomes of hospitalisation for individuals with moderate to profound communication impairment are sub-optimal healthcare, psychological trauma and poor discharge planning (Armitage & Kavanagh, 1998; Balandin et al., 2007; Efraimisson et al., 2004; Hemsley & Balandin 2004).

When ill in hospital, patients are not always in constant and regular contact with family and loved ones and their health management is the responsibility of the hospital staff, including nurses and speech pathologists. Successful communication with the nurses is critical for the patient's wellbeing. If a patient has communication impairments hospitalisation places communication demands on patients and nurses alike. For example, basic needs such as pain relief need to be communicated, along with the development of any medically pertinent symptoms (Hemsley, Balandin, & Worrall, 2012). At a less immediate level, the patient needs to express feelings about being ill and hospitalised, and elicit basic information about the medical condition and plans for its management.

Busy nurses need to be able to manage their time to communicate quickly and effectively with patients and to know how best to communicate with those patients who have difficulty in understanding or communicating verbally (Hemsley et al., in press). At the same time nurses need to understand how to safely manage the mealtimes of patients with swallowing difficulties (Daniels et al., 2000; DeRenzo, 1997). Thus it is important that nurses and speech pathologists work together collaboratively, ensuring that each respects and utilises the other's skills. Nurses know how the patient is managing communicatively on the ward and are usually aware of any communication breakdowns that are occurring, including how the patient's family and friends are coping with any communication difficulties or mealtime management issues. In addition, nurses are likely to notice if the patient is using any communication techniques suggested by the speech pathologist and if these are indeed effective.

One of the challenges facing both nurses and speech pathologists is how best to maintain contact so that communication proceeds smoothly for all concerned. Speech pathology departments in hospitals usually offer both inpatient and outpatient services, so speech pathologists are on the wards regularly. Nevertheless, on a busy ward it is not always easy to maintain cross-disciplinary contact. Nurses need to know how to contact a speech pathologist and to understand the help that speech pathologists can give to nurses. Inviting the speech pathologists to meetings and asking them to make short presentations on some of the different communication disorders commonly seen in hospital and how these are managed may be helpful in building up rapport between the two professions. Similarly, speech pathologists need to understand the ward structure and how to ensure that any communication strategies or particular management programs reach all nursing staff, whatever shift they are working. Thus it is important to develop not only a good working relationship but to maintain open lines of communication so that all stakeholders, including the patient and family members, are informed about how best to manage any communication or mealtime difficulties.

Nurses cannot be expected to be knowledgeable about all forms of communication disability that may occur on a ward, nor do speech pathologists always appreciate how pressed for time nurses may be on a busy ward. Hence it is important that any collaboration is robust enough to allow discussion and a collaborative approach to identify barriers to communication and find acceptable solutions. Such collaborative relationships are built over time, yet around the world there is now evidence that collaborative relationships focusing on communication can be developed and that once established, all, but in particular the patient and family, benefit (Saevareid & Balandin, 2011). Mutual respect, an openness to ideas, a willingness to ask for help, a readiness to consider and indeed offer innovative ideas to solve a problem and preparedness to listen are skills that both nurses and speech pathologists need to bring to any collaboration. Added to this, there is no substitute for getting to know individuals by working with them and learning about what they do.

There is no doubt that communication is critically important in hospital as well as the community. Effective communication makes a hospital stay easier for everyone concerned and will result in better health outcomes for the patient when they return to their community. Nurses and speech pathologists both have much to offer and, together with the patient, are the foundations of a strong collaborative team.

Recommended reading

Miller, C. K., Burklow, K. A., Santoro, K. et al. (2001). An interdisciplinary team approach to the management of pediatric feeding and swallowing disorders. *Children's Health Care, 30*, 201–218.

References

Armitage, S. K., & Kavanagh, K. M. (1998). Consumer-orientated outcomes in discharge planning: a pilot study. *Journal of Clinical Nursing Inquiry, 7*, 74–76.

Australian Institute of Health and Welfare. (2004). *Australia's health 2004*. Canberra: Author.

Balandin, S., Hemsley, B., Sigafoos, J., et al. (2007). Communicating with nurses: The experiences of 10 adults with cerebral palsy and complex communication needs. *Applied Nursing Research, 20,* 56–62.

Beukelman, D. R. (2012). *Augmentative and alternative communication: Supporting children and adults with complex communication needs.* Baltimore: Paul H Brookes.

Daniels, S. K., Ballo, L. A., Mahoney, M., et al. (2000). Clinical predictors of dysphagia and aspiration risk: outcome measures in acute stroke patients. *Archives of Physical Medicine & Rehabilitation, 81*(8), 1030–1033.

DeRenzo, E. G. (1997). Ethical considerations in dysphagia treatment and research: secular and sacred. In B. C. Sonies (Ed.), *Dysphagia: A continuum of care* (pp. 91–106). Gaithersburg: Aspen Publishers.

Efraimisson, E., Sandman, P. O., Hyden, L. C., et al. (2004). Discharge planning: 'fooling ourselves'? — patient participation in conferences. *Journal of Clinical Nursing, 13,* 562–570.

Hemsley, B., & Balandin, S. (2004). Without AAC: The stories of unpaid carers of adults with cerebral palsy and complex communication needs in hospital. *Augmentative and Alternative Communication, 20,* 243–258.

Hemsley, B., Balandin, S., & Worrall, L. (2012). Nursing the patient with complex communication needs: time as a barrier and a facilitator to successful communication in hospital. *Journal of Advanced Nursing, 68*(1), 116–126.

Hemsley, B., Balandin, S., & Worrall, L. (in press). The 'big 5' and beyond: Nurses, paid carers, and adults with developmental disability discuss communication needs in hospital. *Applied Research in Nursing.*

Light, J. C., Beukelman, D. R., & Reichle, J. (Eds.), (2003). *Communicative competence for individuals who use AAC.* Baltimore: Brookes Publishing.

Saevareid, T. J., & Balandin, S. (2011). Nurses' perceptions of attempting cardiopulmonary resuscitation on oldest old patients. *Journal of Advanced Nursing, 67*(8), 1739–1748.

Speech Pathology Australia. (2003). Scope of practice in speech pathology. Retrieved 11 March 2008 from http://www.speechpathologyaustralia.org.au/library/ScopOfPractice.pdf

ROLE OF THE SOCIAL WORKER

Mark Hughes

Nurses and social workers work collaboratively in many health settings, such as hospitals, mental health teams, community health centres and disability and rehabilitation agencies. Depending on the nature of the work and type of multidisciplinary or interdisciplinary team, social workers and nurses can often find themselves undertaking similar tasks and developing strong bonds.

The purpose of social work is to help people achieve optimal health and wellbeing within their own environment, including their family, community and society. In particular, social work is concerned with assisting those who are disadvantaged by underlying social inequalities, such as discrimination on the basis of personal characteristics, identity or group affiliation (e.g. according to ethnicity, gender, sexual identity, age or disability). Thus, social work maintains a commitment to social justice and empowering those who are seen to be excluded from active participation in society (O'Connor et al., 2008).

In Australia qualified social workers have undertaken either a 4-year undergraduate degree or a 2-year qualifying masters degree, which are accredited by the Australian Association of Social Workers (AASW) in relation to a series of professional standards. While many social workers work in health, social workers are also employed in areas such as child protection, income security (Centrelink), housing, employment services, correctional facilities and schools. They could be working in government agencies or any number of non-government organisations ranging from large organisations, such as Uniting Care, through to small agencies employing just a few staff, such as domestic violence shelters. Similarly, the range of social work practice can be quite diverse—from individual case management and counselling, to facilitating group interventions, to community development and social action.

In health settings social workers often draw on a biopsychosocial approach. This approach seeks to go beyond the traditional medical model to address the interplay between biological, psychological, environmental, social and behavioural dimensions of illness and wellbeing (Browne, 2012). A key role for social workers in a health team is carrying out biopsychosocial assessments which complement and inform the assessment/diagnostic tasks of other professionals. These assessments may include an identification of:

- physical and personal care needs arising from the patient's health condition, including capacity in activities of daily living
- emotional needs, such as feelings of safety, privacy, dignity
- psychological needs, including coping skills, self-esteem
- social needs, such as personal and family relationships, nature of social networks, attachment to community
- spiritual needs, such as sense of hope, meaning, purpose in life
- practical needs, including direct assistance, financial resources, housing
- informational needs to facilitate decision making (Howell et al., 2012).

A key concern will be to identify the supports available to the person, the impact of these on the person's wellbeing and the availability of the supports to provide assistance over the longer term. Critical to the effectiveness of the assessment process is forming an effective social work relationship with the client or patient. Social workers seek to 'start where the client is at', rather than impose predetermined assumptions. By building a meaningful relationship people are enabled to disclose sensitive issues (such as previous experiences of abuse or trauma) which can have a significant impact on the person's wellbeing and recovery.

In working with people with disabilities and those living with a chronic illness, social workers play a key role in assisting people to live independently; for example, by mobilising available resources prior to people returning home from hospital. They provide counselling to individuals, helping them adjust to and overcome limitations that might arise from their disability or illness. They work with partners, family members and friends and, in particular, provide support to caregivers and help strengthen caregiving networks. Social workers also advocate and lobby on behalf of clients' rights. For example, social workers may sometimes argue against discharging a patient home until appropriate community resources are put in place. In a study evaluating health professionals' understanding of social workers' contributions in multidisciplinary teams, this advocacy role was not well understood and was sometimes misperceived as being obstructive (Mizrahi & Abramson, 2000).

In the health and disability sectors, social workers often draw on a strengths-based approach, which aims to shift the focus away from a person's problems or deficits towards their capabilities or strengths (Saleebey, 2012). It is argued that too much emphasis on a person's problems (such as their illness or disability) undermines their sense of competence and reduces their humanity to a label or diagnosis. While the approach does not ignore the challenges the individual faces, it recognises their survival capacity and strengths in other areas of their life and tries to emulate or build on these (Munford & Sanders, 2005).

Like other professions, social work has also found much value in the social model of disability, which posits that disability arises not from the individual, but from society's failure to accommodate the diversity of impairments that individuals experience (Oliver, 2009). The focus is on society adjusting to individuals' incapacities rather than vice versa. Disability rights campaigns promote the social model of disability and call for disabled people to exercise more authority in the planning, delivery and evaluation of disability services. The often quoted phrase is 'nothing about us, without us'. Social work, like other professions, has been criticised for imposing expert definitions on disabled people's lives (Beaulaurier & Taylor, 2001). However, recent promotion of partnerships with consumer groups provides opportunities for social workers and other professionals to work alongside clients to support them in gaining more control not just over the services designated to respond to their needs, but also over other aspects of their lives (Postle & Beresford, 2007).

CONCLUSION

Social work has long articulated a commitment to multidisciplinary practice. However, like other allied health professionals, social workers can experience challenges in team work, such as role overlap, differences in terminology and alternative ways of defining patient problems. There may also be power dynamics within teams—possibly reflecting wider social divisions (e.g. gendered labour patterns)—which impact on team members. Sometimes the language of partnership may 'paper over' deeper power conflicts and 'turf wars' between the professions (Longoria, 2005). Nonetheless, these sorts of difficulties are often overcome in everyday practice because optimal multidisciplinary healthcare relies on effective professional relationships that are focused on the needs of the client/patient.

Recommended reading

Barnes, D., & Hugman, R. (2002). Portrait of social work. *Journal of Interprofessional Care, 16*(3), 277–288.

References

Beaulaurier, R. L., & Taylor, S. H. (2001). Social work practice with people with disabilities in the era of disability rights. *Social Work in Health Care, 32*(4), 67–91.

Browne, T. (2012). Social work roles in health-care settings. In S. Gehlert & T. Browne (Eds.), *Handbook of health social work* (2nd ed.). New Jersey: John Wiley.

Howell, D., Mayo, S., Currie, S., et al. (2012). *Psychosocial health care needs assessment of adult cancer patients: a consensus-based guideline. Support Care Cancer.* Published online 13 May 2012, DOI 10.1007/s00520-012-1468-x

Longoria, R. A. (2005). Is inter-organizational collaboration always a good thing? *Journal of Sociology and Social Welfare, 32*(3), 123–139.

Mizrahi, T., & Abramson, J. S. (2000). Collaboration between social workers and physicians: perspectives on a shared case. *Social Work in Health Care, 31*(3), 1–24.

Munford, R., & Sanders, J. (2005). Working with families: strengths-based approaches. In R. Munford, K. O'Donoghue, & M. Nash (Eds.), *Social work theories in action*. London: Jessica Kingsley Publishers.

O'Connor, I., Wilson, J., Setterlund, D., et al. (2008). *Social work and human service practice* (5th ed.). Frenchs Forest: Pearson Education Australia.

Oliver, M. (2009). *Understanding disability: From theory to practice* (2nd ed.). Basingstoke: Macmillan.

Postle, K., & Beresford, P. (2007). Capacity building and the reconception of political participation: a role for social care workers? *British Journal of Social Work*, *37*, 143–158.

Saleebey, D. (2012). The strengths approach to practice: beginnings. In D. Saleebey (Ed.), *The strengths perspective in social work practice* (6th ed.). Boston: Allyn & Bacon.

CHAPTER 3

Vicki Drury
Samar Aoun

Models of care

Learning objectives

When you have completed this chapter you will be able to:

- critically examine existing models of management for long term conditions
- describe and discuss the evidence base that has contributed to the self-management model of care
- describe the fundamental elements of the self-management model of care for people with long-term conditions
- identify opportunities and strategies for applying self-management approaches to the management of diverse long-term conditions
- apply a self-management approach in the delivery of care to people with long-term conditions.

Key words

models of care, self-management, chronic disease, chronic care model, long-term conditions

INTRODUCTION

Caring for populations who are living longer with chronic conditions is undoubtedly the major healthcare challenge of this century for many developed countries (Bodenheimer et al., 2002; Bury & Ink, 2005; Commonwealth of Australia, 2008; Jordan & Osborne, 2007; Lorig et al., 2005). The co-existence of co-morbid long-term conditions is increasing with estimates that more than 80% of elderly people with a long-term condition have two or more co-morbid diseases (Caughey et al., 2008; Wolff, Starfield, & Anderson, 2002). With the global ageing population, the impact of long-term conditions will place a significant burden both on the fiscal costs of healthcare as well as on the healthcare workforce (Brooks, 2008). Internationally many countries have developed strategies to facilitate the development of clear, comprehensive, collaborative approaches to the prevention, detection and management of long-term conditions (Department of Health (UK), 2004; National Health Priority Action Council, 2006). Producing long-term, cost-effective public health impact is now the primary concern for interventions in lifestyle risk modification (Eakin et al., 2007; Foster et al., 2008; Kelly, Menzies, & Taylor, 2003; Lindner, Menzies, & Kelly, 2003; Lindner et al., 2003; VanWormer & Boucher, 2004). However, the development and delivery of an effective strategy to assist people to alter their lifestyle and behaviour has been challenging. People at risk or living with long-term conditions need to develop and continue practising complex self-management strategies to allow them to live a healthier life (Heisler, 2006). Current literature suggests that people with long-term conditions who effectively maintain self-management practices make better use of their health professionals' time, have better self-care and experience clear clinical benefits (Jordan & Osborne, 2007). Thus, there has been a growing popularity and emphasis on promoting formal self-management education programs across the developed world (Jordan & Osborne, 2007; Heisler, 2006). Numerous models of care have arisen in the past decade in an attempt to manage the increasing burden of chronic disease. Common elements exist within all the models as governments adapt them to meet the needs of their populations.

MODELS OF CARE FOR PEOPLE WITH LONG-TERM CONDITIONS

The chronic care model

Evidence suggests that the Chronic Care Model, developed by Wagner et al. (2001) at the McColl Institute in the United States more than a decade ago, is effective across a number of chronic conditions in improving both clinical and behavioural outcomes (Adams et al., 2007; Coleman et al., 2009; Piatt et al., 2006). The key elements in this model viewed as being critical to effective management of patients with long-term conditions are: community resources; the healthcare system; patient self-management; decision support; delivery system redesign; and clinical information systems (Carrier, 2009; Coleman et al., 2009; Wagner et al., 2001). The key principles of the model include empowering people to manage their conditions, providing effective and responsible self-management support and organising community resources to meet the needs of people with long-term conditions (Carrier, 2009; Wagner et al., 2001). A revision of this model in 2003 led to the inclusion of cultural competency, patient safety, care coordination, case management and community policies (Carrier, 2009); however, this model lacks a population health aspect and therefore is limited to impacting on those people with long-term conditions and does not meet the need for a model that is inclusive of health promotion and health prevention (Barr et al., 2003). A recent meta-analysis of 112 studies implementing interventions based on the Chronic Care Model found that interventions that included at least one element from this model were associated with better health outcomes, however they could find no single element that appeared more effective than others (McGettrick & O'Neill, 2006).

The expanded Chronic Care Model

A Canadian team felt that the Chronic Care Model did not meet the needs of health promotion or health prevention clinicians and integrated the Ottawa Charter for Health Promotion determinants with the key elements of the Chronic Care Model enabling the

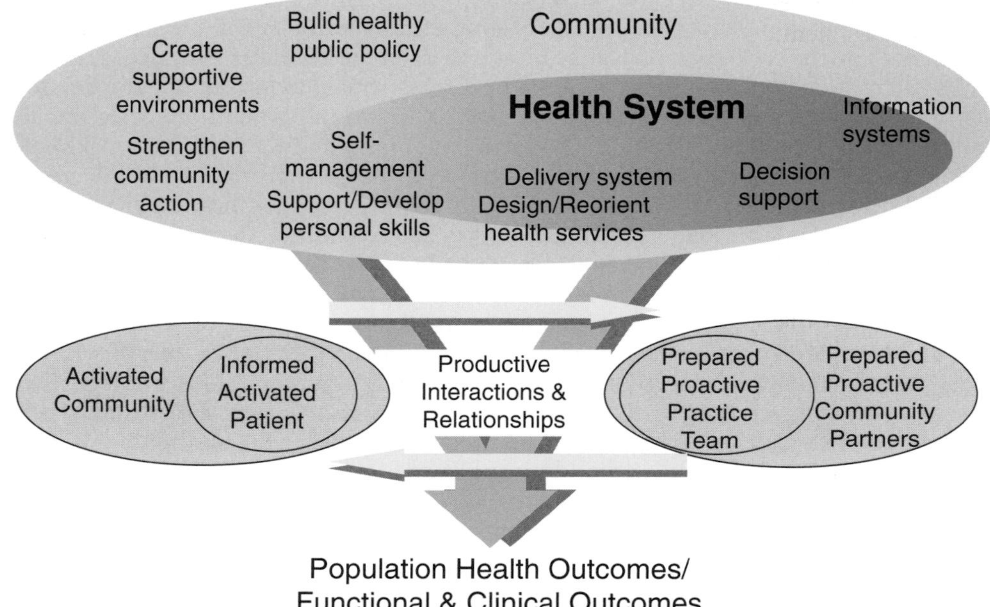

FIGURE 3.1 The Expanded Chronic Care Model. *Note*: from Barr et al., 2003.

inclusion of health prevention, social determinants of health and community participation to be included in work concerning long-term conditions (Barr et al., 2003; Coleman et al., 2009). See Figure 3.1.

Innovative care for chronic conditions model

The World Health Organization (WHO) together with the McColl Institute adapted the Chronic Care Model developing a framework which expanded the community and policy aspects and focused on improving care for people with long-term conditions at three levels: (1) the macro level (policy); (2) the meso level (healthcare organisations and community); and (3) micro (individual and family) (Carrier, 2009; Epping-Jordan et al, 2004). This framework is relevant for both prevention and management of long-term conditions and provides an adaptable foundation to construct or redesign health systems within the local context (Epping-Jordan et al., 2004).

The National Chronic Disease Strategy in Australia

The Australian Government developed the National Chronic Disease Strategy (NCDS) in acknowledgment that the existing system focused on acute, short-term problems. This strategy aims to prevent or delay the onset of chronic diseases; reduce complications; reduce avoidable hospital admission; and implement best practice in the prevention, assessment and management of chronic disease. Adopting a population health approach, the strategy contains four key areas (Geiger-Brown & Trinkoff, 2010):

1 prevention across the continuum
2 early detection and early treatment

3 integration and continuity of prevention and care
4 self-management.

Nationally in Australia the priority health areas for chronic disease are asthma, cancer, cardiovascular disease, diabetes and musculoskeletal conditions. These diseases were highlighted as national priorities due to the excessive burden they place on Australian communities and the ability to minimise the diseases through lifestyle and behavioural changes and modifications within the environment through policy and legislative changes (South Australia Dept. of Health Statewide Service Strategy Division, 2008).

Fundamental to the Australian national strategy to reduce the burden of chronic disease and to improve the ability of individuals to effectively manage their conditions are the concepts of self-management and self-management support (National Health Priority Action Council, 2006).

An overview of the historical development of self-management programs

The two approaches applied to self-management that are most evident in the literature are the Stanford approach which uses peer leaders and is conducted in groups, and the Flinders program which is an individual, clinician-led approach underpinned by cognitive behaviour therapy principles (Government of Western Australia, 2009; Lawn & Schoo, 2010). Both approaches have been credibly evaluated and are extensively used globally (Bodenheimer et al., 2002; Jordan et al., 2008; Lawn et al., 2007; Lorig et al., 2005, 2006).

The first chronic disease self-management program was developed by Kate Lorig and Stanford University in the 1970s. This first program, designed specifically for people with arthritis, became a blueprint for subsequent programs (Lorig et al., 2006). Stanford Patient Education Research Centre, under the leadership of Lorig, continues to develop, deliver and evaluate chronic disease self-management programs to patients and training for healthcare professionals and lay persons with chronic diseases. The Stanford program is a community based, group program which is led by pairs of trained lay people who have a chronic disease themselves (Carrier, 2009; Lorig et al., 2006).

Despite global interest in the Stanford program it was not until 1997 that both Australia and the United Kingdom developed similar programs. The Flinders program in Australia (originally known as the Flinders Model) developed from the SA Health Plus coordinated care trial. The Flinders program involves using designated tools that assist with assessment, goal setting and care planning. Unlike the Stanford program, the Flinders program is an individual program that is initiated and supported by a health professional (Lorig et al., 2001).

In the United Kingdom, the Living with Long Term Illness project was established in 1998. Findings from this project contributed to the Expert Patients taskforce which was established in 1999. The aim of the taskforce was to combine both patient and clinical organisations to develop self-management programs (Carrier, 2009). The current program is planned around three phases: case management; disease management; and self-management support (Bandura, 2005). The Expert Patient Program is a 6-week, lay-led program based on the Stanford program delivered within the National Health Service (Bandura, 2005; Zimmerman, 2000). It was during this period that the focus shifted from the term 'chronic disease' to the more inclusive term 'long-term conditions'.

Although the aforementioned programs provide clinicians with specific guidelines and information, most long-term conditions are responsive to a generic approach to self-management (Jones, 2006; Lawn & Schoo, 2010). Enabling people to accept responsibility for the self-management of their long-term condition is a complex issue that encompasses readiness for change, intrinsic motivation and high self-efficacy (Packer et al., 2009).

The self-management framework

The self-management approach acknowledges that people must cope not only with the disease and the consequences of the disease but also the impact that it has on their life.

Self-management is an approach to the management of a long-term condition that recognises the central role of the person in health promotion, disease prevention and successful management of the disease (Bodenheimer et al., 2002). Self-management is the individual's ability to manage the disease process, the emotional consequences of living with the disease and the changes that occur to daily living as a consequence of the disease (Corbin & Strauss, 1988). In self-management the person with the long-term condition is motivated to take responsibility for their health needs and is supported by health professionals and community services who work collaboratively to assist the individual to manage their chronic illnesses (Jordan et al., 2008).

Evidence shows that programs incorporating self-management skills can enhance health outcomes (Bodenheimer et al., 2002; McMurray et al., 2002). Self-management is both a process whereby education or training is provided to people with chronic illness and an outcome when people with long-term conditions achieve the skills and knowledge to manage the medical, emotional and role aspects of their illness.

The health professional works in partnership with the person providing self-management support and works with the person towards the achievement of common goals.

The literature identifies the following skills as being essential in facilitating self-management support with a person with a long-term condition (Aoun et al., 2009; Battersby et al., 2008; Jones, 2006; Lawn & Schoo, 2010; Warner et al., 2011):

- assessing the person's readiness for change
- using motivational interviewing techniques
- assisting the person to set goals and develop a realistic and achievable action plan
- building self-efficacy.

Assessing readiness for change

It is essential that a person is assessed to determine whether they are motivated to make some changes in their life and also whether they want to take the lead role in managing their long-term condition. Understanding the readiness of a person in relation to changing behaviour affects the way you will communicate and respond to that person using motivational interviewing techniques.

Prochaska and DiClemente (1983) developed a model of behaviour change that provides an easy yet credible method of assessing an individual's readiness for change (Prochaska & Norcross, 2001). In this model it is suggested that people go through a series of changes when altering behaviour. It is acknowledged in the health promotion literature that people are often at different stages of change in relation to adopting self-management strategies (Keefe et al., 2000; Velicer et al., 1995). Furthermore, there is substantial evidence demonstrating that behaviour change is more effective when an individual's stage of change is considered in the development of goals and care planning (DiClemente, Nidecker & Bellack, 2008; Keefe et al., 2000). The transtheoretical model, also known as the Stages of Change, developed by Prochaska and DiClemente in the mid 1970s for use in smoking cessation, is commonly used to determine readiness for change (Burns et al., 2005; Dijkstra et al., 2001; Parchman et al., 2002). In this model 'stage' is a temporal construct that

TABLE 3.1

Transtheoretical model. *Note*: From Prochaska & diClemente, 1983, 1998; Prochaska & Norcross, 2001; Zimmerman, Olsen, & Bosworth, 2000.

STAGE	BEHAVIOUR
Pre-contemplation	The person has no intention of making any changes in the next 6 months. While they may lack motivation, they may also lack the knowledge and skills that enable them to change behaviour.
Contemplation	In this stage the person is contemplating change within the next 6 months. Although aware of the benefits of changing behaviour, ambivalence occurs as the person focuses on the barriers and costs that will occur during the change period.
Preparation	Individuals in this stage are preparing to take action within the next month. They generally have a plan and may have already taken some action towards the change.
Action	The person has made modifications and action is observable and measurable. It is during this stage that ongoing support is essential as relapse is a high risk.
Maintenance	The changes have been made and the risk of relapse is decreasing. Individuals in this stage feel confident that they continue the new behaviour.

signifies when specific changes are likely to occur (Keefe et al., 2000; Prochaska & DiClemente, 1998). Rather than behaviour change being viewed as an event, in this model change is viewed as occurring over time (this is the temporal aspect) with individuals moving through a series of five stages from pre-contemplation, when they have no intention to change, to a final stage of maintenance where they have made changes and have implemented strategies to prevent relapse and sustain the behaviour change (Prochaska & DiClemente, 1998).

The stages of change described in this model are summarised in Table 3.1.

Using motivational interviewing to facilitate behaviour change

In addition to assessing an individual's readiness for change, motivation, barriers to change, attitudes and self-efficacy also need to be assessed. Motivational interviewing has become an accepted communication strategy for working with individuals who do not appear to be ready to change behaviours that may be considered necessary by the healthcare professional (Britt, Hudson, & Blampied, 2004). Motivational interviewing is based on the premise that most people do not enter into a consultation with a health professional ready and willing to make behaviour changes, thus the healthcare professional's role is to assist the individual to explore and resolve their ambivalence about behaviour change. Motivational interviewing differs from other forms of counselling as it is more focused and goal directed. The motivation to change is intrinsic and elicited from the individual. Consequently the gains for the individual are driven by internal needs and goals. Individuals are encouraged and assisted to explore their feelings and concerns about the current behaviour and the potential new behaviour. This often results in ambivalence or mixed feelings whereby the individual weighs up the costs and benefits of changing behaviours. Motivational interviewing is a continuous process of eliciting information from the individual, the provision of information by the healthcare professional and then eliciting information on the individual's understanding of the new information (Resnicow, Davis, & Rollnick, 2006). There are four fundamental phases in motivational interviewing: (1) engaging; (2) guiding; (3) evoking; and (4) planning (Britt et al., 2004; Miller & Moyers, 2006; Rubak et al., 2005; VanWormer & Boucher, 2004). See Table 3.2.

TABLE 3.2
Phases in Motivational Interviewing

PHASE	CLINICIAN'S ROLE AND RESPONSIBILITIES	COMMUNICATION STRATEGIES
Engaging (express empathy)	Build a rapport with the person. Use OARS. Open ended questions. Affirm. Reflective listening. Summarise. Assess the individual's stage of change.	How are things going? What do you want to do next? What are the good things about … and what are the less good things?
Guiding (develop discrepancy)	Explore the values and attitudes held by the individual. Identify goals and break into small achievable and measurable steps. Encourage the individual to identify the benefits and costs to changing behaviour. Allow the individual to form their own argument concerning changing behaviour.	How would you like things to be different? How do you think you could do that? How can I help you achieve that? Who is in your life that would support you making these changes?
Evoking (role with resistance)	The individual has identified a goal aimed at changing behaviour and is motivated to make the change. Use selective eliciting: elicit and selectively reinforce the individual's motivational statements, intention to change and ability to change. Do not argue. Use reflection. Summarise. Affirm the statements made.	It sounds like this is really difficult for you … What is most important to you now? So what you are saying is …
Planning (support self-efficacy)	Identify and set goals using SMART criteria (Bovend'Eerdt, Botell, & Wade, 2009): • specific • measurable • achievable • realistic • timely.	How did you manage something like this in the past? How do you think you could do this?

Goal setting and action planning

Goal setting and action planning are collaborative processes in which the clinician assists the individual to choose a behaviour change goal. Prior to setting goals the clinician has a responsibility to ensure that the individual has adequate information to make an informed choice. Once a goal has been agreed to then an action plan to assist with goal attainment is developed collaboratively (MacGregor et al., 2006; Wagner et al., 2001). To enable both the clinical staff and the individual to be able to measure whether goals have been attained the SMART acronym can be applied (see Table 3.3).

A simple template for setting SMART goals contains the following:

Goal ....

When do I want to achieve it ....

TABLE 3.3

Applying SMART goal. *Note*: From Bourbeau, Nault & Dang-Tan, 2004; Katch & Mead, 2010.

SPECIFIC	Ensure the goal is specific to the problem. Get the person to start with 'my goal is to …'. This will make it specific. Ensure it is unambiguous. Describe goals in simple terms. What do they want to achieve? How will they achieve it? And when will they achieve it?
MEASURABLE	The person needs to be able to determine if they have reached their goal. Write down how it will be measured if they reach their goal. You can also add in a starting point. If the goal is measurable the person will be able to celebrate when they reach their milestone.
ACHIEVABLE	The person needs to be able to think they CAN do this. Ask the following questions: What skills do you need to achieve this? What information and knowledge do you need? What help, assistance or collaboration do you need? What resources do you need? What barriers may block progress? Are you making any assumptions? Is there a better way of doing things? What steps do you need to accomplish your goal?
REALISTIC	The person must be able to expect to attain the goal. Don't allow them to set it too high to satisfy their friends or family nor base their goals on someone else's aspirations. Write down 'I want to accomplish this goal because…'. Is this reasonable? This will keep them motivated.
TIME FRAMED	The person must have a time frame to achieve their goal. This helps them stay focused and minimises procrastination. How long will it take to finish each step in the plan?

How I will achieve it ……………………………………………………………………………………

How I will measure it ……………………………………………………………………………………

Action planning results in a written commitment to action. Action plans are stated in measurable behavioural outcomes so may be developed using SMART goals (Brekke, Hjortdahl, & Kvien, 2001; Marks & Allegrante, 2005). When developing action plans from goals, assist the person to strive for a change that is behaviour specific and always begin when a person has a confidence level of 7 or higher. You can determine the confidence level simply by asking the person on a scale of 0–10, with 10 being confident they can achieve the goal they have set, how confident they are that they will be successful (Jones, 2006; Victorian Government Department of Human Services, 2007). A sample action plan is shown in Box 3.1.

Self-efficacy

Self-efficacy has been found to be essential in the development of self-management skills among people with long-term conditions (Lorig et al., 2006; Warner et al., 2011).

Bandura's social cognitive theory posits that motivation and behaviour are moderated by cognitive, behavioural, personal and environmental factors (Crothers, Hughes, & Morine, 2008). Bandura's seminal work in social cognitive theory termed the interplay between these factors the Triadic Model of Reciprocal Causation and asserts that although each functions as an interacting element they also influence each other bi-directionally (Bandura, 2005). For example, a person's ability to self-manage their illness (behavioural factor) is influenced by how the person is affected (cognitive factors) by institutional policies and processes (environmental factors).

Self-efficacy lies at the heart of Bandura's social cognitive theory (Bandura, 1986; Zimmerman, 2000). Self-efficacy is an individual's belief that they have the ability to achieve in certain situations (Lorig & Holman, 2003). Basically self-efficacy is the 'I can' or

BOX 3.1
Goal-behaviour action plan

Name: Joe Smith **Date:** ....

Phone: ....

The change I want to make is: Stop smoking.

My goal for the next 2 weeks is: To access information from the Quit line; gain support from family and friends; visit my family doctor for additional advice and support.

The steps I will take to achieve my goal are (what, when, where, how much, how often):

- I will identify reasons why I want to quit
- I will create a quit plan
- I will develop strategies to cope with cravings and stress.

The things that could make it difficult to achieve my goal include: Stressful events.

My plan for overcoming these difficulties includes:

- plan to quit at a time when no stressful life events are due to occur
- have a support person that I can seek advice and support from when I am facing challenges.

Support/resources I will need to achieve my goal include:

- friends and family
- family doctor
- Quit line (internet).

My confidence level (scale of 1–10, 10 being completely confident that you can achieve the entire plan): 8.

Review date: .... (insert date for 2 weeks)

Review method: (phone, email, in person): In person with clinician.

'I cannot' belief and reflects an individual's confidence in performing specific tasks. Bandura suggests that individual self-efficacy is acquired through four sources: (1) mastery experience; (2) vicarious experience; (3) social persuasion; and (4) physiological factors (Bandura, 1994; Marks & Allegrante, 2005; Warner et al., 2011).

1 Mastery experience is performing a task successfully. Past experiences that show competence at mastering a similar skill or knowledge related to the skill contributes to a person's confidence in performing a task successfully. Success raises self-efficacy, failure lowers it!
2 Vicarious experience is when a person compares themselves to another person with similar abilities/disabilities and sees the person succeeding. This increases the person's self-efficacy; however, it needs to be noted that where they see the other person failing this will decrease their self-efficacy. In other words, the person thinks 'if they can do it, I can do it too'.
3 Social persuasions refers to either positive encouragement or negative comments. Positive encouragement increases a person's self-efficacy whereas negative persuasions decrease self-efficacy.

4 Physiological factors are our own emotional responses to situations. When a person is in a stressful situation physical symptoms may occur; for example, nausea and sweating. It is not the intensity of the symptoms; rather it is how the person perceives and interprets them. Learning how to effectively manage stress and developing effective coping skills improves a person's self-efficacy.

In essence, self-efficacy involves helping the people to set realistic goals, learn positive self-talk and learn the ability to visualise success. It is an intrinsic belief in your ability to perform a task successfully. Self-efficacy is an important component in self-management and it has been found that behaviour related to self-management is affected by individual self-efficacy (Farrell, Wicks & Martin, 2004; Pearson et al., 2007). Numerous research studies have demonstrated the importance of including self-efficacy in self-management programs across a number of chronic diseases; for example: cardiovascular disease (Katch & Mead, 2010); chronic obstructive pulmonary disease (Bourbeau et al., 2004); chronic kidney disease (Curtin et al., 2008); diabetes (Johnston-Brooks, Lewis & Garg, 2002); ophthalmic disease (Brody, Roch-Levecq, Thomas, Kaplan, & Brown, 2005); and arthritis (Brekke et al., 2001). Consequently self-efficacy is usually incorporated into programs using a range of self-efficacy enhancing strategies such as providing positive reinforcement, support in mastering new skills, modelling of new behaviours and building confidence (Jones, 2006; Marks & Allegrante, 2005).

Self-management support

A key element in self-management is the support and advocacy provided to people and their families to empower them to take a central role in managing their condition, set realistic and achievable goals, making informed decisions about their care and participate in healthy behaviours (Robert Wood Johnson Foundation, 2011; Victorian Government Department of Human Services, 2007). Self-management support involves a partnership between the individual and the health professional where the health professional is the coach and the individual and their carers are the managers of daily care. In this model, the individual, family and carers and health professionals share information, understand the individual's goals and create an action plan that guides care at home as well as in the clinical setting. The principles underpinning self-management support are to work collaboratively to (South Australia Dept. of Health Statewide Service Strategy Division, 2008):

- define the issues
- set goals and problem solve
- provide active, sustained follow-up.

The major difference between this model and the traditional medical model is that the patient is actively involved in their own care and works with the healthcare professional to manage the disease. The healthcare professional is the expert in the disease and the disease process while the patient is the expert about their life. Bodenheimer et al. (2002) describe the role of the healthcare professional as providing support to the individual by assisting them to make informed choices, set their own goals and develop problem-solving skills.

The healthcare professional has a role of support when facilitating self-management with people. Core knowledge and skills essential for healthcare professionals to provide self-management support can be centred around three platforms (National Health Priority Action Council, 2006).

1 Assessment skills; assessing:
   - readiness for change
   - risk factors

- support systems
- self-management ability.

2 Behaviour change skills:
- effective use of motivational interviewing techniques
- understanding of theoretical models of behaviour change
- able to assist individual with goal setting, problem solving and developing action plans.

3 Organisational strategies:
- working in multidisciplinary teams
- applying evidence to practice
- sound knowledge of community resources.

The principles of self-management support as discussed in the literature (Battersby et al., 2008; Harvey et al., 2008; Lorig, 2000; Packer et al., 2009; Vancouver Coastal Health, 2008) include establishing a rapport and eliciting information from the individual about their progress, and the barriers and challenges they have confronted.

It is the role of the healthcare professional to assess the individual's readiness for change and to help them understand and explore the consequences of current behaviours and any ambivalence towards change. These techniques require the healthcare professional to have an understanding of the stages of change as well as motivational interviewing techniques and self-efficacy theory.

It is important to realise and accept that not all people will be ready to change. Pivotal to every self-management program is the development of an interpersonal relationship between the healthcare professional and the individual. This relationship provides a safe environment for the healthcare professional to help the individual to explore ambivalence and concerns, to provide education and help the individual understand their lifestyle and concerns.

PUTTING IT ALL TOGETHER

Theories such as the transtheoretical model, motivational interviewing and the social cognitive theory have long provided a foundation for primary healthcare and health promotion strategies. However, many clinicians and healthcare students are perplexed by the different theories and have difficulties recognising the relationship between theories and how they can be integrated in clinical practice. Table 3.4 demonstrates the interrelationships between the transtheoretical model, motivational interviewing and self-efficacy theory when facilitating self-management of long-term conditions.

In Case Study 3.1 we describe how the self-management framework, including transtheoretical and social cognitive theories, were applied to a community-based project aimed at helping men lose weight (Aoun et al., 2009; Bovend'Eerdt et al., 2009; Farrell et al., 2004; MacGregor et al., 2006).

CONCLUSION

The traditional medical model is not a sustainable model for people with long-term conditions. Self-management models have existed since the 1970s and the current government emphasis on self-management has resulted in a number of programs being developed. Generic self-management principles, however, may be used for any person with a long-term

TABLE 3.4

Integrating Theoretical Concepts. *Note*: From Brody et al., 2005; Curtin et al., 2008; Johnston-Brooks et al., 2002.

THEORIES	STAGE OF CHANGE (TRANSTHEORETICAL MODEL)	CHARACTERISTICS	TECHNIQUES	HEALTH PROFESSIONAL'S ROLE
Motivational interviewing. Social cognitive theory — self-efficacy.	Pre-contemplation	Not thinking about changing anything. May be aware of problems but lack the motivation to make any changes.	Motivational interviewing (Rollnick, Miller, & Butler, 2008) Mastery experience (Bandura, 1986, 2005) Vicarious experience (Bandura, 1986, 2005)	Raise doubt about perceived risks and problems associated with current issue and with changing behaviours. • Ask the client if they want to change this area of their life. • Encourage the client to consider whether changes could improve their lifestyle. At this stage you are encouraging the client to reflect rather than act. • Does the client need further education or resources?
	Contemplation	Not sure whether they want to change or not – ambivalent.		Suggest reasons to change and risks to not changing. Increase the client's self-efficacy for change. • Ask the client if they want to change this area of their life. • Explore changing the behaviour with the client – what effect would changes have on them? Their family? Their friends? What are the pros and cons? • Can you identify some positive outcomes for them to consider?
Motivational interviewing. Social cognitive theory — self-efficacy.	Preparation	Have been trying to change or are planning to act.	Motivational interviewing (Rollnick, Miller, & Butler, 2008). Mastery experience (Bandura, 1986, 2005). Vicarious experience (Bandura, 1986, 2005). Social persuasions (Bandura, 1986, 2005). Psychological symptoms (Bandura, 1986, 2005).	Help the client decide on the best course of action to take to … • Help your client to problem solve. • Identify social support and resources available. • Verify that they have the skills and knowledge to change. • Help them set small goals so that they have a sense of achievement.

(continued next page...)

TABLE 3.4
Integrating Theoretical Concepts — cont'd

THEORIES	STAGE OF CHANGE (TRANSTHEORETICAL MODEL)	CHARACTERISTICS	TECHNIQUES	HEALTH PROFESSIONAL'S ROLE
Motivational interviewing. Social cognitive theory — self-efficacy. Write — action planning.	Action	Practising new behaviour for 3–6 months.	Motivational interviewing (Rollnick, Miller, & Butler, 2008). Action planning (Gibson & Powell, 2004). Mastery experience (Bandura, 1986, 2005). Vicarious experience (Bandura, 1986, 2005). Social persuasions (Bandura, 1986, 2005). Psychological symptoms (Bandura, 1986, 2005).	Support the client to set goals and initiate the change. • Focus on restructuring cues and social support. • Bolster self-efficacy for dealing with obstacles. • Combat feelings of loss and reiterate long-term benefits.
	Maintenance	Continued commitment to sustaining new behaviour. Post-6 months to 5 years.		• Provide ongoing support and follow up. • Give positive reinforcement. • Discuss coping with relapse.
	Relapse	Go back to previous behaviour.		Don't let the client get hindered by relapse; rather, assist them to rekindle their motivation for change. • Help client determine the trigger for relapse. • Re-evaluate motivational readiness and barriers to getting back on track. • Plan coping strategies with your client to deal with triggers and barriers.

CASE STUDY 3.1 Description of intervention

The Waist Disposal Challenge (WDC) is an innovative health promotion intervention implemented at the community level via service clubs (Rotary clubs) and is partly led by volunteer peer support lay leaders, named 'champions'. It targets overweight or obese men at risk of developing chronic diseases. The WDC comprises three levels:

Level 1 consists of training club champions to be peer leaders

Level 2 is a weight loss competition between clubs and the club that achieves the largest reduction in body mass index (BMI) is awarded the 'waist disposal trophy'

Level 3 consists of a lifestyle coaching program using telephone coaching sessions undertaken by health professionals trained as lifestyle coaches.

Application of the transtheoretical model and social cognitive theory

Two conceptual approaches form the basis of the program: the transtheoretical model and social cognitive theory. The transtheoretical model as previously discussed assesses individual readiness to change behaviour while social cognitive theory promotes self-efficacy behaviours and beliefs.

Assessing readiness for change using the transtheoretical model

The transtheoretical model (Nutbeam & Harris, 1998; Zimmerman et al., 2000) posits that people have varying levels of motivation or readiness to change. Accordingly, by using strategies effective for each stage, the program assists participants to move through the different stages of change (Aoun et al., 2009).

As illustrated in Figure 3.2, the education (Level 1) provided by the champions highlighted the advantages of changing health behaviours, particularly for those men in the pre-contemplation phase where individuals may have been resistant to change or unaware of the need to change. The BMI competition (Level 2) facilitated

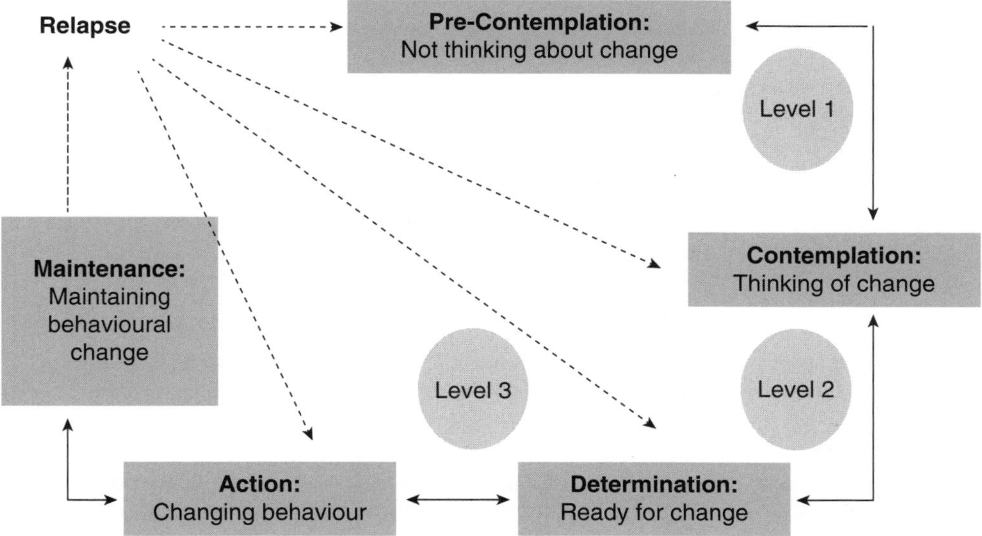

FIGURE 3.2 The impact of the three levels of intervention on the cycle of behavioural change.
Note: From Aoun et al., 2012.

CASE STUDY 3.1 Description of intervention — cont'd

individuals moving from a stage of contemplation where they were aware and open to change to the preparation phase where individuals were ready to change. The individual lifestyle coaching session (Level 3) helped individuals identify barriers, plan action for change and set realistic and achievable goals while also providing positive affirmation and building self-efficacy (Aoun et al., 2012).

Enhancing self-efficacy

An important aspect of the social cognitive theory (Bandura, 1986) is enhancing self-efficacy, the confidence in one's ability to solve difficulties related to behaviour change and in increasing self-regulatory skills including setting goals, solving problems and monitoring and rewarding oneself.

A number of factors were incorporated into the program to enhance self-efficacy behaviours and beliefs.

1. Champions were trained to deliver three educational presentations on nutrition, exercise and other healthy lifestyle habits during normal club meetings. Champions had themselves undertaken the program therefore self-efficacy was built through vicarious experience; that is, individuals were able to view the success of others and believe that they could also achieve the same result.
2. Healthy competition between clubs was fostered through a BMI competition whereby monthly BMI data was put into a computer-based program showing loss across a number of different clubs. This promoted positive encouragement among club members as well as emotional feelings of achievement and pride.
3. Lifestyle coaching adopting motivational interviewing (MI) techniques was provided to participating individuals. As part of this technique, participants were encouraged to talk as much as, or more than, the coaches. Coaches relied primarily on reflective listening and positive affirmations rather than direct questioning, persuasion or advice giving (Alexander et al., 2010; Resnicow et al., 2008). The essence of the coaching sessions was captured in a coaching contract drawn up during each coaching session by the coach (in consultation with the participant). The written contract aimed to provide increased ownership and commitment to self-management by focusing on strategies that assist in reducing weight and achieving other health-related goals.

Key outcomes of the program

93 champions from 52 clubs received the training. 1100 club members received the educational presentations by the champions and 764 participated in the BMI competition. The coaching program was run as a pilot with 40 participants.

The feedback received from the 52 participating Rotary Clubs has been very positive.

- The improvements in champions' knowledge, confidence and skills to perform this role (measured before and after the training program) were significant.
- When delivering the educational sessions, the champions performed equally well if not better than health professionals particularly in motivating their peers to make changes to their diet or increase their physical activity. Club members related well to having one of them act as a champion and as a health resource for their clubs.
- The BMI competition was highly successful with an 82% completion rate.
- The largest individual losses were within the first 6 months of the competition.

CASE STUDY 3.1 Description of intervention — cont'd

- 16 clubs showed significant reductions in BMI ($p < 0.01$), with another 17 clubs showing BMI reductions although not statistically significant, and only three clubs had a slight increase.
- For those who participated in the pilot lifestyle coaching program, they experienced improvements in dietary intake and physical activity, improved quality of life and self-reported wellbeing.
- Participants gave high ratings on how the coaching program had positively affected a number of their lifestyle habits and were very satisfied with the interaction they had with their coaches.
- The vast majority of participants provided feedback that it was a worthwhile program to be involved in and they would definitely recommend it to other clubs.

The champions' comments on the WDC include:

- 'It isn't a short-term thing but a lifetime philosophy we are trying to get across. It is always pleasing to get the positive comments and see the joy on people's faces as they see improvement and get encouragement.'
- 'It's created a very definite awareness of health issues and what we should be doing about what we eat and how or whether we exercise. Members now talk about their weight and what they are doing about it!! Members are now tuned into what is required to keep healthy and that's a good thing.'
- 'We have given a lot of thought to the meals being served at the club, and work with the caterer on a regular basis to ensure that healthy options are available at every club meeting.'

The latest feedback on WDC from *participating members* has been very positive (2011 data).

- 'It generated a lot of energy and good humour to reduce weight.'
- 'It added to the social structure of a meeting.'
- 'Regular weigh-ins were an incentive to controlling diet.'
- 'Some members benefited greatly which was good for their health.'
- 'Maintain the program, it needs to continue.'
- 'Run for a longer period of time.'
- 'This is an excellent program but it needs more publicity spelling out its advantages.'

Implications for practice

This case demonstrates how a relatively simple intervention can be adapted within a group setting in the community. By training peers as the leaders it is cost effective while at the same time self-efficacy is enhanced as the peer leaders transmit values, behaviours and attitudes to others who model their behaviours accordingly.

These concepts can be adapted and implemented into practice individually as well as in a group setting. When any patient with a chronic disease or disability presents to a health professional there is an opportunity to assess readiness to change behaviours, and use motivational interviewing to encourage people to identify and decrease feelings of ambivalence, leading to a motivation to change behaviour. The fundamental constructs to build self-efficacy can be utilised to increase individual confidence that changes can be made and sustained successfully.

Reflective questions

1 With the current move towards self-management for all long-term conditions and disabilities and the evidence supporting this model, why are some health professionals reluctant to move away from the traditional medical model and what can be done at a systems level to facilitate change?

2 With the dispersion of population in Australia and limited access to professional development for many clinicians, what tools could be developed that would facilitate patient engagement with self-management practices and clinician expertise in providing self-management support?

3 If working collaboratively as partners in care is an underlying principle of self-management, what strategies are needed to facilitate patient and clinician behaviour changes and embed this into practice?

condition or disability. In order to embed these principles into the healthcare system, attitudes of both clinicians and the general population need to change and embrace working as partners in care.

Recommended reading

Aoun, S., Osseiran-Moisson, R., Shahid, S., et al. (2012). Telephone lifestyle coaching: Is it feasible as a behavioural change intervention for men? *Journal of Health Psychology, 17*(2), 227–236.

Aoun, S., Osseiran-Moisson, R., Collins, F., et al. (2009). A Self-Management Concept for Men at the Community Level: The 'Waist' Disposal Challenge. *Journal of Health Psychology, 14*(5), 663–674.

Aoun S., Shahid S., Le L., et al. (2012). The role and influence of champions in a community-based lifestyle risk modification program. *Journal of Health Psychology*, published online July 12, 2012, doi:10.1177/1359105312449194

Drury, V., Mackey, S., Tay, P., et al. (2012). A pilot study of the effectiveness of a low vision self-management program for older Singaporeans. *International Journal of Ophthalmic Practice, 3*(5), 189–193.

Lawn, S., & Schoo, A. (2010). Supporting self-management of chronic health conditions: Common approaches. *Patient Education and Counseling, 80*(2), 205–211.

References

Adams, S. G., Smith, P. K., Allan, P. F., et al. (2007). Systematic Review of the Chronic Care Model in Chronic Obstructive Pulmonary Disease Prevention and Management. *Archives of Internal Medicine, 167*(6), 551–561. doi:10.1001/archinte.167.6.551

Alexander, G. L., Mcclure, J. B., Calvi, J. H., et al. (2010). A Randomized Clinical Trial Evaluating Online Interventions to Improve Fruit and Vegetable Consumption. *American Journal of Public Health, 100*(2), 319–326.

Aoun, S., Osseiran-Moisson, R., Collins, F., et al. (2009). A self-management concept for men at the community level: the 'Waist' Disposal Challenge. *Journal of Health Psychology, 14*(5), 663–674. Retrieved May 2, 2013, from http://hpq.sagepub.com/content/14/5/663

Aoun, S., Osseiran-Moisson, R., Shahid, S., et al. (2012). Telephone Lifestyle Coaching: Is It Feasible as a Behavioural Change Intervention for Men? *Journal of Health Psychology*, *17*(2), 227–236. doi:10.1177/1359105311413480

Bandura, A. (1986). *Social foundations of thought and action: a social cognitive theory*. NJ: Prentice-Hall: Englewood Cliffs.

Bandura, A. (1994). Self-efficacy. In V. Ramachaudran (Ed.), Encyclopedia of human behavior (vol. 4, pp. 71–81). New York: Academic Press.

Bandura, A. (2005). The Primacy of Self-Regulation in Health Promotion. *Applied Psychology*, *54*(2), 245–254. doi:10.1111/j.1464-0597.2005.00208.x

Barr, V., Robinson, S., Marin-Link, B., et al. (2003). The Expanded Chronic Care Model: An Integration of Concepts and Strategies from Population Health Promotion and the Chronic Care Model. *Healthcare Quarterly*, *7*(1), 73–82. Retrieved March 12, 2013, from http://www.longwoods.com/product/16763

Battersby, M. W., Ah Kit, J., Prideaux, C., et al. (2008). Implementing the Flinders Model of self-management support with Aboriginal people who have diabetes: findings from a pilot study. *Australian Journal of Primary Health*, *14*(1), 66–74.

Bodenheimer, T., Lorig, K., Holman, H., et al. (2002). Patient self-management of chronic disease in primary care. *The Journal of the American Medical Association*, *288*(19), 2469–2475. doi:10.1001/jama.288.19.2469

Bourbeau, J., Nault, D., & Dang-Tan, T. (2004). Self-management and behaviour modification in COPD. *Patient Education and Counseling*, *52*(3), 271–277. doi:http://dx.doi.org/10.1016/S0738-3991(03)00102-2

Bovend'Eerdt, T., Botell, R., & Wade, D. (2009). Writing SMART rehabilitation goals and achieving goal attainment scaling: a practical guide. *Clinical Rehabilitation*, *23*(4), 352–361. doi: 10.1177/0269215508101741

Brekke, M., Hjortdahl, P., & Kvien, T. K. (2001). Self-efficacy and health status in rheumatoid arthritis: a two-year longitudinal observational study. *Rheumatology*, *40*(4), 387–392. doi:10.1093/rheumatology/40.4.387

Britt, E., Hudson, S. M., & Blampied, N. M. (2004). Motivational interviewing in health settings: a review. *Patient Education and Counseling*, *53*(2), 147–155. doi:10.1016/s0738-3991(03)00141-1

Brody, B. L., Roch-Levecq, A., Thomas, R. G., et al. (2005). Self-management of age-related macular degeneration at the 6-month follow-up: A randomized controlled trial. *Archives of Ophthalmology*, *123*(1), 46–53. doi:10.1001/archopht.123.1.46

Brooks, P. (2008). Managing chronic disease as a team — new models of care delivery. *Diabetes Voice*, *53*, 46–48.

Burns, J. W., Glenn, B., Lofland, K., et al. (2005). Stages of change in readiness to adopt a self-management approach to chronic pain: the moderating role of early-treatment stage progression in predicting outcome. *Pain*, *115*(3), 322–331. doi:10.1016/j.pain.2005.03.007

Bury, M., & Ink, D. (2005). The HSJ debate. Self-management of chronic disease doesn't work. *The Health Service Journal*, *115*, 18–19.

Carrier, J. (2009). *Managing long term conditions and chronic illness in primary care*. Abingdon: Routledge.

Caughey, G., Vitry, A., Gilbert, A., et al. (2008). Prevalence of comorbidity of chronic diseases in Australia. *BMC Public Health*, *8*(1), 221. Retrieved March 12, 2013, from http://www.biomedcentral.com/1471-2458/8/221

Coleman, K., Austin, B. T., Brach, C., et al. (2009). Evidence On The Chronic Care Model In The New Millennium. *Health Affairs*, *28*(1), 75–85. doi:10.1377/hlthaff.28.1.75

Commonwealth of Australia. (2008). *Obesity in Australia, a need for urgent action*. Canberra: Author.

Corbin, J., & Strauss, A. (1988). *Unending work and care: Managing chronic illness at home*. San Francisco: Jossey-Bass Publishers.

Crothers, L., Hughes, T., & Morine, K. (2008). *Theory and cases in school-based consultation: A resource for school psychologists, school counselors, special educators, and other mental health professionals.* New York: Routledge Taylor & Francis Group. Retrieved March 12, 2013, from http://books.google.com/books?id=vKsXLZkKiyIC

Curtin, R. B., Walters, B. A. J., Schatell, D., et al. (2008). Self-efficacy and self-management behaviors in patients with chronic kidney disease. *Advances in Chronic Kidney Disease, 15*(2), 191–205. doi:http://dx.doi.org/10.1053/j.ackd.2008.01.006

Department of Health (UK). (2004). *Improving Chronic Disease Management.* London: Author

DiClemente, C. C., Nidecker, M., & Bellack, A. S. (2008). Motivation and the stages of change among individuals with severe mental illness and substance abuse disorders. *Journal of Substance Abuse Treatment, 34*(1), 25–35. doi:10.1016/j.jsat.2006.12.034

Dijkstra, A., Vlaeyen, J. W. S., Rijnen, H., et al. (2001). Readiness to adopt the self-management approach to cope with chronic pain in fibromyalgic patients. *Pain, 90*(1–2), 37–45. doi:10.1016/s0304-3959(00)00384-5

Eakin, E. G., Lawler, S. P., Vandelanotte, C., et al. (2007). Telephone interventions for physical activity and dietary behavior change: A systematic review. *American Journal of Preventive Medicine, 32*(5), 419–434. Retrieved February 14, 2013, from http://www.sciencedirect.com/science/article/B6VHT-4NMDD5C-D/1/a91f3f20b814ec91c1952a728588a8a9

Epping-Jordan, J. E., Pruitt, S. D., Bengoa, R., et al. (2004). Improving the quality of health care for chronic conditions. *Quality and Safety in Health Care, 13*(4), 299–305. doi:10.1136/qshc.2004.010744

Farrell, K., Wicks, M. N., & Martin, J. C. (2004). Chronic disease self-management improved with enhanced self-efficacy. *Clinical Nursing Research, 13*(4), 289–308. doi:10.1177/1054773804267878

Foster, G., Taylor, S. J. C., Eldridge, S. E., et al. (2008). *Self-management education programmes by lay leaders for people with chronic conditions (Review).* Wiley. doi:10.1002/14651858.CD005108.pub2|ISSN 1469-493X

Geiger-Brown, J., & Trinkoff, A. M. (2010). Is it time to pull the plug on 12-hour shifts?: Part 1. The evidence. *Journal of Nursing Administration, 40*(3), 100–102. doi:110.1097/NNA.1090b1013e3181d0414e. Retrieved January 8, 2013, from http://journals.lww.com/jonajournal/Fulltext/2010/03000/Is_It_Time_to_Pull_the_Plug_on_12_Hour_Shifts__.3.aspx

Gibson, P. G., & Powell, H. (2004). Written action plans for asthma: an evidence-based review of the key components. *Thorax, 59*, 94–99.

Government of Western Australia. (2009). *Self management framework for long-term conditions.* Perth: Western Australia Health Deaprtment.

Harvey, P. W., Petkov, J., Misan, G., et al. (2008). Self-management support and training for patients with chronic and complex conditions improves health-related behaviour and health outcomes. *Australian Health Review, 32*(2), 330–338.

Heisler, N. D. (2006). *Building peer support programs to manage chronic disease: seven models for success.* California: California HealthCare Foundation.

Johnston-Brooks, C. H., Lewis, M. A., & Garg, S. (2002). Self-efficacy impacts self-care and HbA1c in young adults with type 1 diabetes. *Psychosomatic Medicine, 64*(1), 43–51. Retrieved March 12, 2013, from http://www.psychosomaticmedicine.org/content/64/1/43.abstract

Jones, F. (2006). Strategies to enhance chronic disease self-management: How can we apply this to stroke? *Disability and Rehabilitation, 28*(13), 841–847.

Jordan, J. E., & Osborne, R. H. (2007). Chronic disease self-management education programs: challenges ahead. *Medical Journal of Australia, 186*(2), 84. Retrieved March 12, 2013, from http://proquest.umi.com.dbgw.lis.curtin.edu.au/pqdweb?did=1231823111&Fmt=7&clientId=22212&RQT=309&VName=PQD

Jordan, J. E., Briggs, A., Brand, C., et al. (2008). Enhancing patient engagement in chronic disease self-management support initiatives in Australia: the need for an integrated approach. *MJA, 189*(10), s9–s13.

Katch, H., & Mead, H. (2010). The role of self-efficacy in cardiovascular disease self-management: a review of effective programs. *Patient Intelligence, 2*, 33–44.

Keefe, F. J., Lefebvre, J. C., Kerns, R. D., et al. (2000). Understanding the adoption of arthritis self-management: stages of change profiles among arthritis patients. *Pain, 87*(3), 303–313. doi:10.1016/s0304-3959(00)00294-3

Kelly, J., Menzies, D., & Taylor, S. (2003). The Good Life Club: methodology and study design — a discussion. [Special Issue: The Management of Chronic Disease in Primary Care Settings.]. *Australian Journal of Primary Health, 9*(2–3), 186–191.

Lawn, S., & Schoo, A. (2010). Supporting self-management of chronic health conditions: Common approaches. *Patient Education and Counseling, 80*(2), 205–211. doi:10.1016/j.pec.2009.10.006

Lawn, S., Battersby, M. W., Pols, R. G., et al. (2007). The mental health expert patient: findings from a pilot study of a generic chronic condition self-management programme for people with mental illness. *International Journal of Social Psychiatry, 53*(1), 63–74. doi:10.1177/0020764007075010

Lindner, H., Menzies, D., & Kelly, J. (2003). Telephone coach training for health professionals in patient self-management strategies. *Australian Journal of Primary Health, 9*(2–3), 199–207.

Lindner, H., Menzies, D., Kelly, J., et al. (2003). Coaching for behaviour change in chronic disease: a review of the literature and the implications for coaching as a self-management intervention. [Special Issue: The Management of Chronic Disease in Primary Care Settings.]. *Australian Journal of Primary Health, 9*(2–3), 177–185.

Lorig, K. (2000). Self-management education: context, definition, and outcomes and mechanisms. *Chronic Disease Self-Management Conference*, held in Sydney.

Lorig, K. R., Hurwicz, M. L., Sobel, D., et al. (2005). A national dissemination of an evidence-based self-management program: a process evaluation study. *Patient Education and Counseling, 59*(1), 69–79. doi:S0738-3991(04)00332-5 [pii] 10.1016/j.pec.2004.10.002

Lorig, K. R., Ritter, P. L., Laurent, D. D., et al. (2006). Internet-Based Chronic Disease Self-Management: A Randomized Trial. *Medical Care, 44*(11), 964–971 910.1097/1001.mlr.0000233678.0000280203.c0000233671. Retrieved February 12, 2013, from http://journals.lww.com/lww-medicalcare/Fulltext/2006/11000/Internet_Based_Chronic_Disease_Self_Management__A.2.aspx

Lorig, K. R., Ritter, P., Stewart, A. L., et al. (2001). Chronic disease self-management program: 2-year health status and health care utilization outcomes. *Medical Care, 39*(11), 1217–1223. Retrieved February 10, 2013, from http://journals.lww.com/lww-medicalcare/Fulltext/2001/11000/Chronic_Disease_Self_Management_Program__2_Year.8.aspx

Lorig, K., Holman, H. R. (2003). Self-management education: History, definition, outcomes, and mechanisms. *Annals of Behavioral Medicine, 26*(1), 1–7. doi:10.1207/s15324796abm2601_01

MacGregor, K., Handley, M., Wong, S., et al. (2006). Behavior-change action plans in primary care: A feasibility study of clinicians. *The Journal of the American Board of Family Medicine, 19*(3), 215–223. doi:10.3122/jabfm.19.3.215

Marks, R., & Allegrante, J. P. (2005). A review and synthesis of research evidence for self-efficacy-enhancing interventions for reducing chronic disability: implications for health education practice (part II). *Health Promotion Practice, 6*(2), 148–156. doi:10.1177/1524839904266792

McGettrick, K. S., & O'Neill, M. A. (2006). Critical care nurses — perceptions of 12-h shifts. *Nursing in Critical Care, 11*(4), 188–197. doi:10.1111/j.1362-1017.2006.00171.x

McMurray, S., Johnson, G., Davis, S., et al. (2002). Diabetes education and care management significantly improve patient outcomes in the dialysis unit. *American Journal of Kidney Diseases, 40*(3), 566–575.

Miller, W. R., & Moyers, T. (2006). Eight stages in learning motivational interviewing. *Journal of Teaching in the Addictions, 5*(1), 3–17.

National Health Priority Action Council. (2006). *National Chronic Disease Strategy*. Canberra: Australian Government Department of Health and Ageing.

Nutbeam, D., & Harris, E. (1998). *Theory in a nutshell: A practitioner's guide to commonly used therories and models in health promotion.* Sydney: National Centre for Health Promotion.

Packer, T., Drury, V., Ghahari, S., et al. (2009). *Self-management support. An introduction for health professionals.* Perth: Curtin University of Technology.

Parchman, M. L., Pugh, J. A., Noël, P. H., et al. (2002). Continuity of care, self-management behaviors, and glucose control in patients with type 2 diabetes. *Medical Care, 40*(2), 137–144. Retrieved March 14, 2013, from http://journals.lww.com/lww-medicalcare/Fulltext/2002/02000/Continuity_of_Care,_Self_Management_Behaviors,_and.8.aspx

Pearson, M., Mattke, S., Shaw, R., et al. (2007). *Patient self-management support programs: an evaluation. Final contract report (prepared by RAND Health under contract no. 282-00-0005).* Rockville MD: Agency for Healthcare Research and Quality.

Piatt, G. A., Orchard, T. J., Emerson, S., et al. (2006). Translating the chronic care model into the community. *Diabetes Care, 29*(4), 811–817. doi:10.2337/diacare.29.04.06.dc05-1785

Prochaska, J. O., & DiClemente, C. (1983). Stages and processes of self-change of smoking: Toward an integrative model of change. *Journal of Consulting and Clinical Psychology, 51*, 390–395.

Prochaska, J., & DiClemente, C. (1998). Towards a comprehensive, transtheoretical model of change: states of change and addictive behaviors. In W. R. Miller (Ed.), *Applied clinical psychology, Treating addictive behaviors* (pp. 3–24). New York: Plenum Press.

Prochaska, J., & Norcross, J. (2001). Psychotherapy: Theory, Research, Practice, *Training, 38*(4), 443–448.

Resnicow, K., Davis, R. E., Zhang, G., et al. (2008). Tailoring a fruit and vegetable intervention on novel motivational constructs: results of a randomized study. *Annals of Behavioral Medicine: A Publication of The Society of Behavioral Medicine, 35*(2), 159–169.

Resnicow, K., Davis, R., & Rollnick, S. (2006). Motivational interviewing for pediatric obesity: conceptual issues and evidence review. *Journal of the American Dietetic Association, 106*(12), 2024–2033. doi:10.1016/j.jada.2006.09.015

Robert Wood Johnson Foundation. (2011). The Chronic Care Model. Retrieved March 17, 2013, from http://www.improvingchroniccare.org/index.php?p=Self-Management_Support&s=39

Rollnick, S., Miller, W., & Butler, C. (2008). *Motivational Interviewing in Health Care.* New York: Guilford Press.

Rubak, S., Sandbaek, A., Loritzen, T., et al. (2005). Motivational interviewing: a systematic review and meta-analysis. *Br J Gen Pract, 55*(513), 305–312.

South Australia Dept. of Health Statewide Service Strategy Division. (2008). *Chronic disease action plan for South Australia.* Adelaide: Author (ISBN: 9780730899211).

Vancouver Coastal Health. (2008). Chronic Disease Self-Management Support — A practical approach to working with people with chronic disease. Facilitator guide. Vancouver. Retrieved March 17, 2013, from http://www.bcahc.ca/docs/VCH_Guide_Nov1308.pdf

VanWormer, J. J., & Boucher, J. L. (2004). Motivational interviewing and diet modification: A review of the evidence. *Diabetes Educator, 30*(3), 404–419. Retrieved March 17, 2013, from http://www.diabeteseducator.org/ProfessionalResources/Certification/

Velicer, W. F., Hughes, S. L., Fava, J. L., et al. (1995). An empirical typology of subjects within stage of change. *Addictive Behaviors, 20*(3), 299–320. doi:10.1016/0306-4603(94)00069-b

Victorian Government Department of Human Services. (2007). *Diabetes self-management Guidelines for providing services to people newly diagnosed with Type 2 diabetes.* Melbourne: Author.

Wagner, E. H., Austin, B. T., Davis, C., et al. (2001). Improving chronic illness care: translating evidence into action. *Health Affairs, 20*(6), 64–78. doi:10.1377/hlthaff.20.6.64

Warner, L. M., Schüz, B., Knittle, K., et al. (2011). Sources of perceived self-efficacy as predictors of physical activity in older adults. *Applied Psychology: Health and Well-Being, 3*(2), 172–192. doi:10.1111/j.1758-0854.2011.01050.x

Wolff, J. L., Starfield, B., & Anderson, G. (2002). Prevalence, Expenditures, and complications of multiple chronic conditions in the elderly. *Archives of Internal Medicine*, *162*(20), 2269–2276. doi:10.1001/archinte.162.20.2269

Zimmerman, B. (2000). Self-efficacy: An essential motive to learn. *Contemporary Educational Psychology*, *25*(1), 82–91.

Zimmerman, G. L., Olsen, C. G., & Bosworth, M. F. (2000). A 'stages of change' approach to helping patients change behavior. *American Family Physician*, *61*(5), 1409–1416. Retrieved March 17, 2013, from http://proquest.umi.com.dbgw.lis.curtin.edu.au/pqdlink?Ver=1&Exp=02-10-2013&FMT=7&DID=51462503&RQT=309

CHAPTER 4

John Xavier Rolley
Esther Chang
Amanda Johnson

Spirituality and the nurse: engaging in human suffering, hope and meaning

Learning objectives

When you have completed this chapter you will be able to:

- understand spirituality as a key concept of holistic nursing
- appreciate the central role spirituality plays in human living and dying
- appreciate the various religious traditions and the rituals that people and their families bring with them to suffering and illness
- appreciate and recognise the spiritual care role of the nurse in caring for a diverse range of people with chronic illness and/or disability
- reflect on your own spirituality and be conscious of the influence this has on the delivery of nursing care.

Key words

hope, self awareness, spirituality, spiritual care, suffering

Reflective questions

1 Before you read further, spend some time thinking about 'spirituality'. What does this mean to you?

2 What do you think spirituality has to do with nursing?

INTRODUCTION

Before you read another word of this chapter, we invite you to stop for a few minutes and think about the first thoughts, concepts, images and feelings you have when you think about spirituality. Imagine this chapter as a brief journey into this mysterious yet vital aspect of human living and dying. Spirituality is an essential and dynamic phenomenon at work in your life as a person. As a nurse working with people with chronic and complex needs, you will encounter spirituality flowing through their lives.

'Spirituality' is a word loaded with mystery. It has been a source of both comfort and uncertainty. It cannot be touched or tasted, defies attempts at 'pinning it down' to a single definition, cannot be examined by any physical method; yet it flows to connect us in every part of life. This ambiguity in understanding spirituality has led many to use metaphors or word pictures in an attempt to form a better understanding. Such approaches only helps us a little. It is, after all, a mystery. In philosophy, the term is 'metaphysics', meaning it is above and beyond the observable physical world. It is to this mystery we invite you as readers and students to take some time to contemplate this essential component of human experience. For nurses, it is contemplation vital to the health and wellbeing of those for whom they facilitate care. To use a metaphor, the discovery of spirituality is a journey each nurse will take, whether conscious of it or not.

This chapter is placed in the beginning of the book to emphasise the centrality of spirituality in human life. After attempting a definition of spirituality, themes such as suffering, hope and the place of religion and ritual will be discussed. Then, importantly, the chapter turns to the nurse and the importance of spiritual self-knowledge prior to exploring how the nurse can provide spiritually sensitive and safe practice.

As evidenced throughout this book, practice is best founded on principles rather than tasks. In order to assist you to negotiate the concepts of this chapter, two guiding principles for practice are given and integrated into the discussion. They are the importance of nurses to develop:

1 spiritual self-awareness
2 spiritual sensitivity.

Spiritual self-awareness is an essential 'first step' to engaging others' expressions of spirituality. Asking valuable questions of the self is an integral part of this process. Such questions may include: 'What is the meaning and experience of life?', 'What is my/our place in the universe?', 'What drives my sense of hope?' and 'How do I deal with suffering in this life?' Most importantly, how we approach these questions depends on our own sense of values and beliefs.

Spiritual sensitivity, related to cultural sensitivity and safety, is important for nurses and other healthcare professionals in providing care that respects the uniqueness of each person, their contexts of living and significant others, including partners, family and friends. This principle flows from the first principle of self-awareness as respect for one's own unique spiritual perspective. This assists in bridging the interpersonal divide people experience in meeting another person. The bridge between the self and another is then the context where care facilitated through mutual respect leads to healing. It is the basis of person-centred care and the holism.

As you make your way through this chapter, you are asked to pause often. It may be useful to use a journal or diary to note the thoughts and feelings that will inevitably arise. Included in this chapter will be discussion on how to use approaches and tools for reflection on spirituality, both personally and professionally. You are also encouraged to explore these and other techniques to assist in developing a level of spiritual awareness that will assist you to engage meaningfully in the wondrous diversity you face as a nurse in the lives of the people you care for, their significant others, family and friends.

Reflective questions

1 Now that you've read the introduction, do you want to add to your initial reflections?
2 How comfortable are you with your own spiritual awareness?
3 How prepared do you feel to provide spiritual care to people with chronic illness?

SPIRITUALITY: AN ESSENTIAL EXPRESSION OF HUMANITY

Towards a fluid definition of spirituality: it is like 'playing with water'

Spirituality is becoming an important topic of discussion in society in general and healthcare specifically. There is a growing interest in the study of spirituality and nursing with researchers from diverse fields contributing to the debate (Cockell & McSherry, 2012). In particular, there have been studies looking for ways to measure spiritual values and beliefs (Parker, 2006) as well as the development of spirituality and spiritual distress assessment tools for use in clinical settings (Monod et al., 2010). These often aim at determining if a person is experiencing spiritual distress. Fundamental to all this activity is how spirituality is defined and what constructs or concepts underpin the discussion.

The task of defining spirituality has been both contentious and difficult due to its subjective nature (Cooper et al., 2013; Paley, 2008; Chung, Wong, & Chan, 2007), nevertheless it is important for those in healthcare to take up the challenge. When reading on the topic of spirituality keep in mind the spiritual perspectives of the writer or researcher, as well as you, the reader. Each of these perspectives is of central importance. Burkhardt & Nagai-Jacobson state that '... spirituality is a phenomenon that is understood differently depending on the perspective from which it is viewed' (2002, p. 5). There are many interconnected aspects of human life that make defining spirituality so challenging, yet a worthwhile endeavour nonetheless. These include culture, religious background, socioeconomic status, educational level, gender and sexuality. For example, atheists may express spirituality in terms that exclude religion or religious process, while secular humanists may deny the existence of spirituality as a valid element of human experience (McSherry & Ross, 2002). Whatever the perspective, defining spirituality is a complex and subjective process (Cooper et al., 2013); and more importantly an ongoing adventure.

With the above in mind, a simple starting point for this chapter is given by Chung, Wong and Chan as '... the relationship with the self and a dimension beyond the self' (2007, p. 158). In this definition, the two dimensions often associated with spirituality can be seen: the relationship which the individual has with the self, an internal relationship; and that which the person has with an 'other'. 'Other' is a term often used to describe either a divine being, such as a god, or another person. Religious world views are often called upon by individuals in defining how these two relationships are engaged and the extent to which they are experienced. For some, one relationship is internal, the relationship with the self, while the other is external, that is to say, the relationship one has with their God. Other religious traditions perceive both of these as internal relationships: God is within. Whatever approach is taken, including the denial of an external being, every human being faces these two relationships at some level and at some point of time in their lives.

The essence of spirituality appears to be deeply integrated with how people derive and live out meaning in and of life. This includes how the individual defines their 'world view'. By this it is meant that information is gathered from the world around them and through multiple 'filters' such as familial, social, cultural, religious and personal experiences. It is difficult to express this process as a simple concept as it is dynamic and multifactorial (Neff, 2006). As this chapter will discuss, spirituality is a common human experience that sits above and behind personal religious belief and practice.

Swinton and Narayanasamy (2002) argue that spirituality is a universally experienced human phenomenon that is intensely subjective. It is this very subjectivity that underpins the imperative for nurses to act with the deepest respect towards those for whom they care. Inherent in this is a fragility of mystery from which human meaning and spiritual world views are constructed. The bridges over which the self travels in the process of relating to others and the divine are unique. Spirituality is the process of forming the bridge.

Spirituality as connection

Connection is the purpose and process of spiritual experience and expression. This includes the big questions human beings ask about life and its meaning, as well as how relationships impact on the self (Chung et al., 2007). These relationships involve the connections of family, support networks including friends, groups and the community and the divine, in whichever way that is perceived and defined.

'Transcendence' is a term often applied to the role of spirituality in connecting the self to another. This connecting serves to enrich and derive meaning from the relationships that the self touches. In this reaching and touching, relationship is formed and is core to both the human process of relating and caring in nursing (Chang, 2001). The simple touch of compassion towards a person in need can be the source of immense meaning for both the giver and the receiver (Mok & Chiu, 2004). According to Thorup and colleagues (2012, p. 427), 'Care is shaped between the meeting of human beings'. It is in the connection and the intention of the connection that relationship forms: Both the nurse and the person receive as they move beyond themselves and experience 'otherness'. Paradoxically, the otherness is then brought deeply within the self and their sense of self is enriched. The same can be said for negative connection such as abuse. Think of the impact of domestic violence on the victim: diminished sense of self and impaired ability to reconnect meaningfully.

The role of religion in spirituality

Religion and spirituality are often confused with each other, religion being considered equal, conceptually, to spirituality (Barnum, 2011). This is due largely to post–World War II social change and the challenge of the traditional role religion held in the western life (Bash, 2004). With the influx of eastern spiritual traditions into the West, spirituality has been defined in new ways (Bash, 2004) and diverse ways, often giving rise to new religious belief systems and movements. This upheaval in thought has introduced an understandable yet unhelpful confusion to a consideration of the complexities of spirituality.

At one time, being religious and being spiritual were synonymous, as evidenced by the lack of equivalent term to 'spirituality' in the Judeo–Christian religious tradition (Bash, 2004). However, it could be argued that if a person needed to be religious in order to be authentically spiritual, the experiences of many people, including scientists, healthcare professionals, artists, poets, musicians and philosophers, would mean little. Regarding the place of religion, and science in life, Albert Einstein once said, 'Science without religion is lame, but religion without science is blind' (O'Connell & Skevington, 2005).

As discussed earlier, spirituality involves the 'stuff' of life. This does not mean religion does not play an important role in the process of life. Neither does it mean that the person is required to be engaged in a recognised religion (Taylor, 2002). Rather, religion provides a structure for spiritual expression. Religious beliefs may help the individual to construct a view of the world and thereby derive meaning for living their lives (Taylor, 2002). The practice of the religion, then, assists in the reinforcing of those views. (See Table 4.1.)

Some religions are theistic, meaning they hold a central belief in the existence of a god or gods. Others, such as Buddhism, do not believe in a god as such, rather in the process of evolution of each soul toward enlightenment and the release of the need for Karma or purification through reincarnation.

Most religions have complex constructions of the world, how it came about and the place of people in relation to the world. They often prescribe the behaviour of their members regarding these world views, moral values, practice and worship. The Judeo–Christian tradition has a long yet varied history representing two theistic branches of monotheism. Another monotheistic religion, Islam, holds similar beliefs about the value of life and the need for caring for the sick as an extension of belief in God (Rassool, 2000). Furthermore, many of the advances in medicine, science and mathematics prior to the western European Renaissance were due to the work of Islamic scholars (Rassool, 2000). Regardless of the paradigm, it is important to realise that spirituality flows beyond religious structures.

Atheism, on the other hand, while it never describes itself as a religion, has similar albeit opposite beliefs to theism. More recently, there has been an emerging debate about the place of spirituality among those who identify as atheist. Two philosophers have tackled this in the popular press: Alain de Botton and Andre Comte-Sponville. Both argue for an atheism that engages the 'best' of religious traditions, in terms of universal values of love, community, aesthetics, kindness or compassion and ritual (Comte-Sponville, 2006; de Botton, 2012). In their discussion, the notion of spirituality avoids the supernatural and superstitious. This approach is not without criticism from within atheist circles, and serves to remind nurses of the complexity and subjective nature of spirituality. Furthermore, it underscores the need for nurses to avoid categorising clients using 'labels'. Rather, it is vital to respect the individual's complexity and unique perspectives.

The role of ritual in spirituality

Human beings are essentially ritualistic. While the term 'ritual' implies a religious practice, it is seen in broader terms as a human phenomenon. Including religious observances such as going to a sacred space such as a mosque, church or temple, human ritual extends to every part of human existence. Rites of passage in life, such as what we do to connect with another person (for instance, common greetings such as the bow or handshake) and the marking of changes in intimate relationships (such as engagement or betrothal, marriage and death), express milestones in life. Other more mundane examples, such as how people choose their clothes, bathe and eat, as well as celebrate 'special' occasions such as birthdays and anniversaries, and mark grief and loss, speak of the ritual existence humans are living. All these things connect with some sense of meaning in life and ways used to express that meaning. The expression of meaning through ritual can also facilitate gaining greater understanding itself. As such, ritual plays an important role in the lives of those living with chronic illness and/or disabilities and such experiences can bring significant challenge to their sense of self and world view.

Ritual, for the majority of people who identify as being religiously oriented, takes some form of connection with a higher reality or being. Prayer, meditation, corporate forms of worship, spiritual reading and contemplation form the core of most religious expression.

TABLE 4.1
Religious diversity — key points

BELIEF	TYPE OF RELIGION	CORE BELIEFS	CORE PRACTICES
Atheism	Atheistic	• The existence of god cannot be demonstrated. • All of existence can be explained through rational means. • What is yet unexplainable will one day be explainable using rational methods. • There is no life beyond death.	• Various. • Usually humanistic approaches to personal reflection.
Baha'i	Theistic	• God is one. • The various religions of the world are manifestations of the One God. • Baha U'llah, born Mizra Husayn-Ali Nuri, is considered the prophetic fulfilment by Baha'i of Islamic, Christian and other religious traditions. • There is life beyond death.	• Daily prayer. • Pilgrimage. • Reading of holy scriptures.
Buddhism	Atheistic	• Life is a cycle of birth, death and rebirth. • The soul progresses towards enlightenment and the end of the need to suffer. • Nirvana is the ultimate form of being and is essentially absolute unity, or Buddha-hood, with all things. • Various sects have differing approaches to Buddhism with varying beliefs about the existence of deities and the place of ritual.	• Meditation. • Good deeds. • Reading of sacred texts.
Christianity	Theistic	• God is one yet a union of three 'persons': Father, Son and Holy Spirit. • God as creator who is above and beyond the created order. • Jesus as Son of God and Saviour to those who believe. • The word of God is found in the Holy Bible. • The 'Church' as the body of Christ on earth. • One becomes a Christian through baptism. • There is life beyond death. • Many sects which have varying beliefs about these core beliefs and practices.	• Daily prayer. • Reading of the Bible. • Attendance at church services. • The Holy Communion, Eucharist or Mass as the central act of worship for most Christians.

(continued next page...)

TABLE 4.1

Religious diversity — key points — cont'd

BELIEF	TYPE OF RELIGION	CORE BELIEFS	CORE PRACTICES
Hinduism	Polytheistic	• Oldest 'living' religion. • All life is sacred. • God is expressed in many ways and forms. • Life is a cycle of birth, death and rebirth. • Karma is an infinite force for teaching and purifying the soul on its many reincarnations. • People are born into various casts which orders society and is determined by Karma. • There are several sects with devotees focused on the deities associated with them, for example Shivism (Shiva), Krishna Consciousness (Krishna or Vishnu) and Brahmanism (Brahma).	• Meditation. • Attendance at Temple for important feasts and milestones. • The importance of the dharma or teachings found in the many texts such as Vedas, Sutras or sacred writings. • The importance of social conventions regarding caste and family obligations.
Islam	Theistic	• God is one. • God created all things and is above and beyond the created order. • Mohammad is the last and greatest prophet. • The word of God is found in the Quran. • There is life beyond death.	• Daily prayer. • Reading the holy scriptures. • Attending corporate prayer. • Fasting at certain times, including the great fast of Ramadan.
Judaism	Theistic	• God is one. • God created all things and is above and beyond the created order. • There is life beyond death.	• Daily prayer. • Recitation of the Scriptures with emphasis on the Torah or Law.
Shinto	Animistic; Polytheistic	• Japanese indigenous spirituality. • There is life beyond death. • There are several sects.	• Daily reverence of the 'kami' or spirits of the ancestors. • Attendance at special shrine observances.
Sikh	Theistic	• God is one. • God created all things and is above and beyond the created order. • The word of God is found in Guru Granth Sahib or holy scriptures. • Baptism is the way a person becomes a Sikh. • There is life beyond death.	• Daily prayer. • Attendance at festivals and temple events. • Reading of the holy scriptures.

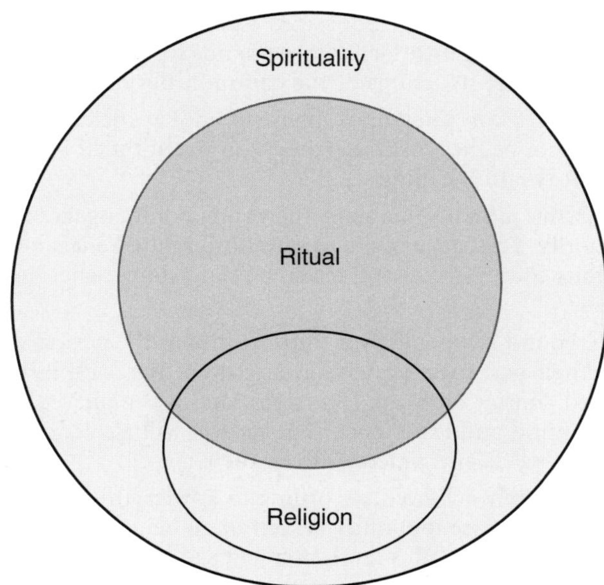

FIGURE 4.1 The relationship between spirituality, religion and ritual.

While debate rages as to the empirically measurable benefits of these activities, many report a deep satisfaction and increased sense of wellbeing through engaging in ritual practice. As such, it continues to be a vital aspect of how human beings gain meaning in life and overcome barriers.

In summary, the concepts of spirituality, religion and ritual can inform and flow into each other. Spirituality is the broader context for both religion and ritual, both of which form expressions of spirituality. This is illustrated in Figure 4.1.

Spiritual development

How human beings develop is a complex process. Developmental psychologists such as Piaget and Erickson have contributed significantly to understanding this phenomenon. As this chapter has argued, the spiritual is indivisible from the physical and therefore undergoes a developmental process. There have been several attempts to posit theories of spiritual, faith or religious development (Streib, 2001; Taylor, 2002). The most significant of these has been Fowler's Stages of Faith Development (Fowler, 1981; Taylor, 2002) and is still acknowledged as one of the leading theories (Hart, Limke, & Budd, 2010). This is a seven-stage model developed following analysis of 400 interviews and is briefly given below (Fowler, 1981). Please note that Fowler defines faith in broad universal terms; that is, the process of finding meaning in life rather than a religious structural definition (Fowler, 1981; Taylor, 2002).

1 *Undifferentiated faith.* Associated with infancy, this stage is related to developing trust, courage, love, hope and mutuality.
2 *Intuitive–projective faith.* A magical and imitative phase linked with early childhood, it is the period when children engage fantasy and beliefs such as the tooth fairy and Santa Claus.

3 *Mythic–literal faith.* The phase of school-aged children up to adolescence, when fantasy is being evaluated against fact with demands for proof. This is also when they learn the values and belief structures of the communities in which they live.
4 *Synthetic–conventional faith.* The typical phase of adolescence in which it is the individual's experience of the world together with the adopted beliefs of their parents that help give identity and meaning.
5 *Individuative–reflective faith.* In this stage the young adult engages in establishing their own spiritual identity. This stage includes questioning the beliefs held in the past by family and religious communities and leads to establishing belief based on their own conceptual process.
6 *Conjunctive faith.* Found in people over mid-life, this is the period where reconciliation of their past together with awareness of the complexities of belief and myth are processed. Fowler (1981, p. 198) states that it is a phase that '... strives to unify opposites in mind and experience'. The person will also connect with others who have divergent beliefs and practices from their own.
7 *Universalising faith.* Rarely achieved, according to Fowler, this level can be described as enlightenment, where an essential unity is seen in all being transcending the need to hold opposing ideas. People at this level often engage in trying to unify society.

Reflective questions

1 Think about your own spirituality. How much has it formed your beliefs, values and views of the world?
2 Reflect on Fowler's stages of faith development. How have you journeyed in your own spiritual developmental path?
3 What impact does it have on your practice?

Fowler's approach is a linear model that has not been without its critics (Streib, 2001). Streib (2001) argues for a more dynamic and open theory. Herein lies a caution regarding linear models: they are limited in that they reduce the process to a series of statements to aid understanding. Whatever system is engaged, it is important to note that spiritual development is not a constant belief but a process of unfolding and becoming. Nowhere is this seen more than when a person is confronted with illness, particularly chronic illness. Here, the individual's very world view is challenged and they must then traverse the paths to a new understanding and meaning.

THE MYSTERY OF SUFFERING: THE EFFECT OF CHRONIC ILLNESS

Finding meaning in suffering

Suffering is a recurrent theme in discussion relating to spirituality and health. It is considered one of the most profound of human experiences and one that the individual must negotiate largely alone (Lohne, 2008). Reed (2003, p. 11) defines suffering as '... a syndrome of some duration, unique to the individual, involving a perceived relentless threat to one or more essential human values, creating certain initially ominous beliefs and a range of related feelings'. Cassell (1991, p. 33), writing what has become a seminal work on the topic, defined suffering as '... the severe distress associated with events that threaten the intactness of the person'. Importantly, this notion of threat to 'intactness' or integrity of a person is not solely reliant on an event but also the perception of what that event means for the individual (Rowe, 2003). For you as the nurse, the 'take home' message found in these two definitions is this: the uniqueness of the person's experience is paramount (Reed, 2003); and suffering has the power to alter an individual's perception of meaning (Cassell, 1991; Rowe, 2003). Suffering confronts the established patterns of life, challenging the one suffering to struggle with finding new meaning. Reich (1989, cited in Taylor, 2002, p. 159) echoes this by saying suffering is '... a frustration to the concrete meaning that we have found in our personal existence'. The concrete nature of meaning exposes the fragility of human world views. Given a significant enough confrontation through an event or perceived consequence of an event, the constructed meaning can crumble. This crumbling is suffering!

Reed (2003) gives four themes related to suffering, including isolation, hopelessness, vulnerability and loss. Isolation is a common experience in suffering (Reed, 2003) and includes the alienation people feel when faced with difficulty in sharing their experiences (Rehnsfeldt & Eriksson, 2004). It can also come about through disruption in normal caring patterns: being cared for and caring for others (Reed, 2003). Hopelessness, experienced as despair or the belief that they are without hope, is a significant experience of those who suffer (Reed, 2003). Through these experiences, it is important to note that the extent to which people experience hopelessness varies with the individual and circumstances, such as in chronic illness, where the feeling may be transitory (Farran, Herth, & Popovich, 1995).

The conflict that chronic illness can engender in a person's life means that ways must be found to make meaning out of the circumstances and consequences to the self. Kralik (2002) describes this as a process of transition that the women in her study experienced from the ordinariness of their perceived world into the turmoil of chronic illness. One study participant said (Kralik, 2002, p. 149):

> ... It doesn't seem to happen the way we'd think it would. Our day of diagnosis seems to take us by great surprise, no matter how long or obvious the road to that point has been. I recall just how quickly it all happened, and how just a few words changed my life forever.

The experience propelled the women into what Kralik (2002) refers to as 'extraordinariness': a profound state of vulnerability and lack of control over the self.

While Kralik and colleagues (2006) describe transition as a psychological process, where the person seeks new meaning, it is important, from the perspective of this chapter, to see the process as being an essentially spiritual one, as it has to do with human meaning-making. Essential to understanding this process is the notion that transition entails progression towards new perceptions, not the return to an older perception (Kralik, Visentin, & van Loon, 2006). The experience renders the notion of 'return' to a previous state impossible, as the person has had to engage in the consequences of the stimulus to their suffering.

How people deal with suffering and thereby gain meaning varies. Again, it depends on their sociocultural context, values and beliefs. These may include behavioural or cognitive or religious approaches (Taylor, 2002). The connections or relationships a person maintains are significant contributors to this process and aid in traversing the experience.

Holding hope

Traversing suffering requires resilience which is born of another human trait: to hold hope. The focus is on a future that is grounded in a perceived reality which is essentially subjective yet vital to life and wellness (Clarke, 2003; Herth, 2000). Without hope, the individual soon loses their emotional connection to life, and death may follow (Clarke, 2003).

Suffering is so confronting due to its effect on the perceived reality of things, to 'lose hope' is to let go of the desire to survive the experience. Losing hope or despairing is the opposite to hope, which, as Fitzgerald Miller (2007, p. 14) states, '... saves persons from the agony of despair'. An Australian philosopher, Zournazi (2002, p. 22), wrote this about hope:

> What does hope involve in everyday life and experience? Imagine you have a friend who is sick or a loved one who is dying: there is a trust that situations or events, even in adversity, have an element that could sustain our belief in the world. This hope has no logical or clear definition to it. It may be the hope that things could be different or the cherishing of life, where courage marks the strength to continue, and where aspects of grief, mourning and death become part of life, and the movement is one away from despair. If we can understand hope as composing life as it emerges, there is the possibility of joy and a hopeful vision for the world.

Hope is not the denial of reality presented by suffering. Rather, it incorporates it into the experience. Farran et al (1995) describe four components to this process: an experiential aspect of appreciating suffering as being a human process; a spiritual/transcendent process where hope and faith are one; a rational thought process giving hope a grounding in the reality of the experience; and a relational process that connects the person to others. In this, hope is a vital human experience that steels the individual on their journey. Nurses, while they cannot 'instil' hope in a person, are instrumental in facilitating the process. Hope is considered an integral concern for nurses (Lohne, 2008).

Families, friends and human connection

Relationships help bring meaning to life, providing it within a context or place for growth and expression (Burkhardt & Nagai-Jacobson, 2002). As social beings, humans need to relate, share, tell stories, hear and be heard, express emotion, love loss and grieve. It is in the nexus of relationships that people come to learn who they are and develop meaning. Isolate an infant, for example, and they run the risk of 'failure to thrive' due to deprivation of interaction, touch and intimacy (Burkhardt & Nagai-Jacobson, 2002). Indeed, it is intimacy between a person, their family, friends and life partner that is essential to survival.

Spirituality is essentially a relationship concept: relationship with the self and with an 'other' or 'others'. Hawkins (1987, cited in Burkhardt & Nagai-Jacobson, 2002, p. 266) said this about the spirituality of relationships:

> When we attempt to lead our spiritual lives apart from the nurture, support and accountability of others, we end up distorting our spiritual growth. The presence of fellow travellers is essential for our growth. We need companionship and communion with others.

Nowhere is this more vital than in illness. Chronic illness, in particular, brings added strains to the person experiencing the illness, let alone the relationships that form their

Reflective questions

1 In what ways have you experienced suffering or seen it in a friend or family member?

2 How do you feel when faced with someone suffering?

3 What are the things that bring you hope?

4 Think about the relationships in your own life. In what ways has each helped you to understand who you are?

CASE STUDY 4.1

Mr Darren Marcs, a 54-year-old man was, 2 weeks prior, diagnosed with end-stage prostate cancer with spread to his regional lymph nodes and metastatic disease to his spine and liver (Grading: T4 N1 M1). He first detected a problem after noting worsening back pain which was not relieved with analgesia. Darren hadn't had any routine prostate screening despite being over the age of 45.

Darren was raised a Roman Catholic yet has not adhered to any religious observance for over the past 25 years and has, since that time, avowed atheism. Darren was divorced 6 years ago in difficult circumstances and of his three children, only one, Michael (aged 22) who is the eldest, has maintained any contact. Darren has requested that his former wife and two remaining children are not told of his diagnosis or prognosis. Darren is in considerable pain which staff are struggling to treat effectively and is showing signs of depression. When he is with his son, Michael, Darren is often teary and observably distressed. Other members of the healthcare team have reported Darren to be 'difficult' and 'prickly' to engage.

Michael approaches you and confides that he is worried about his father's depression. He says his father is deeply afraid of death. Michael, the only member of the family to identify with his father's religious convictions, states he is at a loss as to how to console Darren.

Case study questions

1. Spend some time reflecting on the effects of the disease process on Darren's sense of self, relationships and spirituality.
2. What are some important things to consider when approaching spiritual care for people who identify as being atheist?
3. Is there such a thing as an atheistic spirituality?
4. Reflect on the effect of suffering on Darren's life: What impact is this having on his health?
5. What approaches could you, as the nurse, take to engage Michael in Darren's care?
6. Hold a debate: does atheism automatically preclude a person identifying as a spiritual person?

social fabric. Yet, it is these relationships that are essential to the healing of the person (Taylor, 2002). The role of nurses, then, is to support and role model these healing relationships (Taylor, 2002). You as the nurse, then, becomes one who comes alongside the client and their family; not to replace but enhance.

WHAT DOES SPIRITUALITY HAVE TO DO WITH NURSING?

Challenging the persisting biomedical model

Nursing is a dynamic profession that has experienced rapid change since the time of Florence Nightingale. Integrated with this phenomenon, the broader constructs of health and illness have experienced meteoric development. The medical paradigms founded on rationalism are being challenged while nursing is discovering its heart in more integrated health approaches. The landscape of health and illness in this world is constantly moving, bringing uncertainty and opportunity. Nursing is a key to this process and part of its ongoing resolution.

Nursing is a healthcare profession focused on more than just illness and injury. The World Health Organization (WHO) in its fundamental definition of health recognises that health concerns people's wellbeing rather than the absence of disease (WHO, 1948). What this means for nurses regarding spirituality is complex.

The prevailing healthcare paradigm, particularly in the acute care setting, is the biomedical model. Nursing and health literature is replete with discussion related to the limitations of this approach (Kubsch et al., 2007). For the purpose of this discussion, it is important to focus on how this model sees the individual.

The biomedical model sees the person as a collection of biological processes resulting in life. These processes can be determined by scientific objective measures. An example is the presence of a heartbeat or breathing, both of which can be measured and help to determine the presence of 'life'. In this way, the constituent elements of the person are viewed as separate and distinct (Walker, 2006). This is said to be a reductionist philosophical approach (Harrison-Barbet, 2001; Kubsch et al., 2007). Nurses also engage at this level for example, check for vital signs, carry out procedures and engage in other objective rational assessments. However, defining what it means to be alive is a different challenge.

As discussed earlier in this chapter, spirituality is a human process of finding meaning to life and life experiences. This takes the individual beyond the objective biological determinants of life to the metaphysical (a term that means literally 'beyond or above the physical'). The challenges nurses face when clients, often in distress, ask 'Why is this happening to me?' cannot be answered by citing test results or biological measures of life. Other approaches are necessary.

The imperative of competent spiritual care at the core of nursing does not lie in any sacred or divine calling placed on nurses. Rather, it is the patterns of care that see nurses providing extensive, extended and often intimate support that lie at the heart of this challenge. Herein is the immense opportunity and challenge for nurses to positively affect people's lives.

Nursing the whole being

Nursing theorists have championed the adoption of other models and frameworks for viewing and responding to the human condition (Chung et al., 2007). Taking a humanistic approach, these theories often incorporate the need to approach the person as a complete connected entity: body, mind and spirit. This integration is referred to as 'holism'. As a term, it has been classically defined simply as 'the whole is greater than the sum of its parts' (Kolcaba, 1997). From a health viewpoint, this includes the biological, psychological, sociological and spiritual. The indivisible nature of this union is essential to understanding this concept. It will not do to define holism as a deconstruction of a whole: biological 'bits', psychological 'bits', social 'bits' and spiritual 'bits'. It is by virtue of its integration that holism sits opposite to reductionism (Walker, 2006).

Several nursing theorists engage in integrative notions where the environment, health, the person and nursing converge. The most significant aspect of these notions is the relationships that are formed between the client and the nurse. Easley (2007) describes this in terms of harmony, where the coming together of a conducive environment, the engaging of the client and the nurse, and time, are integral in building the relationship.

Reflective questions

1. How would you describe, in your own words, the role of spirituality as a facilitator for healing?
2. What do you think and believe about holism?
3. Have you ever asked the question, 'Why is this happening to me?'

Spirituality, in this process, forms the integrative force behind nursing care (Taylor, 2002). It involves supporting the individual in their struggle to traverse suffering, find meaning and hold hope. Who the nurse is as a person and how they bring that to their client is equally important (Taylor, 2002). Importantly, this takes intention on the part of the nurse. By that we mean a purposeful choice on the part of the nurse to be present for the person for whom we care (Burkhardt & Nagai-Jacobson, 2002). This underscores the vital role of reflective practice in developing self-knowledge.

THE NURSE AS A WHOLE PERSON: UNCOVERING THE PERSONAL SPIRITUAL ESSENCE

Know thyself!

This famous saying of Socrates, a Greek philosopher who lived circa 470–399 BCE, lies at the heart of being a nurse. How often do nurses ask themselves who they are or what causes them to think and act a certain way? While uncovering answers to such questions takes a lifetime, it is a quest every nurse is encouraged to take. The view that nurses should engage in self-awareness is seen in the literature, particularly described in approaches to educating nurses to engage appropriately in spiritual care (Usher & Holmes, 2006).

The heart of this quest is in understanding the motivators for values, beliefs and resulting actions. It is a journey of discovery about what it is to be human beings living this life. Yet, questions arise as to how this can be engaged. Engaging in reflection is the important thing (Corso, 2012). Bolton (2001) likens those choosing not to engage in reflective practice to the Tennyson poetic character the Lady of Shalott, who, in Bolton's words, is '… cursed only to experience mirror images, weaving them into a tapestry, rather than live her life directly' (p. 114). There is no easy answer other than to say there are as many roads to self-discovery as there are people willing to take the journey.

Several tools exist to assist in engaging this vital process. These include reflective journaling, artwork, meditation, dream analysis, physical movement and ritual. Everyone needs to explore for themselves methods appropriate for their own context. There is no right or wrong way, provided it is authentic to the person's life experience. Two of these techniques are discussed below.

Writing as a tool for reflection

Journalling is a common approach to self-discovery with many potential approaches possible. It is important, if this method is to be used, to have a journal that can be kept confidential in a safe place. Writing for most people is a frightening prospect. The following is a guide to aid the reader in engaging this potentially vital practice, adapted from Bolton (2001), which she refers to as the 'reflective splurge'.

1 Find a space that is quiet and where you will not be distracted for 30 to 40 minutes.
2 Write for about six minutes without stopping — try not to think about the process, just write whatever comes into your head. This is to help get the 'juices' flowing.
3 Pause, reread but do not judge what you have written.
4 Sit quietly again, and focus on what you feel you need to reflect on.
5 Start writing and keep doing so for about 20 to 40 minutes.
6 Spend some time rereading and reflecting on what you have written. Keep the following in mind:
    1 do not worry about grammar, punctuation or spelling
    2 allow reaction and emotion to flow unhindered
    3 remember that what you are writing is your perspective
    4 refrain from judgment.

Writing for reflection takes time. What is more, there will be times when reflective writing will play a large part in life and at other times diminish in significance. The important thing is to engage in the process.

Artwork as a tool for reflection

For people who prefer visual approaches, using one of many artwork genres may be more appropriate. This may include drawing, painting, sculpture or craft work, such as the use of textiles, wood or metal. Instead of words, pictures or symbols may emerge. These will be unique to the individual and become a source of reflection in and of themselves. Wadeson (2000, p. xv), an art therapist, describes the engaging use of art richly.

- It is the legacy of the dying, the plottings of the living and the pain made visible by those in between.
- It is the rivers of separate circumstances, private privations and lonely hauntings flowing together in tides of shifting reflections streaming towards a deep seat of intermingled humanity.
- It is the fixity of the stars in which the evanescent dust of living is coalesced in images.

Using a similar approach to writing, allow yourself to settle in a quiet space that is free from distraction. Choose a medium (painting, drawing, clay, collage or the like) that suits you best. Focus on what it is you want to reflect on and allow it to flow. Again, refrain from judgment. This is a subjective process, but one which can accompany you gently on the journey to deeper understanding. Below is an example of such a work by one of the authors of this chapter, created at a time when he was seeking to understand some personal challenges.

The wounded healer: nurses are human too!

The metaphor of the 'wounded healer' is an archetypal one with links in the sacred stories and myths of many world religions, including Christianity, Buddhism, Hinduism and

Greek mythology (Hall, 1997). The stories coming from those traditions show people with human and divine qualities who experience deep life-shattering trauma, which leads to a journey of wholeness and self-discovery. The result is insight for the healing nourishment of others.

The connection between such mythological beings and nurses may seem strained. The nurse is a human being engaged in promotion of the health and wellbeing of others. The key to understanding the metaphor lies in the humanity of the nurse (Corso, 2012). Here, the person carrying out the role of the nurse is a being living life similarly to those they care for: challenges, joys, frustrations, achievements, routines, relationships, loss, celebration, recreation, illness, sharing and love. These are similar yet different for everyone. Indeed, the common element for both nurse and the client is humanity. Taylor (2002, p. 59) said this regarding the wounded healer: 'What allows wounded individuals to be effective as healers is the recognition of their own woundedness ... the ability to embrace one's woundedness enhances the ability to heal'. This does not mean that the wounded healer projects their brokenness on the clients they care for. Rather, the nurse recognises the need for a continuing process of healing at work within themselves, as a 'healer', as well as the clients they care for (Corso, 2012). The mutuality born of acknowledging the humanity of suffering and healing is the power behind the nurse–client relationship.

The wounded healer archetype highlights to nurses the need for vigilance. Nursing, as a healing art and science, is fraught with potential trauma: suffering can be and is experienced by nurses engaging with people who suffer (Rowe, 2003). Rowe (2003), reflecting on approaches to dealing with suffering, commented that some nurses avoid this potential for suffering by avoiding more personal contact, choosing to adopt a more objective clinical role or they may choose roles that avoid interaction with clients, such as research or education. That is not to say such choices are negative, in and of themselves. Rather, the nurses may be losing the opportunities and rewards that deeper interactions bring (Rowe, 2003).

Essential to the process of dealing with the experience of suffering and healing is the need for openness and safe spaces to explore the challenges. These may entail good mentoring relationships, opportunities for debriefing and reflection. Invariably, these rich experiences will entail personal confrontation of belief systems and values: there is no easy way around these existential 'angsts'. As Rowe (2003) states, suffering is not forever. According to an ancient Hebrew saying, 'This too shall pass'.

Nourishing the spirit of the nurse

Nurses often do not take much time to care for their own spirituality. In order for nurses to provide optimal spiritual care to their patients they need to examine their own life experiences and what meaning this has for them. Thinking about what gives your life meaning and value would assist your spirituality and, in turn, enable you to support your patients. Giving your patient the best spiritual care would mean taking care of your own spiritual needs first (Bell & Troxel, 2001). Following are some suggested approaches to taking care of your spiritual needs:

- finding a quiet time for meditation and reflection
- keeping your own faith traditions
- being with nature
- appreciating the arts
- spending time with those you love
- journalling (Touchy & Zerwekh, 2006, p. 236).

CASE STUDY 4.2

Janet is a registered nurse with 3 years experience in intensive care and a total of 5 years experience since she graduated from university. She is caring for a woman, Phyllis, aged 68 with a long history of chronic respiratory and cardiac illness. Phyllis was brought into hospital by her daughter, Elaine, following deterioration of a bout of influenza. Phyllis has had several admissions in the past 3 months due to either exacerbation of chronic respiratory disease or pulmonary oedema secondary to congestive heart failure.

This admission resulted in Phyllis being admitted to ICU and intubated, requiring full ventilation support. Her admission was characterised by sepsis and multi-organ failure. All attempts at weaning her off ventilation have failed. Her deterioration has been so profound that medical staff feel Phyllis will not survive an extubation. Janet has been appointed as the primary nurse managing Phyllis's care and has been working extensively with the family. Janet understands that the prognosis is not good and has been subtly preparing the family for Phyllis's possible death.

A family conference was called. Elaine, who has been providing the majority of care for Phyllis, and her two other siblings and their partners were in attendance. The healthcare team present included the ICU doctor in charge of her medical care, Janet as the primary nurse caring for Phyllis, the respiratory doctor and a social worker. The ICU doctor spells out Phyllis's medical condition, current treatment, challenges to making any improvement and prognosis. When he suggests that the only alternative left is to extubate, provide medication to keep her comfortable and allow 'nature to take its course', Elaine becomes deeply distressed and lashes out. Elaine refuses to accept that her mother will not recover and '... walk out of this horrid place'. Janet is surprised by Elaine's reaction. She feels she has failed Elaine and her family for not preparing them more adequately for Phyllis's death.

Case study questions

1. What is your initial reaction to Phyllis's situation?
2. Reflect on your own values and beliefs regarding the end of life. You may choose to use techniques discussed earlier in this chapter.
3. Reflect on the two perspectives: Janet, the nurse and Elaine, the daughter and carer.
4. How can a person be 'prepared' for the death of a loved one?
5. What do you feel is an appropriate response for Janet?
6. What is the nurse's role in supporting people's struggle with end-of-life issues?
7. What does this say about the spiritual processes of Janet, Elaine and her family?

Having someone to talk with about your spiritual needs is important. This is especially true for nurses who work with patients and families experiencing grief and loss repeatedly during the trajectory of chronic illness and disability. Following are some personal spirituality questions to promote reflection for nurses (adapted from Newshan, 1988, cited in Touchy & Zerwekh, 2006, p. 236).

- What do I believe in?
- What gives my life meaning?
- What do I hope for?

- Who do I love and who loves me?
- How am I with others?
- What could I change about my relationships?
- Am I willing to heal the relationships which are troubling me?

THE NURSE'S ROLE IN SUPPORTING PEOPLE THROUGH ILLNESS, DISABILITY AND SUFFERING

Considering the value of life and its meaning would help to enhance your spirituality as well as sustain you in supporting your patients and their families' spiritual needs. The nurse needs to have the knowledge and skills in order to conduct a systematic approach in spiritual care when dealing with patients who are suffering from chronic illness and/or disability. A thorough assessment depends on being aware of the spiritual experiences of a patient. It is important that the nurse is committed to a holistic approach to care. To do this the nurses must move beyond observation and enter into conversations with the patients and their families (Cobb, 2001). Nurses need to be aware that their patients may be uncomfortable in disclosing the innermost aspects of self. Fostering disclosure is based on building a trusting and caring relationship between nurse and patient. The ability of the nurse to influence the health and wellbeing of their patients in a positive manner depends on the nurse's capacity to build a caring relationship with the patient.

Listening is one of the most important aspects of a nurse's role in the delivery of spiritual care. When nurses are active listeners they offer support to patients who are seeking meaning of their illness experience. A good listener needs to listen with their heart along with their ears. To be an effective listener it is crucial to give full attention to the person, how they are expressing it and how they are putting it across (Martin-McDonald & Rogers-Clark, 2005). Listening and responding to the spiritual needs and concerns are best conducted in the context of a caring relationship (Touchy & Zerwekh, 2006).

If spiritual care is to be administered with commitment and competence the nurse needs to reflect on what this means in practice and how it can be attained. It is simply an empty gesture in a service philosophy that the spiritual dimension is an important aspect of spiritual care without meaningful actions and provision of relevant resources (Cobb, 2001, p. 107). Spiritual care involves the need for assessment (Chaplain & Mitchell, 2006) and the implementation of a range of interventions, which may include but is not limited to praying with the patient and their family, reading inspirational texts, reminiscing and providing music (Cobb, 2001), using an empathetic manner (Reed, 2003; Touchy & Zerwekh, 2006), symptom management (Touchy & Zerwekh, 2006) and emotional presence. Open-ended questions within the context of the nurse–patient–family relationship can be used to begin a conversation about spiritual matters (Touchy & Zerwekh, 2006, p. 231). Besides listening and giving consideration to the spiritual needs it may be necessary for the patient to be referred to a chaplain or appropriate minister, wherever possible (Chaplain & Mitchell, 2006; Cobb, 2001); or in the case of a person who avows no religion, a support person they trust to assist them in their experience. The nurse should offer to call an appropriate chaplain, or the church, temple, mosque or synagogue for all patients who identify with a specific faith. Spiritual care should not be provided by the nurse in isolation; rather, with the support of a multidisciplinary team that includes a strong spiritual counsellor or chaplain (Chaplain & Mitchell, 2006; Cobb, 2001; Touchy & Zerwekh, 2006, p. 235). 'The best spiritual counsellors are able to listen and offer unconditional love without focusing on evangelism' (Touchy & Zerwekh, 2006, p. 235). The most important

Reflective questions

1 How do you feel spirituality is expressed in nursing those living with chronic illness?
2 What impact does self-reflection on practice have on promoting the nurse's own spiritual process?
3 What must nurses do to ensure they are practising in spiritually sensitive and safe ways when dealing with people suffering from a chronic illness and disability?

consideration is the need for the nurse to respect the individual spiritual perspectives of their patients without imposing the nurse's own personal spiritual views.

CONCLUSION

Nurses often do not take much time to care for their own spirituality. For nurses to provide optimal spiritual care to their patients they need to examine their own life experiences and what meaning this has for them. Suffering and the spirituality experience is unique to the individual and nurses need to understand the influence of various cultures, belief systems and philosophies that affect a person's view of the meaning and value of life. The nurse needs to be accountable and responsible for the sensitive and safe practice of spiritual care for their patients' welfare. Finally, spirituality is more than a domain of health; it resides within the centre of the person's experience of life. For nurses, it forms the glue that holds the healing process together.

Recommended reading

Barnum, B. S. (2011). *Spirituality: the challenges of complexity*. New York: Springer.

Cockell, N., & McSherry, W. (2012). Spiritual care in nursing: an overview of published international research. *Journal of Nursing Management, 20*(8), 958–969.

Comte-Sponville, A. (2006). *The little book of atheist spirituality*. London: Penguin.

Cooper, K., Chang, E., Sheehan, A., et al. (2013). This journal will be published in Sept or Oct of this year.

Taylor, E. J. (2012). *Religion: A critical guide for nurses*. New York: Springer.

References

Barnum, B. S. (2011). *Spirituality: the challenges of complexity*. New York: Springer.

Bash, A. (2004). Spirituality: the emperor's new clothes? *Journal of Clinical Nursing, 13*(1), 11–16.

Bell, V., & Troxel, D. (2001). Spirituality and the person with dementia: A view from the field. *Alzheimer's Care Quarterly, 2*(2), 31–45.

Bolton, G. (2001). *Reflective practice: Writing and professional development*. London: Paul Chapman Publishing.

Burkhardt, M. A., & Nagai-Jacobson, M. G. (2002). *Spirituality: Living our connectedness*. Albany: Delmar.

Cassell, E. J. (1991). *The nature of suffering and the goals of medicine*. New York: Oxford University Press.

Chang, S. O. (2001). The conceptual structure of physical touch in caring. *Journal of Advanced Nursing, 33*(6), 820–827.

Chaplain, J., & Mitchell, D. (2006). Spirituality in palliative care. In J. Lugton & R. McIntyre (Eds.), *Palliative care: The nursing role* (2nd ed.). Edinburgh: Elsevier.

Chung, L. Y. F., Wong, F. K. Y., & Chan, M. F. (2007). Relationship of nurses' spirituality to their understanding and practice of spiritual care. *Journal of Advanced Nursing, 58*(2), 158–170.

Clarke, D. (2003). Faith and hope. *Australasian Psychiatry, 11*(2), 164–168.

Cobb, M. (2001). *The dying soul.* Buckingham: Open University Press.

Cockell, N., McSherry, W. (2012). Spiritual care in nursing: an overview of published international research. *Journal of Nursing Management, 20*(8), 958–969.

Comte-Sponville, A. (2006). *The little book of atheist spirituality.* London: Penguin.

Cooper, K., Chang, E., Sheehan, A., et al. (2013). This journal will be published in Sept or Oct of this year.

Corso, V. M. (2012). Oncology nurse as wounded healer: Developing a compassion identity. *Clinical Journal of Oncology Nursing, 16*(5), 448–450.

de Botton, A. (2012). *Religion for atheists.* London: Hamish Hamilton.

Easley, R. (2007). Harmony: a concept analysis. *Journal of Advanced Nursing, 59*(5), 551–556.

Farran, C. J., Herth, K. A., & Popovich, J. M. (1995). *Hope and hopelessness: Critical clinical constructs.* Thousand Oaks, CA: Sage Publications.

Fitzgerald Miller, J. (2007). Hope: A Construct Central to Nursing. *Nursing Forum, 42*(1), 12–19.

Fowler, J. W. (1981). *Stages of faith: the psychology of human development and the quest for meaning.* San Francisco: Harper & Row.

Hall, J. (1997). Nurses as wounded healers. In S. Ronaldson (Ed.), *Spirituality: the heart of nursing.* Ascot Vale: Ausmed Publications.

Harrison-Barbet, A. (2001). *Mastering philosophy* (2nd ed.). Basingstoke: Palgrave.

Hart, J. T., Limke A., & Budd, P. R. (2010). Attachment and faith development. *Journal of Philosophy and Theology, 35*(2), 122–128.

Herth, K. (2000). Enhancing hope in people with a first recurrence of cancer. *Journal of Advanced Nursing, 32*(6), 1431–1441.

Kolcaba, R. (1997). The primary holisms in nursing. *Journal of Advanced Nursing, 25*(2), 290–296.

Kralik, D. (2002). The quest for ordinariness: transition experienced by midlife women living with chronic illness. *Journal of Advanced Nursing, 39*(2), 146–154.

Kralik, D., Visentin K., & van Loon A. (2006). Transition: a literature review. *Journal of Advanced Nursing, 55*(3), 320–329.

Kubsch, S., O'Shaughnessy, J., Carrick, J., et al. (2007). Acceptance of change in the healthcare paradigm from reductionism to holism. *Holistic Nursing Practice, 21*(3), 140–151.

Lohne, V. (2008). The battle between hoping and suffering: A conceptual model of hope within a context of spinal cord injury. *Advances in Nursing Science, 31*(3), 237–248.

Martin-McDonald, K., & Rogers-Clark, C. (2005). Journeys through illness: Suffering and resilience. In C. Rogers-Clark, K. Martin-McDonald, & A. McCarthy (Eds.), *Living with Illness: Psychosocial Challenges for Nursing.* Sydney: Elsevier.

McSherry, W., & Ross, L. (2002). Dilemmas of spiritual assessment: considerations for nursing practice. *Journal of Advanced Nursing, 38*(5), 479–488.

Mok, E., & Chiu, P. C. (2004). Nurse-patient relationships in palliative care. *Journal of Advanced Nursing, 48*(5), 475–483.

Monod, S. M., Rochat, E., Bula, C. J., et al. (2010). The spiritual distress assessment tool: an instrument to assess spiritual distress in hospitalised elderly persons. *BioMed Central Geriatric, 10*(88). Retrieved August 20, 2012, from http://www.biomedcentral.com/1471-2318/10/88.

Neff, J. A. (2006). Exploring the dimensionality of 'religiosity' and 'spirituality' in the Fetzer Multidimensional Measure. *Journal for the Scientific Study of Religion, 45*(3), 449–459.

O'Connell, K. A., & Skevington, S. M. (2005). The relevance of spirituality, religion and personal beliefs to health-related quality of life: themes from focus groups in Britain. *British Journal of Health Psychology, 10*, 379–398.

Paley, J. (2008). Spirituality and nursing: a reductionist approach. *Nursing Philosophy, 9*(1), 3–18.

Parker, S. (2006). Measuring faith development. *Journal of Psychology and Theology, 34*(4), 337–348.

Rassool, G. H. (2000). The crescent and Islam: healing, nursing and the spiritual dimension. Some considerations toward an understanding of the Islamic perspective on caring. *Journal of Advanced Nursing, 32*(6), 1476–1484.

Reed, F. C. (2003). *Suffering and Illness: Insights for Caregivers.* Philadelphia: F A Davis.

Rehnsfeldt, A., & Eriksson, K. (2004). The progression of suffering implies alleviated suffering. *Scandinavian Journal of Caring Sciences, 18*(3), 264–272.

Rowe, J. (2003). The suffering of the healer. *Nursing Forum, 38*(4), 16–20.

Streib, H. (2001). Faith development theory revisited: The religious styles perspective. *International Journal of the Psychology of Religion, 11*(3), 143–158.

Swinton, J., & Narayanasamy, A. (2002). Response to: 'A critical view of spirituality and spiritual assessment' by P. Draper, W. McSherry (2002). *Journal of Advanced Nursing, 39*, 1–2. *Journal of Advanced Nursing, 40*(2), 158–160.

Taylor, E. J. (2002). *Spiritual care: Nursing theory, research and practice.* New Jersey: Prentice Hall.

Thorup, C. B., Rundqvist, E., Roberts, C., et al. (2012). Care as a matter of courage: vulnerability, suffering and ethical formation in nursing care. *Scandinavian Journal of Caring Sciences, 26*(3), 427–435.

Touchy, T., & Zerwekh, J. V. (2006). Spiritual caring. In J. V. Zerweckh (Ed.), *Nursing care at the end of life: Palliative care for patients and families* (pp. 213–239). Philadelphia: F A Davis.

Usher, K., & Holmes, C. (2006). Reflective practice: what, why and how. In J. Daly, S. Speedy & D. Jackson (Eds.), *Contexts of nursing* (2nd ed., pp. 99–113). Sydney: Elsevier.

Wadeson, H. (2000). *Art therapy practice: Innovative approaches with diverse populations.* New York: John Wiley & Sons.

Walker, K. (2006). On philosophy: nursing and the politics of truth. In J. Daly, S. Speedy & D. Jackson (Eds.), *Contexts of nursing* (2nd ed., pp. 60–72). Sydney: Elsevier.

World Health Organization. (1948). Constitution of the World Health Organization. Retrieved October 10, 2007 from http://www.who.int/governance/eb/who_constitution_en.pdf.

Zournazi, M. (2002). *Hope: New philosophies for change.* Sydney: Pluto Press.

CHAPTER 5

Alan Merritt
Marina Boogaerts

Psychosocial care

Learning objectives

When you have completed this chapter you will be able to:

- recognise the myriad factors that influence a person's experience of illness
- explore ways in which cultural differences between people have an impact on their illness experience and the provision of care
- recognise the features that influence perceptions of quality of life for a person with a chronic illness and disability
- describe the strengths of nurse–patient partnerships in the care for the person with a chronic illness and disability
- identify opportunities and strategies for developing nurse–patient partnerships in clinical practice.

Key words

cultural competence, diversity, empowerment, partnership, person-centred care

INTRODUCTION

This chapter discusses some of the psychosocial issues and implications for a person living with a chronic illness. People have unique and sometimes very complex lives. Chronic illnesses need to be addressed in the context of a person's life and it should be acknowledged that no one knows that life better than the person who lives it. This expertise in one's life is an essential component in forming therapeutic partnerships from which care can be orchestrated.

Notions of recognising the diversity amongst people, including cultural differences, empowerment, collaborative decision making and person-centredness, are essential elements in providing nursing care to people with a chronic illness.

CHRONIC ILLNESS IS A BIT LIKE CRICKET

If chronic illness was a sport it might be test match cricket, while an acute illness might be the 100 metre sprint. These two events have much in common; they are both sport, involve physical competition, include spectators and competitors, have a beginning and an end and have defined rules. They are also very different. Cricket can last for 5 days (and still be a draw) where the sprint can be over in 10 seconds. The analogy works for illnesses in several important ways. One way is that a small error or a tactical decision in the sprint can have immediate and permanent consequences on the result, while in a 5-day test match, there are many twists and turns and it is hard to say that any one error is directly responsible for the outcome and that tactics may be changed many times to respond to the circumstances. In chronic illness, as in cricket, there is time to make decisions, review them and try different approaches without immediate and permanent consequences.

ILLNESS VERSUS DISEASE

Purists will tell you that cricket is more than a sport. They say that it is the sound of leather on willow, white flannel on green fields surrounded by picket fences, good sportsmanship and gentlemanly conduct. It is debatable whether these are really the prominent, defining features, but it is true to say that to a cricket aficionado, there is more to cricket than the game itself. In other words, to cricket lovers, the lived experience of cricket involves more than just the game.

The lived experience for people with a chronic illness involves more than just the disease. It is often the case that when talking about an illness there is an emphasis on a particular disease or condition. This view is perhaps dominant within a Western culture because of the prominence of the biomedical lens through which we observe health-related phenomena (Alonso, 2004). The biomedical model focuses on the structure and functions of the parts of the body and on the pathophysiology of particular medical conditions. Illness, however, is much broader than the features of a particular disease. The notion of illness addresses all the aspects that encompass the lived experience of someone with a chronic disease (Asbring, 2001; Larsen, 2012). In this regard it is important that the lenses through which we look at chronic illness encompass the much broader aspects of the life of the individual.

It is important to recognise factors that affect not only body systems, but also the psychological and social elements of a person's life. This extends to the different perspectives and unique attributions of an individual in response to their chronic illness (Jacobi & Macleod, 2011) and incorporates aspects related to their lives, but external to the disease, such as carers, families and physical environments (McMurray & Clendon, 2011).

In addition, the biomedical model places a strong emphasis on 'curing', which does not fit comfortably with the person with a chronic illness or disability (Fennell, 2003). For these people a cure is usually not possible and any attempts to orient treatment towards a cure may ignore the fuller human experience. There is another parallel to cricket here. In cricket matches, sometimes the aim is not necessarily to win the match but to avoid a loss by eking out a draw.

Caring for someone with a chronic illness is different from caring for someone who needs nursing care for a short period of time and is likely to resume their previous life afterwards. In acute episodes treatment decisions are often made by the healthcare professional as the need for decisive action is often great and the consequences of delay may be profound (Montori, Gafni, & Charles, 2006). There may be little opportunity for patient participation under these circumstances. Patients often adopt the 'sick' role and are happy to follow orders so that they may get well (Montori et al., 2006). In this case the healthcare team, rather than the patient, often takes responsibility for the management of the condition.

In the acute context, the aim of the treatment is to cure the disease and allow life to continue without the illness or condition, while treatment decisions for chronic diseases aim to incorporate the illness into their life, to minimise the impact of the disease and allow participation in life to the fullest extent. Treatment decisions for a person with a chronic illness may not result in 'cure' but may result in healing. Taylor (1995) describes healing as 'progress on a forward path, that moves one closer to a fuller sense of self, whether it be towards improved health or towards a peaceful death' (Taylor, 1995, p. 100).

Ideally, healing occurs within an ongoing partnership between the healthcare team and the person with a chronic illness, the patient taking an active role in setting goals and carrying out the decisions. The partnership between healthcare professionals and patients allows the choices to be revisited and revised on an ongoing basis.

An awareness of the biopsychosocial, cultural and existential experiences associated with chronic illness is useful in order for the healthcare professional to be able to give appropriate and sensitive care (Freeman, 2005). Biopsychosocial factors can be described as the combination of biological (factors affecting the function of the body, related to symptoms and treatment), psychological (thoughts, emotions and behaviour, related to self-concept, body image and sexuality) and social factors (interactions with others, the extent of support and place within a community). Recognising that these factors interact and shape the patient's experience of a chronic illness help us to understand that the experience is unique for each individual. Valuing this unique, lived experience of the person with a chronic illness will assist in moving beyond the biomedically oriented concepts of nursing practice to engage in more holistic approaches.

A PERSON IN THE CONTEXT OF THEIR LIFE

The overall social context within which a person lives includes their cultural background, socioeconomic status, employment, social networks and physical living environment. These are all significant factors in describing the lived experience of someone with a chronic illness. In other words, people come from diverse backgrounds and the lived experience of their life is a unique expression of this.

Each person has unique personal characteristics and circumstances that may inform their response to a chronic illness. Among the personal characteristics that may make one person's response to a chronic illness very different from another's are creativity, life skills, values, world view and the ability to adapt to change (Smith et al., 2008). Among the circumstances that are of influence are the broad range of social factors that make up life in a society. For example, economic aspects of people's lives have implications for individuals, their families and for society; low socioeconomic status and unemployment have been seen to be determinants of ill-health and if a family has a physically or mentally ill family member the risk is multiplied (McMurray & Clendon, 2011).

Our culture plays a large part in determining our perceptions of health, illness and disability. Awareness of cultural diversity and the provision of culturally competent care are very important in caring for people with a chronic illness (Wilson & Grant, 2008). Culture influences our beliefs and values and determines, in large part, our behaviour.

In addition to culture, people have social roles beyond that of simply a person with a chronic illness. There are many roles in life that are essential to describing who we are (Asbring, 2001). A person with diabetes is not only a person with a chronic illness: they may also be a father, a carer, a daughter, a boss, a banker or a cricketer. Who we are is more than the sum of our ills.

Given that these roles describe our different connections with social networks, it is important to consider the people that a person with a chronic illness may have around them in their life. What sorts of relationships do they have with the people that are around them? The presence of people who can provide support to someone with a chronic illness is another factor that influences the lived experience of someone's life (Smith, 2009). It is important to consider what support and care is available to people with a chronic illness, but also to consider what is expected of them.

Carers of people with a chronic illness may need support as well. These people bring valuable knowledge and expertise into the lives of people with chronic illnesses, but it is often the psychosocial needs of the carer that come to the fore in allowing the ill person to be adequately cared for. It is important to recognise the needs of carers as well as the needs of the patient (Rolley, Smith, DiGiacomo, Salamonson, & Davidson, 2011; Miller & Timson, 2004; Öhman & Söderberg, 2004).

Diversity

The concept of diversity is useful when thinking about and caring for people with a chronic illness. The idea simply recognises that people are different from one another and have unique needs. People have different ages, genders, religions and cultural backgrounds. Acknowledging diversity means acknowledging the unique features that influence the lived experience of a person. It is useful to acknowledge the differences and to be aware that the healthcare systems that we work within often do not cater for these unique differences between individuals (Wilson & Grant, 2008).

One of the clearest examples of recognising diversity comes with differences in culture. Culturally competent care involves an awareness of and sensitivity to the differences among people. It involves seeing people not as disadvantaged, but recognising different perspectives and values that may not necessarily be supported in mainstream healthcare systems. Mainstream healthcare systems are based on Western scientific and philosophical ways of thinking, which may not necessarily be reflected in the beliefs and values of other ethnic groups living within the community (Saha et al., 2003).

Developing a culturally competent approach means, firstly, developing an understanding of our own beliefs and values; secondly, recognising and accepting the beliefs and practices of people from other cultures; and, finally, exploring the differences, looking for ways that will enhance access to and provision of healthcare and minimise barriers (Wilson & Grant, 2008; Stein-Parbury, 2009). It is important for nurses to be aware of their own culture and how this may influence what they expect of their patients, as well as of themselves as nurses.

Cultural and linguistic factors affect access to and delivery of services (McMurray & Clendon, 2011). People from culturally and linguistically diverse backgrounds may have limited or no ability to speak, read or write in English. They may be reluctant or unable to access services, make a complaint or ask for help, and local models of service provision may be unfamiliar. In addition, people from different cultural backgrounds may have unresolved issues relating to past experiences and trauma.

All aspects of the healthcare system are developed to cater for the needs of the English-speaking majority. Simple things like signs and posters in a range of community languages

CASE STUDY 5.1

Part 1

Joan is a 69-year-old woman. She was born in Holland and moved to Australia with her parents and older brother and sister when she was 10 years old. They moved to Australia for what her father termed 'a better life'. He was a manual labourer who was attracted by perceptions of the Australian people, the climate and the promise of work on big new infrastructure projects. He was a very strict man who, although he loved his children, found it difficult to express this. As a result his children saw him as stern and unapproachable. Joan's mother deferred to her husband. She was a loving mother who was always at home for her children.

As a child Joan experienced asthma, particularly in the springtime, but despite this was an active child with a keen interest in sport. She played hockey in winter and women's cricket in summer and was an avid follower of the local football team.

Joan's mother died suddenly when Joan was 16 and she remembers this as a very difficult time. She remembers seeing her father cry for the first time and remembers how strange this seemed to her. Joan took on many of her mother's roles, being the only one of her siblings left at home. She left school at this time and took on the role of caring for the household.

Through a social function at the football club, Joan met Fred, one of the community's players and they formed a romance which led to them being married when Joan was 20. Joan and Fred moved into a small house close to her father and she continued to be a faithful daughter, preparing meals that she left for him.

Joan and Fred soon had three children, Michael, William and Deborah. Fred worked in the bank.

Fred was offered a promotion which required the family to move to the city. With her father's blessing, the family moved and set up their home in the new, much bigger and busier environment.

The family was happy in their new home and the children grew up and moved away. Fred died of a sudden heart attack soon after he retired.

Joan moved out of the big family home and lives in a comfortable flat by herself. The children live interstate but visit regularly.

Joan has noticed that her legs are a bit swollen at times and that the skin has become darker. Her legs are not really sore but it feels good when she sits in her recliner chair and puts them up for a while. Recently Joan bumped her leg just above her ankle and tore the skin. The small wound has not healed and actually seems to be getting bigger. Her friends tell her it needs to get some sun on it to dry it out. She says to herself that if it persists another week, she will see her local doctor about it.

1. Consider the factors that may influence Joan's life. What factors are mentioned here?
2. What other factors may there be?
3. Considering the factors that make Joan's life unique that you have uncovered already, how do you think she would respond to having a chronic illness?

and the use of interpreters each time they are needed are valuable contributors to culturally diverse care. Culturally competent care is much more than this, however, and looks more deeply at the unique perspectives of all people.

The meaning a person gives to aspects of health and illness is influenced by culture. For example, some groups of people may believe that illness or disability is a form of punishment. Attitudes to disability, mental health, ageing and illness in general are determined by culture and it is important to understand that everybody has a culture. Culture also influences the expectations patients may have about the relationship between themselves and the healthcare professional (Stein-Parbury, 2009). The partnership approach may be very unfamiliar for people who believe that treatment is the responsibility of the healthcare professional and it is inappropriate or disrespectful to question a health professional about aspects of care.

In order to interact effectively with people from different cultural backgrounds nurses need to be aware of their own culturally influenced values (Stein-Parbury, 2009). When nurses are aware how they are influenced by their own culture they then can listen and respond appropriately to their patients' cultural viewpoints in an environment of trust and respect. This requires nurses to appreciate multiple perspectives on health and to think outside the biomedical orientation of healthcare.

While we have discussed culturally appropriate care, it is useful to extend the idea to embrace other differences among people. Age, gender and spiritual diversity can be recognised in a similar way.

MODELS

You have seen that people are different and are influenced by a wide range of factors. Chronic illnesses are also very different and the course of an illness may be very different for each individual. A person with a chronic illness will go through many changes throughout the course of their illness. The way people adapt to their illness or disability has been extensively researched and models of psychosocial adaptation to chronic illness and disability have been developed.

Chronic illness models or frameworks describe the experience of adaptation, deterioration and rehabilitation and refer to the impact of the illness on all involved. They can be described as a dynamic process that integrates elements such as the patient's past experience and coping and cognitive ability, as well as the patient's social networks, their environment and the availability of resources (Livneh & Parker, 2005). In this dynamic process 'most individuals appear to move toward renewed personal growth and functional adaptation' (Livneh & Parker, 2005, p. 18).

Two models will be mentioned here. Both models are useful as they provide an opportunity to be person-centred in our healthcare delivery.

The Corbin and Strauss illness trajectory model

The 'illness trajectory', developed by Corbin and Strauss, offers a model whereby the goals of the person with a chronic illness and the healthcare provider can be viewed in the context of a long journey. The journey is shown in different phases of the chronic illness experience for the patient. At different times along the trajectory, different elements of care will come to the fore.

The trajectory is non-linear and people may skip phases or return to previous phases more than once. The trajectory model describes the goals of treatment according to each phase. For example, in the stable phase the goal of care is to maintain stability and usual

TABLE 5.1

Trajectory phases. *Note*: Copyright Ruth Bernstein Hyman, PhD.

PHASE	DEFINITION	GOAL OF MANAGEMENT
Pre-trajectory	Genetic factors or lifestyle behaviours that place an individual or community at risk for the development of a chronic condition.	Prevent onset of chronic illness.
Trajectory onset	Appearance of noticeable symptoms, includes period of diagnostic work-up and announcement by biographical limbo as person begins to discover and cope with implications of diagnosis.	Form appropriate trajectory projection and scheme.
Stable	Illness course and symptoms are under control. Biography and everyday life activities are being managed within limitations of illness. Illness management centres in the home.	Maintain stability of illness, biography and everyday life activities.
Unstable	Period of inability to keep symptoms under control or reactivation of illness. Biographical disruption and difficulty in carrying out everyday life activities. Adjustments being made in regimen with care usually taking place at home.	Return to stable.
Acute	Severe and unrelieved symptoms or the development of illness complications necessitating hospitalisation or bed rest to bring illness course under control. Biography and everyday life activities temporarily placed on hold or drastically cut back.	Bring illness under control and resume normal biography and everyday life activities.
Crisis	Critical or life-threatening situation requiring emergency treatment or care. Biography and everyday life activities suspended until crisis passes.	Remove life threat.
Downward	Illness course characterised by rapid or gradual physical decline accompanied by increasing disability or difficulty in controlling symptoms. Requires biographical adjustment and alterations in everyday life activity with each major downward step.	To adapt to increasing disability with each major downward turn.
Dying	Final days or weeks before death. Characterised by gradual or rapid shutting down of body processes, biographical disengagement and closure and relinquishment of everyday life interests and activities.	To bring closure, let go and die peacefully.

life activities, while in the crisis phase the goal is to avert the specific threat to the person's life. Table 5.1 describes the phases and goals of care.

Each person has a unique experience of the trajectory. One of the ways in which the trajectory model is useful in clinical practice is that it helps patients and nurses discuss the needs and goals at particular times in a person's life (Burton, 2000b). Every person will experience the trajectory in different ways. The model provides opportunities for conversations between individuals and healthcare workers about the illness that, in turn, may lead to a shared understanding of a person's unique trajectory experience. It also allows insight into the illness in terms of the goals and work of both clients and clinicians (Allen, Griffiths, & Lyne, 2004).

CASE STUDY 5.1

Part 2

Joan's leg wound has not changed for the better. When she visits her doctor, he recognises it as most likely to be a venous leg ulcer caused by problems with the venous circulation to the legs. He advises Joan on some lifestyle changes that she could make including keeping her leg up on a stool when she is sitting down and perhaps taking a zinc supplement. He also asks her not to put the leg out in the sun and explains that we now know that this is not the best thing. He also makes a referral to the community nursing service to assess and dress the wound. Many of his patients are visited by the community nurses and he has come to know the strengths of what they can provide and how the disciplines of nursing and medicine can complement one another. He knows that they have particular expertise in wound management and access to a wide range of dressing products that may be helpful.

Prior to visiting the doctor Joan has been dressing the wound herself. She has some gauze from the chemist and has cut a crepe bandage into smaller sections to hold the gauze squares in place. The wound is quite moist and she has to change the dressing several times a day.

She doesn't like to go out because of this and feels that others will notice the wound or the wound seepage and think that she doesn't care for herself.

1 Thinking of the shifting perspectives model, does Joan see herself with a leg ulcer as well or ill?
2 How does Joan's view of herself influence her behaviour?

Paterson's 'shifting perspectives model'

The 'shifting perspectives model' (Paterson, 2001) recognises that at times the person with a chronic illness will see themselves as well, with the illness in the background, while at other times see themselves as unwell, with the illness in the foreground. The shift from the perspective that the person is fundamentally well may be precipitated by, for example, symptoms, complications or an impending specialist appointment. It will shift back again once symptoms are controlled and the illness is no longer to the fore. A person's perceptions of their chronic illness will change according to their needs and situation in a pendular fashion, and consequently the person's perception of himself or herself as well or ill (Livneh & Parker, 2005).

This approach to an illness serves a useful function as, when a person sees themselves as well, their behaviour is likely to include activity that increases participation in life activities and promote interaction and self esteem, while when a person sees themselves as unwell, they are likely to engage in behaviours that decrease the effects of ill health or that will re-establish the healthy frame (Paterson, 2001). These activities include attending specialist appointments, taking medication and generally engaging with recommended health regimens.

QUALITY OF LIFE

We have established that the emphasis in approach in chronic illness is not focused on curing but rather maximising a person's capacity to engage in life or to increase the quality of their life. Since the goal of care is to increase quality of life, it would be useful to explore what quality means.

Yoon (cited in Cartwright & Parker, 2005) describes psychosocial factors contributing to quality of life as including good physical health, financial stability, positive family dynamics and cohesiveness, strong social support networks, maintenance of optimal level of cognitive functioning, personal control and prevention of depression.

In a public health context, quality-of-life measures such as 'burden of disease' attempt to quantify the experience of chronic illness. They make use of the notions of years of life lost and years of healthy life lost due to disability to calculate 'disability adjusted life years' (Lopez et al., 2006). This may be useful in a public health context where such measures may be used to plan strategic responses to particular illnesses, but the approach has been met with criticism from advocacy groups as it is thought that it devalues the significance of some conditions (Ackland & Catford, 2006).

Other research has made use of a more qualitative approach in describing the lived experience of people with a chronic illness. Qualitative methodologies such as interviews, focus groups or surveys, which may feature quality-of-life scales, are used to describe quality of life in terms of the lived experience of people (Grypdonck, 2006).

Diagnosis of a chronic illness can bring about feelings of grief and loss. Even in early stages of some conditions, when one may feel relatively well, there can often be strong feelings of loss. Some factors that influence the length and intensity of grief are the amount of social support available, the nature and significance of other life stressors and the perception of lost opportunities due to the illness (Schultz & Bruce, 2005). Other common psychosocial features that emerge related to this are depression, stress and powerlessness (Öhman, Söderberg, & Lundman, 2003).

Some chronic illnesses or disabilities, such as paraplegia, are visible, while others, such as diabetes, are not. Having a chronic illness or disability may subject the patient to unfair treatment from others on the basis of their illness, whether it is noticeable or not. Therefore, in many cases, patients with chronic illnesses may not disclose their conditions from fear of being stigmatised (Joachim & Acorn, 2000).

In fact, people with a chronic illness or disability will often actively conceal the physical signs of their condition. This process is seen when people try to conform to what they see as being 'normal' by attempting to hide the illness or disability from others (Joachim & Acorn, 2003). Chronic illness affects not only the patient but may be seen as an intrusion into family life. Families often use the same strategy and attempt to maintain characteristics of 'normal' family life (Gregory, 2005).

Rather than normalisation, the process of adaptation is seen to be more useful in bringing about reintegration into life. New limitations imposed by the chronic illness are integrated into the new sense of 'normal', bringing about a more realistic and constructive set of circumstances. Adaptation is an ongoing task that can be facilitated and supported by nurses and other caring professionals.

PRINCIPLES OF CARE

A major challenge for people living with a chronic illness is dealing with uncertainty. There is uncertainty before and at the time of diagnosis, uncertainty about how the illness will progress and uncertainty about the unpredictable course of their illness (Burton, 2000a).

In the early stages of an illness, clients may rely on the professional knowledge provided by the nurse, but with time the patient becomes the expert and learns about the illness as they live with it. At this time the focus of nursing care shifts and is centred on

CASE STUDY 5.1

Part 3

The community nurse, Sarah, visits Joan at home. She conducts a thorough health history, meticulously completing the admission form. Sarah then assesses the wound. In her eyes it has all the clinical signs of a venous ulcer. It is moist, has irregular edges and there is brown staining of the skin around the wound edges and lower leg. In order to be clear, she performs a Doppler ultrasound, to see if there is evidence of arterial involvement. She knows that her treatment decisions depend on being very sure of Joan's peripheral vascular status. Sarah notes to herself that when she gets back to the office she will ring the GP and suggest he makes a referral to the vascular specialist for more thorough investigations. In the meantime she dresses the wound conservatively, keeping Joan's comfort in mind.

Over the next few weeks Sarah visits regularly to dress the wound. Joan is happy with the arrangement and quite likes Sarah's visits.

Soon, Joan visits the vascular specialist and venous insufficiency is confirmed and arterial disease is ruled out. Sarah is very pleased about this as it means that she can feel comfortable about applying compression therapy, which she knows will help heal the wound.

A four-layer bandaging system is commenced and Sarah announces that she won't need to come quite as often anymore and that this type of dressing may be left in place for a week. Joan is sceptical and notes to Sarah how tight it feels and that she worries about how hot it is going to get. She also makes comment about how bulky it is. Sarah carefully explains the reasons for compression therapy and clearly explains how it works. She assesses Joan's understanding by giving her opportunities to ask questions and reiterate her understanding in her own words. Sarah is confident that the education she has provided is thorough and adequate.

Joan is still sceptical about the bulk, tightness and heat but feels it's important to do what the doctor says.

This quietly drives Sarah crazy as she is the one working with Joan, but she recognises that for some people, there is a perception of authority that rests with the doctor. She reflects that she is lucky to have such a good working relationship with a GP who recognises nursing's unique contribution to patient care.

CASE STUDY 5.1

Part 4

Joan dislikes the compression bandaging immensely. She feels that the size of the dressing is totally out of proportion to the size of the wound. She understands what Sarah has explained but feels that the dressing is so noticeable by others. For a time Joan won't leave the house and has taken to wearing tracksuit trousers when her usual dress is to wear a skirt. She is particularly annoyed that her lawn bowling shoes don't fit over the dressing.

empowerment, supporting self-management, collaborative decision making and healing partnerships.

It is important to acknowledge that a person's lived experience will be unique because of the unique perspectives and experiences they have. We know this as a person-centred approach.

Partnership

The person with a chronic illness has the best information possible about what it is like to live with their condition. They may not describe it in terms of the medical language that we are used to, but living with something that is around all the time will teach them a lot about it. They will know what makes them feel better or worse, what time of day is most difficult and what strategies make particular activities easier (Campling & Sharpe, 2006). This information is vital in articulating the goals of care and developing a plan to address these (Schoot et al., 2005).

There are a variety of reasons that may inhibit a person from talking openly about their illness and disclosing the true ways in which their illness affects their life. Among these reasons are inadequate trust and fear of hospitalisation or other treatments. They may not want to be seen as complaining or they may be frightened about the prospect that something that is effective may be withdrawn (Hallett et al., 2000).

The nurse has a different sphere of expertise, which is useful in other ways. Nurses bring with them experience, clinical evidence and an understanding of the pathophysiology of conditions and treatments (Carter et al., 2004). This information is also vital in developing a plan of care.

Nurses have to be mindful, however, about making assumptions about the lived experience of the patient. The nurse's experience and knowledge may suggest that a particular approach or strategy is acceptable because it has worked in the past, only to find that it is not acceptable to the patient. In this case the nurse's experience can, in a way, present a barrier to care rather than a useful addition to the relationship. Sometimes the nurse has to 'unknow' some of the things from past experience or take care with assumptions in order to be an effective partner in care (Munhall, 1993). Unknowing means looking at each person's experience as new and unique.

By combining the expertise from both parties into a healing partnership and developing the therapeutic relationship, it is likely that quality of life for that person will be enhanced. The partnership relies on reflective listening and the validation of your patient's emotions (Jonsdottir, Litchfield, & Pharris, 2004). From this, information may be given, perhaps some myths or misunderstandings can be addressed, or perhaps a compromised plan of care can be attempted. This cannot be done effectively without recognising the broader social context of the patients' lives (Carter et al., 2004).

Values and beliefs are unique to each individual and will affect the decisions and choices we make in life. Nurses need to be aware of their own personal values and beliefs in order to create a climate of respect and regard for patients (Stein-Parbury, 2009). Sometimes the therapeutic relationship can take a long time to build and some interventions may take a long time to be established and effective. Therefore, it is important to avoid unrealistic expectations of a 'normal' time frame and process of emotional or physical healing (Fennell, 2003).

Compliance

The term 'compliance' is often used in the context of the goals and strategies of health interventions. It may imply a power relationship and that the 'non-compliant' person is

CASE STUDY 5.1

Part 5

Over the next 2 months Sarah visits Joan every week and applies the dressing. They have arranged a weekly Wednesday morning routine where Joan removes the bandaging layers, places them in a bag and cleans her wound in the shower. After the shower she covers the wound with a clean pad and waits for Sarah to arrive. When Sarah arrives, she looks at the old dressings and applies a new one.

The wound is not healing; in fact it seems to be getting worse. Joan is becoming frustrated and inpatient with Sarah and the treatment.

Sarah is concerned as the evidence suggests that Joan is having the correct treatment for her condition.

Sarah asks questions of Joan to try and work out what's going on. Reluctantly Joan admits that a couple of hours after Sarah leaves, she adjusts the dressing in order to fit her shoes on.

Sarah feels frustrated and annoyed that Joan is not complying with the treatment.

the person who is not doing 'what I say she should do'. Non-compliance has a negative connotation associated with control and power (Murphy & Canales, 2001). The concept of non-compliance fails to acknowledge the range of factors that may influence patients' decisions. If agreed-upon goals are negotiated as acceptable to both patient and nurse and the patient is given the support and resources to work towards them, non-compliance will seldom occur (Russell et al., 2003).

Given the increasing awareness of the negative implications of the term 'compliance', alternative terms such as 'adherence' or more recently 'concordance' have gained popularity. This terminology readjusts the implications slightly by using less power-laden language, but even these terms suggests that people should 'stick' to doing what is asked of them regardless of the factors influencing their life (Bissonnette, 2008). Thinking about approaches to caring for people in terms of agreed-upon goals is useful regardless of whether we are talking about compliance or adherence.

The diabetic client who eats what he wants and doesn't give himself injections is non-compliant with his diet and medications. It is important to recognise that there is no law against people making decisions that impact adversely on their health. This is sometimes very difficult for the nurse to accept but is true nonetheless (Playle & Keeley, 1998). A more useful approach than the labelling of 'non-compliant' patients may be to develop the therapeutic relationship and find out the reasons underlying particular patterns of behaviour (Van Hecke, Grypdonck, & Defloor, 2009).

On the other hand, where a person is cognitively unable to make a reasoned, informed decision about their healthcare, as may be the case for people with, for example, dementia or some mental illnesses, ensuring compliance may be exactly the approach that is called for. In this case it may be right and reasonable for the healthcare professional to make unilateral decisions related to a person's treatment (Vuckovich, 2010). Great care must be taken with this approach, however.

Person-centredness

A patient-centred approach changes the communication between the nurse and the patient, giving greater importance to the point of view of the patient than is the case in one-sided relationships. When the nurse is seen as the holder of all knowledge in the nurse–patient relationship, there is an unequal power base, which may lead to the expectation that the patient will do what the nurse says. In an empowering partnership the nurse is not the provider of care but has a role in 'being with' the patient (Brown, McWilliam, & Ward-Griffin, 2006). The nurse can assist the patient to explore, decide upon and evolve their role as partners in care.

Collaborative decision making

Probably the most important first step in a therapeutic relationship is to agree on the goals of intervention. Something that is acceptable to the nurse may be unacceptable to the patient and vice versa. For example, a nurse may believe that compression bandaging is likely to heal a leg ulcer within a relatively short period of time, but this might mean that the person cannot wear her bowling shoes or the feeling of tightness causes discomfort. If the nurse cannot negotiate interventions that are acceptable to both parties, it is unlikely that the intervention will work.

Goals may be healing of a wound, control of symptoms or regaining a level of functioning that allows that person to engage in a particular activity. Once the goal is established, the nurse and patient can work out the most acceptable way of attaining the goal. Using the nurse's experience and knowledge of strategies combined with the person's understanding of their own life, some strategies can be decided upon and implemented (Van Hecke et al., 2009).

Self-management

One of the most powerful and practical approaches to the management of chronic illness is self-management. Self-management involves the patient taking responsibility for the management of their condition in their daily life (Nolan & Nolan, 1999). That means the patient takes on a new role, the role of a consumer of healthcare. The patient actively seeks information to understand the illness or disability and to learn new skills. The patient becomes an active and informed participant in the relationship with healthcare providers and makes decisions based on best available evidence, personal preference and availability of resources. The patient then actively integrates chronic illness self-management into their lives (Audulv, Asplund, & Norbergh, 2012). Self-management may give the patient a sense of control and may be a process to bring back order into their life (Kralik, Koch, Price, & Howard, 2004). The role of the nurse is to support self-management and the role of the patient is to do the care.

Holistic care

Holistic care is performed when the range of factors that may influence the patient's decision making are acknowledged. Understanding what the patient experiences is essential in delivering therapeutic care. Patients and nurses share a common sense of humanity (Taylor, 2005). Through 'ordinariness' the nurse can connect with the patient. The patient values the shared humanity and at the same time acknowledges the nurse's knowledge and skills — this leads to the formation of a therapeutic relationship with mutual benefits that facilitates healing (Taylor, 2005).

Empowerment

One of the roles of the nurse is to empower the patient so that they can manage their own care. This may be addressing some structural barriers to self-care or providing information or education to the patient and their carers (Oudshoorn, 2005). Empowerment is not a division of labour, describing what the nurse will and will not do, or what the patient should or should not do, but a discourse that results in self-efficacy.

What happens when a nurse believes that a person should assume responsibility for some aspect of care but the person believes the nurse should do it? One common example is in the self-administration of subcutaneous injections. In a biomedically influenced world, it is a common perception that the administration of medications via this route must be performed by a medically focused health professional. This can be quite a challenge to a newly diagnosed diabetic. How do these conflicts get resolved?

In a collaborative partnership between person and clinician it is the development of the therapeutic relationship, including trust and good communication skills, that brings about positive health outcomes and the resolution of conflicting expectations. Understanding and acceptance of their patient's fears and uncertainties will inform the nurse of ways in which they can strategically address the fears to bring about acceptable outcomes. In short, talking about things helps. It allows the nurse to understand and empathise with the patient's point of view and to address the specific concerns in ways that acknowledge the fears (Clarke, Hanson & Ross, 2003).

Sometimes it is a part of the nurse's role to facilitate engagement with the multidisciplinary team. Sometimes this might involve advocacy — speaking on the patient's behalf and representing their needs and wishes (Vaartio, Leino-Kilpi, Salanterä, & Suominen, 2006). A more significant and lasting contribution is the one that is made when a patient has the knowledge, resources and self-belief to speak for themselves. This is where the true value of empowerment lies.

One of the things that differentiates a chronic illness from an acute illness is that there is a longer timeframe involved (Montori et al., 2006). This is true in both the urgency of decisions and the development of partnerships. Often decisions in an acute context need

CASE STUDY 5.1

Part 6

Sarah feels troubled by Joan's admission and can't understand why she wouldn't adhere to the recommended treatment. She thinks 'if she would just persist with the treatment for a couple of months she might not need a dressing at all'. Sarah wonders why this would be the case and recognises that Joan has been dressing her leg herself for quite some time without Sarah knowing about it. She realises that she has been doing a lot of telling, but not a lot of listening.

She recognises that she has missed out on developing a therapeutic relationship with Joan and that this is the first thing she needs to work on. After all, Joan has to live with the leg ulcer all the time and will be the person that is in the best position to understand the way it impacts on her life. Sarah resolves that at the next visit, she will backtrack a bit and spend some time talking to Joan about what's going on and maybe talk about what goals they could set and work towards together.

CASE STUDY 5.1

Part 7

At the next visit, the nurse asks Joan if it is okay to spend a bit more time to talk about her care. Fortunately, Joan doesn't have any pressing engagements or appointments and says that it is all right. Sarah can only imagine what Joan must be thinking given her previous dogmatic stance, but she is grateful to have the opportunity to have this conversation. She shares her concerns and the questions that she has asked herself with Joan.

She begins by acknowledging that Joan clearly knows what is important and what she is capable of. She congratulates her on her perseverance and the changes in diet and lifestyle that she has undertaken and says that she knows that it's not an easy thing to do. She goes on to say that she has cared for many different people with leg ulcers and, while everyone is different, she has a good understanding of some of the challenges and possibilities that Joan might come across.

She suggests that in their therapeutic relationship from this point forward the emphasis is on what she can do to support Joan. She promises to listen to what she has to say and to work with her towards what she needs.

'How has it been for you so far?' she asks.

Joan answers, 'I hate this thing. I feel unclean all the time and I worry that people will think I can't look after myself.'

'Why didn't you tell me how you felt?' asked Sarah.

'Well, since we're being honest here — you were very bossy and in fact I did tell you but you weren't really interested.'

Sarah was a bit taken aback by Joan's words, but could see how her actions could be interpreted. She acknowledged Joan's feelings and explained that she really did want to help and that her expertise was in wound management. Sarah said, 'What I am not expert in is your life. I think we need to work together a bit more and I'll try not to come across as too bossy.'

Sarah wanted to know how the dressing was for Joan and wanted to understand why she took it off. She says, 'I know you told me the dressing was bulky, hot and tight. Was this why you took it off? There isn't much we can do about those things, but if it's too much, would you like to try something else?'

Joan recognised Sarah's genuine interest in working together.

'No, I can handle those things really, it's just that I can't fit my shoes on. I take it off on Wednesdays so that I can wear my shoes for bowls. I'm careful though, I cover the wound and look after it and I put the bandages back on when I get home.'

Sarah didn't realise the extent of Joan's interaction with the wound and was very surprised that the dressing was totally removed less than two hours after it was applied.

Joan was the captain of her lawn bowling team and they were currently winning the regional championship. Joan loved bowling, loved the competitive nature of the sport and had many good friends in and around the bowling club. For Joan, wearing her bowling shoes was a higher priority than wearing her bandages.

CASE STUDY 5.1 — cont'd

She said she didn't tell Sarah about it as she was worried she would be in trouble.

They both felt that this frank conversation allowed them to start working together.

They were able to develop goals that drew on Sarah's expert knowledge of wound management and also on Joan's expert knowledge of her life, resources and capacities.

In the end it was a simple matter of rearranging the timing of the visits. Joan still took the bandage off prior to going to lawn bowls, put on a temporary dressing which Sarah prepared and taught her how to apply, and went bowling. In the afternoon, when she returned home, Sarah applied the full four layer compression bandage system. It was able to stay on for almost a whole week. Both Sarah and Joan acknowledged that the system wasn't perfect, but they also both felt that it was good middle ground. Joan's wound did begin to heal and they both found this very reassuring.

to be made quickly, with immediate and permanent consequences, while in a chronic illness they can be made over a longer period and revised with less immediate consequences. Equally, the partnership between the nurse and the person with a chronic illness may develop slowly over a number of episodes and goals negotiated over time, while in an acute context this is seldom possible.

Patients may like to talk about their experience. This type of storytelling is one way in which people can make meaning of an illness and their lives (Kralik, Telford, Price & Koch, 2005; Telford, Kralik & Koch 2006). By listening to their stories and finding out what is important to them, clinicians can facilitate a shared understanding of the needs of their patients (Hyden, 1997). Giving time and permission to ask questions and seek answers and assistance enhances the partnership (Kralik, 2002). These activities will help patients to incorporate the illness into their life and attach meaning to their illness, which may affect their coping and adaptation in positive ways (Caress et al., 2001).

It is interesting to note that along with suffering comes adaptation and resilience, giving up old versions of self and establishing a new identity. Sometimes having a chronic illness can be seen as a very positive thing in someone's life. Many people say that their life is richer for the new perspectives that they have attained or that they learned things about themselves that they did not know prior to their illness. Examples may be appreciating things that were taken for granted, like the beauty in a sunrise or time spent with children, or recognising one's own strength through completing some very difficult rehabilitation. These things may also be true for nurses who work with people with a chronic illness.

CONCLUSION

People lead very complex lives and no one knows that life better than the person living it. Psychosocial care for the person with a chronic illness depends on the clinician's skill and attitudes in recognising the value of what people know about themselves and their life and working alongside them towards relevant, shared goals. Therapeutic relationships and partnerships provide a foundation where nurses and patients can work together towards

CASE STUDY 5.1

Part 8

Four months later when Sarah comes to visit for the last time, Joan gives her a card and a box of chocolates to share with the team. This will be the last visit unless a new need arises. They have worked together to arrive at a place where Joan feels safe and comfortable with her care. Joan is applying moisturiser to her leg and has bought stockings that have a degree of compression.

Sarah learnt something very valuable about herself and how she might at times be perceived. She learnt about the success that can be had through working towards shared goals. She also learnt quite a bit about lawn bowls.

Reflective questions

1 Think about your own culture. Does your culture influence your perception of health and illness?

2 Consider patients you have cared for — can you identify times when the patient's perceptions of their chronic illness changed according to their needs and situation?

3 The psychosocial needs of the carer also need to be considered — how can you support the carer of someone with a chronic illness?

maximising a person's capacity to engage in life in a meaningful way and minimising the adverse impacts of their illness. Recognising diversity, supporting self-management and empowering people to engage with healthcare systems and other aspects of life are important person-centred strategies that are applied within the partnership to bring about good health outcomes and quality in life.

Recommended reading

Jacobi, S., & Macleod, R. (2011). Making sense of chronic illness — a therapeutic approach. *Journal of Primary Health Care, 3*(2), 136–141.

Lubkin, I., & Larsen, P. (2012). *Chronic Illness: Impact and interventions* (8th ed.). Boston: Jones and Bartlett Publishers.

McMurray, A., & Clendon, J. (2011). *Community health & wellness: Primary health care in practice* (4th ed.). Chatswood, NSW: Elsevier Australia.

Stein-Parbury, J. (2009). *Patient & person: Interpersonal skills in nursing* (4th ed.). Chatswood, N.S.W: Churchill Livingstone Elsevier.

Van Hecke, A., Grypdonck, M., & Defloor, T. (2009). A review of why patients with leg ulcers do not adhere to treatment. *Journal of Clinical Nursing, 18*, 337–349.

References

Ackland, M., & Catford, J. (2006). Measuring population health status in Australia. In H. Keleher & B. Murphy (Eds.), *Understanding health: A determinants approach* (pp. 70–96). Melbourne: Oxford University Press.

Allen, D., Griffiths, L., & Lyne, P. (2004). Understanding complex trajectories in health and social care provision. *Sociology of Health & Illness, 26*(7), 1008–1030.

Alonso, Y. (2004). The biopsychosocial model in medical research: the evolution of the health concept over the last two decades. *Patient Education and Counseling, 53*(2), 239–244. doi: 10.1016/s0738-3991(03).00146-0.

Asbring, P. (2001). Chronic illness — a disruption in life: Identity-transformation among women with chronic fatigue syndrome and fibromyalgia. *Journal of Advanced Nursing, 34*(3), 312–319.

Audulv, A., Asplund, K., & Norbergh, K. (2012). The integration of chronic illness self-management. *Qualitative Health Research, 22*(3), 332–345.

Bissonnette, J. (2008). Adherence: a concept analysis. *Journal of Advanced Nursing, 63*(6), 634–643. doi:10.1111/j.1365-2648.2008.04745.x.

Brown, D., McWilliam, C., & Ward-Griffin, C. (2006). Client-centred empowering partnering in nursing. *Journal of Advanced Nursing, 53*(2), 160–168.

Burton, C. R. (2000a). Living with stroke: A phenomenological study. *Journal of Advanced Nursing, 32*(2), 301–309.

Burton, C. R. (2000b). Re-thinking stroke rehabilitation: The Corbin and Strauss chronic illness trajectory framework. *Journal of Advanced Nursing, 32*(3), 595–602.

Campling, F., & Sharpe, M. (2006). *Living with a long-term illness; the facts.* New York: Oxford University Press.

Caress, A., Luker, K. A., & Owens, R. G. (2001). A descriptive study of meaning of illness in chronic renal disease. *Journal of Advanced Nursing, 33*(6), 716–727.

Carter, H., MacLeod, R., Brander, P., et al. (2004). Issues and innovations in nursing practice: Living with a terminal illness: Patients' priorities. *Journal of Advanced Nursing, 45*(6), 6–11.

Cartwright, C., & Parker, V. (2005). Ageing, health and illness. In C. Rogers-Clark, A. McCarthy & K. Martin-McDonald (Eds.), *Living with Illness* (pp. 54–69). Sydney: Elsevier.

Clarke, A., Hanson, E., & Ross, H. (2003). Seeing the person behind the patient: Enhancing the care of older people using a biographical approach. *Journal of Clinical Nursing, 12*(5), 697–706.

Corbin, J. (2001). Introduction and overview: Chronic illness and nursing. In R. Hyman & J. Corbin (Eds.), *Chronic illness: Research and theory for nursing practice* (pp. 4–5). New York: Springer.

Fennell, P. (2003). *Managing chronic illness using the four-phase treatment approach.* Hoboken, New Jersey: John Wiley and Sons.

Freeman, J. (2005). Towards a definition of holism. *British Journal of General Practice, 55*(511), 154.

Gregory, S. (2005). Living with chronic illness in the family setting. *Sociology of Health & Illness, 27*(3), 372–392.

Grypdonck, M. (2006). Qualitative health research in the era of evidence-based practice. *Qualitative Health Research, 16*(10), 1371–1385.

Hallett, C. E., Austin, L., Caress, A., et al. (2000). Community nurses' perceptions of patient 'compliance' in wound care: A discourse analysis. *Journal of Advanced Nursing, 32*(1), 115–123.

Hyden, L. (1997). Illness and narrative. *Sociology of Health and Illness, 19*(1), 48–69.

Jacobi, S., & Macleod, R. (2011). Making sense of chronic illness — a therapeutic approach. *Journal of Primary Health Care, 3*(2), 136–141.

Joachim, G., & Acorn, S. (2000). Stigma of visible and invisible chronic conditions. *Journal of Advanced Nursing, 32*(1), 243–248.

Joachim, G., & Acorn, S. (2003). Life with a rare chronic disease: The scleroderma experience. *Journal of Advanced Nursing, 42*(6), 598–606.

Jonsdottir, H., Litchfield, M., & Pharris, M. D. (2004). The relational core of nursing practice as partnership. *Journal of Advanced Nursing, 47*(3), 241–248.

Kralik, D. (2002). Issues and innovations in nursing practice: The quest for ordinariness: transition experienced by midlife women living with chronic illness. *Journal of Advanced Nursing, 39*(2), 146–154.

Kralik, D., Koch, T., Price, K., et al. (2004). Patient involvement in clinical nursing: Chronic illness self-management: taking action to create order. *Journal of Clinical Nursing, 13*, 259–267.

Kralik, D., Telford, K., Price, K., et al. (2005). Women's experiences of fatigue in chronic illness. *Journal of Advanced Nursing, 52*(4), 372–380.

Larsen, P. (2012). Chronicity. In I. Lubkin & P. Larsen (Eds.), *Chronic Illness: Impact and interventions* (8th ed., pp. 3–22). Boston: Jones and Bartlett Publishers.

Livneh, H., & Parker, R. (2005). Psychological adaptation to disability: Perspectives from chaos and complexity theory. *Rehabilitation Counselling Bulletin, 49*(1), 17–28.

Lopez, A., Mathers, D., Ezzati, M., et al. (2006). Global and regional burden of disease and risk factors, 2001: Systematic analysis of population health data. *The Lancet, 367*(9524), 1747–1757.

McMurray, A., & Clendon, J. (2011). *Community health & wellness: primary health care in practice* (4th ed.). Chatswood, NSW: Elsevier Australia.

Miller, J., & Timson, D. (2004). Exploring the experiences of partners who live with a chronic low back pain sufferer. *Health & Social Care in the Community, 12*(1), 34–42.

Montori, V. M., Gafni, A., & Charles, C. (2006). A shared treatment decision-making approach between patients with chronic conditions and their clinicians: The case of diabetes. *Health Expectations, 9*(1), 25–36.

Munhall, P. L. (1993). 'Unknowing': Toward another pattern of knowing in nursing. *Nursing Outlook, 41*(3:May–Jun), 125–128.

Murphy, N., & Canales, M. (2001). A critical analysis of compliance. *Nursing Inquiry, 8*(3), 173–181.

Nolan, M., & Nolan, J. (1999). Rehabilitation, chronic illness and disability: The missing elements in nurse education. *Journal of Advanced Nursing, 29*(4), 958–966.

Öhman, M., & Söderberg, S. (2004). The experiences of close relatives living with a person with serious chronic illness. *Qualitative Health Research, 14*(3), 396–410.

Öhman, M., Söderberg, S., & Lundman, B. (2003). Hovering between suffering and enduring: The meaning of living with serious chronic illness. *Qualitative Health Research, 13*(4), 528–542.

Oudshoorn, A. (2005). Power and empowerment: Critical concepts in the nurse-client relationship. *Contemporary Nurse, 20*(1), 57–66.

Paterson, B. L. (2001). The shifting perspectives model of chronic illness. *Journal of Nursing Scholarship, 33*(1), 21–26.

Playle, J. F., & Keeley, P. (1998). Non-compliance and professional power. *Journal of Advanced Nursing, 27*(2), 304–311.

Rolley, J., Smith, J., DiGiacomo, M., et al. (2011). The caregiving role following percutaneous coronary intervention. *Journal of Clinical Nursing, 20*(1/2), 227–235. doi: 10.1111/j.1365-2702.2009.03104.x.

Russell, S., Daly, J., Hughes, E., et al. (2003). Nurses and 'difficult' patients: Negotiating non-compliance. *Journal of Advanced Nursing, 43*(3), 281–287.

Saha, S., Arbelaez, J. J., & Cooper, L. A. (2003). Patient–physician relationships and racial disparities in the quality of health care. *American Journal of Public Health, 93*(10), 1713–1719.

Schoot, T., Proot, I., Meulen, R. T., et al. (2005). Recognition of client values as a basis for tailored care: The view of Dutch expert patients and family caregivers. *Scandinavian Journal of Caring Sciences, 19*(2), 169–176.

Schultz, C., & Bruce, E. (2005). Living with loss and grief. In C. Rogers-Clark, A. McCarthy, & K. Martin-McDonald (Eds.), *Living with illness: Psychological challenges for nurses* (pp. 128–142). Sydney: Elsevier.

Smith, B. W., Dalen, J., Wiggins, K., et al. (2008). The brief resilience scale: Assessing the ability to bounce back. *International Journal of Behavioral Medicine, 15*(3), 194–200.

Smith, P. (2009). The family caregiver's journey in end-of-life care: recognizing and identifying with the role of carer. *International Journal on Disability & Human Development, 8*(1), 67–73.

Stein-Parbury, J. (2009). *Patient & person: interpersonal skills in nursing* (4th ed.). Chatswood, NSW: Churchill Livingstone Elsevier.

Taylor, B. (1995). Nursing as healing work. *Contemporary Nurse, 4*(3), 100–106.

Taylor, B. (2005). Health, wellness, illness, healing and holism, and nursing. In C. Rogers-Clark, A. McCarthy & K. Martin-McDonald (Eds.), *Living with illness: Psychological challenges for nurses* (pp. 97–113). Sydney: Elsevier.

Telford, K., Kralik, D. & Koch, T. (2006). Acceptance and denial: implications for people adapting to chronic illness: literature review. *Journal of Advanced Nursing, 55*(4), 457–464.

Vaartio, H., Leino-Kilpi, H., Salanterä, S., et al. (2006). Nursing advocacy: how is it defined by patients and nurses, what does it involve and how is it experienced? *Scandinavian Journal of Caring Sciences, 20*(3), 282–292.

Van Hecke, A., Grypdonck, M., & Defloor, T. (2009). A review of why patients with leg ulcers do not adhere to treatment. *Journal of Clinical Nursing, 18*, 337–349.

Vuckovich, P. (2010). Compliance versus adherence in serious and persistent mental illness. *Nursing Ethics, 17*(1), 77–85. doi:10.1177/0969733009352047.

Wilson, D., & Grant, J. (2008). Culturally competent partnerships with communities. In K. Francis, Y. Chapman, K. Hoare, et al. (Eds.), *Community as partner: Theory and practice in nursing* (Australia/New Zealand, ed., pp. 113–127). Broadway, NSW: Lippincott Williams & Wilkins Pty Ltd.

CHAPTER 6

Lynne S. Giddings
Dianne E. Roy

Stigmatisation of people living with a chronic illness or disability

Learning objectives

When you have completed this chapter you will be able to:

- identify and name examples of stigmatising processes that could lead to stereotyping, labelling and 'othering' of people who live with chronic illness and/or disability
- use self-reflexive questioning to assist in deconstructing situations that may marginalise and discriminate against people who live with chronic illness and/or disability
- develop strategies to identify, name and challenge stigmatising processes experienced by people who live with chronic illness and/or disability
- apply specific principles of nursing practice to avoid stigmatising people who live with chronic illness and/or disability
- become 'part of the solution' to prevent the marginalisation and discrimination of people who live with chronic illness and/or disability.

Key words

discrimination, health disparities, marginalisation, stereotyping, stigma

INTRODUCTION

This chapter focuses on the concept of stigma and related processes, such as stereotyping, labelling and othering, and their effects on people who live with chronic illness and/or disability. Such processes not only affect individuals, families and their communities, but also contribute to disparities in healthcare. For the purposes of this chapter we focus our discussion on how nurses can challenge these stigmatising processes in the context of working with people with chronic illness and/or disability. We acknowledge that the 'isms', such as racism, sexism, heterosexism and classism, also intersect within the healthcare context. It is also important to acknowledge the distinction between chronic illness and disability. Illness is caused by disease whereas disability is created within societal structures (Oliver, 2009) which includes the processes that happen 'when one group of people create barriers by designing a world only for their way of living, taking no account of the impairments other people have'(Ministry of Health, 2001, p. 3). When these terms are used synonymously it is difficult to challenge the stigmatising processes that make invisible the different needs of people living with an impairment (but not an illness) who experience disability. After exploring issues relating to nurses and the processes of stigma and the value of using the social model of disability to guide self-reflexive practice, we will discuss various principles of nursing care using fictitious case study scenarios.

NURSES AND STIGMA

Stigma, defining people as abnormal if they do not meet an expected norm, is related to being different; it pervades all levels of society and crosses all cultures. We are all affected by it, we are all part of the problem but we can also make ourselves part of the solution. Nurses who care for people who live with chronic illness and/or disability are well positioned to challenge the everyday processes of stigmatisation. Through the naming of the processes and their effects, possibilities for conscious action are opened up at the personal, professional and socio-political levels. One of the first principles as healthcare providers is to 'know ourselves' in relation to who we are in the world so that we are able to deconstruct (identify and name) the stigmatising processes that lead to marginalisation and discrimination of others.

Knowing ourselves

Many nurses believe that they treat everyone the same and/or they are not privileged or oppressed in any way. We challenge this position as we believe that all of us contribute to disparities within society and the healthcare system. If we start with the premise that we all use stigmatising processes and are all affected by them, then we can get somewhere with challenging them. We offer here some self-reflexive questions that can assist nurses to care effectively for people who are different from themselves, such as those who live with chronic illness and/or disability. These questions have been informed by the work of Porter (1996), Maeve (1998), Smith (1999) and Giddings (2005a).

1 Am I acknowledging my position of power and privilege in relation to the people with impairments and/or disabilities whom I work alongside or care for?
2 Am I actively trying to understand and accept the validity of each individual's experience?
3 Am I recognising the expertise/developing expertise of people in living with their illness and/or disability?
4 Am I working with and supporting the personally developed strategies for self-management of people living with chronic illness and/or disability?

Self-reflexive approaches to nursing practice are grounded in respect and regard for people. They help position nurses as potential advocates and social activists by making visible stigmatising processes such as stereotyping, labelling and othering, and their outcome: social isolation, powerlessness and health disparities. (See Table 6-1.) These processes and

TABLE 6.1
Definitions of stigmatising processes

STIGMATISING PROCESS	DEFINITION
Stereotyping	Involves categorising and prejudging (prejudice) individuals based on an oversimplified set of beliefs about the nature and characteristics of particular groups.
Labelling	The application of negative stereotypes by naming individuals and their identified group as problematic.
Othering	The social construction of people with certain characteristics into named groups that are viewed as 'different' in some way from what is widely believed in society to be 'normal'.

outcomes are complex and interlink to produce a society in which some people and groups within certain contexts are privileged and others are marginalised and discriminated against. Of course, how one views these processes depends on where one is standing. Those people who are privileged by belonging to a dominant cultural/social group, such as being male, white, heterosexual, middle-class and able, may not be able to 'see' that just belonging to a mainstream group can advantage them in relation to others. Conversely, those people who are identified as belonging to a group that is marginalised within society may effectively internalise the dominant cultural attitudes and so believe them to be true (Giddings, 2005a; Johnson, 2006); they have an acquired social consciousness or false consciousness so they self-fulfil or act out the stereotypical behaviour (Giddings, 2005b). For example, a person who is living with diabetes may self-label as 'a diabetic' or may accept a 'sick role' of unnecessary dependency. All groups within society, including the disabled community, marginalise and discriminate from within. For example, a person who is able to articulate their experiences and needs (able-disabled) may privilege themselves to speak for those who live with both intellectual and physical impairment and are less able to speak for themselves (disabled-disabled). Such discriminatory processes can inadvertently be supported by otherwise sound and beneficial policies such as the New Zealand Disability Strategy (Ministry of Health, 2001) by creating an assumption that 'one size fits all'.

In the broadest terms, we are arguing that people coming into the healthcare system, no matter what their difference, need to be culturally safe; that is, receive effective and safe nursing practice (Nursing Council of New Zealand, 2011; Papps, 2005). Nurses need to not only be aware and sensitive to the effects of stigmatising processes within society and the healthcare system, but also have a social consciousness that enables action by developing strategies for implementing change: working with, not against (Giddings, Roy & Predeger, 2007; Roy & Giddings, 2012); naming not blaming; and deconstructing power relations rather than passively accepting the status quo (Giddings, 2005b; Johnson, 2006).

Deconstructing (identifying, naming and challenging) societal stigmatising processes

Even today it is not uncommon to hear stigmatising or othering terms used to describe people who live with chronic illness and/or disability. For example, people are sometimes described as being 'handicapped', 'crippled', 'retarded', 'suffering from', 'mongoloid' or 'wheelchair-bound'. They may also be labelled by their condition, for example 'arthritic', 'diabetic', 'lunatic', 'asthmatic', 'spastic', 'quadriplegic' or 'epileptic'. Identifying such labelling is one of the first steps in challenging the processes of stigmatisation. It can assist in making stereotypes and related health disparities visible and open to critique. Nurses need to be aware, however, that many people living with chronic illness and/or disability may wish to conceal and keep their condition secret in an attempt to pass as 'normal'. These attempts, though a protective response to the marginalising and discriminatory practices within society, feed into their hidden nature and make them difficult to challenge. It is important to challenge stigmatising processes as they not only have negative effects for the individual living with chronic illness and/or disability, but also for their family, friends and community, and can even extend to those who care for them. Within nursing itself, for example, there are processes that marginalise and discriminate. Nursing educational programs often exclude people with disabilities (Carroll, 2004; Sin & Fong, 2008) and nurses living with chronic illness and/or disability often report difficulties with maintaining employment and/or achieving promotion (Giddings, 1997; Sin & Fong, 2008; Wallis, 2004; Wallis, 2006; Weiss, 2005).

Self-reflexive practice that identifies, names and challenges stigmatising processes can be guided by the social model of disability first described by Oliver (1990; 2009). It was specifically developed in the 1980s to address 'issues of oppression and discrimination of disabled people, caused by institutional forms of exclusion and by cultural attitudes embedded in social practices' (Terzi, 2004, p. 141). The model has been extensively reviewed, critiqued and used to inform research, policy and practice (see for example, Dowling, 2006; Ministry of Health, 2001; Mitra, 2006; Oliver, 2009; Scullion, 2010; Shakespeare, 2008; Shakespeare & Watson, 1997; Terzi, 2004; Thomas, 2001; Tregaskis, 2002). Within this model it is argued that people, as individuals, live with impairments. Concomitantly (Oliver, 1996, p. 33):

> Disability is all the things that impose restrictions on disabled people; ranging from individual prejudice to institutional discrimination, from inaccessible public buildings to unusable transport systems, from segregated education to excluding work arrangements, and so on. Further, the consequences of this failure do not simply and randomly fall on individuals but systematically upon disabled people as a group who experience this failure as discrimination institutionalised through society.

The social model of disability moves the problem of disability away from the individual to society. The onus is on society, therefore, to adapt and cater for the needs of individuals and families who live with chronic illness and/or disabilities (Webb & Tossell, 1999). A recent case in New Zealand highlighted institutional discrimination against families who provide specific disability-related care for their 'adult disabled children' (Human Rights Commission, 2012, p. 1 of 3). Although the adult aged children, all living with significant impairments, were assessed by the Ministry of Health as requiring this care, policy stated that only non-family members could be paid (Human Rights Commission, 2012). Families providing disability-related care successfully challenged this policy by employing human rights legislation. A Human Rights Review Tribunal concluded in 2010 that the policy was discriminatory under the Human Rights Act (New Zealand Statutes, 1993) 'as it is unlawful to discriminate against someone because of their status as a family member' (Human Rights Commission, 2012, p. 1 of 3). The Ministry appealed the decision through the High Court and the Court of Appeal. Both courts, however, upheld the decision with the High Court noting that the Ministry's policy was at odds with the New Zealand Disability Strategy (Ministry of Health, 2001). In June 2012, the Ministry capitulated and agreed to pay parents as caregivers.

Presented in Case Study 6.1 are common scenarios that can help you explore the principles of nursing care that can guide your self-reflexive practice in relation to identifying, naming and challenging stigmatising processes while caring for and working with people who live with chronic illness and/or disability.

CASE STUDY 6.1

Serena (32 years) and her partner Nigel (30 years) have been living with her parents, Muriel and Keith, in their large suburban home for the last 2 years. They are in the process of moving into a place of their own in the inner-city. Serena works full-time as a case manager for a family carer support organisation and Nigel as an architect for the city council. Serena was born with spina bifida and has paralysis of her lower body and uses a wheelchair; Nigel has lived with diabetes (Type 1) since he was 16 years old. Adding to the complexity of the family situation, Muriel has lived with multiple sclerosis for nearly 20 years.

Part 1

Serena and Nigel frequently go to the movies, often enjoying a coffee or meal before the show. Although the local theatre is accessible for wheelchairs, the cafés and restaurants in the area have narrow doorways and often steps. Once making it into a café, Serena then has to negotiate her wheelchair to a table, often a difficult task. Recently, on Nigel's birthday when they were ordering a coffee, the person behind the counter looked down at Serena, then turned to Nigel and asked, 'What type of coffee does she want?'

Nigel replied, 'You can ask her.'

The young woman leaned over the counter and talking slowly and loudly asked, 'What—type—of—coffee—do—you—want?'

Serena replied, 'I do not have a hearing impairment and I would like a trim latte with two sugars, please. My partner will have a double shot long black, no sugar. And while we are at it, we will have two pieces of that delicious-looking apple cake, thanks.'

While they were consuming the coffee and cake, Serena chuckled and said, 'What if the practice nurse catches you eating *that*, Nigel?'

Nigel laughed and replied, 'She would be shocked, I'm sure. She just doesn't seem to understand that sometimes on a special occasion, one just has to have it.'

Serena needed to go to the toilet. The café's toilet facilities were outside, down some steps and near the storeroom. Such inaccessibility necessitated that she wait until they reached the movie theatre. Although the theatre has two wheelchair-accessible toilets, they are both situated in the women's and men's toilet areas respectively. As Serena requires assistance with toileting, no matter which they choose they often receive disapproving looks from other patrons. Nigel reflects on the irony posed by such situations given his work as an architect.

Part 2

Nigel injured his leg while playing club rugby. He was transported to the Emergency Department (ED) by ambulance with a suspected fracture of the tibia. With the focus on his acute injury, his belongings, including his medication and blood glucose meter, were left behind in the changing rooms. He alerted the ambulance staff to the fact he has diabetes (Type 1). They immediately tested his blood glucose level (BGL), which was found to be within normal range at 5.2 mmol/L. On arrival at ED, Nigel was triaged and sent to the acute area for further assessment. Soon after, he began to feel strange and experienced a tingling sensation around his mouth; symptoms he recognised as signalling the beginning of a hypoglycaemic episode. He pressed the

CASE STUDY 6.1 — cont'd

call bell which was eventually answered by a nurse. Nigel told the nurse he was experiencing a 'hypo' and requested some food or glucose tablets. He explained that his 'gear' had not come with him so he could not self-test. The nurse checked his chart. She said that as his BGL was 5.2 mmol/L only half an hour earlier, treatment was not necessary. Nigel explained that he had been playing rugby and because of his accident had not had his planned snack at half-time. He knew his BGL had dropped and that he must have some glucose or food immediately. The nurse replied that he was not allowed anything to eat because of his injury, but she would do a repeat BGL to see if it was low. The nurse left the room. Ten minutes later another nurse escorting Serena to Nigel's bedside found him semi-conscious, sweating profusely and tachycardic. She immediately called for emergency assistance.

Part 3

In anticipation of their move, Serena changed her primary care provider from the health centre she had attended since childhood to an inner-city practice belonging to the same Primary Health Organisation. Prior to the move, she checked out the accessibility of the building and the clinic, and arranged for her health records to be transferred. In due course, Serena made an appointment for a routine cervical smear. On arrival she was informed by the nurse that the clinic's height adjustable examination table was broken and she was unsure when it would be fixed. As Serena was unable to transfer to a regular height examination table, the nurse offered to arrange a home visit so Serena could have the smear taken on her own bed. Serena accepted the offer. Two weeks later she was surprised to receive an invoice for $120. She immediately phoned the practice. On asking why it was so high, she was told by the practice manager that 'this is the standard charge for a home visit'. Serena explained what had happened, but the practice manager said there was nothing she could do. Serena asked to speak to the nurse. On asking what was the standard cost for a smear, the nurse replied '$20'. Serena pointed out that the home visit resulted from the fact that the equipment was malfunctioning and asked why she should pay more than other women for this preventative health service. The nurse paused, then replied, 'Oh, I see your point. I'm sorry; I have never thought of it that way before. I agree, you shouldn't be asked to pay more than other women. I will take this case to the practice management team meeting tomorrow morning.'

Next morning at the meeting, members of the management team initially expressed surprise when the issue was raised, as surely it only required the equipment to be repaired. The nurse argued that the issue was broader and similar situations may arise when the practice is not able to provide equitable services for people living with disability. Following robust discussion, the team came to agreement that the charge was discriminatory and would be changed and that a policy review was required. The nurse offered to draft a document that could be circulated to extend the discussion to include other practices in their primary health organisation.

Part 4

Serena's mother, Muriel, had elective surgery for a hysterectomy. She was admitted to a four-bed room in a surgical unit. The morning following surgery when the nurse finished checking her wound, he stressed to Muriel the importance of walking soon after surgery and instructed her to walk to the end of the ward and back. Some time later the nurse returned and asked Muriel if she had been for her walk. Muriel shook

CASE STUDY 6.1 — cont'd

her head, but before she could explain, the nurse loudly remarked, 'I don't know why some people can't help themselves', and left the room.

Sally in the neighbouring bed chortled, 'Well, that was a good telling-off.'

Muriel responded, 'Actually, I live with multiple sclerosis and would have been lucky to make it to the door prior to my surgery, let alone now!'

Silence hung between them.

Part 5

For a number of years Muriel has been on the committee of a local community action group. Six months previously the committee were notified that their meeting room, which had been made available at no cost, was to be demolished. Finding a new no-cost or low-cost venue proved difficult. Eventually one was found, but access was via two flights of stairs. With Muriel's increasing level of physical impairment access was prohibitive to her attending meetings. Still keen to be actively involved on the committee, she put her name forward for the position of treasurer. The position had been notoriously hard to fill and Muriel knew that she had the skills and could do the work from home, thanks to computer and internet technology. Being treasurer, she reasoned, meant she could continue her contribution to the group without attending the meetings in person. She withdrew her nomination, however, when it became clear that this was not acceptable to all members of the committee.

At the recent annual general meeting no nominations were received for treasurer. On the incoming committee, however, was a nurse who, on hearing of Muriel's earlier self-nomination, challenged the processes that excluded her from the position. The nurse successfully argued that there were options, including the treasurer's work being done electronically and communicated via emails as Muriel had suggested or, in the longer term, applying for funding so the committee could pay for a venue that is accessible to everyone.

Part 6

Serena received a call at work from Kerry, a woman who cares for her adult aged son who lives with severe physical and intellectual impairments resulting from a rare congenital condition. Kerry was seeking advice on what day-service options might be available for her son, Malcolm. He had recently been made redundant following the closure of the facility where he had worked for 5 years in a supported environment. The chances of him finding another job within his capability were limited. Kerry expressed concern that since Malcolm had not been going to work each day, he had lost contact with his friends and colleagues. She struggles to get him out of the house. Kerry said:

> Going to work meant so much more to him than the money; it was his life. It gave structure to his day and the opportunity to be with his friends. And even though he couldn't focus on a task for more than a few minutes at a time, when he completed one of his jobs he had a real sense of pride. The money didn't really matter to him. And then of course there is the impact on my life. I am just so tired and life is so much more of a juggle than before. I used to be able to have a bit of a break when he was at work and get some things done. Like now I can only go to the supermarket at night when my daughter can come and be with her brother because he can't be left alone. And if I take him, then we have to endure people staring when his behaviour becomes socially unacceptable — which is quite often. Honestly, Malcolm going to work is what got me through the week; sort of re-charged my batteries.

PRINCIPLES OF NURSING PRACTICE IN CARING FOR PEOPLE LIVING WITH CHRONIC ILLNESS AND OR/DISABILITY

Work with people in context

The stories of people who live with chronic illness and/or disability may have some similarities, but each person's journey is unique (Giddings et al., 2007; Kralik, 2010). Rather than generalising experiences with the risk of stereotyping, such as 'the difficult arthritic in cubicle three', nurses need to work within the context of the person's everyday life.

Working with the person in context means getting to know them and their families and how they live with, or are learning to live with, their chronic illness and/or disability. It means supporting the person to develop their capacity and capability to self-manage. Nursing decisions can then be guided by what the person needs and perceives as working uniquely for them. The nurse needs to be ready to step in and help by offering suggestions, strategies and support, and at times taking over care; they also need to be ready to step back when not required (Giddings et al., 2007).

Historically, nursing practice has been underpinned by a biomedical approach to care with a focus on the individual, pathophysiology and cure. This model, though successful in treating acute diseases and acute events within chronic illnesses, is limited for general use in the overall management of chronic illness and/or disabilities (Pincus, 2000). As well as having a sound knowledge of pathophysiology and protocols of care informed by contemporary chronic care approaches, nurses need to be self-reflexive so they are constantly alert to when they are 'taking over', labelling or using generalised norms and beliefs about how someone should behave or act.

Nursing care based on a social model of disability and chronic care approaches can complement the biomedical model in such a way that the expertise and resourcefulness of people living with chronic illness and/or disability are more easily recognised and valued. This involves nurses working consciously in partnership with their clients and supporting self-management, rather than always taking control and prescribing strategies (Giddings et al., 2007). Nurses need to recognise that 'Each day, [people] decide what they are going to eat, whether they will exercise and to what extent they will consume prescribed medicines' (Bodenheimer et al., 2002, p. 2470). The question is not whether people self-manage their chronic illness and/or disability, but how? The focus should be on supporting a person's right to self-determination in self-management decisions (Roy, Mahony, Horsburgh, & Bycroft, 2011). This serves to empower them to act rather than accept the status quo of health disparities and discrimination. This was evident when Serena challenged the charge for the home visit that enabled her to have a cervical smear (Case Study 6.1, part 3). Although maybe unintentional, this form of institutional discrimination, embedded in policy, could have created a barrier to Serena accessing appropriate health services.

If nurses use self-reflexive questioning while working with a client, they will remain alert to when they are making stereotypical assumptions that could stand in the way of their giving contextualised care. They will also be more likely to see and name such assumptions when played out in society. Take, for example, the barista who assumed, because Serena used a wheelchair, that she had hearing and cognitive impairments (Case Study 6.1, part 1). Each time such incidences are named and challenged within the healthcare system and society generally, the world becomes a safer place for those who are different from the mainstream in some way.

Working effectively with the person in context involves developing therapeutic relationships to enable communication processes and comprehensive assessments that are appropriate to the person's situation. People living with chronic illness and/or disability are mostly hospitalised when receiving treatment for an acute exacerbation or a co-morbid condition. Knowledge of a person's situation and of the possibility of co-morbidity is essential for comprehensive assessment and delivery of effective care of the person in context, whether in the community or in hospital (O'Brien, Wyke, Guthrie, Watt, & Mercer, 2011; Roy & Giddings, 2012). The nurse caring for Muriel following her hysterectomy, for example, did not contextualise his care (Case Study 6.1, part 4). In insisting Muriel walk to the end of the ward and back, he based his care on expected norms, perhaps the prescribed clinical pathway. In a study of 20 people with osteoarthritis and co-morbidities undergoing total knee joint replacement, Williams, Dunning and Manias (2007) found that little regard was given to the person's co-morbidities; instead they were expected to conform to and recover 'at the rate specified by the clinical pathway' (p. 250). In Muriel's case, good assessment skills and an understanding of her unique context would have enabled the nurse to recognise her co-morbidities. Muriel could have then been encouraged to mobilise in a way that prevented post-operative complications and promoted recovery but was within her ability. Instead, the care offered marginalised Muriel, labelling her 'non-compliant' and not wanting to 'help herself' in her recovery.

Nurses need to adapt to the ever-changing client context. Client care cannot be prescribed by strict clinical protocols that ignore the ever-changing nature of a person's experience. Nurses need to be flexible and open to being guided by the self-knowledge of their clients while being vigilant to signs of tension or change. Many chronic illnesses, such as multiple sclerosis and rheumatoid arthritis, are characterised by periods of exacerbation and remission of disease activity, when there may be a need for hands-on nursing care. Age and life stage, along with the ebb and flow of relationships and family life, also impact on the experience (Roy & Giddings, 2012). The impact on Kerry's life, for example, when Malcolm was made redundant (Case Study 6.1, part 6) demonstrates the complexity and ripple effects within the family of living with chronic illness and/or disability that go beyond the pathophysiological.

There may not always be the need for direct nursing care when working with people living with chronic illness and/or disability, but nurses must remain aware of and work with the ever-changing client context. They need to continually challenge stigmatising processes that get in the way of contextualising care.

Recognise and value expertise and resourcefulness

Nurses need to recognise and work with the expertise/developing expertise of their clients. This is essential for effective care (Giddings et al., 2007; Roy, 2001; Roy & Giddings, 2012). Over time, people and their families who live with the daily reality of chronic illness and/or disability develop self-knowing as well as effective strategies for self-management and care. These strategies are not only informed through the person–health professional relationship but also through social and media sources such as family, friends, magazines and the internet. Nigel demonstrated expertise when he recognised the beginning of a hypoglycaemic episode (Case Study 6.1, part 2). He based this on his self-knowledge developed through having experienced similar episodes over the past 14 years. Had the nurse recognised and valued his expertise and self-knowing, the subsequent emergency situation may have been avoided.

Recognising and valuing the unique expertise of the person is empowering to both parties in the person–health professional relationship. There is a fine balance between stepping in and holding back in offering care that requires nurses to know their clients in context. This balance can only be achieved by establishing processes of negotiation, with two-way communication within an ongoing therapeutic relationship that is mutually respectful of each other's expertise (Koch, Jenkin, & Kralik, 2004; Toombs, 2004). Such a relationship, which enhances the person's highly tuned knowing of themselves, can make the difference between effective and ineffective care and self-management (Giddings et al., 2007; Roy & Giddings, 2012; Roy et al., 2011). At a societal level it is essential that people living with chronic illness and/or disability are included in decision-making processes and that their expertise is valued, listened to and acted upon when plans are made for provision of services, design of buildings and so forth. Nurses, too, need to take responsibility, not only in advocating for this client group, but also in becoming politically active. The nurse (Case Study 6.1, part 3) advocated for Serena when she took the issue of the charge for the home visit to the practice management team meeting. She demonstrated political action when she broadened the issue to one of equity for all people living with a disability.

Support rights to self-determination

Nurses have an important role in providing education and care that is not only appropriate and timely, but also presented in a way that respects a person's right to self-determination. For example, nurses, along with other health professionals, are often required to prescribe and reinforce what a person should or should not do in living with a chronic illness and/or disability, such as giving guidance about appropriate dietary modifications to people with diabetes. The techniques and strategies suggested may at times, however, be at odds with the person's everyday reality. There are always tensions between what people 'should do', 'can do' or 'choose to do' (Roy, 2001; Roy et al., 2011). Rather than setting rigid protocols, nurses need to respect their client's self-determination by acknowledging and working with such tensions. They can talk with the person about how they might realistically and individually incorporate dietary modification (for example) into their everyday lives, establishing a pathway for success, not failure. Such strategies would incorporate 'what matters most' and enable them to live positively with the inevitable tensions. For example, when Serena and Nigel were at the cafe (Case Study 6.1, part 1), Nigel chose to have a piece of cake, in spite of the dictatorial voice of the practice nurse ringing in his ears. On this occasion 'what mattered most' was Serena and Nigel's celebration, not his dietary adherence. Nigel knew this was a special occasion and that the consequence would be close monitoring of his blood glucose levels and possible increase of his next insulin dose. He also probably knew it was not something he would do every day if he wished to avoid long-term complications.

Be aware of the potential for social isolation

Nurses need to remain vigilant in relation to their clients' overall wellbeing. Numerous studies have shown that people living with chronic illness and/or disability experience loneliness and social isolation (see for example, Lindsay, Gow, Vanderpyl, Logo & Dalbeth, 2011; Rokach, Lechcier-Kimel, & Safarov, 2006; Schur, 2002; Rokach, 2012). They are less likely to socialise with friends outside the home or to be involved in religious, recreational or any other groups or activities (Schur, 2002). Research by Alpass and Neville (2003) found that it was social isolation not their chronic illness that led to depression in older men. Participants in Lindsay et al.'s (2011) study who were living with gout reported experiencing both physical and social isolation.

Social isolation and loneliness in many instances results from the disabling effects of discrimination and marginalisation that limit opportunities for such things as travel, socialising and employment. These situations continue to exist despite the ratification of the United Nations Convention on the Rights of Persons with Disabilities (2006) in New

Zealand and Australia in 2008 and legislation such as the Disability Discrimination Act 1992 (Australian Statutes, 1992) and the Human Rights Act 1993 (New Zealand Statutes, 1993) aimed at 'abolishing discrimination against people living with disabilities and to encourage equal opportunities for people in all areas' (Varnham, 2004, p. 48).With the loss of employment, Malcolm experienced increased social isolation and loneliness (Case Study 6.1, part 6). When he was made redundant, he lost not only his salary but also structure to his day, contact with his friends and doing work that re-enforced his sense of self-worth.

Societal attitudes that do not value contributions made in different ways by people who are differently able can contribute to the social isolation. Similarly, many people living with chronic illness and/or disability are unable to find paid employment, often due to the inflexibility of workplace practices and the attitudes of employers. Labour force statistics show significantly lower employment rates for people living with chronic illness and/or disability than the general population (Statistics New Zealand, 2008). This is significant given that unemployment has been shown to have a strong association with ill health and depression (Keller-Olaman, Williams, Knight, & McGee, 2004).

Nurses need to work with individuals and families in strategising ways to offset the possibility of social isolation. They also need to be aware of the increased potential for depression in people who live with chronic illness and/or disability. Referral to other providers may be necessary for the individual and other family members. Being mindful of possible barriers to inclusion, challenging these and seeking new or different ways of doing things are actions nurses can take within their work situations or within the broader community. The nurse elected to the community action group committee (Case Study 6.1, part 5) demonstrated such action in suggesting short- and long-term solutions to overcome the barriers excluding Muriel from participation on the committee, concomitantly reducing the risk of social isolation.

CONCLUSION

Nurses who work with people living with chronic illness and/or disability can act to maintain the status quo of marginalisation and discrimination (do nothing) or challenge it (do something). Nurses who use the social model of disability and incorporate self-reflexive practice in their approach to care can challenge their own positions of privilege and take actions that uncover the often hidden processes of stigmatisation of their clients. They need to continually challenge stigmatising processes within the clinical setting, their communities, in the media and within their own social milieu. Actions can be at a:

- personal level: being alert to stigmatising processes such as stereotyping, labelling and othering
- professional level: working with people in context; recognising and valuing their expertise and resourcefulness; supporting their rights to self-determination and remaining mindful of the risks of social isolation
- socio-political level: making visible and challenging stigmatising practices that marginalise and discriminate against people with chronic illnesses and/or disabilities.

> You say the little efforts that I make will do no good: they never will prevail to tip the hovering scale where justice hangs in balance. I don't think I ever thought they would. But I am prejudiced beyond debate in favour of my right to choose which side shall feel the stubborn ounces of my weight. (Overstreet, *Hands laid upon the wind* (1955, p. 15), cited in Johnson, 2006, p. 136)

Reflective questions

1. How can self-reflexive questioning assist you in reviewing your positions of power and privilege in relation to people living with chronic illness and/or disability?
2. How can you become more aware of actions that unintentionally marginalise and discriminate against people in your work and social contexts?
3. How can you challenge everyday situations in nursing practice where people who live with chronic illness and/or disability are marginalised and discriminated against?

Recommended reading

Giddings, L. S. (2005). Health disparities, social injustice, and the culture of nursing. *Nursing Research*, *54*(5), 304–312.

Giddings, L. S. (2005). A theoretical model of social consciousness. *Advances in Nursing Science*, *28*(3), 224–239.

Giddings, L. S., Roy, D. E., & Predeger, E. (2007). Women's experience of ageing with a chronic condition. *Journal of Advanced Nursing*, *58*(6), 557–565. doi: 10.1111/j.1365-2648.2007.04243.x

Oliver, M. (2009). *Understanding disability: From theory to practice* (2nd ed.). Basingstoke, UK: Palgrave Macmillan.

Roy, D. E., & Giddings, L. S. (2012). The experiences of women (65–74 years) living with a long-term condition in the shadow of ageing. *Journal of Advanced Nursing*, *68*(1), 181–190. doi: 10.1111/j.1365-2648.2011.05830.x

References

Alpass, F. M., Neville, S. (2003). Loneliness, health and depression in older males. *Aging & Mental Health*, *7*(3), 212–216.

Australian Statutes. (1992). *Disability Discrimination Act*. Australia: Australia Statutes.

Bodenheimer, T., Wagner, E. H., & Grumbach, K. (2002). Improving primary care for patients with chronic illness. *The Journal of the American Medical Association*, *288*(14), 1775–1779.

Carroll, S. M. (2004). Inclusion of people with physical disabilities in nursing education. *Journal of Nursing Education*, *43*(5), 207–212.

Dowling, M. (2006). Translating theory into practice? The implications for practitioners and users and carers. *Practice*, *18*(1), 17–30. doi: 10.1080/09503150600576751

Giddings, L. S. (1997). *In/visibility in nursing: stories from the margins*. Denver, USA: Doctoral thesis, University of Colorado.

Giddings, L. S. (2005a). Health disparities, social injustice, and the culture of nursing. *Nursing Research*, *54*(5), 304–312.

Giddings, L. S. (2005b). A theoretical model of social consciousness. *Advances in Nursing Science*, *28*(3), 224–239.

Giddings, L. S., Roy, D. E., & Predeger, E. (2007). Women's experience of ageing with a chronic condition. *Journal of Advanced Nursing*, *58*(6), 557–565. doi: 10.1111/j.1365-2648.2007.04243.x

Human Rights Commission. (2012). Parents as Caregivers' case: Background information. Retrieved April 14, 2013 from http://www.hrc.co.nz/2012/parents-as-caregivers-case-background-information

Johnson, A. G. (2006). *Privilege, power, and difference* (2nd ed.). New York: McGraw-Hill.

Keller-Olaman, S., Williams, S., Knight, R., et al. (2004). The self-rated health of women in midlife: A cross-sectional and longitudinal study of a New Zealand sample. *New Zealand Journal of Psychology, 33*(2), 68–77.

Koch, T., Jenkin, P., & Kralik, D. (2004). Chronic illness self-management: locating the 'self'. *Journal of Advanced Nursing, 48*(5), 484–492.

Kralik, D. (2010). Future directions. In D. Kralik, B. Paterson, & V. Coates (Eds.), *Translating chronic illness research into practice* (pp. 199–204). Oxford, UK: Wiley-Blackwell.

Lindsay, K., Gow, P., Vanderpyl, J., et al. (2011). The experience and impact of living with gout: a study of men with chronic gout using a qualitative grounded theory approach. *Journal of Clinical Rheumatology: Practical Reports on Rheumatic and Musculoskeletal Diseases, 17*(1), 1–6. doi: 10.1097/RHU.0b013e318204a8f9

Maeve, M. K. (1998). A critical analysis of physcian research into nursing practice. *Nursing Outlook, 46*(1), 24–28.

Ministry of Health. (2001). *The New Zealand Disability Strategy: Making a World of Difference whakanui oranga*. Author. Retrieved May 4, 2013, from http://www.odi.govt.nz/nzds/

Mitra, S. (2006). The capability approach and disability. *Journal of Disability Policy Studies, 16*(4), 236–247.

New Zealand Statutes. (1993). *Human Rights Act*. New Zealand: New Zealand Statutes.

Nursing Council of New Zealand. (2011). Guidelines for cultural safety, the Treaty of Waitangi and Maori health in nursing education and practice (rev. ed.). Retrieved May 4, 2013, from http://www.nursingcouncil.org.nz/download/97/cultural-safety11.pdf

O'Brien, R., Wyke, S., Guthrie, B., et al. (2011). An 'endless struggle': a qualitative study of general practitioners' and practice nurses' experiences of managing multimorbidity in socio-economically deprived areas of Scotland. *Chronic Illness, 7*(1), 45–59. doi: 10.1177/1742395310382461

Oliver, M. (1990). *The politics of Disablement: A sociological approach*. New York: St. Martin's Press.

Oliver, M. (1996). *Understanding Disability: From theory to practice*. New York: St. Martin's Press.

Oliver, M. (2009). *Understanding Disability: From theory to practice* (2nd ed.). Basingstoke, UK: Palgrave Macmillan.

Papps, E. (2005). Cultural safety: Daring to be different. In D. Wepa (Ed.), *Cultural safety in Aotearoa New Zealand* (pp. 20–27). Auckland, NZ: Pearson Education New Zealand.

Pincus, T. (2000). Challenges to the biomedical model: are actions of patients almost always as important as actions of health professionals in long-term outcomes of chronic diseases? *Advances in Mind-Body Medicine, 16*(4), 287–294.

Porter, S. (1996). Men researching women working. *Nursing Outlook, 44*(1), 22–26.

Rokach, A. (2012). Loneliness updated: an introduction. *The Journal of Psychology, 146*(1–2), 1–6. doi: 10.1080/00223980.2012.629501

Rokach, A., Lechcier-Kimel, R., & Safarov, A. (2006). Loneliness of people with physical disabilities. *Social Behavior & Personality: An International Journal, 34*(6), 681–699.

Roy, D. E. (2001). *The Everyday Always-thereness of Living with Rheumatoid Arthritis*. PhD Doctoral thesis, Auckland, New Zealand: Massey University.

Roy, D. E., & Giddings, L. S. (2012). The experiences of women. (65–74 years). living with a long-term condition in the shadow of ageing. *Journal of Advanced Nursing, 68*(1), 181–190. doi: 10.1111/j.1365-2648.2011.05830.x

Roy, D. E., Mahony, F. M., Horsburgh, M. P., et al. (2011). Partnering in primary care in New Zealand: clients' and nurses' experience of the Flinders Program™ in the management of long-term conditions. *Journal of Nursing and Healthcare of Chronic Illness, 3*(2), 140–149. doi: 10.1111/j.1752-9824.2011.01088.x

Schur, L. (2002). The difference a job makes: The effects of employment among people with disabilities. *Journal of Economic Issues, 36*(2), 339.

Scullion, P. A. (2010). Models of disability: their influence in nursing and potential role in challenging discrimination. *Journal of Advanced Nursing, 66*(3), 697–707. doi: 10.1111/j.1365-2648.2009.05211.x

Shakespeare, T. (2008). Debating disability. *Journal of Medical Ethics, 34*(1), 11–14. doi: 10.1136/jme.2006.019992

Shakespeare, T., & Watson, N. (1997). Defending the social model. *Disability & Society, 12*(2), 293–300.

Sin, C. H., & Fong, J. (2008). 'Do no harm'? Professional regulation of disabled nursing students and nurses in Great Britain. *Journal of Advanced Nursing, 62*(6), 642–652. doi: 10.1111/j.1365-2648.2008.04633.x

Smith, L. T. (1999). *Decolonizing Methodologies: Research and indigenous peoples.* London/Dunedin: Zed Books/University of Otago Press.

Statistics New Zealand. (2008). *Disability and the Labour Market in New Zealand in 2006.* Wellington, New Zealand: Author. Retrieved May 4, 2013, from http://www.stats.govt.nz/browse_for_stats/health/disabilities/disability-and-the-labour-market-in-nz-2006.aspx

Terzi, L. (2004). The social model of disability: A philosophical critique. *Journal of Applied Philosophy, 21*(2), 141–157.

Thomas, C. (2001). Medicine, gender, and disability: disabled women's health care encounters. *Health Care for Women International, 22*(3), 245–262.

Toombs, S. K. (2004). 'Is she experiencing any pain?': disability and the physician-patient relationship. *Internal Medicine Journal, 34*, 645–647.

Tregaskis, C. (2002). Social model theory: the story so far … *Disability & Society, 17*(4), 457–470.

United Nations. (2006). Convention on the Rights of Persons with Disabilities. Retrieved May 4, 2013, from http://www.un.org/disabilities/convention/conventionfull.shtml

Varnham, S. (2004). Current developments in Australia. *Education & the Law, 16*(1), 47–59.

Wallis, L. (2004). Positive support. *Nursing Standard, 18*(29), 22.

Wallis, L. (2006). Rights for equals. *Nursing Standard, 20*(39), 78–79.

Webb, R., & Tossell, D. (1999). *Social issues for carers: Towards positive practice* (2nd ed.). London: Arnold.

Weiss, B. (2005). Disabilities don't stop these nurses. *RN, 68*(1), 45–48.

Williams, A., Dunning, T., & Manias, E. (2007). Continuity of care and general wellbeing of patients with comorbidities requiring joint replacement. *Journal of Advanced Nursing, 57*(3), 244–256.

CHAPTER 7

Tinashe Dune

Sexuality in chronic illness and disability

Learning objectives

When you have completed this chapter you will be able to:

- comprehend the multifactorial issues of the topic
- relate to the way people may experience changes to their sexuality due to chronic illness and/or disability
- explore the resources available
- articulate clinical scenarios where intervention is necessitated
- comprehend alterations to quality of life for this group of people.

Key words

chronic illness, disability, sexuality, sexual health, sexual wellbeing

INTRODUCTION

The purpose of this chapter is to explore how adults may experience changes to their sexuality when living with chronic illness and/or disability. The topic is vast because sex and sexuality are complex areas of human experience across the lifespan. Issues of sexuality for children or adolescents with chronic illness and/or disability are not explored in this chapter. To structure our exploration of the topic, we draw on research data to understand the biological, psychological and social impact on sex and sexuality when people are living with chronic illness and/or disability. We also discuss promotion of sexual health and wellbeing as well as identify the implications for nursing practice.

Sexual expression is a part of life, and of course sex is important because it means that the human species can propagate! Satisfaction with sexual relationships is important to quality of life (Robinson & Molzahn, 2007). Even though sex and sexual expression is a fundamental part of life, it may be a taboo topic for conversation by many people. This may be even more so for adults with chronic conditions and/or disability, because sex is often associated with beauty and physical fitness; therefore people with a visible disability or illness may be perceived by others to be non-sexual (Dune & Shuttleworth, 2009). People with disability or illness, however, are sexual beings and often have to overcome uninformed judgments and attitudes in addition to personal and physiological barriers to sex and sexuality (Dune, 2012a). For example, disability and illness may result in many physical and psychological changes to movement, bodily sensations, abilities to communicate, continence, behaviour, relationships and sexual functioning. These changes may affect sexuality, body image and the feelings that people have about themselves (Kralik & Telford, 2006). In addition, symptoms such as pain and fatigue, and prescribed treatments and medicines, may also affect sexual desire and sexual function (Dune, 2012b). For people with chronic illness and/or disability, sex can be a source of comfort, intimacy and pleasure when illness has changed so many aspects of life (McInnes, 2003). People with chronic illness and disability can experience problems with arousal, lubrication, fear, position, exacerbating pain, low confidence, performance worries and relationship problems (Kaufman, 2010) and also difficulties when initiating new relationships. Although the physical demands of sexual activity can be high, few chronic illnesses require restriction of sexual activity (Nusbaum, Hamilton, & Lenahan, 2003) but rather may require rethinking, trialling and adapting to changed approaches (Kaufman, 2010; Kralik & Telford, 2006). The range of problems and people's preferences for help suggest that multidisciplinary intervention is required (Dune, 2012c).

Effective nursing care has as its foundation the health worker understanding the whole body, yet the topic of sexual health for people with illness and/or disability may be a neglected element within the scope of holistic nursing care (Haboubi & Lincoln, 2003; Ho & Fernandez, 2012). Certainly training in sexual health is limited (Nusbaum et al., 2003). Sexuality and sexual functioning is a nursing concern because it is an important aspect of a person's sense of wellbeing and quality of life. While health workers may not be able to affect the progression or physiological impact of chronic illness, they may be able to make a difference to people by affirming and validating the issues people experience and providing supportive advice and navigation towards resources (Dune, 2012c; Kong, Wu & Loke, 2009). Health workers may need to work with people to access information or participate in conversation about sexuality with people who are learning to live with an altered body as a consequence of illness or disability. It is important, however, that health workers who may need to counsel people on this topic are comfortable with talking about sex and sexuality (Dunning, 2005; Julien, Tom & Kline, 2010).

BACKGROUND

The dialogue reported in this chapter has come from a research program that has been conducted over the past decade and compiled from multiple inquiries with people learning to live with chronic illness and/or disability. Much of the dialogue has been extracted from a study that aimed to understand how people learn to incorporate chronic illness and/or disability into their lives. Daily email conversations between the first author and 35 women and 17 men who live with long-term illness took place during a 2-year period (2003–05) using a facilitated, private electronic mail (email) discussion list.

The decision to use email came from our knowledge about some of the consequences of illness that people living with chronic conditions confront in their lives. Challenges such as fatigue, pain, decreased socialisation and decreased mobility may limit attendance at groups or participation in one-to-one interviews. The use of email enabled the collaborative process of data generation and data analysis to occur concurrently and frequently, and enabled longitudinal research with people living with chronic illness to describe the processes involved with 'moving on' or transition. This inquiry has reinforced electronic discussions as one research method for gaining understandings longitudinally (Kralik et al., 2005; Kralik, Price, Warren, & Koch, 2006).

Transition encompasses people's responses during a passage of change. Life and living involve transitional processes (Kralik, Visentin, & Van Loon, 2006). A transitions approach to disruptive life events such as chronic illness creates a focus on what is changing, how we experience those changes and how we can respond. It is not a focus on the illness or disease. Times of transition can be very difficult periods in people's lives. People experience transition when one chapter of their life is over and another begins. They look for ways to move through the turmoil to create some order in their lives by reorienting themselves to new situations (Berger, 2008). Transition may also provide people with the opportunity to review their life, get rid of some old baggage and find new ways of living. Transition can involve testing new ways through trial and error living, doing and being (Kralik, Visentin, & Van Loon, 2006).

During frequent email conversations, participants communicated about events and experiences in their everyday lives. The impact of illness on sexuality was a topic of conversation as participants explored ways to live with an altered sense of sexuality. Stories told often persuaded people to revisit their own stories as new understandings emerged through listening and reflecting on the lives of others in the group. It was evident that chronic illness and/or disability can have profound impact on the individual and partner and the effects can be multifactorial (Esmail, Huang, Lee, & Maruska, 2010).

DEFINING THE TERMS

There have been many definitions of the terms 'sex', 'sexuality', 'sexual health' and 'sexual wellbeing'. Some writers suggest there have been no adequate definitions that can be broadly utilised in healthcare (Batcup & Thomas, 1994; Harrison, 1999). Sex has been defined as 'sexual activity such as sexual intercourse' (Roe & May, 1999) and sexuality as 'an individual's self-concept which is shaped by their personality and societal upbringing' (Evans, 2000). The term sexuality is a broad concept which has many meanings. For example, according to the American Psychological Association (2012) sexuality is a process with three stages: (1) desire (an interest in being sexual); (2) excitement (the state of arousal that sexual stimulation causes); and (3) orgasm (sexual pleasure's peak). Taken on its own, this definition limits sexuality to a model of function and possible dysfunction (similar to the medical model used in Western healthcare systems) which overlooks the psychological, social, cultural and dynamic nature of human sexuality and sexual wellbeing (American Psychological Association, 2012). In order to acknowledge the complex and expansive nature of human sexuality, some scholars and educators describe sexuality as an array of human experiences that includes family relationships, dating, physical development, sexual behaviour, sexualisation, sensuality, reproduction, gender and body image (Planned Parenthood of the Southern Finger Lakes, 2012).

Furthermore, some sexuality educators use a model called the circles of sexuality. This model includes five interconnected circles which represent five broad areas of sexuality: sensuality, intimacy, sexual identity, sexual health and reproduction and sexualisation. In this model, sexuality is represented as much more than sexual arousal, intercourse and orgasm. This way of thinking about sexuality highlights the importance of all the feelings, thoughts and behaviours associated with being a certain gender, being attracted to someone or being in a loving or intimate relationship (deFur, 2012). According to this model, sexuality — and its many elements — is a fundamental and natural part of being human for people of all ages. So, while defining sexuality can be difficult, it is nevertheless present throughout the lifespan. Notably, Schalet (2004) asserts that sexuality is 'the expression of an age-blind desire for meaningful intimacy and connection with others'.

As mentioned, a key aspect of sexuality is sexual health. Although the term sexual health is also expansive and complicated, definitions are generally in agreement with one another. For the purposes of this chapter, sexual health — as defined by the World Health Organization (2012) — is:

> a state of physical, mental and social well-being in relation to sexuality. It requires a positive and respectful approach to sexuality and sexual relationships, as well as the possibility of having pleasurable and safe sexual experiences, free of coercion, discrimination and violence.

In order to maintain sexual health, healthcare providers and institutions must play an important role. However, if older people are not acknowledged as sexual or having sexuality, programs designed to address the sexual health needs of older people will not be successful — to the detriment of their overall sexual wellbeing (Minichiello & Hawkes, 2011).

Given that sex, sexuality and sexual health are complementary concepts, how does sexual wellbeing factor in and what does it mean? Similar to the term 'sexual health', sexual wellbeing is the healthy and satisfactory experience of one's sexuality (Dune, 2011). The meanings of the terms 'sex' and 'sexuality' are closely linked and by citing these definitions we do not suggest that it is the same for all people. On the contrary, sex and sexuality experiences, meanings, wellbeing and understandings change throughout the lifespan and as a result of different experiences.

Sexual activity continues across the lifespan yet older people may be perceived as being incapable of a sexual relationship and therefore not requiring support, advice or education in this area (Shuttleworth, Russell, Weerakoon & Dune, 2010; Wallace, 2005). Sexual health needs are often a delicate balance of emotional and physical issues, and those seeking advice may be worried and concerned about misconceptions. For instance, upbringing, belief imprinted in the formative years and societal values are deterrents to older people requesting advice, as it is not necessarily the 'done thing', and that this negative stereotype is supported in the media, where ageing and sexuality are not positively portrayed (Farell & Belza, 2012; Nelson, 2005).

Sexual development and sexual identity evolve throughout the lifespan. However, many factors shape the sexual attitudes and needs of individuals, which may alter at times throughout the lifespan in response to given circumstances (Coleman, 2012; Gott & Hinchliff, 2003). For example, people who have a past history of sexual abuse or assault may interpret sexuality differently (Van Loon & Kralik, 2006). When chronic illness becomes a part of people's lives, surgical intervention and medical treatments may result in their appearance being altered and symptoms such as pain, stiffness, fatigue and depression may change the way they feel about their sexual selves (Dune, 2012b). We asked people living with chronic illness and disability what sexuality meant to them.

Garry was living with chronic fatigue and in his response he linked sexuality to gender. He thought sexuality was how 'you feel about yourself as a man and confidence in how others perceive you as a desirable person'. He later added that 'sexuality is the physical and emotional attributes that are considered gender-specific'.

Donna shared how sexuality includes 'affection, willingness to tune in to a partner's emotions, for example, if there is a need to talk about something or not talk about something, touch, hugs, loyalty and love'. She perceived sexuality to be linked to 'sensuality of movement, hand gestures, a lovely smile, a flick of the hair, sunlight striking shining hair, sudden bursts of unexpected humour'.

Olivia was learning to live with a neurological condition that had impacted significantly on her life. In her response she identified that sexuality was linked with her sense of self:

> It's part of my whole being that I feel very much connected to. My sexuality is me. How I dress, how I relate, alone and/or with others, it's connected to my interests, my politics, my work. The connection varies in intensity and positivity. It's connected to how I feel about myself physically, intellectually and emotionally. It's influenced by the current context and the external dynamic. It's a moving feast.

THE IMPACT OF CHRONIC ILLNESS AND/OR DISABILITY ON SEXUALITY AND SEXUAL HEALTH

The effects of chronic illness and/or disability on sexuality and sexual health can be classified as biological, psychological and social (Parish, 2002; McInnes, 2003; Yee & Sundquist, 2003). Biological or physical factors that affect sexuality and sexual health are those that are associated with the illness, disability or treatments. Examples may be reduced cardiovascular or pulmonary function, fatigue and pain. Surgical procedures and treatments may result in altered function and/or appearance. Psychological factors relate to changed relationships, depression, anxiety and grief associated with loss and change associated with chronic illness and/or disability. Social factors relate to challenges such as stigma and how others perceive people with illness and disability (Esmail, Darry, Walter, & Knupp, 2010). While these factors will be discussed separately, they are entwined in the realities of everyday life for people with chronic illness. We will now discuss these factors in more detail.

Biological impact

Sexual dysfunction is caused by different conditions, with even more differences between men and women. The desire and capacity to engage in sexual activity can be affected by illness and disability in multiple ways through neurological, vascular and endocrine systems (Berman & Bassuk, 2002; Nusbaum et al. 2003) and as a consequence symptoms such as pain and fatigue may be prioritised in people's lives (Kralik, Koch, & Eastwood, 2003). In addition, the effects of medications and treatments (McInnes, 2003) and surgical intervention can also affect an individual's capacity and desire to engage in sexual activity (Emilee, Ussher, & Perz, 2010).

There is a lot of importance placed on a sexually functioning body and the popular ideal is for people to be thin, fit and healthy (Dune & Shuttleworth, 2009). The reality, however, is that people have an assortment of body shapes, and illness and/or disability can further reshape the human body, which can affect a person's sexuality significantly, as Bronwyn explains:

> I'm afraid I do not feel like a sexual being at all anymore. Anything to avoid it. I feel so guilty about this, particularly as my husband is so understanding and never pressures me. But I feel I am being unfair, not fulfilling his needs. Most of the time I just hate this body so much and feel like I'd be contaminating him to do it. It is so rare that not even a spark of interest in sexual activity enters my brain, which is, after all, the most important sex organ.

The biological or physical impact of illness and disability can cause significant change in a person's life, as Karen revealed:

> The thing I was most bitter and angry about and the thing that made my grieving so painful was the loss of my physical abilities, lifestyle and quality of life. Like the ability to walk without pain and with a 'normal' gait, to run, skip, hop, jump, do aerobics, play squash, be spontaneous. The ability to control my bladder … to feel with my feet and achieve orgasm.

When illness or treatments made visible changes it was evident that those changes dominated the illness experience. People perceive that a beautiful, sexual body is a body without illness. Raelene explained:

> I don't like the visible changes [rheumatoid arthritis] has caused … muscle wastage, oversized knuckles, distorted fingers, turned-in knee and not to mention the scars from joint replacements. Rarely will I look at myself in a full-length mirror (I don't like what I see) because every time I do I notice another change in my body. As you can see, my feelings towards my body have changed dramatically. It's not me the person I dislike, it's the body. I think I feel this way because I feel powerless to stop the changes. Prior to the visible changes, I was more accepting of my body, despite the pain, as I couldn't see the destruction that was happening within.

Karen described how her changed body altered the meaning of sexual activity because illness forced changes to both sexual activity and her response to intimacy:

> Constant pain, spasticity, areas of numbness and hypersensitivity now mean touch that was once pleasurable is now unpleasant or not felt and positions that I once enjoyed are now painful. Much of the dialogue around sex that used to be erotic and sensual is now focused around ensuring I am as comfortable as possible and negotiating the difficulties imposed by a body that does not function properly.

As with other life activities, the person who is learning to live with chronic illness and/or disability may have to make adaptations in their life. For example, sexual activity may be less spontaneous and require planning in order to prepare for issues such as fatigue, pain, breathlessness and bowel and bladder evacuation, as the nerves servicing the reproductive organs can be impaired, leading to changes in sexual functioning. Slowed arousal time, reduced libido or desire and altered orgasmic response are not uncommon experiences. Fatigue also dampens sexual desire (Webber et al., 2011). Men with illness or disability may experience erectile dysfunction (a common problem that can have serious physical and psychological effects — also known as impotence) or difficulty due to physiological factors or medication that may respond to further investigations. Some people with illness and disability may need to learn to incorporate prosthesis or another permanent intervention such as an indwelling urinary catheter into their lives and sexual activity. Adaptations to be made may include trying different positions during sex activity, expanding their sexual repertoire or a partner playing a more active role. Masturbation may enable experimentation with changing bodily sensations. It can be important for people with an illness or disability that impairs the neurological system to identify areas of the body that allow sensation and to use those areas to augment sexual expression (Nusbaum et al., 2003). Other forms of sexual expression may also be used. This may call for experimentation and alternative methods of pleasuring. Assistive devices may be useful for some people (Kaufman, 2010) — these can be purchased discreetly by mail order.

Psychological impact

Media images portray traditional images of stereotypical male and female roles and what may define the gender role. For example, males are often portrayed as active, physically tough and in positions of status and power while females are often portrayed as attractive, fashion-conscious and fulfilling domestic or caring roles. Sexuality is often associated with being young, good-looking and socially in demand. Men and women experience these messages as pressure to be and act in accordance with these images, even though most people do not fit these impossible standards. These images do not reflect the reality of what it is to be a man or a woman. They reflect a very narrow understanding and, in doing so, neglect the diversity of sexuality. Yet alongside these images, people may feel inadequate and different (Dune & Shuttleworth, 2009). As a woman in a lesbian relationship, Donna described her resistance to conform to popular images:

> I ignore the pressure to act and be a certain way. I find many of the advertising images boring but admire the physical beauty of some people, for example David Beckham, the face of Catherine Zeta-Jones or the attraction of Bruce Willis. Advertising images are always extremely heterosexual, although some androgynous looking models do appear in ads and movies and homosexuality is camped up, so that it is rare for the general public to see images of normal people who happen to be homosexual. I like my own style. I enjoy doing what I want to do, for example not always having to wear make-up when going out. The lifespan has become shorter and wasting life on trying to be something the media or other people want is a waste of my precious time.

Chloe drew comparisons with her life, abilities and body image before illness to illustrate the impact of chronic disease:

> Once I was able to do it all, raise my kids, work full-time and run the house. Illness gradually took away my ability to do so and now I'm no longer able to work at all. I'm grateful my children were in their teens before I became really ill, but find illness impacts on my ability to do the things I feel I should be able to manage with my grandchildren. I used to dance and moved gracefully. Now I often move like a ruptured duck … when either the elbow crutch or walking stick is needed. Hardly the best way to look one's feminine best.

Chronic illness and disability changes the dynamics of relationships (Esmail, Darry, Walter, & Knupp, 2010; Kralik et al., 2001). Karen reflected on the difficulty of coming to terms with the changes within her relationship:

> For years I struggled to keep doing all the things I had done prior to illness because I feared my partner's realisation that I was becoming less of a partner in the relationship. Accepting my need to increasingly depend on my partner for some things has been one of the hardest things I've had to come to terms with, and for him too I think. Although he is very supportive he has had to change his perception of me as a partner as well. I am not able to contribute to this relationship in the way that I used to but I still want to be seen as an equal partner. Managing to maintain my personal power in a relationship alongside increasing disability is a very fine line to tread and one I am constantly grappling with.

Changes to sexuality for some people because of illness and disability may mean managing their partner's sexual needs at a time when illness is causing turmoil in their lives (Dune, 2012b). Jan was dependent on her partner and a formal carer to assist with activities of daily living. When she reflected about the ways a neurological illness had reshaped her sexuality she spoke of how important it was for her to be together with her partner. She longed for him to embrace her. Sex had been an important and enjoyable part of her life before illness and disability. Her dependency made her feel vulnerable, and she revealed how she was now a passive sexual partner and she would 'lie back whilst he gets on with it' with little pleasure experienced. Jan excused her partner's sexual self-interest because she felt that it was one way she was able to contribute to their relationship and provided an opportunity for physical closeness.

Pre-existing relationship issues may be exacerbated by the challenges of illness. For some people their lover may become their carer. Some people may prioritise aspects of illness or disability or for other reasons may not feel like being sexually active and may avoid being sexual with their partner. Other research participants perceived it was the changes in their sexual desires that negatively affected relationships. Loss of sexual desires and the inability to meet their partner's sexual needs created friction within the relationship and was a barrier to effective communication about changing sexual needs and desires. Participants talked about feelings of guilt about elements of illness that were beyond their control such as changes to their appearance or a change to physical sensation. Hanna revealed, '... unhealthy as it is, I have built up an amazing retinue of avoidance strategies. I do not like myself for this'.

Within many relationships there may not be a common dialogue around sexuality. This reflects on the broader societal attitudes to sexuality, which foster discomfort in talking about the topic. This can be very difficult if dialogue between partners around sex and sexuality has not previously existed.

> Having [this illness] has certainly had an impact on my sexuality and in the early days affected my relationship with my partner. I was depressed and I could not stand anyone touching me, let alone feel like being intimate. My partner took this to be that I was pushing him away. The antidepressants I take have had the side effect of causing me to be unable to climax ... [Our relationship] has never got back to how it used to be.

Communication is an important component in all relationships (Di Guilio, 2003; Dune, 2012a; Esmail, Munro, & Gibson, 2007). When a disability or illness exists, it becomes important that partners and individuals are given the opportunity to discuss thoughts, feelings, needs, wants and how they can mutually satisfy each other. How do people begin to talk about sex and sexuality if they have not done so before? Health workers may assist by initiating discussion in a matter-of-fact but sensitive way, and letting people know that sexuality is considered to be an important aspect of their health. Garry reflected:

> I try to let my partner know what is needed and listen to my partner's needs. It becomes even more important that I am fully aware of how my illness is affecting my partner. This can be difficult as I am not always fully aware of any problems, so when I am able I try to be as attentive as possible.

Social impact

Sometimes our ideals and values about sexuality and disabilities have to do with unwritten rules (Simon & Gagnon, 1986, 1987, 2003). In our society, we judge harshly those who break rules about sexuality and sexual behaviour. Unfortunately, most of the rules are not formally taught, are learned incidentally and vary according to the age, situation and culture. The person with illness or disability may need to incorporate many changes into their lives (Kralik et al., 2001). Some of those changes may include traditional gender roles that were previously valued and are a defining factor for a person's identity (Simon & Gagnon, 1986, 1987, 2003). Illness or disability may affect a person's ability to continue to perform those roles in a way that they value (Esmail et al., 2007). For example, it may no longer be possible to play sport, wear certain clothing or undertake paid work. A person may not be able to move as they once did. Pain or fatigue might affect their energy levels and limit their activities. These effects can lead people to feel that they are not leading a valued life. Chronic illness and disability can provide an opportunity for individuals to redefine what is important to them as Janice revealed:

> My looks had changed from the normal look before chronic pain took its toll to the woman I am today. I have had to relearn self-esteem, self-love, self-worth. If I didn't love myself how could I expect others to love me? Once I relearned this I smiled more, I had more confidence

> and I had regained my positive attitude. Easier to love this person than one who was always complaining of pain.

Gender (being male or female) is closely linked to roles and not being able to fulfil certain familiar roles can feel threatening. Reliance by a traditionally less dominant partner may be intimidating and frightening, causing tension, anxiety and distress. Garry considered how illness had affected his gendered roles.

> The symptoms of illness combined with side effects of medications can reduce your self-image of being a male. The normal range of man-type activities becomes reduced and I went through a long stage of feeling less of a man. I have gone through this phase until I learned to accept that the limitations placed upon me by my illness/medication are now a part of me and the realisation that if you cannot change something then you may as well learn to live with it. I still have occasions when I feel 'inferior' to other men but these have less impact on me.

The judgment of others can have a significant impact on how people perceive themselves and people with chronic illness and/or disability often need to develop ways to protect themselves from those judgments.

> I try to ignore others and what I imagine they are thinking. At one time I would try to keep up the activities of a normal male, like doing all the heavy work. It took me some time to learn that I must not be concerned if others perceive me as weak because I have limited abilities. This learning process was mostly enforced on me as I continued having bad physical after-effects from doing things.

Sometimes, in the face of negative reactions, people with chronic illness and/or disability learn ways to protect themselves. Evident in our responses is that we hold to certain principles in maintaining self-worth.

> I have almost given up telling people of my health problems. Even those who know me best, outside my immediate family, have no concept of this type of illness. I have gotten tired of the blank looks and unbelieving looks.

People with illness and/or disability may become socially withdrawn if they think they are judged by others. People who are gay or lesbian and living with disability and/or chronic illness may be reluctant to disclose and discuss issues regarding their sexuality. Research has reported that lesbian women and gay men were reluctant to seek care when they had health concerns because of past negative experiences with the health sector (Stover, 2011). It can also be difficult for people whose illness or disability is not visible or whose condition may be treated with suspicion or has social stigma attached such as people living with chronic pain or HIV.

IMPLICATIONS FOR HEALTH PRACTICE

If sex and sexuality is often a taboo subject for people, why should health workers raise this issue with people? (Haboubi & Lincoln, 2003; Minichiello & Hawkes, 2011) The assumption that people with chronic illness or disability are non-sexual can present a barrier to people gaining information and having open discussion about a major aspect of their life (Miller & Marini, 2007). Health workers have a significant role to play in addressing barriers to sexual fulfilment that are a result of disability, chronic illness and treatments. Nurses express their concern over their role in this field:

> You are so concerned about the other problems they are coming in with that you're not really concerned with sexuality.

The constant contact that health workers have with clients provides them with the opportunity to facilitate communications about sexuality and to ensure that sexuality is accorded the same priority as other health issues. In doing so, a foundation of acceptance and respect for the whole person is established, which provides people with permission to ask questions or seek assistance with sex and sexuality issues. However, Guthrie (1999) found that when interviewed on this topic nurses cited a lack of time and heavy workloads as principal reasons why they did not discuss sexual health issues with their clients. The report also shows that nurses use tactics such as routinising behaviours, distancing and avoidance to prevent initiation of discussion. Karen shared her experiences:

> Loss of bladder control undermines my sense of competence and freedom in the world. To feel safer about having sex without being incontinent I need to follow a routine before and after sex, which interrupts the flow of emotions involved in arousal and intimacy. I would love to be able to just go with my feelings at the time but I'm afraid to … the embarrassment of being incontinent during sex is too great a risk. I would hate the shame of it. I had the good fortune of meeting a continence nurse who approached the subject of sexuality with me in a safe and comfortable manner. Through exploration of the difficulties I was experiencing with sexual activity and the suggestion of helpful strategies … I managed to resume a level of sexual activity that I previously thought was lost forever. I have an endless well of gratitude within me for that continence nurse.

The acknowledgment of the sexual aspect of a person by a health worker and the willingness to assist in this area is extremely affirming for people who are coming to terms with the effects of disability and/or chronic illness. Examples of interventions are provided in Case Studies 7.1 and 7.2. Sexuality is a sensitive and value-laden area, and individuals range in both their attitudes and their comfort levels with regard to sexuality. It is important that health workers develop an awareness of their own values about sex and sexuality in order to facilitate open communications (Earle, 2001). Creating a comfortable environment and using lay sexual terms are effective ways of communicating about sexuality (Bitzer, Platano, Tschudin, & Alder, 2007; Dune, 2012c; Haboubi & Lincoln, 2003). Ashley described the relationship he would like to have with his health team:

> I have the right to be treated as a person with a medical condition, rather than a medical condition. While part of me is broken, I am still a valuable person, and should be treated as one. This is my medical condition and I know how it affects me more than anybody else — so while guidance and information does help, the final decisions on how to manage my condition must be mine. To maintain my sense of being 'in control', I must be in charge — but with the guidance and assistance of people (including my health team) around me.

We have revealed that the ways people respond to illness, disability and sexuality are diverse but central to their wellbeing. Despite this, only a minority of people receive help for sexual concerns. For example, a Danish study found that only 10% of men with diabetes attending a clinic had been provided the opportunity to discuss sexuality, even though the effects of diabetes on erectile function are widely known (Jensen, 1996). People who participated in the inquiries reported in this chapter would have benefited from health professionals who were prepared to confront and explore sexuality issues and their relationship to other aspects of their lives. This confirms the findings of other authors (Lindau et al., 2010; Rosen et al., 2004) which indicate that clients would welcome health workers initiating discussion about the impact of illness on sexuality.

Bitzer and colleagues (2007) suggests that health workers may assist clients to communicate about the way sexual feelings are affected by illness by developing confidence in their own ability to listen and respond. Conversations can commence with the promotion of sexual health. Health promotion may include talking about acting within one's own value system to prevent unplanned pregnancies, seeking early prenatal care, or avoiding contracting or transmitting sexually transmitted disease. Health-promoting behaviours such as self breast and testicular examination and regular check-ups are responsible ways to identify potential problems. With knowledge of resources and services in the sexuality health area people can be facilitated towards expanded opportunities for appropriate assistance and support. A health worker might say during a conversation with a client, 'Many people with your condition find they have some sexual concerns … is this area a concern for you?' The client may have been wanting the topic of sex and sexuality to be raised. Of course, the health worker should also be prepared if the person does not respond. It may be, however, that the door has been opened for conversation to occur at a later time.

Although ageing (even in healthy individuals) may contribute to changes in the sexual dynamics of a relationship, a number of treatment modalities are available, both psychological and medical. Doctors and other healthcare providers are expected to be able to manage the sexual health issues of their patients. Even those who are not trained experts in sexual health can provide help simply by minimally expanding what they are already trained to do: first, assess and evaluate; second, treat and/or refer. Simply initiating a discussion of sexual concerns is often the most valuable component of treatment for couples. By asking about sexuality the healthcare provider informs the patient that it is appropriate to discuss sexual problems in that setting and validates self-perception as a sexual being. It is hard to provide an effective intervention, regardless of the type of treatment, if there is no mention of a problem (Bitzer et al., 2007).

Despite our sexually enlightened culture, many people hold onto fairly restrictive and conservative views of what is 'appropriate' and 'normal' (Miller & Marini, 2007). Therefore, appropriate intervention may involve helping people to redefine 'normal' sexual activity. Change does not have to be extreme for couples to notice significant improvement in sexual fulfilment. It may be something as simple (but often not considered) as suggesting that couples engage in sexual activity in the morning when pain and fatigue is less rather than late in the evening when there is a greater likelihood of fatigue. Options can also include using different positions and using pillows as needed. It can be important to talk with people about establishing ways of communicating about sexual need and desire. This is important in light of progressive illness where some adjustment or change may be constant. Communication itself can be seductive, enticing and sexual. Effective communication in everyday life is also important for the quality of the overall relationship, which is also critical to couples' sexual lives.

CONCLUSION

This chapter has only 'touched' on the broad topic of sexuality. However, in every clinical contact it is important for people living with illness and/or disability to feel that their concerns and experiences are affirmed. Discussing issues of sex and sexuality can be difficult, so health workers should create time and space for discussion to take place with clients. Sexuality is such an integral part of people's lives and is essential for their sense of health and wellbeing. When illness forces changes to the way people live and experience their lives, they will most likely experience changes to their sexuality. Physical symptoms may also have impact upon the ways they engage in sexual activity, yet research has shown that people who live with chronic illness place considerable emphasis on staying connected to a sense of their sexuality. It is important that health workers do not assume that sexuality no longer matters or that people do not relate to it because of illness or disability and that they embrace opportunities for people to talk about sexuality. This not only acknowledges a person as a sexual being but also affirms them as a whole person.

CASE STUDY 7.1

Alex is a 22-year-old with severe spastic quadriplegic cerebral palsy, which was diagnosed when he was 2. Alex has always lived with a carer. First with his mother and stepfather, then in the fully accessible residential building at the university where he completed his undergraduate studies in law and was provided with living support from nurses within the university's attendant care program. After university, Alex's mother (who was his primary carer when he lived at home) passed away and he now lives in an aged care facility as it is the only place equipped to meet his health needs in his community. He requires daily assistance with all activities of daily living, including eating, bathing, getting dressed, getting out of bed and getting into bed. On Facebook he sees that his peers from university are dating, travelling and trialling employment options. Alex is the youngest resident in the aged care facility and has little opportunity for interaction with his peers or non-facility residents.

In discussion with the nursing staff he expresses that his poor sense of self and limited potential to participate in intimate relationships has diminished his sense of belonging and purpose and jokes that the world would be better off without him.

Discussions with Alex's stepfather, who pays for his stay at the aged care facility, uncover that he does love Alex and wants him to be around his peers and engage in intimate relationships but believes that it is up to Alex to make it happen. According to Alex's stepfather, living with a severe disability moves a player from the field and onto the bench.

Issues identified by the nurse in collaboration with Alex and his stepfather:

- tight muscles and joints
- difficulty communicating — speech impairment
- diminished sense of self
- diminished sense of purpose
- diminished sense of belonging
- lack of sexual and relationship intimacy.

Collaborative assessment between the nurse, Alex and his stepfather led to:

- a physical assessment which identified acute muscle and joint tightness resulting in scoliosis and discomfort
- medication review (GP/local pharmacist) to relieve limb spasticity and encourage mobility
- weekly physiotherapy session to relieve limb spasticity and encourage mobility
- review of the communication/interaction between healthcare providers and Alex and his stepfather
- allowing Alex access to the aged care facility accessible vehicle which can be scheduled ahead of time if Alex would like to attend events with his peers outside of the facility
- allowing Alex a more relaxed care provision schedule if he would like to participate in activities with peers or have a guest visit him at the aged care facility.

Alex was keen to be allowed these privileges but was warned that he too had to make an effort to connect with his peers online and in person in order to avoid feeling helpless and social withdrawal.

CASE STUDY 7.1 — cont'd

Collaborative plan of care:

- meet with aged care facility counsellor to discuss weekly events, feelings and accomplishments
- medication daily to relax the muscles
- referred to physiotherapy for pool exercises to increase mobility and flexibility
- occupational therapy referral to assess for adaptive device modifications or other equipment.

At the next appointment the plan of care was reviewed:

- Alex felt he had improved his social skills by talking with the counsellor weekly
- muscle tension reduced
- weekly pool exercises reduced pain and mobility and limb flexibility increased
- Alex used the accessible vehicle once a month to visit friends he had made while at university.

Alex was markedly less self-loathing and melancholic but admitted that others' perceptions of chronic illness and disability were a constant challenge in his efforts to relate to his peers socially and sexually. Alex did however feel more relaxed about communicating about his abilities and making social and sexual 'overtures' towards others. Alex's stepfather began to invite Alex to his monthly football club outings at the local ex-servicemen's club. Alex was happy to be invited and have the opportunity to connect with his stepfather and other club members. Doing so reduced the fear and stigma of disability in the group and those around them. The Cerebral Palsy Foundation provides support and social opportunities for Alex and his peers with and without disabilities to interact and learn from one another.

CASE STUDY 7.2

Sienna is a 30-year-old woman who was involved in a motor vehicle accident. The car in which she was a passenger was travelling at a speed of 160 km per hour at the time of the accident. Sienna was thrown from the car and suffered a partial spinal cord injury (L2–4). Partial sensation remained in thighs and groin but bladder and bowel control was lost.

At the time of her accident Sienna was engaged to Billy (not involved in the accident) who subsequently and spontaneously ended the relationship. A year after Sienna's most pressing health issues were under control she began seeing Frank. Frank is interested in having children and has asked Sienna if they could start trying to conceive. Sienna has not given him her answer as she is unsure about her ability to conceive, carry a child to term or parent as these aspects following her injury were never discussed.

Sienna was originally admitted for continence management. Urinary incontinence was a major concern, despite the fact that she performed clean self intermittent catheterisation (CSIC) twice daily. Initial visits were challenging because Sienna seemed preoccupied and reluctant to talk about her personal and/or sexual life.

CASE STUDY 7.2 — cont'd

Sienna eventually began to trust and build rapport with the nurse and began discussing some of her thoughts and feelings as she questioned her womanhood (including fertility and parenting). She was particularly concerned that being in a wheelchair meant that she was not the best partner for Frank and would not be a good parent to potential children. She was devastated because:

- her first partner had left her without explanation
- she is unsure of her womanhood
- she is worried that she will be a bad parent
- she does not want to disappoint Frank.

Sienna felt that she was not a 'real' woman if she could not be a mother or partner. She had always wanted children and her own family but perceived that it was now out of the question because since her accident her sexuality and potential to have a family was never discussed with family or healthcare providers. Sienna decided to find resources online but was left confused by positive as well as negative anecdotal experiences from parents with spinal cord injury. She longed to talk to someone knowledgeable before she decides what to tell Frank.

Collaborative plan of care developed with Simon:

- review oral fluid intake (mainly soft drink or coffee)
- implement routine bowel management — Movicol daily
- continue CSIC
- consent to a medication review
- weekly discussions with a sexual health nurse who has worked with parents with disability.

After one month Sienna said that she had become more comfortable with the idea of parenting with a disability. She decided that she want to try to conceive a child with Frank on the condition that he help her organise a group for parents with disabilities in their local community. A few months after the establishment of the group, which met once a month at the local community centre, Sienna discovered she was pregnant. Sienna shared the news with her parents and thought they would be excited. Instead, they were concerned and asked her how she was going to deal with a baby who was incontinent when she herself continued to have continence issues.

During the first trimester of her pregnancy Sienna and Frank continued running the parents with disabilities group to which they invited knowledgeable guest speakers who provided accurate information and advice about parenting, relationships, sexuality and health. Sienna also invited her parents to sit in at the meetings. Sienna felt more capable as a partner and parent when she was supported and acknowledged by those close to her and in her community as valuable and worthy.

Reflective questions

1. What is sexual health?
2. What are the prevalent barriers people with chronic illness and/or disability experience in regards to sexual health and wellbeing?
3. How can healthcare workers help to promote and facilitate sexual health and wellbeing for people with chronic illness and/or disability?

Acknowledgment: The author would like to thank Debbie Kralik and Norah Bostock for their contribution to this chapter.

Recommended reading

Kralik, D., & Telford, K. (2006). 'A stranger in my own body': body image and chronic illness. In F. Columus (Ed.), *Body image*. Hauppauge, NY: NOVA Science Publishers.

Miller, E., & Marini, I. (2007). Female sexuality and spinal cord injury. In A. Orto & P. Power (Eds.), *The psychological and social impact of illness and disability* (Chapter 11, pp. 176–193). New York: Springer Publishing.

Dune, T. M. (2012). Sexuality and physical disability: exploring the barriers and solutions in healthcare. *Sexuality and Disability*, *30*, 247–255.

Bitzer, J., Platano, G., Tschudin, S., et al. (2007). Sexual counseling for women in the context of physical diseases: A teaching model for physicians. *The Journal of Sexual Medicine*, *4*(1), 29–37.

Kaufman, M. (2010). *The Ultimate Guide to Sex and Disability: For All of us Who Live with Disabilities, Chronic Pain, and Illness*. Berkeley, CA: Cleis Press.

References

American Psychological Association (2012). *Sexuality*. Retrieved July 14, 2012, from www.apa.org/topics/sexuality/index.aspx.

Batcup, D., & Thomas, B. (1994). Mixing the genders: an ethical dilemma. How nursing theory has dealt with sexuality and gender. *Nursing Ethics*, *1*(1), 43–52.

Berger, R. J. (2008). Agency, structure, and the transition to disability: A case study with implications for life history research. *The Sociological Quarterly*, *49*(2), 309–333.

Berman, J., & Bassuk, J. (2002). Physiology and pathophysiology of female sexual function and dysfunction. *World Journal of Urology*, *20*(2), 111–118.

Bitzer, J., Platano, G., Tschudin, S., et al. (2007). Sexual counseling for women in the context of physical diseases: A teaching model for physicians. *The Journal of Sexual Medicine*, *4*(1), 29–37.

Coleman, E. (2012). Sexual Health Across the Lifespan. In *2012 National STD Prevention Conference*. CDC.

deFur, K. (2012). Getting to the good: Adopting a pleasure framework for sexuality education. *American Journal of Sexuality Education*, *7*(12), 146–159.

Di Giulio, G. (2003). Sexuality and people living with physical or developmental disabilities: a review of key issues. *Canadian Journal of Human Sexuality*, *12*(1), 53–68.

Dune, T. M. (2011). *Making sense of sex with people with cerebral palsy* (PhD Thesis). Sydney, Australia: The University of Sydney.

Dune, T. M. (2012a). Understanding experiences of sexuality with cerebral palsy through sexual script theory. *International Journal of Social Science Studies, 1*(1), 1–12.

Dune, T. M. (2012b). Sexual expression, fulfilment and haemophilia: reflections from the 16th Australian and New Zealand Haemophilia Conference. *Haemophilia, 18*(3), e138–e139.

Dune, T. M. (2012c). Sexuality and physical disability: Exploring the barriers and solutions in healthcare. *Sexuality and Disability, 30*, 247–255.

Dune, T. M., & Shuttleworth, R. P. (2009). 'It's just supposed to happen': The myth of sexual spontaneity and the sexually marginalized. *Sexuality and Disability, 27*(2), 97–108.

Dunning, T. (2005). *Nursing Care of Older People with Diabetes.* Oxford: Blackwell Publishing.

Earle, S. (2001). Disability, facilitated sex and the role of the nurse. *Integrative literature reviews and meta-analysis, 36*(3), 433–440.

Emilee, G., Ussher, J. M., & Perz, J. (2010). Sexuality after breast cancer: a review. *Maturitas, 66*(4), 397–407.

Esmail, S., Darry, K., Walter, A., et al. (2010). Attitudes and perceptions towards disability and sexuality. *Disability & Rehabilitation, 32*(14), 1148–1155.

Esmail, S., Huang, J., Lee, I., et al. (2010). Couple's experiences when men are diagnosed with multiple sclerosis in the context of their sexual relationship. *Sexuality and Disability, 28*(1), 15–27.

Esmail, S., Munro, B., & Gibson, N. (2007). Couple's experience with multiple sclerosis in the context of their sexual relationship. *Sexuality and Disability, 25*(4), 163–177.

Evans, D. (2000). Speaking of sex: the need to dispel myths and overcome fears. *British Journal of Nursing, 9*(10), 650–655.

Farrell, J., & Belza, B. (2012). Are older patients comfortable discussing sexual health with nurses? *Nursing Research, 61*(1), 51.

Gott, M., & Hinchliff, S. (2003). Barriers to seeking treatment for sexual problems in primary care: A qualitative study with older people. *Family Practice, 20*(6), 690–695.

Guthrie, C. (1999). Nurses' perceptions of sexuality relating to patient care. *Journal of Clinical Nursing, 8*(3), 313–321.

Haboubi, N., & Lincoln, N. (2003). Views of health professionals on discussing sexual issues with patients. *Disability and Rehabilitation, 25*(6), 291–296.

Harrison, T. (1999). The sexual male. In T. Harrison, K. Dignan (Eds.), *Men's Health* (Chapter 4, pp. 63–76). London: Elsevier.

Ho, T. M., & Fernández, M. (2012). Patient's sexual health: do we care enough? *Journal of Renal Care, 32*(4), 183–186.

Jensen, S. (1996). Sexual dysfunction and diabetes mellitus. A six year follow-up study. *Archives of Sexual Behaviour, 15*, 271–284.

Julien, J. O., Thom, B., & Kline, N. E. (2010). Identification of barriers to sexual health assessment in oncology nursing practice. In *Oncology Nursing Forum* (*Vol. 37*, No. 3, pp. 186–190). Oncology Nursing Society.

Kaufman, M. (2010). *The Ultimate Guide to Sex and Disability: For All of us Who Live with Disabilities, Chronic Pain, and Illness.* Berkeley, CA: Cleis Press.

Kong, S. K. F., Wu, L. H., & Loke, A. Y. (2009). Nursing students' knowledge, attitude and readiness to work for clients with sexual health concerns. *Journal of Clinical Nursing, 18*(16), 2372–2382.

Kralik, D., Koch, T., & Eastwood, S. (2003). The salience of the body: transition in sexual self-identity for women living with multiple sclerosis. *Journal of Advanced Nursing, 42*(1), 11–20.

Kralik, D., Koch, T., & Telford, K. (2001). Constructions of sexuality for midlife women living with chronic illness. *Journal of Advanced Nursing, 35*(2), 180–187.

Kralik, D., Price, K., Warren, J., et al. (2006). Issues of using email group conversations as data for nursing research. *Journal of Advanced Nursing, 53*(2), 213–220.

Kralik, D., & Telford, K. (2006). 'A stranger in my own body': body image and chronic illness. In F. Columus (Ed.), *Body Image*. Hauppauge, NY: NOVA Science Publichers.

Kralik, D., Visentin, K., & Van Loon, A. (2006). Transition: a literature review. *Journal of Advanced Nursing, 55*(3), 320–329.

Kralik, D., Warren, J., Price, K., et al. (2005). The ethics of research using electronic mail discussion groups. *Journal of Advanced Nursing, 52*(5), 537–545.

Lindau, S. T., Tang, H., Gomero, A., et al. (2010). Sexuality among middle-aged and older adults with diagnosed and undiagnosed diabetes. A national, population-based study. *Diabetes Care, 33*(10), 2202–2210.

McInnes, R. (2003). Chronic illness and sexuality. *Medical Journal of Australia, 179*(16), 263–266.

Miller, E., Marini, I. (2007). Female sexuality and spinal cord injury. In A. Orto, P. Power (Eds.), *The Psychological and Social Impact of Illness and Disability* (Chapter 11, pp. 176–193). New York: Springer Publishing.

Minichiello, V., & Hawkes, G. (2011). *A ripe old age: The joy of sex later in life (just don't forget the condoms). The Conversation*. Retrieved May 3, 2013, from http:/theconversation.edu.au/a-ripe-old-age-the-joy-of-sex-later-in-life-just-dont-forget-the-condoms-1969

Nelson, T. D. (2005). Ageism: Prejudice against our feared future self. *Journal of Social Issues, 61*(2). doi: 10.1111/j.1540-4560.2005.00402.x

Nusbaum, M., Hamilton, C., & Lenahan, P. (2003). Chronic illness and sexual functioning. *American Family Physician, 67*, 347–354, 357.

Parish, K. (2002). Sexuality and haemophilia: connections across the life-span. *Haemophilia, 8*, 353–359.

Planned Parenthood of the Southern Finger Lakes. (2012). *What is sexuality anyway?* Retrieved July 14, 2012, from www.plannedparenthood.org/ppsfl/what-sexuality-anyway-2480.htm

Robinson, J. G., & Molzahn, A. E. (2007). Sexuality and quality of life. *Journal of Gerontological Nursing, 33*(3), 19.

Roe, B., May, C. (1999). Incontinence and sexuality: findings from a qualitative perspective. *Journal of Advanced Nursing, 30*(3), 573–579.

Rosen, R. C., Fisher, W. A., Eardley, I., et al. (2004). The multinational Men's Attitudes to Life Events and Sexuality (MALES) study: I. Prevalence of erectile dysfunction and related health concerns in the general population. *Current Medical Research and Opinion, 20*(5), 607–617.

Schalet, A. (2004). Must we fear adolescent sexuality? *Medscape General Medicine, 6*(4). Retrieved May 3, 2013, from http://www.ncbi.nlm.nih.gov/pmc/articles/PMC1480590/

Shuttleworth, R., Russell, C., Weerakoon, P., et al. (2010). Sexuality in residential aged care: A survey of perceptions and policies in Australian nursing homes. *Sexuality and Disability, 28*(2), 187–194.

Simon, W., & Gagnon, J. H. (1986). Sexual scripts: Permanence and change. *Archives of Sexual Behavior, 15*(2), 97–120.

Simon, W., & Gagnon, J. H. (1987). A sexual scripts approach. In J. H. Geer & W. T. O'Donohue (Eds.), *Theories of Human Sexuality* (pp. 363–383). London: Plenum Press.

Simon, W., & Gagnon, J. H. (2003). Sexual scripts: Origins, influences and changes. *Qualitative Sociology, 26*(4), 491–497.

Stover, C. M. (2011). *Exploring Healthcare Experiences of Lesbian, Gay, and Bisexual College Students Using Community-Based Participatory Research: A Dissertation*. University of Massachusetts Medical School. Graduate School of Nursing Dissertations. Paper 21. Retrieved date: May 3, 2013, from http://escholarship.umassmed.edu/gsn_diss/21

Van Loon, A., & Kralik, D. (2006). A capacity building process for women with a history of child sexual abuse. *Australian Journal of Primary Health*, *12*(2), 167–176.

Wallace, M. (2005). Sexuality. *Urologic Nursing*, *25*(5), 373–375.

Webber, K., Mok, K., Bennett, B., et al. (2011). If I am in the mood, I enjoy it: an exploration of cancer-related fatigue and sexual functioning in women with breast cancer. *The Oncologist*, *16*(9), 1333–1344.

World Health Organization. (2012). *Sexual health*. Retrieved July 14, 2012, from www.who.int/topics/sexual_health/en/

Yee, L., & Sundquist, K. (2003). Older women's sexuality. *Medical Journal of Australia*, *178*(16), 640–642.

CHAPTER 8

Jennifer Evans
Susan Gallagher

Developmental and intellectual disability

Learning objectives

When you have completed this chapter you will be able to:

- explain the differences and similarities between developmental disabilities and intellectual disabilities
- Identify some of the challenges associated with nursing a person with a developmental or intellectual disability and their family
- examine the nurse's role in promoting independence for people with developmental and intellectual disabilities and their families
- explore quality-of-life issues for people with developmental and intellectual disabilities and their families
- describe and discuss the role of community and the principle of inclusion for people with developmental and intellectual disability.

Key words

intervention, developmental disability, family/carer, intellectual disability, quality of life

INTRODUCTION

Disability is a generic term used to describe any limitation that restricts everyday activity. Disability is a part of life and almost everyone will experience being impaired at some stage during their life either temporarily or permanently. Twenty per cent of people in Australia reported that they had a disability in the 2007 Australian Bureau of Statistics *Survey of disability, ageing and carers*, however, the number of people with disabilities is growing due to ageing populations. The World Health Organization (WHO, 2011) reports a global increase in chronic health conditions associated with disability. There is a wide range of causative factors involved and the disabilities are equally varied, ranging from mild to severe. Many individuals will require some degree of support and assistance throughout their lives. This need for long-term care can alter the expectations and dynamics of family life and be the catalyst for change and considerable stress.

This chapter presents some key issues for people with developmental and intellectual disability and their families, such as the effect that altered mobility and fatigue have on the activities of daily living and the way in which body image affects an individual's quality of life. The role of education for individuals and their families and carers is also highlighted. The principle of practice that is central to this chapter is the promotion of independence for these individuals and their families. It is imperative that each individual be as free as possible from the influence and control of others to make the everyday decisions and experience the highs and lows of life that the rest of society take for granted.

THE CHALLENGES OF DEFINITION

It can be difficult to determine a precise and widely accepted definition of the terms developmental and intellectual disability. Terminology in this area is updated when new information becomes available or when there are changes in clinical practice and societal attitudes. For example, in 2007, the American Association on Mental Retardation, the world's oldest organisation representing professionals in developmental disabilities, changed its name to the American Association on Intellectual and Developmental Disabilities (AAIDD). The name change occurred because the term 'intellectual and developmental disabilities' was thought to be less stigmatising than 'mental retardation', 'feeble mindedness' and other terminology that has been used in the past. Speaking on the name change, Dr Taylor, then editor of the journal *Intellectual and Developmental Disabilities*, explained that (Prabhala, 2007):

> Anyone who believes that we have finally arrived at the perfect terminology will be proven wrong by history. I am sure that at some future point we will find the phrase intellectual and developmental disabilities to be inadequate and demeaning.

There have also been developments in defining intellectual disability in Australia over the past decade, and we have moved closer to the International Classification of Functioning, Disability and Health (ICF) conceptual framework. According to ICF, endorsed by the WHO and used in Australia, 'disability' is an umbrella term for impairment, activity limitation and participation restriction, as influenced by environmental factors.

- Impairments are 'problems of body function or structure such as significant deviation or loss'.
- Activity limitations are 'difficulties an individual may have in executing activities' (core activities are defined as self-care, mobility and communication).
- Participation restrictions are 'problems an individual may experience in involvement in life situations' (school, employment).
- Environmental factors 'make up the physical, social and attitudinal environment in which people live and conduct their lives' (WHO, 2001).

A developmental disability can be further described as a severe, chronic disability that begins any time from birth through to the age of 21 and is expected to last for a lifetime. Developmental disabilities may be cognitive, physical or a combination of both and may cause serious limitations in everyday activities of life, including self-care, communication, learning, mobility or being able to work or live independently (National Association of Councils on Developmental Disabilities, 2012).

Generally it can be said that a person is regarded as having an intellectual disability if they have low intellectual functioning and significant limitations in adaptive behaviour and the condition is present from childhood (defined as under age 18).

Current disability policy in Australia espouses a multidimensional approach that includes assessment of the need for support as one of the components and classifications of disability (Australian Institute of Health and Welfare [AIHW], 2008). The support approach assesses the specific needs of an individual and then recommends strategies, services and supports that will optimise the functioning of that person. The AAIDD recommends that an individual's need for supports be analysed in at least nine key areas, such as human development, teaching and education, home living, community living, employment, health and safety, behaviour, social activities and protection and advocacy (AAIDD, 2013).

There are also difficulties in defining what exactly is meant by the term 'physical disability'. The ICF recognises that most human bodies function in a standard way and that for some individuals there are limitations in this standard operation. The ways in which these limitations affect the individual going about the activities of daily living are also recognised. The context of the individual's living arrangements is also considered by the ICF when determining the degree of disability that is being experienced by the individual (WHO, 2001). When all of these factors are taken into consideration, the definition of physical disability endorsed by the ICF is a condition where a person experiences significant deviation or loss in their body function or structure that results in physical limitations in their physical activity that may affect their participation in life, depending on the context within which they live.

In Australia, another way of categorising disabilities is by 'disability groups'. These groups, such as 'intellectual disability' and 'physical disability', are based on underlying health conditions, limitations in activity and participation and related to environmental factors. They are recognised in the area of disability as well as in legislative and administrative contexts. Australian disability administrators, peak bodies, people with disabilities and service providers use disability groups as a basis for describing groups of people with similar experiences of disability and patterns of impairments, activity limitations, participation restrictions and related environmental factors (AIHW, 2010).

An issue that further complicates the accurate definition of developmental disability is that of dual diagnosis. Dual diagnosis refers to the coexistence of intellectual disability and psychiatric disorder. Treatment can be difficult for this group of individuals for a variety of reasons. There seems to be inadequate knowledge about psychopathology in people with intellectual disability among caregivers and common deficits such as communication, processing skills, cognitive functioning and social skills sometimes present barriers to appropriate care. Werner and Stawski (2012) found that in order for care to improve within the developmental disability area, not only the knowledge and competence of practitioners, but also their attitude towards people with a developmental disability needs to progress from the current level. They describe a self-perpetuating cycle of poor training leading to poor treatment of individuals with developmental disability and then poor training for the next generation of psychiatrists (p. 301). It seems that education that relates directly to the caring of people with disability is given little attention in the undergraduate educational curriculums for many of the health professions. Frequently the topic is left as a postgraduate specialty that is not undertaken by the majority of healthcare workers. Even though people with intellectual disability are entitled to access all specialist services as needed, there seems to be a lack of expertise in this area and people with intellectual disability and a concurrent mental health problem may not be diagnosed and therefore left to cope as best they can without appropriate care.

FACTORS THAT CONTRIBUTE TO THE DEVELOPMENT OF DEVELOPMENTAL AND INTELLECTUAL DISABILITY

Causes

For many people with disability, especially those with an intellectual disability, the precise cause remains uncertain. There have been many attempts to classify the causes of disability and the number of different systems used reflects the ambiguous nature of aetiologies, which can be affected by the environmental and personal attributes of the people involved.

The system of classification chosen here relates to the timing of the primary causal factor.

Congenital

Congenital causes include disabilities and disorders that are present from conception or develop during pregnancy. Included in this category are chromosome disorders (e.g. Down syndrome) and genetic disorders (e.g. phenylketonuria, haemophilia).

Prenatal

During pregnancy the fetus is vulnerable to environmental influences, many of which are likely to result in a variety of disabilities. This category includes the connection between maternal nutrition and fetal development, the drugs and other potentially harmful substances taken during pregnancy (e.g. nicotine and cigarette smoking) and the effects of maternal illness and disease (e.g. malnutrition, rubella) during pregnancy.

Perinatal

There have been many advances in the care provided for mothers and their babies in recent times due in part to technological advances, improved birthing management and sophisticated neonatal care. Even so, the time during and immediately following birth is crucial for a baby to avoid any influences that may result in disability. Examples of conditions caused by perinatal influences include brain damage during birth and asphyxia.

Postnatal

Disability during the postnatal period is the result of a wide variety of possible causes. Among these are physical injury following an accident, ingestion of poisonous substances and infection such as encephalitis.

Prevention

By identifying and understanding the causes of disability wherever possible, appropriate supports and actions can be provided to limit or reduce the risk factors. We can approach the prevention of disability from the perspectives of primary, secondary and tertiary prevention.

Primary prevention is aimed at preventing disability from occurring. Strategies employed to reduce the chance of disability include the promotion of health and nutrition, adequate education about pregnancy and antenatal care, genetic counselling programs, government campaigns (e.g. anti-smoking campaigns), immunisation programs and legislation requiring the wearing of seat belts in cars and bike helmets when riding bikes.

Secondary prevention is aimed at limiting the impact of a disability once detected. Examples of this type of prevention include early intervention education programs for children with disability and the commencement of diet restrictions for children who have specific disorders of metabolism (e.g. phenylketonuria).

Tertiary prevention is aimed at reducing the impact that an established disability has on an individual by providing adequate services to support the individual, for example individually designed employment programs, pension benefits, provision of access ramps.

The environment in which a person lives and works has a great impact on the way a person is able to go about their daily business. The WHO (2011) released a report including a section highlighting barriers commonly encountered. These include inadequate policies and standards that fail to take into account the needs of people with disabilities, negative attitudes and misconceptions that lessen a person's opportunities to education, employment or social participation, lack of provision or problems with service delivery, inadequate funding and lack of consultation with the person who has a disability. These barriers add to the disadvantages experienced by people with disabilities.

ALTERED MOBILITY AND FATIGUE

The necessity for disability to be considered within the context of the environment, individual factors and the requirement for tailored supports has been presented previously. Adaptive behaviour can be described as the collection of conceptual, social and practical skills that people have learned so they can function in their everyday lives. Some examples of practical skills include personal activities of daily living such as eating, dressing, mobility and hygiene requirements.

It is important for people with disabilities to be as independent as possible in their activities of daily living since their independence contributes to both their own self-esteem and society's perception of their worth as a person. The autonomous performance of daily living activities empowers individuals and assists them to be included and valued in the community. Despite an increase in public awareness about the difficulties people with disabilities face in their everyday life, hardships continue. Hoenig, Landerman, Shipp and George (2003) conducted a study to identify factors associated with activity restriction among wheelchair users. They found that mobility limitations and environmental barriers were associated with restricted participation in diverse activities outside the home. Similarly, Ryan, Grant, Dall, Gray, Newton and Granat (2009) found that people who experienced chronic back pain had a lower level as well as an altered pattern of physical activity compared with matched controls in their study.

A number of screening tools have been developed to assess the adaptive behaviours of people with developmental and intellectual disabilities. These include the Australian Developmental Behaviour Checklist (DBC), the Adaptive Behaviour Scale and Scales of Independent Behaviour. The DBC is commonly used in Australia at present and consists of a 96-item checklist that is completed by parents or other primary carers, reporting behavioural and emotional problems in children and young people with intellectual or developmental disability over a 6-month period. The items were independently derived from a study of the medical files of 7000 children with an intellectual disability and adolescents seen in a developmental assessment clinic.

The DBC (2012) provides scores at three levels.

1 Total behaviour problem score — an overall measure of behavioural and emotional problems.
2 Five sub-scales (derived from factor analysis) — disruptive or antisocial behaviour, self-absorbed behaviour, communications disturbance, anxiety problems and social relating problems.
3 Individual behaviour items — indicates the prevalence and severity of individual symptoms.

BODY IMAGE

Body image or self-concept may be defined as a relatively stable set of perceptions that individuals hold about themselves. Self-esteem is the degree to which people regard themselves favourably. Both body image and self-esteem begin to develop shortly after birth and continue throughout life. As a person grows and is confronted with the challenges presented through the usual developmental periods, the body image adjusts. If a person at any age loses a body function that has always been taken for granted, it is common to go through a grieving process. Kübler-Ross (1969) first described the process of a person adjusting to change in their body by outlining the following stages: shock and denial, anger, bargaining, depression and acceptance. The loss of body function can affect a person's feelings about their whole body image.

Australian society today values youth, athletic bodies, sporting attainment and physical fitness (Taleporos & McCabe, 2005). There is no shortage of support for this ideal in the media. Socially unacceptable appearance and behaviours, such as impaired mobility, dribbling and spasm, are sometimes displayed by individuals with disabilities and remind us all of our own mortality, so disabilities are to be avoided as much as possible. Graf, Blankenship and Marini (2009) asked people with spinal cord dysfunction about their experiences of living with a disability. They described two extremes. In some instances they are ignored, forgotten and unacknowledged while at other times they describe being the centre of unwanted attention and being stared at in public. This societal view of disabilities as personal tragedy assumes that individuals with a disability could not be happy or feel good about themselves. Abdul, the man in Case Study 8.1, can challenge this view by presenting himself as an independent man getting on with his life. He is simply making the most of his attributes and finding ways to overcome his deficits in much the same way as any other person.

A number of studies have been undertaken that shed some light on the relationship between disability and self-esteem. Studies undertaken to determine the impact of disability on a person's self-esteem have found that the participants with more severe physical disabilities had lower levels of body esteem than their able-bodied counterparts (Taleporos & McCabe, 2005; Howes, Edwards, & Benton, 2005). Taleporos and McCabe (2005) explained this finding by the 'high level of sociocultural pressures within western society to conform to the ideal of the "body beautiful"' (p. 646). Paterson, McKenzie and Lindsay (2012) found the greater perception of stigma was related to lower self-esteem. This suggests that if an individual has a poor self-esteem, the greater the likelihood of being stigmatised and vice versa.

People with physical disability who required assistance from others were also more likely to express feelings of lower body esteem. This was particularly the case for men, whose body esteem dropped more than women's as the need for assistance increased (Taleporos & McCabe, 2005). They suggested that this might mean that physical disability may have more impact on men's body image than women's. Clearly these findings have implications for health professionals, who need to ensure and maintain a person's independence for as long as possible. Indeed Larner (2005) stated that nurses are in the key position to influence the psychological outcome of rehabilitation due to their 24-hour contact and intimate involvement with treatment regimens.

While people with disabilities expressed lower esteem relating to aspects such as muscular strength, agility and general body, this finding did not apply to other aspects of disability. The duration of disability was not found to be related to body esteem, nor was a person's face (Taleporos & McCabe, 2005). This might be explained by the sample of the study that comprised mainly people with spinal cord injury and multiple sclerosis, which would have little involvement of the face. The duration of the disability may also be explained by the participant being able to overcome some of the difficulties posed by a new injury so that they regain their independence.

Shields, Murdoch, Dodd, & Taylor (2006) conducted a review of articles measuring self-concept of children with cerebral palsy and compared this with the self-concept of children without disabilities, using the domains of self-concept, social acceptance, athletic competence, scholastic competence and behavioural conduct. They found that adolescent females with cerebral palsy may have a lower self-concept in the domains of social acceptance, physical appearance and athletic and scholastic competence compared with that of adolescent females without disabilities. They concluded that it was not possible, generally, to assume that people with cerebral palsy have a lower global self-concept than those without the disability.

We have seen that both the causes and the effects of disability can be very broad and sometimes difficult to diagnose. For parents, first the suspicion and then the growing awareness that their child has a disability is very stressful. Graungaard and Skov (2006) found that the communication process between health professionals and parents during the diagnostic period was of great importance and seemed to influence the way they coped with their child later. Also important was the stated diagnosis, because this gave parents something tangible to regain some predictability and control in their life. Unfortunately Graungaard and Skov (2006) reported that most parents were critical and dissatisfied with their early experiences with health professionals.

The impact that having a child with a disability or caring for a person with a disability has on the carer's self-esteem has been considered in the literature. Even though raising children without a disability involves many challenges, for those parents who do have a child with a disability, they can expect to add the responsibility of providing long-term care for their child, facing additional medical expenses and experiencing stigma (Wong, Wong, Martinson, Lai, Chen, & He, 2004). The increased physical and psychological stresses many of these parents face can result in higher levels of stress and lower self-concept (Todd & Jones, 2005; Hassall, Rose, & McDonald, 2005).

Tam and Cheng (2005) explored the self-concepts of parents with a child of school age with a severe intellectual disability and found that they generally had a lower concept of self than parents of children who did not have a disability. The parents reported that the most stressful aspect of caring for their child included conflicts with the family. This is consistent with other research findings linking adequate support with lower levels of stress in mothers of children with disabilities (Hassall et al., 2005). Koshti-Richman (2009) found that parents of children with disabilities frequently put the needs of the child before their own. This results in the parent sometimes being deprived of an adequate night's sleep or eating a balanced meal.

Case Study 8.1 highlights some of the issues relating to altered mobility and self-esteem for a young man and his family.

CASE STUDY 8.1

Abdul is a 23-year-old man who has cerebral palsy with spastic quadriplegia. He uses an electric wheelchair for mobility and attends part-time work in a supported environment. He lives in the family home with both parents and five older siblings. Abdul has difficulty swallowing food and drink and has been hospitalised several times due to aspiration which has led to pneumonia. Abdul is able to speak but he takes a long time to form the words and is sometimes difficult to understand. The community nurse visits the home twice each week to assist with bathing, toileting and pressure area care.

Questions

1 How can the nurse ensure that Abdul obtains sufficient nutrition?
2 What documentation would need to accompany Abdul if admitted to hospital?
3 What community groups or activities are available to Abdul's parents?

QUALITY OF LIFE

The Commonwealth Disability Services Act 1986 and the United Nations Standard Rules on the Equalisation of Opportunities for Persons with Disabilities (UN, 1994) both require quality of life data to guide and assist with the provision of services for people with disabilities. The regulations under the Disability Services Act 1986 include seven principles and 14 objectives. Principle 4 states:

> People with disabilities have the same rights as other members of Australian society to services which will support their attaining a reasonable quality of life.

The concept of what exactly constitutes quality of life has been controversial, given that the provision of adequate physical environment (shelter, clothing, meals etc.) may not in itself provide quality of life; nor may the provision of a positive social environment. Schalock is a well-known and respected researcher and author on such matters and currently describes quality of life as a:

- '*sensitising notion* that gives us a sense of reference and guidance from the individual's perspective, focusing on the person and the individual's environment
- *unifying theme* that provides a framework for conceptualising, measuring and applying the quality-of-life construct
- *social construct* that is being used as an overriding principle to enhance an individual's wellbeing and to collaborate for programmatic, community and societal change' (Schalock, 2004, p. 205)

This definition illustrates that quality of life is a balance of both physical and social environments that focuses on the individual's needs and wants.

The delivery of services for people with disabilities may be hampered because some people might be unable or find it difficult to evaluate aspects of quality of life regarding the effectiveness and/or quality of the service provided. McVilly, Burton-Smith and Davidson (2000) examined concurrence between a subject's self-reported quality of life and assessments of their quality of life made by proxies who were either a close relative or someone acting in a supportive role similar to that of a family member. The findings

CASE STUDY 8.2

Scott is a 6-year-old child with an intellectual disability. He lives with his parents and 10-year-old sister and has reached his developmental milestones later than others. Eight weeks ago, he started at the local primary school where he has been observed hitting and pushing other children in the playground. In class, the teacher has noted that he is disruptive to other students and finds it difficult to attend to the set task. Scott's teacher has seen him staring into space at times and says it is hard to gain his attention at these times. When asked, his parents confirmed that this behaviour also occurs at home and they do not know how to manage him. His sister is embarrassed by his behaviour at school and is being teased by her peers and comes home most days in tears.

Questions

1. When working with children such as Scott, why is it important to have a general understanding of behaviour management?
2. What support is available for the family of Scott in the community?
3. What investigations would you suggest for Scott?

endorsed the use of standardised approaches such as the *Comprehensive quality of life scale for adults* (Deakin University, 1997) for proxy-based measures of quality of living. The confirmation of the usefulness of proxy-based measures has been supported more recently. The Evaluation of Quality of Life Instrument (EQLI) was found to be valid by Nota, Soresi and Perry (2006). The EQLI was designed to elicit from staff of health and social care services assessments of the level of satisfaction experienced by adults with an intellectual disability.

The concept of family quality of life is a relatively recent extension of quality of life in the field of intellectual and developmental disability and shifts the focus of quality of life from an individual to the family unit (Rillotta, Kirby, Shearer, & Nettelbeck, 2012). The quality of life for families is important since much of the care and support for people with intellectual and developmental disability is provided by the family unit.

INTERVENTIONS TO ATTAIN COMPLIANCE

With the increase of children being born with a developmental and/or intellectual disability (D/ID) and living into older age, there is increasing demand in all areas of service provision. People with D/ID have different levels of health and education requirements across the lifespan (Brown & Parmenter, 2011). Nurses involved in providing care and treatment for people with D/ID often encounter difficulties in certain situations where the treatment may be complex, requiring many hospital admissions and/or extended community nursing. Neurological conditions, low frustration levels, an inability to communicate effectively, unfamiliar people and environment, pain, fear and anxiety and parent and/or carer attitudes can lead to behaviour that prevents or reduces intervention compliance.

Utilising communication and listening skills, reflection and critical analysis of the situation leads to good practice in supporting children, adolescents and adults with D/ID in their treatment experience (Williamson, 2004). Nurses should be aware that providing care for a person with D/ID may take place in a variety of settings such as the home, school, hospital, group home, residential facility or nursing home, where many variables within these environments may have a positive or negative impact on intervention compliance.

To meet the challenge of caring for children and adults with D/ID in a variety of settings, nurses need to be able to gather data that will then be used to meet their needs and promote independence. Using the basic principles of assessing, planning, implementing and evaluating intervention (APIE) will help to ensure that individual and objective nursing care can be provided.

During the assessing and planning phase the nurse should consider that children, adolescents and adults with D/ID have emotional and behavioural needs that will change over time. Nurses should understand that, like the non-disabled population, people with D/ID have needs, desires, dreams and differences. Understanding this will facilitate a cooperative relationship between the nurse, the person with a disability and their family or carer, providing a greater opportunity for adherence to intervention requirements (Dokken & Ahmann, 2006). This will also ensure that all interventions are planned to meet individual needs; for example, strategies that may work for a 3-year-old boy with an autistic disorder are unlikely to be effective for a 9-year-old girl functioning in the moderate range of intellectual disability with Down syndrome or a 50-year-old man with severe intellectual disability and a seizure disorder.

It is also beneficial that the nurse include the following key principles of basic human rights (Disability Services Act 1993, No 3): independence, choice and inclusion when planning any intervention. Using these principles demonstrates the nurse's value of people with disability and their families or carers, and also assists in structuring intervention that will lead to compliance through the development of a trusting relationship and mutual respect (Chen & Boothroyd, 2006).

Many people with D/ID have problems that affect their ability to be independent in all activities of daily living. For example, Abdul has neuromuscular problems as a result of cerebral palsy (CP). Hoon and Tolley cited in Batshaw (2012) describe cerebral palsy as 'a group of chronic motor disorders that result from malformation or injury of the developing brain … impairments associated with CP are variable and non-progressive but permanent' (p. 424). Many children and adults with CP live in the community with their parents and/or carers. However, some children and adults continue to reside in government-funded or private residential facilities.

The attainment of intervention compliance for people with multiple disabilities such as CP may be affected by living arrangements, education of family or carers and health professionals due to poorly coordinated services, gaps in services and social disadvantage (Ross & Parkes, 2004).

By using the principles of APIE nurses can determine parents' and carers' concerns, such as their confidence in feeding, toileting, using adaptive equipment appropriately, managing wheelchairs and correct positioning techniques. The most common health issue for admission to hospital for people with multiple disabilities are respiratory problems often related to aspiration of food and/or fluids, usually due to poor feeding and positioning techniques (Barks & Shaw, 2011; Murphy, Hoff, & Jorgenson, 2006).

Teaching appropriate skills, being supportive and providing parents and carers with positive feedback will help to develop their skills, and confidence in these areas will make them more likely to follow intervention requirements for their child. The outcome for the child or adult is that they will feel more secure, their comfort will be enhanced and there will be less time spent in hospital.

Many parents/carers have had negative hospital experiences and are concerned that nursing and allied health staff aren't able to care appropriately for their children with D/ID during a hospital admission. This is not an uncommon issue and it is not without much consideration that parents voice their concern. Parents in this situation fear that their criticism of poor previous treatment may create more complications and barriers (Samuel, Hobden, LeRoy, & Lacey, 2012) with service providers. This parental concern is evident in the study by Prezant and Marshak (2006) where 121 parents of children with disabilities were asked how they viewed helpful actions by service providers. Data analysis produced ten categories of helpful actions identified by parents and listed them in order of frequency: performed their job well; supported parent and child; encouraged inclusion; enhanced self-esteem of child; had high expectations of child; went beyond 'required' job duties; taught parents; organised necessary accommodation for child; engaged in advocacy; and learned from parents (p. 35). In this study some parents viewed actions by professionals as helpful, but many found them to be obstructive. Although this is a small study it was evident that these parents want a relationship with their child's health or educational professional that reciprocates 'respect, collaboration, communication and information sharing' (p. 31).

To ensure intervention compliance within the hospital environment it is important that the nurse collaborates with the child's parents in developing an individual care plan that will address the child's needs and identify the type of help that is required. This care plan can be updated at regular intervals by parents and other health professionals and brought with the child whenever he/she is admitted to hospital (Thurgate, 2006). This approach will reassure parents that nurses, doctors and other allied health professionals will be better informed about their child and his/her healthcare needs across their lifespan.

Putting this into practice will require the nurse to allocate appropriate time during the admission process to ensure that an individual's assessment covers all aspects of care. This assessment can be guided by the questions in Table 8.1.

Using this assessment information (Thurgate, 2006) the nurse will be able to plan effective intervention by liaising with other health professionals such as physiotherapists, speech therapists and occupational therapists to ensure better outcomes associated with hospitalisation.

The process for gaining intervention compliance from children with challenging behaviour involves patience, a non-judgmental approach, tolerance and an understanding of the D/ID and related behaviour disorders. The findings of a pilot study on families of children with autism conducted by Hall and Graff (2010) stressed that 'nurses can take the lead in promoting a partnership between parents and health professionals by sharing information …' (p. 201).

Autism usually appears in early infancy and early childhood and is thought to have neurological and genetic origins. The American Psychiatric Association's Diagnostic and Statistical Manual defines autism spectrum disorder as a group of developmental disabilities that affects social and communication skills (American Psychiatric Association, 2000). Towbin, Mauk and Batshaw (2012) describe children with autism spectrum disorder (ASD) as showing difficulties in social situations, verbal and non-verbal communications, interactive and pretend play and behavioural abnormalities, such as odd mannerisms or body movements and ritualistic behaviour.

According to Bailey, Hare, Hatton and Limb (2006) there is a large proportion of people with intellectual disabilities who have challenging behaviours, for example self-injury, verbal and physical aggression and stereotypical behaviour. The impact of this behaviour limits or prevents access to the community for the person with D/ID, their family or carers.

In a study by Bailey et al. (2006) they found that care staff felt sad, hopeless, helpless, frustrated, guilty and angry towards the person with an intellectual disability and challenging behaviour. These negative emotions lead to care staff using negative behaviours such as restraint and avoidance in an effort to manage the situation. Feldman, Atkinson,

TABLE 8.1

Information needed for continuity of care. Note: Adapted from Thurgate (2006).

COMMUNICATION	Does the child verbalise? Have any special words? If non-verbal how do they communicate — eye point, sign, switches or other forms of communication? How may their behaviour communicate if they are bored, need a pad change or are tired?
BREATHING	What is the child's normal breathing pattern? Do they have physiotherapy or an exercise routine?
MAINTAINING A SAFE ENVIRONMENT	Does the child have epilepsy? What are the seizures like? Is there a known trigger? Does the child have an emergency protocol? What medication is the child on? If mobile, are they safe on their feet? If non-mobile, what equipment do they require?
NUTRITION	How is the child fed? If enterally, what is their mouth care routine? Have they got a spare gastrostomy tube? If orally, what consistency do they like their food? Do they participate (e.g. hand-over-hand feeding)?
CARE OF SKIN	Undertake a skin assessment. How frequently is the child moved? Do they have a particular routine?
DRESSING	Does the child need assistance? Total, partial or just needs verbal encouragement? Give the child choice.
BODY TEMPERATURE	Does the child have poor temperature control?
PAIN	How does the child react if they are in pain — cry, grizzle or fidget? What other behaviours may indicate that the child is in pain?
SLEEP	What is the child's normal routine? How is the child positioned? What is the environment like? Does the child have a comforter? Is the child turned or changed during the night?
TOILETING	Is the child continent — do they have any special signs or words for the toilet? Is the child incontinent — do they wear different pads during the day and at night? Does the child's behaviour change if they require a pad change? Is the child intermittently catheterised or learning to self-catheterise? How often does the child have their bowels open? Does the child have a bowel regimen?
RELIGION	Does the child have a religious or spiritual affiliation? How does this affect their care?
PLAY/SCHOOL/ACTIVITIES	What activities does the child enjoy and not enjoy doing? Does the child have a special comforter? What sort of sensory activities does the child participate in?
SENSORY ABILITY	What is the child's vision and hearing like? Do they wear glasses or a hearing aid?
PARENTAL/CARER COMFORTING	How does the parent comfort the child when they are distressed?

Foti-Gervais and Condillac (2004) looked at whether people with intellectual disabilities received formal or informal interventions for their challenging behaviour. They discovered that the majority of people had no formal intervention plans leading to a lack of '(1) input from a qualified professional; (2) a written intervention plan; (3) organised caregiver training and supervision; and (4) formal monitoring and evaluation of implementation, outcomes ...' (p. 66).

Continuing research in this area has shown that there is a higher risk for young people with an intellectual disability than for their peers with a non-intellectual disability for a range of behavioural, emotional and diagnosed psychiatric disorders. Emerson, Robertson and Wood (2005) found that children and adolescents with intellectual disabilities are now having more attention directed towards their emotional and behavioural needs than in previous years.

Mottram and Berger-Gross (2004) studied the effectiveness of a classroom behavioural intervention program on children with acquired brain injury and disruptive behaviour. These children displayed inattention, excesses of non-compliance, aggression and deficits in self-management, social and academic skills. The program was based on operant techniques using a token economy with response cost, program rules and mystery motivators. Staff involved in the program were surprised that one of the children with 'autistic-like presentation' (p. 140) showed a good improvement as his level of disruptive behaviour fell to within normal limits and remained stable throughout the intervention.

Functional behavioural assessment (FBA) is effective because it is both descriptive and provides positive support which has led to better interventions for people with severe behavioural problems. Functional analysis is the experimental assessment of behaviour that can be used to develop interventions. It requires the observer to identify and record causal relationships that exist in the environment that occur before and after the target behaviour (Ling & Mak, 2012).

Depending on how severely affected they are, children with autism spectrum disorder (ASD) usually don't comply with intervention programs. They aren't usually 'in touch' with people or their environment and encouraging them to participate in activities can be frustrating and challenging. Connecting to these children is made even more difficult, as many have communication deficits, little to no eye contact and stereotypical behaviour. Research into early identification and early intervention of ASD, a neurodevelopmental disorder, continues to be a challenge. However, Boyd, Odom, Humphreys and Sam (2010) stress that continuing research is important as it has shown that children have better outcomes if they are diagnosed early and followed-up with intervention with motor, sensory and behavioural programs.

Parental responsibility for the 24-hour care of a child with ASD can be overwhelming. If parents and/or carers aren't given the education and support required they will not be able to fulfil their role in their child's intervention programs. Giarelli, Souders, Pinto-Martin, et al. (2005) developed an intervention pilot study for parents of children who had received a recent diagnosis of ASD. The main purpose of this pilot study was to:

- refine a parent-focused nursing intervention for parents of children with ASD
- modify and revise intervention protocol for a larger study
- test the effects of post-diagnosis nursing intervention.

'The intervention consisted of 3 hours of individualised advanced practice nursing care for parents by telephone and in the home' (Giarelli et al., 2005, p. 394). This included assessment of functional status of the child; for example behaviour, nutrition, sleep, speech and language needs. Assessment of the family included persistent family barriers to implementation of the treatment plan and child behaviour management. Instruction provided information and reinforcement to continue effective behaviour management; the treatment involved problem solving, psychological support, encouragement and ongoing revision of the treatment plan. A positive result from this small study ($n = 31$) was that the participating families appreciated their experience. However, the authors stressed that a three-hour intervention protocol didn't provide sufficient time to cover all the issues for these families.

Challenging behaviour is complex, and according to Matson, Neal, Fodstad and Hess (2010) early identification of the relationship between socialisation and challenging behaviour is necessary to achieve a better understanding leading to more informed treatment. Challenging behaviour may be reinforced by more than one reinforcer within the child's environment. Functional analysis identifies these reinforcers, enabling the nurse to develop a behavioural intervention that can be followed by parents in the home and other social settings.

The development of a home or residential program begins with an assessment. The nurse as part of the multidisciplinary team will need to discuss the initial assessment of the child with the parents and the team. This consultation will help to build trust and rapport with the family/carers as they are active participants in the intervention program and vital to its success. Principles that will help to develop the nurse's practice in assessing, planning for behaviour intervention and evaluation of individual behaviour modification programs are listed in Box 8.1.

Once the initial assessment has been concluded the nurse can arrange to observe and record the child's behaviour in the home environment. The effective collection of data will determine whether the intervention will be successful for the child and their family.

Using the observational method, functional analysis, requires the nurses to record the observable aspects of the child's behaviour that occurs before and after the target behaviour, for example hitting others. The ABC approach (in Box 8.2) is a useful tool for gathering information on behaviour as it happens.

All behaviour can be assessed utilising the ABC approach. If the behaviour is rewarded by a positive consequence, for example when a child gets something they want, it is more likely to increase in frequency. However, should the behaviour not be positively rewarded

BOX 8.1

Assessment of children with challenging behaviours (Source: Giarelli et al., 2005.)

A holistic assessment is needed and should cover the following areas:

- Medical history including psychological history.
- Child's living arrangements — family and/or carers?
- Quality of life — what are the positive aspects of the child's life?
- In what ways are the child's needs being met?
- Can the child communicate independently?
- Has the child's behaviour been described?
- What behaviour modification strategies have/or are being used?
- Is close observation necessary to prevent injury to self or others?
- Document data and use for planning intervention.
- If more specific assessment is required, what other members of the health team should be included?

BOX 8.2
The ABC approach

- What happens before the behaviour (antecedents)? Antecedents are things or events that set the scene for the behaviour to occur; for example, Scott's behaviour responds to antecedents that have been learned and therefore can be changed.
- The behaviour that is observed.
- What happens after the behaviour (consequences)?

then the frequency of that behaviour over time will decrease (Lovell, 2011). It is also important to look at what aspects in the home or residential environment can be changed to facilitate the intervention.

Using the ABC approach will enable the nurse to view the child's behaviour in context. The nurse will need to note that any emotional and/or behavioural problem should not be viewed as the child's alone. It is important to know how the child interacts with his or her environment.

Therefore, it may be that the child's behaviour is a successful way for him to get what he wants from the environment. Recording the chain of events in this manner will enable the nurse to change those aspects of the child's environment that may then lead to a change in his behaviour.

The following is an example of the first day of observing a child in his home environment and this is what the nurse observes and records:

Antecedent: the child is playing with his toys on the floor of the lounge room. His older sister comes into the room and accidentally kicks over the toys.

Behaviour: the child starts to cry and hit his sister.

Consequence: the child's mother rushes over to hold his hands, restraining him from hitting his sister. She tells his sister that she should know better, making her pick up the toys and put them back in place. The child's mother speaks calmly to him, as she waits for his sister to replace the toys. The child stops crying when his toys are back in place; his mother lets go of his hands.

In this observation the nurse records that the child's mother makes an attempt to communicate with him during this event. The nurse also records that the child hits his sister for scattering his toys; however, the child isn't told not to hit his sister. More observations would need to be done in the home environment before an intervention program could be planned and implemented.

FAMILY AND CARERS

The impact on the parents when a child is born with D/ID may be devastating. Parents are in shock and are unable to face the reality of the situation. They suffer the loss of their dreams for a 'normal' child and experience the feeling of 'falling apart' and an inability to cope with the stressors related to this diagnosis.

Parental reactions usually follow these stages:

- denial — it can't be happening to us
- projection of blame — it's your fault, it's the doctor's fault

- fear — how are we going to manage, what will happen to our child in the future?
- guilt, mourning or grief — for the loss of their dream, the development of chronic sorrow
- withdrawal — no one can help
- rejection — I don't want to see the baby
- acceptance — may take time.

Parents of children with D/ID move through the above stages in a circular motion and may over time either develop adequate coping mechanisms or have a negative outlook and remain in the grieving stage. How they cope is dependent on the practical support that is available from family, friends, their cultural aspects and health professionals who are well trained in the area (Choi, Yong, & Young, 2011). Financial security, social life and availability of resources to assist the child and family are paramount in helping families to cope.

It is important for the nurse to understand how the family/carer adjusts and copes with a child who has a lifelong disability. To achieve this goal nurses should follow these steps when talking with family members and carers:

- body language — be relaxed
- be attentive — show that you are interested
- don't be judgmental — consider your responses
- expect and tolerate silences, tears, anger and other emotions
- look at positive and negative feelings and the content from the family/carer's viewpoint
- empathise rather than sympathise
- discuss practical day-to-day issues in being a parent and providing 24-hour care for their child
- discuss the family's/carer's long-term expectations for their child
- support the family/carer through various stages across the lifespan.

Nurses need to provide accurate information on the following areas to help the child's family make informed decisions about their future:

- child's disability and the phases of normal development
- agencies that provide training and consultation for families/carers
- availability of health and related services
- early intervention and other educational programs
- legal protection and advocacy services
- respite care and availability of financial support
- community-based living (Betz et al., 2004).

Generally, people with D/ID are living longer and sharing a life expectancy similar to that of the general population, so Abdul and Scott can expect to live into older age. This increased life expectancy is attributed to advances in technology and better preventative healthcare, resulting in the decreased development of secondary problems related to their D/ID. Betz et al. (2004) recommend that healthcare professionals gain a better understanding of service needs for the D/ID population by developing research studies that will ensure that evidence-based services are available to meet the lifelong needs of these people and their families and carers.

Reflective questions

1. What strategies can nurses use to ensure that people with D/ID are provided with appropriate care when admitted to hospital?
2. What do nurses need to know to be able to communicate effectively with the family or carer of a person with D/ID?
3. How can nurses help the community to develop positive attitudes towards people with D/ID?

EDUCATION OF THE PERSON AND FAMILY

In Case Study 8.2 it is evident that education will have an important role in Scott's development. For many children with D/ID this may begin with early intervention programs (Birkin, Anderson, Seymour, & Moore, 2008) progressing to preschool, and then on to special primary and/or high school. Some children with D/ID, depending on their academic and functional ability, may be able to attend mainstream school with support from specially trained teacher aides and, depending on their health status, the school nurse. At age 18, school finishes and parents and carers need advice on what is available for their adult child. Some may be able to go on to further education facilities that provide support for people with disabilities and others (see Case Study 8.1) may find work in areas that offer a supported work environment. Through work support programs there is the opportunity for people with D/ID to find work in the wider community (Disability Services Australia, 2007).

The nurse and other health professionals will continue to provide health education and support for the family or carer, which includes the long-term management and treatment of problems related to the child's disability across their lifespan.

CONCLUSION

Caring for people with D/ID and their families and carers is challenging for nurses. The case studies on Abdul and Scott have attempted to illustrate how people with D/ID and their families are affected in all aspects of their lives. Parents and carers have the 24-hour responsibility for their children and should be included in care planning at all times. It should be remembered that, for many people with D/ID, family members are very involved in the care and decision-making process even into their adult lives. Nurses need to acknowledge and utilise the knowledge and skills of these parents and carers as they are involved in the ongoing therapy and education programs for their children. Developing a collaborative relationship with parents and carers will help to ensure that the needs of their children will be met over their lifetime. Nurses need more professional development in this area to be able to provide advanced practice and work more effectively with parents, carers and the multidisciplinary team.

Recommended reading

Batshaw, M. L. (2012). *Children with Disabilities* (7th ed.). Baltimore: Paul H Brookes Publishing Co.

Giarelli, E., Souders, M., Pinto-Martin, J., et al. (2005). Intervention pilot for parents of children with autistic spectrum disorder. *Journal of Pediatric Nursing, 31*(5), 389–399.

Glasson, E. J., Sullivan, S. G., Hussain, R., et al. (2005). An assessment of intellectual disability among Aboriginal Australians. *Journal of Intellectual Disability Research, 49*(8), 626–634.

Hall, H. R., & Graff, C. J. (2010). Parenting challenges in families of children with autism: A pilot study. *Issues in Comprehensive Pediatric Nursing, 33*, 187–204.

Smyth, C. M., & Bell, D. (2006). From biscuits to boyfriends: the ramifications of choice for people with learning disabilities. *British Journal of Learning Disabilities, 34*(4), 227–236.

References

American Association on Intellectual and Developmental Disabilities. (2013). *Frequently asked questions on intellectual disability and the AAIDD definition*. Retrieved May 6, 2013, from http://www.aaidd.org/content_185.cfm

American Psychiatric Association. (2000). *Diagnostic and Statistical Manual of Mental Disorders* (4th ed., text rev.). International version. Washington DC: Author.

Australian Bureau of Statistics. (2007). *Survey of disability, ageing and carers, Australia: Summary of findings*. Canberra: Author.

Australian Institute of Health and Welfare. (2008). *Disability in Australia: trends in prevalence, education, employment and community living*. Cat. no. AUS103. Canberra: Author.

Australian Institute of Health and Welfare. (2010). *National community services data dictionary*. Version 6. Cat.no. HWI 109 Canberra: Author. Retrieved March 20, 2010, from http://www.aihw.gov.au/publication-detail/?id=6442468386

Bailey, B. A., Hare, D. J., Hatton, C., et al. (2006). The response to challenging behaviour by care staff: emotional responses, attributions of cause and observations of practice. *Journal of Intellectual Disability Research, 50*(3), 199–211.

Barks, L., & Shaw, P. (2011). Wheelchair Positioning and Breathing in Children with Cerebral Palsy: Study Methods and Lessons Learned. *Rehabilitation Nursing, 36*(4), 146–152, 174.

Batshaw, M. L. (2012). *Children with Disabilities* (7th ed.). Baltimore: Paul H Brookes Publishing Co.

Betz, C. L., Baer, M. T., Poulsen, M., et al. (2004). Secondary analysis of primary and preventative services accessed and perceived service barriers by children with developmental disabilities and their families. *Issues in Comprehensive Paediatric Nursing, 27*, 83–106.

Birkin, C., Anderson, A., Seymour, F., et al. (2008). A parent-focused early intervention program for autism: Who gets access? *Journal of Intellectual & Developmental Disability, 33*(2), 108–116.

Boyd, B. A., Odom, S. L., Humphreys, B. P., et al. (2010). Infants and toddlers with autism spectrum disorder: early identification and early intervention. *Journal of Early Intervention, 32*(2), 75–98.

Brown, R. L., & Parmenter, T. R. (2011). Challenges of Residential and Community Care: An analysis and appraisal of supported living programs across the lifespan (Editorial). *Journal of Intellectual Disability Research, 55*, Part 8, 719.

Chen, H. J., & Boothroyd, R. A. (2006). Caregiver's level of trust in their children's health care providers. *Journal of Child and Family Studies, 15*(1), 57–70.

Choi, E. K., Yong, J. L., & Young, L. (2011). Factors associated with emotional response of parents at the time of diagnosis of Down syndrome. *Journal for Specialists in Pediatric Nursing, 16*, 113–120.

Commonwealth of Australia. (1986). *Disability Services Act 1986*. Canberra: Author.

Deakin University. (1997) *Comprehensive quality of life scale for adults*. (5th ed.). (ComQol-A5). Retrieved May 6, 2013, from http://www.deakin.edu.au/research/acqol/instruments/comqol-scale/comqol-a5.pdf

Developmental Behaviour Checklist. (2012). *Monash University*. Retrieved March 20, 2012, from http://www.med.monash.edu.au/spppm/research/devpsych/dbc.download/dbc-info-package.pdf

Disability Services Australia. (2007). *Life to live*. Retrieved May 6, 2013, from http://www.dsa.org.au/life_site/text/education/index.html

Dokken, D., & Ahmann, E. (2006). The many roles of family members in 'Family-Centred Care' — Part 1. *Paediatric Nursing, 32*(6), 562–565.

Emerson, E., Robertson, J., & Wood, J. (2005). Emotional and behavioural needs of children and adolescents with intellectual disabilities in an urban conurbation. *Journal of Intellectual Disability Research, 49*(1), 16–24.

Feldman, M. A., Atkinson, L., Foti-Gervais, L., et al. (2004). Formal versus informal interventions for challenging behaviour in persons with intellectual disabilities. *Journal of Intellectual Disability Research, 48*(1), 60–68.

Giarelli, E., Souders, M., Pinto-Martin, J., et al (2005). Intervention pilot for parents of children with autistic spectrum disorder. *Journal of Pediatric Nursing, 31*(5), 171–187.

Graf, N. M., Blankenship, C. J., & Marini, I. (2009). One hundred words about disability. *Journal of Rehabilitation, 75*(2), 25–34.

Graungaard, A., & Skov, L. (2006). Why do we need a diagnosis? A qualitative study of parents' experiences, coping and needs, when the newborn child is severely disabled. *Child: care, health and development, 33*(3), 296–307.

Hall, H. R., & Graff, J. C. (2010). Parenting challenges in families of children with autism: A pilot study. *Issues in Comprehensive Pediatric Nursing, 33*, 187–204.

Hassall, R., Rose, J., & McDonald, J. (2005). Parenting stress in mothers of children with an intellectual disability: the effects of parental cognitions in relation to child characteristics and family support. *Journal of Intellectual Disability Research, 49*(6), 405–418.

Hoenig, H., Landerman, L. R., Shipp, K. M., et al. (2003). Activity restriction among wheelchair users. *Journal of American Geriatrics Society, 51*(9), 1244–1251.

Hoon, A. H., Jr., & Tolley, F. (2012). In M. L. Batshaw (Ed.), *Children with Disabilities* (7th ed.). Baltimore: Paul H Brookes Publishing Co.

Howes, H., Edwards, S., & Benton, D. (2005). Male body image following acquired brain injury. *Brain Injury, 19*(2), 135–147.

Koshti-Richman, A. (2009). Caring for a disabled child at home: parents' views. *Nursing Children and Young People, 21*(6), 19–21.

Kübler-Ross, E. (1969). *On Death and Dying*. New York: Macmillan.

Larner, S. (2005). Common psychological challenges for patients with newly acquired disability. *Nursing Standard, 23*(19), 33–39.

Ling, C. Y. M., & Mak, W. W. S. (2012). Coping with challenging behaviours of children with autism: effectiveness of brief training workshop for frontline staff in special education settings. *Journal of Intellectual Disability Research, 56*(3), 258–269.

Lovell, I. C. (2011). Understanding and working with challenging behavior. *Learning Disability Practice, 14*(2), 32–38.

Matson, J. L., Neal, D., Fodstad, J. C., et al. (2010). The relation of social behaviours and challenging behaviours in infants and toddlers with autism spectrum disorders. *Developmental Neurorehabilitation, 13*(3), 164–169.

McVilly, K. R., Burton-Smith, R. M., & Davidson, J. A. (2000). Concurrence between subject and proxy ratings of quality of life for people with and without intellectual disabilities. *Journal of Intellectual & Developmental Disability, 25*(1), 19–39.

Mottram, L., & Berger-Gross, P. (2004). An intervention to reduce disruptive behaviours in children with brain injury. *Pediatric Rehabilitation, 7*(2), 133–143.

Murphy, N. A., Hoff, C., & Jorgenson, T. (2006). Costs and complications of hospitalizations for children with cerebral palsy. *Paediatric Rehabilitation, 9*(1), 47–52.

National Association of Councils on Developmental Disabilities. (2012). *What are developmental disabilities?* Retrieved March 27, 2012, from http://www.nacdd.org/about-nacdd/what-are-developmental-disabilities.aspx

Nota, L., Soresi, S., & Perry, J. (2006). Quality of life in adults with an intellectual disability: the Evaluation of Quality of Life Instrument. *Journal of Intellectual Disability Research, 50*(5), 371–385.

NSW Disability Services Act. (1993) No 3 Retrieved May 6, 2013, from http://www.legislation.nsw.gov.au

Paterson, L., McKenzie, K., & Lindsay, B. (2012). Stigma, social comparison and self esteem in adults with an intellectual disability. *Journal of Applied Research in Intellectual Disabilities, 25*, 166–176.

Prabhala, A. (2007). Mental retardation is no more — new name is intellectual and developmental disabilities. *AAIDD news (American Association in Intellectual and Developmental Disabilities)*. Retrieved May 24, 2007 from http://www.aamr.org/About_AAIDD/MR_name_change.htm

Prezant, F. P., & Marshak, L. (2006). Helpful actions seen through the eyes of parents of children with disabilities. *Disability & Society, 21*(1), 31–45.

Rillotta, F., Kirby, N., Shearer, J., et al. (2012). Family quality of life of Australian families with a member with an intellectual/developmental disability. *Journal of Intellectual Disability Research, 56*(1), 71–86.

Ross, A., & Parkes, J. (2004). Making doors open: caring for families of children with severe cerebral palsy. *Paediatric Nursing, 16*(5), 14–18.

Ryan, C. G., Grant, P. M., Dall, P. M., et al. (2009). Individuals with chronic low back pain have a lower level, and an altered pattern, of physical activity compared with matched controls: an observational study. *Australian Journal of Physiotherapy, 55*, 53–58.

Samuel, P. S., Hobden, K. L., LeRoy, B. W., et al. (2012). Analysing family service needs of typically underserved families in the USA. *Journal of Intellectual Disability Research, 56*(1), 111–128.

Schalock, R. L. (2004). The concept of quality of life: what we know and do not know. *Journal of Intellectual Disability Research, 48*(3), 203–216.

Shields, N., Murdoch, A., Dodd, K. J., et al. (2006). A systematic review of the self concept of children with cerebral palsy compared with children without disability. *Developmental Medicine & Child Neurology, 48*, 151–157.

Taleporos, G., & McCabe, M. P. (2005). The relationship between the severity and duration of physical disability and body esteem. *Psychology and Health, 20*(5), 637–650.

Tam, S. F., & Cheng, A. (2005). Self-concepts of parents with a child of school age with a severe intellectual disability. *Journal of Intellectual Disabilities, 9*(3), 253–268.

Thurgate, C. (2006). Living with disability: Part 3 Communication and care. *Paediatric Nursing, 18*(5), 38–44.

Todd, S., & Jones, S. (2005). Looking at the future and seeing the past: The challenge of the middle years of parenting a child with intellectual disabilities. *Journal of Intellectual Disability Research, 49*, 389–404.

Towbin, K. E., Mauk, J. E., & Batshaw, M. L. (2012). Pervasive developmental disorders. In M. L. Batshaw (Ed.), *Children with Disabilities* (7th ed.). Baltimore: Paul H Brookes Publishing.

United Nations. (1994). *Standard Rules on the Equalization of Opportunities for Persons with Disabilities*. Retrieved May 6, 2013, from www.un.org/disabilities/default.asp?id=26

Werner, S., & Stawski, M. (2012). Knowledge, attitudes and training of professionals on dual diagnosis of intellectual disability and psychiatric disorder. *Journal of Intellectual Disability Research, 56*(3), 291–304.

Williamson, A. (2004). Improving services for people with learning disabilities. *Nursing Standard, 18*(24), 43–51.

Wong, S. Y., Wong, T. K. S., Martinson, I., et al. (2004). Needs of Chinese parents of children with developmental disability. *Journal of Learning Disabilities, 8*, 141–158.

World Health Organization. (2001). *International classification of functioning, disability and health*. Geneva: Author.

World Health Organization. (2011). *Summary. World report on disability*. Geneva: Author.

CHAPTER 9

Clint Douglas

Management of chronic pain

Learning objectives

When you have completed this chapter you will be able to:

- recognise the scope and impact of chronic pain in Australia
- discuss the relevance of a biopsychosocial model of chronic pain for persons with chronic illness and disability
- identify key components of pain assessment
- acknowledge the central role the person with chronic pain takes in the management of their health
- identify a range of therapies available for the management of chronic pain.

Key words

chronic pain, disability-related pain, biopsychosocial model, pain assessment, pain management

INTRODUCTION

Pain is a common and often under-recognised problem among people with chronic illness and disability. For example, accumulating evidence demonstrates that pain is a prominent component of most of the specific chronic diseases discussed in this volume. Recent surveys have found pain is prevalent among people with stroke (Klit, Finnerup, Overvad, Andersen, & Jensen, 2011), multiple sclerosis (Douglas, Wollin, & Windsor, 2008a), chronic obstructive pulmonary disease (Bentsen, Rustoen, & Miaskowski, 2011), chronic heart failure (Evangelista, Sackett, & Dracup, 2009), chronic kidney disease (Davidson, 2003), inflammatory bowel disease (Schirbel et al., 2010), diabetes (Bair et al., 2010), HIV/AIDS (Namisango et al., 2012) and cancer (van den Beuken-van Everdingen et al., 2007). A consistent finding across these studies is that individuals often report multiple types of pain and a significant subset experience moderate-to-severe pain intensity on a daily basis. Once pain develops, it often becomes a chronic problem across the illness trajectory. For example, a comprehensive review of symptom prevalence in end-stage cancer, AIDS, heart disease, COPD and renal disease revealed pain was found among more than 50% of people for all five conditions (Solano, Gomes, & Higginson, 2006). As the life expectancy of individuals with chronic illness has increased, observations of the prevalence of pain problems over the entire disease course without reversible causes suggests disability-related pain is often best conceptualised as a chronic pain condition (e.g., Marcus, Kerns, Rosenfeld, & Breitbart, 2000).

The clinical significance of chronic pain in the context of a disabling disease is underscored by the negative impact of pain on functioning. Chronic pain can cause severe physical, emotional, social and economic problems for affected individuals and their significant others. The general pain literature has documented the profound effects that chronic pain has on mood, personality and social relationships, as well as the concomitant experiences of depression, sleep disturbance and decrease in overall function (e.g. Turk et al., 2008). Much less is known about the specific impact of pain on physical and psychosocial functioning among people who already have a physical disability. Although there are significant gaps in the literature, the available evidence indicates that chronic disability-related pain is associated with poorer adjustment and reduced quality of life, independent of the effects of the disease itself (e.g. Douglas et al., 2009; also see reviews by Ehde et al., 2003; Ehde & Hanley, 2006). Taken together, these findings suggest chronic disability-related pain warrants further research and clinical attention as a significant problem in its own right.

This chapter is written for nurses and other health professionals as a broad overview of a complex topic. It briefly reviews the scope and nature of chronic pain with a particular focus on chronic pain secondary to chronic illness and disability. It argues the relevance of a biopsychosocial model of chronic disability-related pain and discusses the important role of some key psychosocial factors in shaping the pain experience. Key components of pain assessment and the array of therapies that are available are also briefly outlined.

CHRONIC PAIN DEFINED

The most oft-cited definition of pain in the literature and that accepted by the International Association for the Study of Pain (Merskey, 1986, p. 51) is:

> Pain is an unpleasant sensory and emotional experience associated with actual or potential tissue damage or described in terms of such damage.

This definition underscores the inherent subjectivity of pain and acknowledges the importance of emotional as well as sensory factors in the pain experience. It also highlights that although pain is usually considered as a warning signal of actual or potential tissue damage, pain can occur in the absence of tissue damage, even though the experience may be described as if the damage has occurred.

The most widely accepted and clinically useful definition of pain, however, was developed by a leading nursing expert on pain, Margo McCaffery (1968), who wrote (p. 95):

> Pain is whatever the experiencing person says it is, existing whenever he says it does.

In evolutionary terms, *acute pain* can be understood as an important biological protective mechanism to warn the body of injury or disease. It directs immediate attention to the situation, promotes reflexive withdrawal and fosters other actions that prevent further damage and enhance healing. Acute pain usually stops long before healing has occurred, which may take days or a few weeks.

In contrast, *chronic pain* persists constantly or intermittently past the normal time of healing and serves no biological purpose. It refers to pain that persists for extended periods of time (i.e. months or years), that accompanies a disease process, or that is associated with an injury that has not resolved within an expected time (Turk & Melzack, 2011). The mechanisms underlying the transition from acute to chronic pain include a complex interaction of physiological, emotional, cognitive, social and environmental factors. One of the most salient contributors to the pathophysiology of chronic pain is the neuroplasticity of the nervous system which refers to the ability of neurons throughout the peripheral and central nervous systems to change their structure and function because of nociceptive input. Recognising that chronic pain is perpetuated by factors that are both pathogenetically and physically remote from the originating cause, Siddall and Cousins (2004) have argued that chronic pain should be recognised as a disease entity in its own right.

Although pain problems are often classified by duration, another approach is to categorise pain problems based on underlying mechanisms. *Nociceptive* (physiological) pain is sustained by ongoing activation of the sensory system that subserves the perception of noxious stimuli. It implies the existence of damage to somatic or visceral tissues sufficient to activate the nociceptive system (Pasero & McCaffery, 2011). *Neuropathic* (pathophysiological) pain is sustained by a set of mechanisms that is driven by damage to, or dysfunction of, the peripheral or central nervous systems (Pasero & McCaffery, 2011). Neuropathic pain problems are common in diseases affecting the nervous system such as multiple sclerosis, diabetes mellitus and herpes zoster. It may also result from surgery or trauma to nervous tissue.

THE SCOPE AND IMPACT OF CHRONIC PAIN

Chronic pain is a major health problem in our communities that exacts a substantial social and economic burden on both the affected individual and society. Blyth and colleagues' (2001) seminal Australian prevalence study ($n = 17543$) found that approximately one in five people experience chronic pain (defined as pain experienced every day for 3 months in the 6 months prior to interview), with an overall prevalence of 17.1% for men and 20% for women. These findings are consistent with international data. For example, a World Health Organization (WHO) survey of primary care patients in 15 countries reported that 22% of patients reported persistent pain (Gureje, 1998).

The MBF Foundation report *The High Price of Pain,* conducted by Access Economics (2007) using epidemiological data from the University of Sydney Pain Management Research Institute, estimated that around 3.2 million Australians (1.4 million men and 1.7 million women) experience chronic pain (not including children or adolescents). This is projected to increase to 5 million by 2050 as Australia's population ages. The economic impact of chronic pain on the Australian community is also significant — costing approximately $34.3 billion annually, or $10 847 per person with chronic pain — making it the nation's third most costly health problem (Access Economics, 2007).

For most of those affected, the presence of chronic pain compromises all aspects of their lives and the lives of their significant others. It is a major cause of physical and psychosocial disability, leading to loss of employment, interference with daily activities, emotional distress and depression and social isolation from family and friends (Dworkin & Breitbart, 2004). Enduring pain can create a sense of hopelessness and helplessness, increasing the risk of suicide (Tang & Crane, 2006). Wallis's (2005) words capture the pervasive impact of chronic pain (p. 46):

> Chronic pain is a thief. It breaks into your body and robs you blind. With lightning fingers, it can take away your livelihood, your marriage, your friends, your favourite pastimes and big chunks of your personality. Left unapprehended, it will steal your days and your nights until the world has collapsed into a cramped cell of suffering.

The increasing burden of pain and resources devoted to its treatment, as well as the growing insight by clinicians that pain affects the person as a whole, has seen the rapid development of a large body of literature on pain and quality of life (QOL). Niv and Kreitler's (2001) comprehensive review of this broad area of research draws several key conclusions about the impact of pain on QOL. The first and major conclusion supported by a great number of studies is that pain has a significant adverse effect on QOL. This effect is very strong and exists despite different kinds of pain, diseases, cultures and individuals. Second, the effect is pervasive and is manifested in many domains of life. The domains most affected are the physical, followed by the emotional, social and cognitive functioning. Third, the degree and kind of impact on QOL was shown to depend on features of pain such as its duration, intensity, present activation and salience of affective and evaluative components, as well as on the disease that contributes to modulating the meaning of the pain and on characteristics of the patients themselves, demographic and psychological.

Given the evidence cited here about the scope and impact of chronic pain, it might be expected that pain would be well treated. Unfortunately, this is not the case. In the Australian context, Cousins (2012) provides evidence that pain has long been underestimated by health professionals and sufferers poorly served and stigmatised by previous healthcare approaches which have lagged behind the advances and recommendations of the time. Part of the problem, Cousins suggests, has been the absence of data on the prevalence of pain and the associated costs of treatment which have conspired to make pain almost invisible as a national health priority.

It is also particularly difficult for people with chronic pain to obtain effective care and support because chronic pain is poorly understood by the general community, including many health professionals. The growing evidence base and theoretical insights into chronic pain have been translated into practice with limited success across the healthcare system. The next section deals with these important conceptual issues.

UNDERSTANDING CHRONIC PAIN SECONDARY TO DISABILITY

Over the past half-century researchers have developed several theoretical perspectives of chronic pain (see e.g. Novy, Nelson, Francis, & Turk, 1995) and there is an extensive literature examining the utility of these models. Much of this work, however, has focused on individuals suffering from chronic non-malignant pain as a primary condition (e.g. chronic low back pain, headaches). In contrast, very little has been written about the experience of chronic pain secondary to a disabling disease, despite pain being a prominent characteristic of many chronic diseases and its potential to compound distress and disability (Ehde et al., 2003). This is particularly the case for rehabilitation populations such as people with multiple sclerosis, spinal cord injury and cerebral palsy. Little is known, for example, about how pain contributes to disability, distress and QOL in these populations. Few studies have examined the psychosocial aspects of pain in these groups. Only relatively recently have researchers begun to explore the utility of psychological approaches to chronic pain conditions related to chronic diseases such as arthritis, cancer and sickle cell disease (Keefe, Abernethy, & Campbell, 2005).

A major contributor to the current state is the failure of the prevailing biomedical model of pain to provide an adequate conceptualisation of chronic pain complicating disability. Although the dominant theoretical model in the chronic pain literature is a biopsychosocial model, most health professionals and lay persons continue to view disability-related pain from a traditional biomedical model (Keefe et al., 2005). According to this view, chronic pain is a symptom of underlying disease activity that can be treated only by identifying and correcting underlying tissue pathology. Psychological and social factors are viewed as reactions to pain such that once the underlying disease is successfully treated, the associated psychosocial complications will disappear. While this model has proved useful in producing a number of important insights into pathophysiological mechanisms and the development of pharmacological treatments for clinical pain, it falls short when faced with the complexity of chronic pain (Turk & Flor, 1999).

Investigators' loyalty to the biomedical model can in part be attributed to the prevalent assumption that chronic pain secondary to chronic illness and disability is uniquely different to chronic pain as a primary condition. The putative distinction between these conditions implies that, since they are unique, the principles that are important to each differ and thus they should be viewed and treated differently. This distinction is based primarily on the belief that disability-related pain is closely tied to disease activity or tissue damage, whereas the association between reports of pain and tissue damage in people with chronic pain as a primary condition is of lower magnitude and, in some cases, largely nonexistent. Thus, researchers concerned with disability-related pain have attempted to explain it in terms of disease activity and pathological pain mechanisms. Conversely, in the literature on chronic pain as a primary condition, greater attention is given to the role of psychosocial and environmental contributors to pain. These divergent literatures reflect the theoretical perspectives of researchers based on the presumed aetiology of chronic pain.

Consistent with this view, Campbell and colleagues (2003, p. 400) point to the fundamentally different assumptions relating to pain based on its putative aetiology. They maintain that, in disease-related pain:

> ... persistent pain is believed to be more strongly linked to peripheral factors, psychosocial factors are considered to be less important and treatments that primarily alter peripheral, nociceptive input are often effective.

Yet where chronic pain is the primary condition, they assert that (p. 401):

> ... persistent pain is believed to be more strongly linked to changes in the central nervous system, psychosocial factors are considered to play a major role and psychopharmacological treatments that alter depression are often effective in pain management.

Clinical approaches to the treatment of disability-related pain also reflect the dominance of a biomedical paradigm. The literature demonstrates that health professionals have tended to focus on physical modalities of treatment to the exclusion of psychosocial interventions (Ehde & Jensen, 2004; Keefe et al., 2005). Conventional methods of pain management consist of empirically-based pharmacological, surgical and other physical interventions aimed at eliminating the cause of the pain. Medical interventions alone, however, often fail to effectively treat individuals with chronic pain and carry with them the potential for iatrogenic complications (Turk, Wilson, & Cahana, 2011).

Recognising that chronic pain and disability are not only influenced by tissue pathology but also by psychological and social factors, multidisciplinary interventions for chronic pain have become more accepted with various comprehensive approaches and have rapidly increased in number over the last few decades. There is strong evidence that multidisciplinary pain programs which attend to the role of psychosocial contributors to pain are effective in populations where chronic pain is the primary condition (Gatchel & Okifuji, 2006). What has not been argued so cogently, however, is that even when a disease process is identifiable and treatable, psychosocial factors remain central to the development and perpetuation of chronic pain and may provide fruitful targets for intervention. There is a notable absence of research examining the effectiveness of multidisciplinary pain programs for chronic disability-related pain.

It could be argued, therefore, that although over the past few decades a major paradigm shift has occurred in the conceptualisation of chronic pain from a biopsychosocial perspective, pain experienced by individuals with a disability continues to be understood largely from a traditional biomedical model, despite its inherent limitations. Instead, an integrative model of chronic pain which attends to the multiple physical, psychosocial and behavioural factors involved is a more useful perspective to guide the study, assessment and treatment of disability-related pain.

TOWARDS A BIOPSYCHOSOCIAL MODEL OF CHRONIC DISABILITY-RELATED PAIN

Despite the intuitive appeal of a biomedical conceptualisation of disability-related pain, the assumption that there exists a simple one-to-one relationship between tissue pathology and pain has been convincingly refuted in the general pain literature. Pain — regardless of its presumed aetiology — is always more than a simple sensation. It is a subjective, perceptual experience that involves the person as a whole. Disease or tissue injury is only one, albeit a significant, contributor to the experience of pain. Over time, it is far more likely that psychosocial and behavioural factors interact with tissue damage to influence adjustment to pain (Turk, 1996). Thus it is argued here that disability-related pain may best be viewed from a biopsychosocial perspective which seeks to incorporate the interrelationships among physical, psychological and social factors and the changes that occur among these relationships over time.

Biopsychosocial theorists draw attention to the distinction between disease and illness in understanding chronic pain (Gatchel, Peng, Peters, Fuchs, & Turk, 2007). Whereas the biomedical model has focused on disease, an objective, disruptive biological event caused by pathological, anatomic or physiological changes, the biopsychosocial model instead emphasises illness (Engel, 1977). Illness is defined as the human experience of symptoms and suffering, resulting in physical discomfort, emotional distress, functional limitations and psychosocial disruption (Larsen, 2013). It refers to how the individual, family members and the social network around them receive and respond to the consequences of the symptoms.

The distinction between disease and illness is analogous to that of nociception and pain (Gatchel et al., 2007). Nociception is a physiological phenomenon that involves activation of sensory transduction in nerves by thermal, mechanical or chemical energy impinging on specialised nerve endings. The nerves involved convey information about tissue damage to the CNS, but such sensations are not yet considered pain until they are subjected to higher order psychological and cognitive processing that involves appraisals. Hence, *nociception* is a sensory process with nociceptive stimuli *capable* of producing pain. *Pain*, however, is a subjective, perceptual experience that results from the nociceptive input and is modulated on a number of different levels in the CNS (Turk & Monarch, 2002). This conception of pain is consistent with the IASP definition of pain discussed earlier which

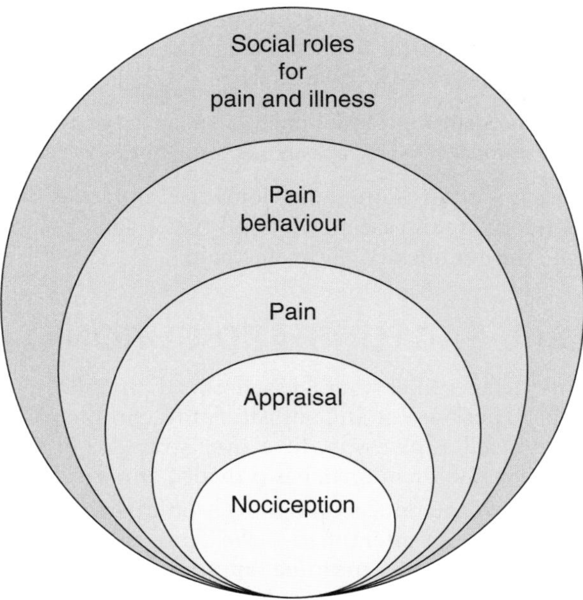

FIGURE 9.1 Biopsychosocial model of pain. *Note*: From Turk & Burwinkle (2006, p. 647).

highlights that nociception may be necessary for pain to occur, but it is not sufficient to account for pain as a clinical phenomenon, which is always a perceptual experience.

The biopsychosocial model thus focuses on the illness experience, attending to the multiple factors that both contribute to and are affected by pain. It builds on Melzack and Wall's (1965) gate-control theory of pain perception which focused primarily on the neurophysiology of pain by emphasising the influence of psychosocial and behavioural components of chronic pain. The conceptual view of the biopsychosocial model is presented in Figure 9.1. This nested circles model demonstrates the interdependent relationships among processes that culminate in the person's perception of pain and overt pain behaviours. For example, biological factors may initiate and maintain nociceptive input, psychological factors influence the appraisal and perception of pain and social factors shape the person's behavioural responses.

Several key assumptions characterise the biopsychosocial model of pain, as championed by Turk and colleagues (Turk, 1996; Turk & Flor, 1999). A central premise of the model is the multidimensional nature of chronic pain. From this perspective, pain is never solely somatically or psychologically based. Instead, the model posits that neurobiological, psychological and sociocultural factors interact to contribute to the development and perpetuation of pain. According to the model it is this dynamic and reciprocal interplay among biomedical, psychosocial and behavioural factors that produces the individual's subjective experience of, and responses to, pain. Nociceptive stimulation, for example, can cause biological, psychological and social changes that, in turn, affect future responses to pain. Moreover, psychological and social mechanisms can modulate nociceptive input and the response to treatment (Turk, 1996). The model also explicitly acknowledges that during the evolution of a pain problem, the relative weighting of physical, psychological and social factors may shift. Thus, although biomedical contributors may initiate the report of pain and predominate during the acute phase, over time psychosocial factors play an increasingly important role in the maintenance of and adjustment to pain (Turk, 1996).

In brief, the biopsychosocial conceptualisation of pain comprises three major elements: (1) integrated action; (2) reciprocal determinism; and (3) development and evolution (Turk, 1996). It holds that pain (Turk, 1996, p. 24):

> ... is a complex amalgam maintained by an interdependent set of biomedical, psychosocial, and behavioural factors, whose relationships are not static but evolve and change over time.

This can be contrasted with the dominant biomedical model of disability-related pain, whose emphasis on underlying disease activity and tissue damage alone is too narrow in scope to accommodate the complexity of chronic pain.

PSYCHOSOCIAL FACTORS AND CHRONIC PAIN

The biopsychosocial model identifies several psychosocial variables, in particular, as having a prominent role in the experience of and adjustment to chronic pain including attitudes and beliefs about pain as well as pain-specific coping strategies (Turk, 1996; Turk & Flor, 1999). Research on these variables, in turn, has provided empirical support for the model.

As active processors of information, people with chronic pain develop underlying beliefs, attitudes and assumptions in an attempt to make sense of their pain condition. These include attributions about the cause, meaning, appropriate treatment of pain, as well as perceptions of control over pain and personal coping efficacy (Thorn, 2004). Although certain beliefs may be adaptive and promote positive adjustment, others are likely to contribute to heightened pain, distress and disability. A large and growing body of research shows that pain-related beliefs are strongly associated with various measures of pain severity, physical and psychosocial functioning (Douglas, Wollin, & Windsor, 2008b; DeGood & Cook, 2011), as well as response and adherence to multidisciplinary pain treatments (Jensen, Turner, & Romano, 2007). For example, beliefs that one does not have control over pain, that pain signifies harm and that one is disabled by pain are particularly problematic for people with chronic pain; increases in self-efficacy beliefs for managing pain appears beneficial (Ehde & Jensen, 2010). These beliefs, appraisals and expectancies held by individuals regarding the possible consequences of pain and their abilities to deal with them are hypothesised to affect functioning directly by influencing mood as well as indirectly by influencing coping efforts (Jensen, Turner, Romano, & Karoly, 1991).

Faced with ongoing pain, individuals also learn and utilise a variety of strategies to help them cope or deal with their pain (Keefe, Rumble, Scipio, Giordano, & Perri, 2004). Pain coping is defined as purposeful cognitive and behavioural efforts to manage or negate the negative impact of pain (Jensen et al., 1991). Much of the pain literature broadly classifies coping strategies as active or passive. In general, studies have found active coping strategies (efforts to function in spite of pain or to distract oneself from pain, such as activity or ignoring pain) to be associated with adaptive functioning and passive coping strategies (withdrawal or surrendering control to an external source, such as resting or medication use) to be related to greater pain and depression (Boothby, Thorn, Stroud, & Jensen, 1999). Interestingly, although maladaptive strategies are strongly associated with negative outcomes, adaptive strategies generally show only modest correlations with positive outcomes (Geisser, Robinson, & Riley, 1999).

One specific maladaptive coping response that has consistently demonstrated robust associations with virtually all pain outcomes investigated is termed catastrophising. It refers to 'a method of cognitively coping with pain characterised by negative self-statements and overly negative thoughts and ideas about the future' (Keefe, Brown, Wallston, & Caldwell, 1989, p. 51). Greater endorsement of catastrophic thinking when in pain has been consistently associated with higher levels of pain, distress and disability among diverse populations (Ehde & Jensen, 2010; Keefe et al., 2004). Research findings concerning the relationship between other specific pain coping strategies and adjustment to chronic pain have been somewhat more inconsistent (Boothby et al., 1999). When significant associations are found, greater use of coping self-statements is generally related to positive adjustment, whereas hoping, pain-contingent rest and wishful thinking are frequently associated with greater dysfunction. Ignoring pain, reinterpreting pain and distraction/diverting attention in contrast, rarely predict functioning among people with chronic pain (Boothby et al., 1999).

Attention to the social environment is another important component of the biopsychosocial model, particularly perceived social support and the role of solicitous responses of significant others to pain. It draws on operant conditioning principles that emphasise the role that pain-contingent social responses such as solicitous responses to demonstrations of pain and disability (e.g. offers to take over tasks or encouragement to become less active) may play in the perpetuation of chronic pain. While perceived general social support has found to be associated with positive functioning among persons with chronic pain, solicitous responses to pain behaviours from spouses and family members tend to be associated with greater pain and disability (Kerns, Rosenberg, & Otis, 2002; Schwartz, Jensen & Romano, 2005).

Although there is a large body of evidence to support a biopsychosocial model in understanding and treating chronic pain as a primary condition, only recently have researchers begun to examine its utility among persons with disability-related pain. Jensen and colleagues' (2011) recent systematic review of psychosocial factors and adjustment to chronic disability-related pain identified 29 studies investigating these variables among people with spinal cord injury, acquired amputation, cerebral palsy, multiple sclerosis and muscular dystrophy. Strong and consistent associations between psychosocial factors and adjustment to pain were observed in all disability groups including: (1) catastrophising cognitions; (2) task persistence, guarding and resting coping responses; and (3) perceived social support and solicitous responding social factors. Pain-related beliefs were significantly associated with adjustment for all groups, except persons with acquired amputation. Consistent with the general pain literature, the belief that one can control pain and its effects was found to be associated with positive outcomes, whereas the beliefs that one is necessarily disabled by pain, others should be solicitous (and take care of the patient) when in pain and that pain is an indication of physical damage were associated with poorer adjustment. Taken together, these findings support the importance of psychosocial factors as significant predictors of pain and functioning in persons with physical disabilities. They also suggest the possibility that interventions targeting these variables would reduce the negative impact of chronic disability-related pain.

STIGMA AND CHRONIC PAIN

The broader social context of the individual also profoundly shapes the chronic pain experience. This is an understudied area of chronic pain, with few Australian studies on this topic (Nielsen, Foster, Henman & Strong, 2012; Tollefson, Usher & Foster, 2011). One of the most important social aspects from the perspective of people with chronic pain is the stigmatisation of chronic pain. Frequently the person with chronic pain faces not only the negative personal impact of pain, but also the potent social dilemma of not being believed or having their experience delegitimised by others. Indeed, it is the very nature of chronic pain — its invisibility, its subjectivity, its challenge to the biomedical paradigm — that is deeply problematic for the sufferer (Heshusius, 2009). Pain simply cannot be proved or disproved. In contrast to the visible manifestations of disease, pain is privately experienced, demonstrable to others only through the individual's self-report or other non-verbal pain behaviour. As one author with chronic pain explains so well (Heshusius, 2009, p. 14):

> We appear normal. That is our liability. One can wince and moan only for so long. There comes a point where giving expression to one's pain takes energy one no longer has. One becomes quiet and pain becomes internalised ... Also, wincing and moaning when in acute pain are instinctive behaviours to which others respond with sympathy. When it becomes clear the pain will not go away, others may feel helpless. They may start to think you are exaggerating. They may be overwhelmed. They change the subject. The person in pain withdraws. You try to keep your composure, to stay coherent, not fall apart. Others will see exhaustion and depression in your face before they see pain.

The invisibility and often lack of known physical basis for chronic pain frequently invites speculation and judgments from others about its legitimacy. In the past this has led to labelling of individuals as fraudulent when they claim pain over time for which there is no medical explanation. This stigma, attached to those who report pain without an identifiable pathological basis, occurs in part because their illness falls outside of the socially sanctioned biomedical model of healthcare (Jackson, 2005). If medicine is unable to identify and treat the pain, either the person may be seen to be exaggerating for secondary gain, or the pain is attributed to psychogenic causes. Cohen, Quintner, Buchanan, Nielsen and Guy (2011) call for health professionals to critically reflect on their own, often inadvertent, potential to contribute to the stigmatisation of people with chronic pain when they adopt this dualistic thinking inherent in the biomedical model of pain.

Interestingly, despite their known medical diagnosis, the stigma of chronic pain has also been found to be central to the pain experience of people with physical disabilities (Douglas, Windsor, & Wollin, 2008). In contrast to visible impairments, pain problems may be dismissed or discredited by friends, family, co-workers and others. People with physical disabilities are often particularly aware of the contested nature of their pain experience during encounters with healthcare providers (Douglas et al., 2008; Yorkston, Johnson, Boesflug, Skala, & Amtmann, 2010). From their perspective, pain is often trivialised by healthcare providers as a natural or expected part of their disease, or dismissed altogether. Over time, people with disabilities tend to keep pain hidden from others to avoid negative responses and the threat of stigma (Douglas et al., 2008; Dudgeon, Gerrard, Jensen, Rhodes, & Tyler, 2002).

In the clinical setting, pain problems may be overlooked among people with chronic illness and disability given the myriad of other symptoms experienced. However, clinicians should not discount the problem of pain in persons with other, more obvious impairments. It is important that clinicians acknowledge and validate the person's report of pain and allow enough time during interactions to discuss pain and pain-related concerns. Health professionals should also be cognisant that people with chronic disabling conditions may be reluctant to disclose or discuss their pain problems. Dudgeon and colleagues (2002) recommend that it may help some clients if the practitioner normalises pain by stressing that it is a common problem in people with physical disabilities. Chapter 5 also provides some excellent strategies to prevent stigma when working with people with chronic illness and disability.

Case Study 9.1 is a story of Paul's experience with chronic back pain taken from a phenomenological study of the experience of chronic illness in rural Australia (Tollefson et al., 2011). His was a long story of struggle for recognition and compensation. The story deals with trust, belief, self-stigma and emotions of fear and anger associated with chronic back pain.

CASE STUDY 9.1

Paul was on sickness benefits and had ceased work. He lived outside a regional city in Victoria and was booked in to have an operation in Melbourne. Before he was due to go to Melbourne the Department of Social Security sent him a letter, requiring him to present at the local office of the Department of Social Security on 9 April, which was a Friday. So, wanting everything to be right for the family while he was away, he went into the Department on the preceding Monday.

He was in the queue and recognised another man in the queue, whom he knew to be a 'bludger'. He wanted to appear different from this man but how could he? — his back pain was not obvious to those around him. Paul resigned himself to the fact that he and the man looked remarkably similar. 'I am here because I am sick,' he cried inwardly, with enough passion to make his heart race and his back ache.

He shuffled from side to side, trying to ease the pain. There were no chairs anywhere; he could not take a walk around because he would lose his place and have to start queuing all over again.

After over half an hour, which seemed an eternity, his turn came. He held his letter out to the clerk behind the glass-fronted counter and before he could open his mouth to give the prepared apology for presenting earlier than the day stipulated in the letter, it was snatched from his outstretched hand. It disappeared under the hole in the glass screen. The clerk glanced at the letter and with a resigned look on his face said in a singsong tone, 'This says to bring it in on Friday'.

'I know,' Paul replied mirroring his tone, 'but Friday is Good Friday. There won't be anyone here.' Paul knew he had irritated the man.

'Well, you can't bring it in today.'

'That is okay,' Paul said, 'when shall I bring it in?'

The clerk thought about this and said, 'Tuesday after.'

Now the frustration was beginning to well up inside Paul. He described it, 'The pain in my back was like two hard bricks pressing down, my stomach ached and my teeth were clenched.' He really wanted to cry but that was unthinkable — that, or reach through the glass hole and throttle his tormentor. People were shifting in the queue behind Paul. He explained that he was going away to Melbourne on Sunday.

'Well, take it to an office in Melbourne,' the clerk responded.

'I will be in hospital,' Paul replied. 'Gotcha!' he thought. 'Can I bring it here on Thursday?' he asked.

'No,' was the clerk's belligerent reply.

Paul asked for the manager but there was not one. He tried asking for the clerk's name but he would not give it to him. Paul felt that the people in the queue were enjoying the scene; he had to give up but before he did so he clenched his fist tightly and shot it towards the clerk's jaw. Stopping just at the glass, he opened both hands and placed them flat on the glass which divided them. The man looked scared and Paul was ashamed, defeated, disgusted and so angry. His hands slipped slowly down the glass and dejectedly he walked to his rickety old ute for the 20 km jolting journey through the bush with nothing to offer his family.

The concept of legitimation is bound up with trust. Challenges in patient-provider interactions in the management of chronic pain in primary care have been identified, including insufficient knowledge of pain management, time constraints, differing goals and attitudes concerning treatment, and debate surrounding the use of opioids for chronic pain (Frantsve & Kerns, 2007; Matthias et al., 2010). Specialist multidisciplinary pain management services have arisen over the past four decades to support general practitioners (GPs) in the care of individuals with chronic pain. Yet Hogg and colleagues' (2012) Australian survey found there are long waiting times for an initial appointment at many publicly funded pain management services, with a median wait of 150 days, and several services reported a waiting time of over a year. By comparison, of the 20% of the population reporting chronic pain, less than 0.2% will gain access to a specialist service in any given year. For Australians living outside capital cities, the proportion who gain access is even lower (Hogg, Gibson, Helou, DeGabriele, & Farrel, 2012).

Indeed, it was many years after Paul first sought medical attention for his chronic back pain that a diagnosis was eventually made and surgery offered as a last resort. However, to retain the person's trust, health professionals need to be seen to be exploring all options to find a diagnosis and treatment. This eventually adds to the financial burden of chronic pain and demoralisation as a diagnosis and cure remains elusive. If a cure or full explanation of the pain is unavailable, people search through their own lives to come up with some sort of explanation for the pain. Accidents, hereditary weaknesses, childhood illnesses and normal ageing are used to give meaning to the pain within the person's life (Richardson, Ong, & Sim, 2006).

Much of the care of those who live with chronic pain falls onto the person with pain and their family. Community nurses, GPs and, where available, the heath professionals in specialised pain clinics are increasingly recognising the need for supportive and educative models of care for people with chronic pain in the community so that they do not feel they are reliant on services that are not readily available or do not exist. People who live in rural and remote areas often have to rely on the very limited resources of the healthcare system in their area, as travel is often too traumatic and expensive to contemplate (Tollefson & Usher, 2006). People who live with chronic pain are also occasionally admitted to hospital or will present at community health centres or general practices for conditions other than their chronic pain. Chronic pain will complicate their treatment requiring all health professionals to have an understanding of chronic pain.

CULTURAL DETERMINANTS OF THE EXPERIENCE OF CHRONIC PAIN

Culture is significant in shaping beliefs about pain, in dictating acceptable pain behaviour and giving meaning to the pain experience. Thus culture affects the individual's perception, report and expression of pain. Pain assessment and management strategies put in place can easily fail if cultural considerations are not addressed between the individual and health professional. For example, some important pain cues for central Australian Aboriginal people that may be misinterpreted by non-Indigenous health professionals during pain assessment include: silence, physically lying on their side with eyes averted, feigning sleep (using 'centring' to control the pain experience), head turned away or hiding their head/body under a blanket on questioning, a slight upward nod of the head with downcast eyes when asked if in pain and the whispered response 'paining, Sister' (Fenwick, 2006; Fenwick & Stevens, 2004).

There is a paucity of research examining the pain experience of Australian Aboriginal and Torres Strait Islander people. McGrath's (2006) qualitative study in Australia's

Northern Territory explored issues associated with pain management for rural and remote Aboriginal peoples. A key finding was the importance of those involved in pain management being aware of the complexity of cultural relationship rules that determine who should and should not be directly involved in providing physical care. It also found that Aboriginal peoples may have a higher threshold of pain and are less likely to report pain, especially the men, who do not wish to appear weak. Pain management is influenced by the cultural concerns of 'pay back' and 'blame'. There is also a mistrust of mainstream medicine, stemming from a lack of understanding of clinical notions of pain relief, fear of the administration, side effects and ramifications of medications, and fear that Western pain medications will speed up the dying process and inhibit the passing on of traditional knowledge and secrets that occurs during end-of-life. Developing relationships built on trust between health professionals and Aboriginal peoples is reported as the most important strategy for overcoming such fears.

Davidhizar and Giger's (2004) review of the literature on caring for people in pain from diverse cultural backgrounds recommends several key strategies to assist in culturally appropriate assessment and management, namely: (1) utilising assessment tools to assist in measuring pain; (2) appreciating variations in affective response to pain; (3) being sensitive to variations in communication styles; (4) recognising that communication of pain may not be acceptable within a culture; (5) appreciating that the meaning of pain varies between cultures; (6) utilising the knowledge of biological variations; and (7) developing a personal awareness of values and beliefs that may affect responses to pain. This last recommendation is particularly important. Fenwick (2006) suggests that non-Indigenous nurses working within rich cultural environments need to listen to Indigenous people and respect the differences that exist. Health professionals need to adopt culturally safe pain assessment strategies and wherever possible defer to the person with chronic pain or their family and friends for cultural interpretations. Wherever possible, help should be sought from professionals with inside understanding of cultural norms; an obvious example is Indigenous health workers in Australia.

ASSESSMENT OF CHRONIC PAIN

A biopsychosocial assessment of chronic pain is the key to developing an effective management plan. Assessment begins with a comprehensive pain history (using the PQRST mnemonic) including provoking/palliative factors, quality, region (location) and radiation, severity and temporal pattern (onset, duration, pattern) for each individual pain problem. Evaluation of psychosocial factors such as pain beliefs and coping strategies, mood and social interactions is undertaken. Assessment of the impact of pain on functioning and QOL is also an essential component to direct treatment. Finally, a physical assessment should be completed focusing on neurological and musculoskeletal body systems.

This section provides only a brief introduction to some key pain assessment tools. For a comprehensive review of chronic pain assessment please refer to Turk and Melzack's (2011) excellent text.

Pain rating scales

Pain intensity — a quantitative estimate of the severity or magnitude of perceived pain — is without a doubt the most salient dimension of pain and a variety of pain rating scales have been developed to measure it. Most of these tools are highly correlated with each other and therefore they can be used in most situations (Jensen & Karoly, 2011). What is important is that the assessment tool is selected based on the individual's needs (e.g.

developmental, cognitive, language and cultural factors) with consideration of the particular strengths and weaknesses of each tool.

The numerical rating scale (NRS) is the most widely used measure of pain intensity in clinical practice. A NRS asks the client to rate their pain from 0 to 10 (an 11-point scale) or 0 to 100 (a 101-point scale), with the understanding that the 0 represents one end of the pain intensity continuum ('no pain') and the 10 or 100 represents the other extreme of pain intensity ('pain as bad as it can be'). Clients simply state or circle the number on written versions of the scale that best represents their pain intensity by asking: 'On a scale of 0 to 10, with 0 being no pain and 10 being the worst possible pain you could imagine, where would you rate the pain you are experiencing right now?' The reliability and validity of the NRS is well established (Jensen & Karoly, 2011) and is easily administered. Based on their review of measures, Pasero and McCaffery (2011) recommend a combined NRS and faces scale as the preferred pain rating scale in most clinical settings.

A verbal descriptor scale (VDS) simply consists of a list of adjectives describing different levels of pain intensity. Clients are asked to read over the list of descriptors and choose the word that best describes their pain intensity on the scale. A simple and clinically useful example is no pain, mild, moderate and severe pain (scored numerically from 0 to 3).

The visual analogue scale (VAS) consists of a 10 cm horizontal line, representing a continuum of pain intensity, with verbal descriptors at each end (e.g. 'no pain' to 'pain as bad as it can be' or 'worst possible pain'). The client is asked to indicate which point along the line best represents their pain intensity. The distance measured from the 'no pain' end to the mark made by the client is the pain intensity score. The VAS is commonly used in research as a measure of pain intensity.

The faces pain scale is another tool that was originally developed for children but has been found to be useful and popular among adults, especially those with cognitive or communication difficulties. Facial pain scales include cartoon faces (e.g. Wong-Baker FACES Pain Rating Scale; Wong & Baker, 1988), hand-drawn realistic depictions (e.g. The Faces Pain Scale — Revised; Hicks, von Baeyer, Spafford, van Korlaar & Goodenough, 2001) and photographs of actual children in distress (e.g. Oucher Scale; Beyer, Denyes, & Villarruel, 1992). The Wong-Baker FACES pain rating scale, for example, contains 6 cartoon faces (from 'smiling' to 'crying') and is recommended for persons aged 3 years and older. An explanation is given to the client that each face is a person who feels happy because he has no pain (hurt) or sad because he has some or a lot of pain. Instructions are read to the client and they are asked to choose the face that best describes their pain intensity.

Quality

Unidimensional measures of pain intensity alone do not capture the other qualitative aspects of pain. Asking the client to describe the quality of their pain using their own words is important. Providing a list of possible descriptors can sometimes be helpful if clients find it difficult to do this.

Although used more for research than clinical practice, the McGill Pain Questionnaire (MPQ) (Melzack, 1975) provides a measure of the sensory, affective and evaluative aspects of the pain experience, based on the gate-control theory. It consists of 78 pain descriptors which are categorised into 20 groups evaluating the major dimensions of pain quality. Clients are read each list of descriptors and may select one word from each group if applicable to their pain. Each of the 78 words has been assigned a rank value within its group. From this data, it is possible to derive a Pain Rating Index (PRI) for the sensory, affective, evaluative and miscellaneous subscales, as well as a total PRI (Melzack, 1975). The psychometric properties of the MPQ have been well established and the MPQ is often utilised as a gold standard against which to validate pain measures (Katz & Melzack, 2011).

The types of words chosen can also provide valuable information about the underlying pain mechanisms. For example, it has been demonstrated clinically that individuals with neuropathic pain are significantly more likely to use particular sensory adjectives (e.g. electric-shock, burning, tingling, cold, pricking and itching) to describe their pain. A Short-Form MPQ (Melzack, 1987) has been developed and recently expanded and revised as the Short-Form MPQ–2 (Dworkin et al., 2009), capable of discriminating neuropathic and non-neuropathic pain. Other specifically designed measures such as the Neuropathic Pain Scale (Galer & Jensen, 1997) can be useful when a neuropathic component is suspected.

Onset and duration

Information should be elicited about the onset, duration and pattern of pain. When did the pain begin? How long has it lasted? Does it occur at the same time each day? How often does it recur? Is it intermittent or constant?

Location

To assess pain location, the client is asked to describe or point to all areas of discomfort. Pain sites can be documented on a body diagram. A pain drawing consists of outline drawings of the human body, front and back, on which the participant indicates the location of pain by shading the painful area (see Case Study 9.2).

Exacerbating/relieving factors

The client is asked to describe provoking factors, such as physical movement or position, certain activities or environmental factors. For example, with a ruptured intervertebral disc, the low back pain and radiation down the leg is usually aggravated by bending over or lifting objects. When exacerbating factors are identified, it is easier to plan interventions to prevent pain from occurring or worsening.

People with chronic pain have usually tried a number of pain management techniques so it is informative to know whether the client has found effective ways of relieving pain, including drug and non-drug pain management techniques. These strategies can then be incorporated into the management plan if appropriate.

Impact of pain

An assessment of the impact of pain on QOL domains is particularly useful to determine treatment priorities. Several pain assessment instruments incorporate most of the relevant questions and can help standardise pain assessment. The Brief Pain Inventory (BPI; Cleeland, 1989), for example, is a widely used measure of pain severity and interference for clinical and research purposes (see Figure 9.2). It is relatively short, easy for patients to complete and is sensitive to changes in pain over time or in response to treatment. The BPI scale assesses the extent to which pain interferes with mood, walking, general activity, work, relations with other people, sleep and enjoyment of life. Using validated, brief screening tools such as the BPI is useful for identifying problems which can then be more comprehensively assessed by the nurse and/or referred for specialist assessment and management.

Brief Pain Inventory

Date___ /___ /___ Time: ________

Name:__________ __________ __________
Last First Middle Initial

1) Throughout our lives, most of us have had pain from time to time (such as minor headaches, sprains and toothaches). Have you had pain other than these everyday kinds of pain today?
1. Yes 2. No

2) On the diagram, shade in the areas where you feel pain. Put an X on the area that hurts the most.

Right Left Left Right

3) Please rate your pain by circling the one number that best describes your pain at its **worst** in the past 24 hours.

0 1 2 3 4 5 6 7 8 9 10
No pain — Pain as bad as you can imagine

4) Please rate your pain by circling the one number that best describes your pain at its **least** in the past 24 hours.

0 1 2 3 4 5 6 7 8 9 10
No pain — Pain as bad as you can imagine

5) Please rate your pain by circling the one number that best describes your pain on the **average.**

0 1 2 3 4 5 6 7 8 9 10
No pain — Pain as bad as you can imagine

6) Please rate your pain by circling the one number that tells how much pain you have **right now.**

0 1 2 3 4 5 6 7 8 9 10
No pain — Pain as bad as you can imagine

7) What treatments or medications are you receiving for your pain?

____

____

8) In the past 24 hours, how much **relief** have pain treatments or medications provided? Please circle the one percentage that most shows how much relief you have received.

0% 10 20 30 40 50 60 70 80 90 100%
No relief — Complete relief

9) Circle the one number that describes how, during the past 24 hours, pain has **interfered** with your:

A. General activity

0 1 2 3 4 5 6 7 8 9 10
Does not interfere — Completely interferes

B. Mood

0 1 2 3 4 5 6 7 8 9 10
Does not interfere — Completely interferes

C. Walking ability

0 1 2 3 4 5 6 7 8 9 10
Does not interfere — Completely interferes

D. Normal work (includes both work outside the home and housework)

0 1 2 3 4 5 6 7 8 9 10
Does not interfere — Completely interferes

E. Relations with other people

0 1 2 3 4 5 6 7 8 9 10
Does not interfere — Completely interferes

F. Sleep

0 1 2 3 4 5 6 7 8 9 10
Does not interfere — Completely interferes

G. Enjoyment of life

0 1 2 3 4 5 6 7 8 9 10
Does not interfere — Completely interferes

FIGURE 9.2 Brief Pain Inventory. *Note*: From: Pasero & McCaffery (2011, Form 3-2, p. 53).

Pain diaries

Pain diaries are also effective tools to assess the peaks and troughs of pain, identify triggers and to determine the effectiveness of treatments (see Figure 9.3). A common problem is that people fail to fill them out or complete them just before an appointment 'for the nurse'. The client and family should receive explanations of the purpose of using the pain diary, along with information about how and when to complete the diary. The discussion also helps the nurse to establish the degree to which the person is committed to collecting the information.

There is increasing clinical and research interest in the use of electronic pain diaries (e.g. digital pens, palmtop computers, mobile phones) to improve compliance and satisfaction. Research thus far suggests electronic pain assessment measures are preferable compared with traditional paper and pencil measures, yet there are some notable barriers such as cost, hardware and software requirements, concerns about confidentiality, respondent burden and modifying the behaviour of clients and providers (Marceau, Smith, & Jamison, 2011). Further research is needed to examine the effectiveness of electronic pain assessment over and above standard practices.

MANAGEMENT OF CHRONIC PAIN

People with chronic pain generally refer themselves to GPs who now act as agents for a broad range of conventional and complementary specialists to manage chronic pain. The majority of nurses become involved in the care of people with chronic pain when it affects function or psychological wellbeing to such an extent that independence in activities of living or self-care needs are adversely affected. These nurses take a supportive and educative role to enable people with chronic pain to adopt positive self-management strategies that maximise their independence.

There are nurse practitioners who specifically work with people who are referred to pain clinics and there are specialist nurses who work with people with conditions that are particularly associated with chronic pain, for example people with cancer and specialists in oncology nursing, or people with long-term angina and specialists in cardiac rehabilitation nursing. These nurses work in multidisciplinary teams and have extended knowledge of chronic pain and skills in the assessment, therapy and evaluation of pain management. While nurses play a critical role, the management of chronic pain is essentially in the hands of individuals and support for them comes from a range of health professionals whose roles can overlap to a large degree in the offering and delivery of a person-centred philosophy of healthcare service. People with chronic pain and their families are the primary managers of chronic pain — including that caused by cancer — as treatment has shifted from the hospital to the outpatient department or GP surgery to the home.

While many of the specific treatment options for chronic pain are outlined below, there are some important generic principles of practice that are relevant to all health professionals working with people with chronic pain. Unruh and Harman (2002) provide an excellent discussion of these guiding principles which are summarised in Box 9.1. The reader is encouraged to reflect on their past experience of working with clients with chronic pain as a health professional or student — or perhaps personal experience of pain and interaction with health professionals — and consider how these principles might facilitate therapeutic intervention.

Effective communication and a trusting relationship are fundamental to helping the person in pain to achieve their goals. It is vital for nurses to give opportunities for people to talk about their pain and pain-related concerns, validate their experiences and provide

Pain Control Diary: Patient Example

This is a record of how your pain medicines are working. Please keep this record until you and your nurse/doctor find the dose and frequency of medicine that provides satisfactory pain relief for you most of the time. After that, you only need to keep this record when you have problems related to your pain medicines.

Name: *Martin* Date: *Friday*

GOALS Satisfactory pain rating: *3* Activities: *sleep through the night; walk around the house*

Analgesics: *ibuprofen 400 mg 8 am, 2 pm, 8 pm; duloxetine 30 mg 8 am, 8 pm; MS Contin 100 mg 8 am, 8 pm; MSIR 30 mg every 2 hours if needed*

My pain rating scale:

0 1 2 3 4 5 6 7 8 9 10

0 = No pain; 5 = Moderate pain; 10 = Worst possible pain

Directions: Rate your pain before you take pain medicine and 1 to 2 hours later.

Time	Pain Rating	Pain Medicine I Took	Side Effects (drowsy? upset stomach?)	Other
12:15 am	*6*	*30 MSIR*	*No*	
3	*6*	*30 MSIR*		*can't sleep*
5:15	*6*	*30 MSIR*		
8	*6*	*30 MSIR* *+ ibaprofen* *+ MS Contin 100 mg* *+ dulonetine*		*staying in bed*
10	*5*			*talk with nurse*
10:30	*6*	*MSIR 45 mg* *MS Contin 30 mg*		
12:30 pm	*3*			*planning to nap*

If pain is greater than *5*, or if you have other problems with your pain medicine, call:

Nurse: Name/phone *C. Adams 555-1234*

Doctor: Name/phone *Janes 555-4321*

FIGURE 9.3 Pain diary. *Note*: From Pasero & McCaffery (2011, Form 3-11, pp. 116–17).

CASE STUDY 9.2

The following case study is an example of a nursing assessment of an individual with chronic disability-related pain drawn from research on the impact of pain on the quality of life of people with multiple sclerosis (Douglas et al., 2009).

History

Mrs L is a 41-year-old married woman living in south-east Queensland, who presents with worsening pain in her hands. She has secondary progressive multiple sclerosis diagnosed 2 years ago. Mrs L was employed as an office worker, but was unable to continue working because of increasing pain and fatigue.

Mrs L reports pain and fatigue as her worst MS-related problems. She has minor difficulties with memory and speech. There is some upper extremity involvement with difficulty with zips, handling small coins and washing her hair. She also reports bladder incontinence and sexual dysfunction.

Current medications for pain include Avonex® (interferon beta-1a), Zoloft® (sertraline) and Neurontin® (gabapentin).

Pain characteristics

- Using a 0–10 numerical rating scale Mrs L reported her pain was 2/10 on assessment. Over the past 2 weeks Mrs L rates her pain as 10/10 at its worst, 2/10 at its least and 8/10 on average.
- Mrs L indicated she experiences pain in both hands and right leg, shown on the pain drawings below.
- She completed the McGill Pain Questionnaire and endorsed the following: sensory descriptors were flickering, shooting, lancinating, cramping, searing, hurting and taut; affective descriptors were exhausting, terrifying, punishing and wretched; evaluative descriptor chosen was unbearable; miscellaneous descriptors chosen were radiating, numb, freezing and torturing.
- She describes the pain as constant over the past year and a half.
- Provoking factors identified were heat, stress and friction. She manages her pain best by controlling the temperature (keeping cool) and avoiding stress.

Psychosocial responses to pain

- On the Pain Beliefs and Perceptions Inventory, Mrs L endorses beliefs about pain constancy and pain permanence, but scores low on beliefs about self-blame or that pain is a mystery.
- The Coping Strategies Questionnaire was administered and scores demonstrate frequent use of catastrophising, praying/hoping and ignoring pain, low scores for coping self-statements or increasing behavioural activities and no use of reinterpreting pain or diverting attention.
- Her perceived self-efficacy was low with perceived control over pain scored as 1/6 and ability to decrease pain 2/6 on the CSQ.

Impact of pain

- Mrs L completed the Brief Pain Inventory pain interference scales (0 = does not interfere, 10 = completely interferes) indicating: mood 5/10, walking 0/10, general activity 8/10, work 10/10, relations with other people 3/10, sleep 3/10 and enjoyment of life 5/10.

CASE STUDY 9.2 — cont'd

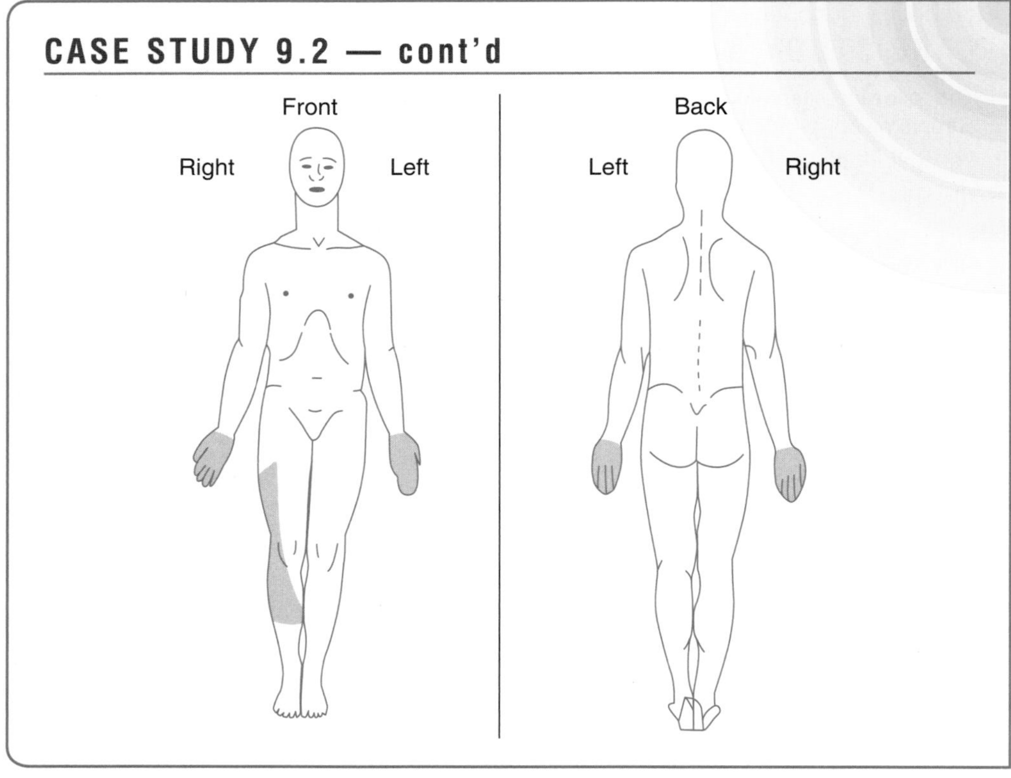

BOX 9.1
Generic principles of practice

Note: From Unruh & Harman (2002), Box 8.2, p. 152.

- Believe the client's description of her or his pain and suffering.
- Treat acute pain aggressively.
- Always assess the client's pain and its impact on daily life before planning intervention.
- Avoid 'leaps to the head' to explain the client's pain.
- Determine whether the primary goal of intervention is pain reduction or improvement in function.
- Incorporate evidence-based decision-making into practice.
- Combine medical, pharmacological, cognitive behavioural, occupational and physical strategies.
- Understand and correct misconceptions about the use of pain medication and addiction risks.
- Recognise that a positive response to a cognitive behavioural intervention does not mean that the client's pain has a psychological cause.
- Help the client to make long-term lifestyle changes.
- Involve the client's family whenever possible.
- Recognise dual responsibilities and obligations.
- Create a positive therapeutic milieu.
- Conduct an ethical practice.
- Participate in research, education and professional pain associations.

interventions that enable self-management. Good communication with the multidisciplinary team and mutual respect for their specialist contributions is also essential. Developing a trusting, therapeutic relationship with the person involves accepting the person's report of pain, actively listening, displaying empathy and using effective verbal and non-verbal communication skills.

Education about the illness, its manifestations, diagnostic studies and the treatment regimen can assist to diminish anxiety, reduce stress and assist the person to cope with ongoing pain, self-manage the pain, enhance feelings of control and adhere to the treatment plan (Richardson, Adams, & Poole, 2006). As always, it is important to evaluate the person's knowledge levels before starting. Partners, friends and lay carers are important players in the management of chronic pain and can assist the person with chronic pain by supporting their coping strategies and not undermining their skills. This support is encouraged when the partners are included in the pain management education and they are supported to learn the principles of self-management. Close communication about the pain experience between partners is supportive (Newton-John & Williams, 2006). Negative impacts on the relationship include friction between the partners, resentment, decrease in intimacy and ultimately erosion of the relationship, which can end in separation and divorce (Sofaer-Bennett, Holloway et al., 2007). Sofaer-Bennett, Walker et al. (2007) also found that personal friendships wane as pain interferes with visiting, social outings and movement. Holidays become a pleasure of the past, and planned activities are frequently cancelled due to pain.

Management should be directed towards addressing the impact of pain on QOL domains affected, particularly mood and sleep. People with chronic pain are often depressed and there is evidence that treatment with antidepressants and psychological therapies can be effective (Holmes, Christelis, & Arnold, 2012). Sleep disturbance is also frequently a problem, contributing to irritability and difficulty with relationships (Call-Schmidt & Richardson, 2003). Sleep promotion interventions such as teaching the individual and partner about the need for stimulus control, progressive muscle relaxation and sleep hygiene measures are the first-line management strategies. Sleep hygiene measures include establishing a sleep routine, environmental control, limiting caffeine and alcohol (and, for some, fluids) during the evening, establishing the bedroom as a sleep room (not for reading, working or hobbies), physical comfort (temperature, perhaps a warm bath just prior to bedtime, planning analgesia so the effects are peaking at the time of falling asleep) and promoting relaxation. If these are ineffective, the assistance of the multidisciplinary team must be sought for such additional measures as hypnotic medication, biofeedback and cognitive behavioural therapy (Zelman, Brandenberg, & Gore, 2006).

TREATMENT OPTIONS

Treatment options for chronic pain broadly include: pharmacological approaches; interventional techniques including nerve blocks, surgery, implantable drug-delivery systems and spinal-cord stimulators; exercise and physical rehabilitation; psychological treatments; interdisciplinary treatment; and complementary and alternative treatments. It is beyond the scope of this chapter to provide a detailed discussion of each of these treatments and the reader should consult recent reviews by Turk, Wilson and Cahana (2011) and Portenoy (2011) on the management of chronic non-cancer and cancer pain. Based on their comprehensive review, Turk and others draw the sobering conclusion that overall, present treatment options for chronic non-cancer pain result in modest improvements at best. Given these findings management should include dialogue with the client about realistic expectations of pain relief and a need to bring the focus to improvement of function.

Management often necessitates use of a blend of different approaches based on the individual's response to treatment.

Analgesics

There are three classes of analgesics: non-opioids (paracetamol, non-steroidal anti-inflammatory drugs [NSAIDs]), opioids and adjuvant drugs. The WHO analgesic pain ladder is a well-known treatment model developed for people with cancer pain, but broadly relevant to other acute and chronic pain problems (WHO, 2007). The three steps of the analgesic ladder address different pain intensities beginning with a non-opioid analgesic such as paracetamol or an NSAID and possibly an adjuvant, then adding so-called 'mild' opioids such as codeine and eventually 'strong' opioids such as morphine. Administration of analgesics should be orally whenever possible and around the clock rather than as needed. Adjuvant analgesics are drugs that have a primary indication other than pain but are analgesic for some painful conditions. They include drugs such as anticonvulsants, antidepressants, sodium channel blockers or muscle relaxants. Older people taking these adjuvants, even in small doses, should be carefully monitored for their effect and side effects.

Pharmacological management of chronic pain is a complex area and beyond the remit of this chapter. The reader is referred to Pasero and McCaffery's (2011) classic pain management text for a comprehensive review of pharmacological management. Nurses are required to understand the actions and side effects of all analgesics in a medication regimen and to help the recipient and carers obtain and use this information in the safe and efficient administration and storage of the medicine. Contemporary technology is moving at a fast pace and it is now possible, as illustrated in Case study 9.3, to have 'state of the art' administration technology at home and beyond to ensure continuous administration of opioids.

The greatest barriers to adequate and timely pain management for people with chronic pain remain those fears and misconceptions that have been reported for decades, such as the side effects of opioids, fear of addiction and the belief that pain indicates disease progression (Pasero & McCaffery, 2011). Family caregivers who have good pain management knowledge are less influenced by these beliefs and are better able to manage pain levels (Vallerand, Collins-Bohler, Templin, & Hasenau, 2007). Discussing each aspect of their pain management with the person and their significant others, and ensuring a good understanding of the basics of self-care, prepares the person to better manage their chronic pain.

Non-drug interventions

Non-pharmaceutical interventions can bring relief from chronic pain and give people a sense of control. Relaxation therapy, cutaneous stimulation such as heat and cold, massage, guided imagery, music therapy, self-hypnosis and biofeedback are some examples.

Kerns, Sellinger and Goodin (2011) provide a critical review of the broad domain of psychological interventions for chronic pain including self-regulatory, behavioural, cognitive behavioural and acceptance and commitment therapy. Cognitive behavioural therapy is an effective approach for assisting people to manage their pain. The primary aims of cognitive behavioural therapy are to help patients to alter beliefs that are detrimental to their self-management of the pain; monitor their thoughts, emotions and behaviours and link these to environmental events, pain, emotional distress and psychosocial difficulties; develop and maintain effective and adaptive ways of thinking, feeling and responding; and perform behaviours that assist them to cope with pain, emotional distress and psychosocial difficulties (Adams, Poole, & Richardson, 2006). Interventions that influence the person's cognition, such as education, reassurance, coping strategy training, stress management, cognitive restructuring, distraction, problem solving, changing pain behaviours, increasing physical activity, goal setting and pacing are all part of cognitive behavioural therapy (Richardson, Adams, & Poole, 2006).

People living with chronic pain often fear that they will increase the pain and cause further damage by movement and exercise; or that there is an underlying pathology that has not yet been discovered. Reassurance and education can assist the person to understand the fallacy of these beliefs and develop more realistic strategies, such as exercise and pacing to prevent further deterioration in their physical capabilities. Acceptance that chronic pain is not curable or not even explainable is difficult and the individual with chronic pain needs professional as well as personal support to come to this acceptance.

Complementary therapies

People who suffer from chronic pain are increasingly turning to complementary and alternative therapies. The philosophical orientation of these therapists is opposite to the reductive stance taken by conventional Western medicine. They take a holistic perspective and treat, according to their particular tradition, the person rather than the causative pathology. The emphasis is on total wellbeing rather than the control or, some would say, masking of symptoms, in this particular case pain. Of course as the sciences of complementary therapy and Western medicine advance, their boundaries overlap. Indeed, in many general practices medical practitioners and complementary therapists work from the same centre. Some registered nurses also bring their expertise in complementary therapies to the management of chronic pain and have led research in developing an evidence base for these approaches.

Given the increasing use of complementary therapies for chronic pain, health professionals require knowledge about the use and effectiveness of these specific practices so that they can assist clients to make informed, evidence-based decisions about these therapies. The reader is referred to Tan and colleagues' (2007) systematic review of the effectiveness of commonly used complementary therapies for chronic pain.

CASE STUDY 9.3

This case study is used to show a typical professional approach to diagnosis and treatment of a person with chronic pain. It illustrates the importance of therapeutic communication and a holistic approach. The breakthrough in the management of this person is accurate diagnosis of the cause of the pain and pharmaceutical therapy associated with an understanding of the emotional turmoil of the person involved. The nursing role is a combination of diagnosis, support and education and continuing evaluation.

Social history

Mr B, a 69-year-old retired man living in north Queensland, is married with four grown children. His wife is very supportive of Mr B's condition. He does not drink or smoke and has no significant family history.

Relevant medical history

Depression, anxiety, hypogonadism.

CASE STUDY 9.3 — cont'd

Presenting problem

Mr B presented to a neurologist for investigation of left arm paraesthesia and dysthesia of left thigh — chronic radiculopathy (spinal nerve root disease). He was diagnosed at that time with multiple sclerosis following positive results on Magnetic Resonance Imaging (MRI) and lumbar puncture. Prior to diagnosis Mr B developed recurrent left upper quadrant abdominal pain. This was diagnosed as pancreatitis and led to a distal pancreatectomy for a possible lesion on the tail of the pancreas with multiple subsequent operations for removal of collections. Sepsis followed.

This pain was extensively investigated in 1994, when Mr B had CT scans and endoscopic retrograde cholangio-pancreatography as well as pancreatic biochemistry tests. All resulted in 'no abnormality detected'. Mr B was admitted to a private hospital for investigation of severe back pain a short time later.

Mr B was depressed to the point of considering suicide. His medications at this stage were:

- Baclofen 20 mg BD
- Prozac 20 mg daily
- Kapanol 50 mg BD
- Pethidine 150 mg intramuscularly PRN Q4H
- Maxalon 10 mg PRN 4/24.

An epidural catheter was inserted with an infusion of Marcain 0.25% and Fentanyl to provide pain relief. The catheter remained in situ for 7 days before it was removed. It was believed that the pain may have been the result of spinal cord lesions. Following this admission Mr B was transferred to the public hospital for implantation of an intrathecal catheter with a drug delivery pump. The overall goal was to reach a therapeutic level of drug administration where pain was kept at an acceptable level. Post-operatively some technical complications occurred while titrating the dose (an intrathecal pump will not eliminate all pain, but with it working at a therapeutic rate the pain will be decreased to a manageable level). Pain management strategies developed in conjunction with allied health staff experts in pain management were implemented. As part of the team approach to his pain management Mr B was referred to a clinical psychologist. During his consultations it was uncovered that Mr B was grieving for the 'life' he had lost and his altered relationship with his wife. He felt that his condition was causing his relationship to break down because his wife needed to take on more of the day-to-day running of the household. He mourned the loss of responsibility and control that he had had at work prior to the chronic pain. He felt he could no longer make a difference at work.

By 2002, the pain was no longer at a manageable level and the intrathecal pump dose per day was titrated to 3.0 mg/day of morphine with clonidine added. Clonidine has an analgesic effect mediated at the alpha$_2$-adrenergic sites, which are located in the dorsal horn of the spinal cord (Pasero & McCaffery, 2011). Binding to these receptor sites activates the endogenous inhibitory pathway and pain is diminished.

CASE STUDY 9.3 — cont'd

The prescription was changed numerous times and Mr B experienced exacerbations of his multiple sclerosis, which required admission into hospital or bolus doses of the morphine/clonidine that were programmed into the intrathecal pump by the pain management specialist. Mr B has now been on a stable dose of 11.5 mg/day of morphine, although he continues to experience some leg pain. MRI results show compromise of the bilateral neural foraminae at L5–S1.

The attending gastroenterologist now believes that Mr B's presenting pain may never have been pancreatic pain but was much more likely to have been associated with the onset of multiple sclerosis. Although Mr B's pain levels have increased over the past 10 years, he has used many positive management strategies to deal with it. With the assistance of his GP and the pain management team he has been able to travel extensively around Australia by pre-arranging his pump refills in other centres across the country. Mr B has learned to manage his chronic disability-related pain and is enjoying a full life.

CONCLUSION

Chronic pain is a common problem experienced among persons with chronic illness and disability. Despite significant gaps in the literature, the available evidence demonstrates the negative impact of pain on QOL, over and above the effects of the disease itself. It was argued here that the biopsychosocial model offers the most heuristic approach to chronic disability-related pain. From this perspective it is the person in pain, rather than the underlying disease process, that is the focus of assessment and management.

Chronic pain is also invisible to others. Health professionals are encouraged to routinely screen for pain problems during each interaction with persons with physical disabilities. Elicitation of a pain problem should prompt a comprehensive pain assessment as well as the need to assess its potential impact on the person's QOL. Many of the strategies for adequately managing and adapting to chronic pain are educational — self-management, coping skills, knowledge of the condition and effective use of analgesia — and registered nurses have a significant role in this education (Tollefson et al., 2011). Timely referral to and collaboration with specialist pain management services will also enhance the care of people with chronic pain and ensure they receive the best available therapies.

Reflective questions

1 Pain is an under-recognised and under-treated problem among people with disabilities. Why do you think this is so? What are the potential barriers?

2 Revisit Case study 9.2 and determine the clinical priorities in this case. What strategies could you utilise to promote the client's self-management of pain in this situation?

3 What are your experiences of working with people with chronic pain as a student or health professional? Did you feel adequately prepared? What knowledge gaps have you identified that require further study?

Acknowledgment: This chapter was adapted from the previous edition based on the work of Joanne Tollefson, Karen Piggot and Mary FitzGerald. Any errors or omissions are the author's own.

Recommended reading

Nicholas, M., Molloy, A., Tonkin, L., et al. (2011). *Manage your pain: Practical and positive ways of adapting to chronic pain*. Sydney: ABC Books.

Pasero, C., & McCaffery, M. (Eds.). (2011). *Pain assessment and pharmacologic management*. St. Louis: Mosby Elsevier.

Portenoy, R. K. (2011). Treatment of cancer pain. *Lancet, 377*, 2236–2247.

Turk, D. C., & Melzack, R. (Eds.). (2011). *Handbook of pain assessment* (3rd ed.). New York: Guilford Press.

Turk, D. C., Wilson, H. D., & Cahana, A. (2011). Treatment of chronic non-cancer pain. *Lancet, 377*, 2226–2235.

References

Access Economics. (2007). The high price of pain: the economic impact of persistent pain in Australia. Report by Access Economics Pty Limited for MBF Foundation in collaboration with University of Sydney Pain Management Research Institute. Retrieved May 2, 2013, from http://www.bupa.com.au/staticfiles/BupaP3/Health%20and%20Wellness/MediaFiles/PDFs/MBF_Foundation_the_price_of_pain.pdf

Adams, N., Poole, H., & Richardson, C. (2006). Psychological approaches to chronic pain management: part 1. *Journal of Clinical Nursing, 15*, 290–300.

Bair, M. J., Brizendine, E. J., Ackermann, R. T., et al. (2010). Prevalence of pain and association with quality of life, depression and glycaemic control in patients with diabetes. *Diabetic Medicine: A Journal of the British Diabetic Association, 27*, 578–584.

Bentsen, S. B., Rustoen, T., & Miaskowski, C. (2011). Prevalence and characteristics of pain in patients with chronic obstructive pulmonary disease compared to the Norwegian general population. *The Journal of Pain, 12*(5), 539–545.

Beyer, J. E., Denyes, M. J., & Villarruel, A. M. (1992). The creation, validation, and continuing development of the Oucher: A measure of pain intensity in children. *Journal of Pediatric Nursing, 7*(5), 335–346.

Blyth, F., March, L., Brnabic, A., et al. (2001). Chronic pain in Australia: a prevalence study. *Pain, 89*(2–3), 127–134.

Boothby, J. L., Thorn, B., Stroud, M. W., et al. (1999). Coping with pain. In R. J. Gatchel & D. C. Turk (Eds.), *Psychosocial factors in pain: critical perspectives*. New York: Guilford Press.

Call-Schmidt, T. A., & Richardson, S. J. (2003). Prevalence of sleep disturbance and its relationship to pain in adults with chronic pain. *Pain Management Nursing, 4*(3), 124–133.

Campbell, L. C., Clauw, D. J, & Keefe, F. J. (2003). Persistent pain and depression: a biopsychosocial perspective. *Biological Psychiatry, 54*, 399–409.

Cleeland, C. S. (1989). Measurement of pain by subjective report. In C. R. Chapman & J. D. Loeser (Eds.), *Issues in pain measurement*. New York: Raven Press.

Cohen, M., Quintner, J., Buchanan, D., et al. (2011). Stigmatization of patients with chronic pain: the extinction of empathy. *Pain Medicine (Malden, Mass.), 12*, 1637–1643.

Cousins, M. J. (2012). Unrelieved pain: a major health care priority. *Medical Journal of Australia, 196*(6), 373–374.

Davidhizar, R., & Giger, J. N. (2004). A review of the literature on care of clients in pain who are culturally diverse. *International Nursing Review, 51*, 47–55.

Davidson, S. N. (2003). Pain in hemodialysis patients: prevalence, cause, severity, and management. *American Journal of Kidney Diseases, 42*(6), 1239–1247.

DeGood, D. E., & Cook, A. J. (2011). Psychosocial assessment: comprehensive measures and measures specific to pain beliefs and coping. In D. C. Turk & R. Melzack (Eds.). *Handbook of pain assessment* (3rd ed.). New York: Guilford Press.

Douglas, C., Windsor, C., & Wollin, J. (2008). Understanding chronic pain complicating disability: finding meaning through focus group methodology. *The Journal of Neuroscience Nursing: Journal of the American Association of Neuroscience Nurses, 40*(3), 158–168.

Douglas, C., Wollin, J., & Windsor, C. (2008a). Illness and demographic correlates of chronic pain among a community-based sample of people with multiple sclerosis. *Archives of Physical Medicine and Rehabilitation, 89*, 1923–1932.

Douglas, C., Wollin, J., & Windsor, C. (2008b). Biopsychosocial correlates of adjustment to pain among people with multiple sclerosis. *The Clinical Journal of Pain, 24*(7), 559–567.

Douglas, C., Wollin, J., & Windsor, C. (2009). The impact of pain on the quality of life of people with multiple sclerosis: a community survey. *International Journal of Multiple Sclerosis Care, 11*(3), 127–136.

Dudgeon, B. J., Gerrard, B. C., Jensen, M. P., et al. (2002). Physical disability and the experience of chronic pain. *Archives of Physical Medicine and Rehabilitation, 83*, 229–235.

Dworkin, R. H., & Breitbart, W. S. (Eds.). (2004). *Psychosocial aspects of pain: a handbook for health care providers*. Seattle: IASP Press.

Dworkin, R. H., Turk, D. C., Revicki, D. A., et al. (2009). Development and initial validation of an expanded and revised version of the Short-Form McGill Pain Questionnaire. (SF-MPQ-2). *Pain, 144*, 35–42.

Ehde, D. M., & Hanley, M. A. (2006). Pain in patient groups frequently treated by physiatrists. *Physical Medicine and Rehabilitation Clinics Of North America, 17*, 275–285.

Ehde, D. M., & Jensen, M. P. (2004). Feasibility of a cognitive restructuring intervention for treatment of chronic pain in persons with disabilities. *Rehabilitation Psychology, 49*, 254–258.

Ehde, D. M., & Jensen, M. P. (2010). Coping and catastrophic thinking: the experience and treatment of chronic pain. In D. David, S. J. Lynn & A. Ellis (Eds.), *Rational and irrational beliefs: research, theory, and clinical practice*. New York: Oxford University Press.

Ehde, D. M., Jensen, M. P., Engel, J. M., et al. (2003). Chronic pain secondary to disability: A review. *The Clinical Journal of Pain, 19*, 3–17.

Engel, G. L. (1977). The need for a new medical model: a challenge for biomedicine. *Science, 196*, 129–136.

Evangelista, L. S., Sackett E., & Dracup K. (2009). Pain and heart failure: unrecognised and untreated. *European Journal of Cardiovascular Nursing: Journal of the Working Group on Cardiovascular Nursing of the European Society of Cardiology, 8*(3), 169–173.

Fenwick, C. (2006). Assessing pain across the cultural gap: Central Australian Indigenous peoples' pain assessment. *Contemporary Nurse, 22*(2), 218–227.

Fenwick, C., & Stevens, J. (2004). Post operative pain experiences of central Australian Aboriginal women. What do we understand? *Australian Journal of Rural Health, 12*(1), 22–27.

Frantsve, L. M., & Kerns, R. D. (2007). Patient-provider interactions in the management of chronic pain: current findings within the context of shared medical decision making. *Pain Medicine (Malden, Mass.), 8*, 25–35.

Galer, B. S., & Jensen, M. P. (1997). Development and preliminary validation of a pain measure specific to neuropathic pain: the Neuropathic Pain Scale. *Neurology, 48*, 337–338.

Gatchel, R. J., & Okifuji, A. (2006). Evidence-based scientific data documenting the treatment and cost-effectiveness of comprehensive pain programs for chronic nonmalignant pain. *The Journal of Pain, 7*, 779–793.

Gatchel, R. J., Peng, Y. B., Peters, M. L., et al. (2007). The biopsychosocial approach to chronic pain: scientific advances and future directions. *Psychological Bulletin, 133*(4), 581–624.

Geisser, M. E., Robinson, M. E., & Riley, J. L. (1999). Pain beliefs, coping, and adjustment to chronic pain: let's focus more on the negative. *Pain Forum, 8*, 161–168.

Gureje, O. (1998). Persistent pain and well-being: a World Health Organization study in primary care. *JAMA: The Journal of the American Medical Association, 280*, 147–151.

Heshusius, L. (2009). *Inside chronic pain: an intimate and critical account.* New York: Cornell University Press.

Hicks, C. L., von Baeyer, C. L., Spafford, P. A., et al. (2001). The Faces Pain Scale — revised: toward a common metric in pediatric pain measurement. *Pain, 93*(2), 173–183.

Hogg, M. N., Gibson, S., Helou, A., et al. (2012). Waiting in pain: a systematic investigation into the provision of persistent pain services in Australia. *Medical Journal of Australia, 196*(6), 386–390.

Holmes, A., Christelis, N., & Arnold, C. (2012). Depression and chronic pain. *Medical Journal of Australia Open, 1*(Suppl 4), 17–20.

Jackson, J. E. (2005). Stigma, liminality, and chronic pain: mind-body borderlands. *American Ethnologist, 32*(3), 332–353.

Jensen, M. P., & Karoly, P. (2011). Self-report scales and procedures for assessing pain in adults. In D. C. Turk & R. Melzack (Eds.), *Handbook of pain assessment* (3rd ed.). New York: Guilford Press.

Jensen, M. P., Moore, M. R., Bockow, T. B., et al. (2011). Psychosocial factors and adjustment to chronic pain in persons with physical disabilities: a systematic review. *Archives of Physical Medicine and Rehabilitation, 92*, 146–160.

Jensen, M. P., Turner, J. A., & Romano, J. M. (2007). Changes after multidisciplinary pain treatment in patient beliefs and coping are associated with concurrent changes in patient functioning. *Pain, 131*, 38–47.

Jensen, M. P., Turner, J. A., Romano, J. M., et al. (1991). Coping with chronic pain: a critical review of the literature. *Pain, 47*, 249–283.

Katz, J., & Melzack, R. (2011). The McGill Pain Questionnaire: development, psychometric properties, and usefulness of the long form, short form, and short form-2. In D. C. Turk & R. Melzack (Eds.), *Handbook of pain assessment* (3rd ed.). New York: Guilford Press.

Keefe, F. J., Abernethy, A. P., & Campbell, L. C. (2005). Psychological approaches to understanding and treating disease-related pain. *Annual Review of Psychology, 56*, 601–630.

Keefe, F. J., Brown, G. K., Wallston, K. A., et al. (1989). Coping with rheumatoid arthritis pain: Catastrophizing as a maladaptive strategy. *Pain, 37*, 51–56.

Keefe, F. J., Rumble, M. E., Scipio, C. D., et al. (2004). Psychological aspects of persistent pain: current state of the science. *The Journal of Pain, 5*, 195–211.

Kerns, R. D., Rosenberg, R., & Otis, J. D. (2002). Self-appraised problem solving and pain-relevant social support as predictors of the experience of chronic pain. *Annals of Behavioral Medicine: A Publication of the Society of Behavioral Medicine, 24*, 100–105.

Kerns, R. D., Sellinger, J., & Goodin, B. R. (2011). Psychological treatment of chronic pain. *Annual Review of Clinical Psychology, 7*, 411–434.

Klit, H., Finnerup, N. B., Overvad, K., et al. (2011). Pain following stroke: a population-based follow-up study. *PLoS ONE, 6*(11), e27607. doi: 10.1371/journal.pone.0027607

Larsen, P. D. (2013). Chronicity. In I. M. Lubkin & P. D. Larsen (Eds.), *Chronic illness: impact and interventions* (8th ed.). Burlington: Jones & Bartlett.

Marceau, L. D., Smith, L. D., & Jamison, R. N. (2011). Electronic pain assessment in clinical practice. *Pain Management, 1*(4), 325–336.

Marcus, K. S., Kerns, R. D., Rosenfeld, B., et al. (2000). HIV/AIDS-related pain as a chronic pain condition: implications of a biopsychosocial model for comprehensive assessment and effective management. *Pain Medicine (Malden, Mass.)*, *1*(3), 260–273.

Matthias, M. S., Parpart, A. L., Nyland, K. A., et al. (2010). The patient-provider relationship in chronic pain care: providers' perspectives. *Pain Medicine (Malden, Mass.)*, *11*, 1688–1697.

McCaffery, M. (1968). *Nursing practice theories related to cognition, bodily pain, and man-environment interactions*. Los Angeles: University of California Students' Store.

McGrath, P. (2006). 'The biggest worry'... research findings on pain management for aboriginal peoples in Northern Territory, Australia. *Rural and Remote Health*, *6*, 549.

Melzack, R. (1975). The McGill Pain Questionnaire: major properties and scoring methods. *Pain*, *1*, 277–299.

Melzack, R. (1987). The Short-Form McGill Pain Questionnaire. *Pain*, *30*, 191–197.

Melzack, R., & Wall, P. D. (1965). Pain mechanisms: a new theory. *Science*, *150*, 971–979.

Merskey, H. (Ed.). (1986). Classification of chronic pain syndromes and definitions of pain terms. *Pain*, (Suppl 3), S1–S225.

Namisango, E., Harding, R., Atuhaire, L., et al. (2012). Pain among ambulatory HIV/AIDS patients: Multicenter study of prevalence, intensity, associated factors, and effect. *The Journal of Pain*, *13*(7), 704–713.

Newton-John, T. R., & Williams, A. C. (2006). Chronic pain couples: perceived marital interactions and pain behaviours. *Pain*, *123*, 53–63.

Nielsen, M., Foster, M., Henman, P., et al. (2012). 'Talk to us like we're people, not an X-ray': the experience of receiving care for chronic pain. *Australian Journal of Primary Health*, http://dx.doi.org/10.1071/PY11154

Niv, D., & Kreitler, S. (2001). Pain and quality of life. *Pain Practice*, *1*, 150–161.

Novy, D. M., Nelson, D. V., Francis, D. J., et al. (1995). Perspectives of chronic pain: an evaluative comparison of restrictive and comprehensive models. *Psychological Bulletin*, *118*, 238–247.

Pasero, C., & McCaffery, M. (Eds.). (2011). *Pain assessment and pharmacologic management*. St. Louis: Mosby Elsevier.

Portenoy, R. K. (2011). Treatment of cancer pain. *Lancet*, *377*, 2236–2247.

Richardson, C., Adams, N., & Poole, H. (2006). Psychological approaches to chronic pain management: part 2. *Journal of Clinical Nursing*, *15*, 1196–1202.

Richardson, J. C., Ong, B. N., & Sim, J. (2006). Is chronic widespread pain biographically disruptive? *Social Science and Medicine*, *63*, 1573–1585.

Schirbel, A., Reichert, A., Roll, S., et al. (2010). Impact of pain on health-related quality of life in patients with inflammatory bowel disease. *World Journal of Gastroenterology*, *16*(25), 3168–3177.

Schwartz, L., Jensen, M. P., & Romano, J. M. (2005). The development and psychometric evaluation of an instrument to assess spouse responses to pain and well behavior in patients with chronic pain: the Spouse Response Inventory. *The Journal of Pain*, *6*, 243–252.

Siddall, P. J., & Cousins, M. J. (2004). Persistent pain as a disease entity: implications for clinical management. *Anesthesia & Analgesia*, *99*(2), 510–520.

Sofaer-Bennett, B., Holloway, I., Moore, A., et al. (2007). Perseverance by older people in their management of chronic pain: a qualitative study. *Pain Medicine (Malden, Mass.)*, *8*(3), 271–280.

Sofaer-Bennett, B., Walker, J., Moore, A., et al. (2007). The social consequences for older people of neuropathic pain: a qualitative study. *Pain Medicine (Malden, Mass.)*, *8*(3), 263–270.

Solano, J. P., Gomes, B., & Higginson, I. J. (2006). A comparison of symptom prevalence in far advanced cancer, AIDS, heart disease, chronic obstructive pulmonary disease and renal disease. *Journal of Pain and Symptom Management*, *31*(1), 58–69.

Tan, G., Craine, M. H., Bair, M. J., et al. (2007). Efficacy of selected complementary and alternative medicine interventions for chronic pain. *Journal of Rehabilitation Research and Development, 44*(2), 195–222.

Tang, N. E. Y., & Crane, C. (2006). Suicidality in chronic pain: a review of the prevalence, risk factors and psychological links. *Psychological Medicine, 36*, 575–586.

Thorn, B. E. (2004). *Cognitive therapy for chronic pain*. New York: Guilford Press.

Tollefson, J., & Usher, K. (2006). Chronic pain in the rural arena. *The Australian Journal of Rural Health, 14*, 134–135.

Tollefson, J., Usher, K., & Foster, K. (2011). Relationships in pain: the experience of relationships to people living with chronic pain in rural areas. *International Journal of Nursing Practice, 17*, 478–485.

Turk, D. C. (1996). Biopsychosocial perspective on chronic pain. In R. J. Gatchel & D. C. Turk (Eds.), *Psychological approaches to pain management: a practitioner's handbook*. New York: Guilford Press.

Turk, D. C., & Burwinkle, T. M. (2006). Coping with chronic pain. In A. Carr & M. McNulty (Eds.), *The handbook of adult clinical psychology: an evidence-based practice approach* (pp. 627–688). London: Routledge.

Turk, D. C., Dworkin, R. H., Revicki, D., et al. (2008). Identifying important outcome domains for chronic pain clinical trials: an IMMPACT survey of people with pain. *Pain, 137*(2), 276–285.

Turk, D. C., & Flor, H. (1999). Chronic pain: a biobehavioral perspective. In R. J. Gatchel & D. C. Turk (Eds.), *Psychosocial factors in pain: critical perspectives*. New York: Guilford Press.

Turk, D. C., & Melzack, R. (2011). The measurement of pain and the assessment of people experiencing pain. In D. C. Turk & R. Melzack (Eds.), *Handbook of pain assessment* (3rd ed.). New York: Guilford Press.

Turk, D. C., & Monarch, E. S. (2002). Biopsychosocial perspective on chronic pain. In D. C. Turk & R. Gatchel (Eds.), *Psychological approaches to pain management: a practitioner's handbook* (2nd ed.). New York: Guilford Press.

Turk, D. C., Wilson, H. D., & Cahana, A. (2011). Treatment of chronic non-cancer pain. *Lancet, 377*, 2226–2235.

Unruh, A. M., & Harman, K. (2002). Generic principles of practice. In J. Strong, A. M. Unruh, A. Wright & G. D. Baxter (Eds.), *Pain: a textbook for therapists*. Edinburgh: Churchill Livingstone.

Vallerand, A. H., Collins-Bohler, D., Templin, T., et al. (2007). Knowledge of and barriers to management in caregivers of cancer patients receiving homecare. *Cancer Nursing, 30*(1), 31–37.

van den Beuken-van Everdingen, M. H. J., de Rijke, J. M., Kessels, A. G., et al. (2007). Prevalence of pain in patients with cancer: systematic review of the past 40 years. *Annals of Oncology, 18*, 1437–1449.

Wallis, C. (2005). The right (and wrong) way to treat chronic pain. *Time*, February 20. Retrieved August 23, 2012, from http://www.time.com/time/magazine/article/0,9171,1029836,00.html

Wong, D. L., & Baker, C. M. (1988). Pain in children: comparison of assessment scales. *Pediatric Nursing, 14*(1), 9–17.

World Health Organization. (2007). *Analgesic Ladder*. Geneva: Author. Retrieved August 28, 2012, from www.who.int/cancer/palliative/painladder/en/

Yorkston, K. M., Johnson, K., Boesflug, E., et al. (2010). Communicating about the experience of pain and fatigue in disability. *Quality of Life Research: An International Journal of Quality of Life Aspects of Treatment, Care and Rehabilitation, 19*, 243–251.

Zelman, D. C., Brandenberg, N. A., & Gore, M. (2006). Sleep impairment in patients with painful diabetic peripheral neuropathy. *The Clinical Journal of Pain, 22*(8), 681–685.

CHAPTER

10

Julie Pryor
Kate O'Reilly
Melissa Bonser
Gillian Garrett

Rehabilitation for the individual and family

Learning objectives

When you have completed this chapter you will be able to:

- conceptualise rehabilitation as a personal journey undertaken by persons experiencing disability, their family and friends
- understand the importance of rehabilitation interventions across the continuum of care
- discuss the relevance of the International Classification of Functioning, Disability and Health (World Health Organization, 2001) to nursing practice in acute, specialty inpatient rehabilitation and community settings
- design, deliver and evaluate person-centred nursing care in line with the International Classification of Functioning, Disability and Health
- set mutually agreed short-term SMART goals with patients.

Key words

brain injury, disability, goal setting, rehabilitation, spinal cord injury

INTRODUCTION

Following injury or illness, many persons embark on a rehabilitation journey, an 'individual, active and dynamic process' (Barnes & Ward, 2000, p. 6) aimed at regaining control over their bodies and their lives (Ozer, 1999). Rehabilitation can differ significantly from one person to another and may extend over a person's lifetime (Pagulayan, Temkin, Machamer, & Dikmen, 2006). Because of emotional, physical and sometimes cognitive assault, a person's awareness of this intensely personal journey can evolve over a protracted period as impairments associated with the injury or illness may not be apparent to the person for some time. Furthermore, each person's journey is unique in that the experience of injury or illness is assigned personal significance in accordance with the individual's context (Donnelly, Donnelly, & Grohman, 2005). Family members, friends and colleagues also embark on a journey of their own as they seek to make sense of what has happened and integrate this into their lives.

Nursing's role in rehabilitation begins at the person's first point of contact with health services and rehabilitation informs all nursing decision making thereafter. Rehabilitation requires all healthcare professionals to possess, and act upon, an awareness of how what does and does not happen today affects the person's desired tomorrow (Plaisted, 1978). As such, rehabilitation is more than a series of intermittent interventions done to patients by health professionals (Pryor, 2005). It is a continuous process that:

- is underpinned by patient enablement (Burton & Gibbon, 2006)
- requires active patient participation (Pryor, 2005)
- is enhanced by a self-management approach (McPherson, Brander, Taylor, & McNaughton, 2001) that fosters a *can do* attitude and the preservation of self-esteem (Hickey, 2009a).

Rehabilitation is about adaptation, reconstruction of self identity and developing a sense of a new normal (Ellis-Hill, 2011; Levack, Kayes, & Fadyl, 2010). As such, theories of learning and change as well as health and illness models are central to rehabilitation.

REHABILITATION AS AN INTERVENTION

Rehabilitation is a health strategy aimed at enabling human functioning. As an 'educational, problem-solving process' (Wade, 2005, p. 814), rehabilitation is different from, but related to, preventative, curative and supportive strategies (Stucki, Cieza, & Melvin, 2007). While rehabilitation is commonly understood to be about the return of physical function, Pryor and Dean (2012) point out that *re* in rehabilitation can also mean *to do again*; this creates opportunities for *doing in different ways*; for example, washing one's body using different techniques and equipment. This is particularly important when return to a previous level of function is not likely, either in the short term or at all.

In rehabilitation there is a strong emphasis on the restoration of individual functioning and independence, as evidenced in the following definition from a highly reputable source:

> Rehabilitation means a goal-oriented and time-limited process aimed at enabling an impaired person to reach an optimal mental, physical and/or social functional level, thus providing her or him with the tools to change her or his own life (United Nations, 2006).
>
> Habilitation, on the other hand, is support for a person to attain new skills. This term is used in reference skill development in people born with disability (Habilitation Benefits Coalition, 2011; United Nations, 2012).

Rehabilitation was initially practised on a large scale during World War II to get injured servicemen back to the field of combat (Smith, 2005). While initially thought of as the third phase of medicine (Rusk, 1960), rehabilitation is now understood as an important component of healthcare across the continuum of care. This has come about as awareness of the benefits of rehabilitation as an intervention and service type has grown. As a consequence, rehabilitation is provided to persons experiencing functional performance limitations associated with a wide range of illnesses and injuries as well as limitations associated with the ageing process.

Rehabilitation is a complex intervention (Cameron, 2010), using two different, but equally important, types of rehabilitation interventions. One is support and the other is treatments (Wade, 2005); support conserves function by maintaining existing abilities and preventing new or further disability, while treatments are about restoring function (Pryor, 2012). Ward, Barnes, Stark and Ryan (2009) explain how treatments are designed to reduce activity limitations, assist with new skill development or alter the physical and/or social environment to enable participation. In Australia, the National Stroke Foundation's (2010) guidelines for acute, sub-acute and long-term management of stroke include a wide range of rehabilitation interventions. While healthcare professionals provide treatments and supports, rehabilitation goals cannot be achieved without active patient participation in rehabilitation activities. Most importantly, rehabilitation services need to remember that a person's physical, mental, emotional, social and spiritual needs impinge on each other (Ellis-Hill, Payne, & Ward, 2008) and address all aspects of a person's rehabilitation.

Research provides insight into what is valued by users of rehabilitation services and in so doing assists service providers to focus more on personal biographies. See Table 10.1 for examples of the findings of such studies.

Taking these characteristics into account, rehabilitation as an intervention or a service focuses on:

- maintaining and restoring functioning
- promoting health and wellbeing
- preventing and minimising disability (Australasian Rehabilitation Nurses Association, 2002; Williams & Pryor, 2010).

TABLE 10.1

Examples of findings of studies about what rehabilitation service users value. *Note*: Reprinted by permission from Macmillan Publishers Ltd: Spinal Cord 45:260–274. Experience of rehabilitation following spinal cord injury: a meta-synthesis of qualitative findings by Hammell K W (2007).

STUDY DETAILS	SUMMARY OF FINDINGS
Cott (2004) Qualitative study using focus groups with 33 rehabilitation clients (spinal cord injury, *n* = 3; acquired brain injury, *n* = 4; chronic obstructive pulmonary disease, *n* = 5; stroke, *n* = 7; and arthritis and/or joint replacements, *n* = 14).	Rehabilitation patients in this study valued rehabilitation services that were characterised by: 1 individualisation of programs to the needs of each patient in order to prepare them for life in the real world 2 mutual participation with health professionals in decision-making and goal-setting 3 outcomes that are meaningful to the patient 4 sharing of information and education that is appropriate, timely and according to the patient's wishes 5 emotional support 6 family and peer involvement throughout the rehabilitation process; and 7 coordination and continuity across the multiple service sectors (p. 1418).
Hammell (2007) Qualitative meta-synthesis of eight papers (seven studies) involving rehabilitation patients with spinal cord injury.	Important dimensions of rehabilitation from the patient's perspective were: 1 staff who make patients feel valued as people 2 peers, with spinal cord injury 3 programs that prepare them for life in the real world outside of hospital 4 rehabilitation settings that do not resemble institutions and do not use standardised rehabilitation programs 5 rehabilitation programs that adequately address sexual needs.

In this context, the terms functioning and disability are defined in the World Health Organization (WHO) International Classification of Functioning, Disability and Health (ICF) (WHO, 2001). However, one must remember that a person experiencing disability also retains many abilities (Mastos, Miller, Eliasson, & Immes, 2007). Therefore, an integral component of rehabilitation is to nurture preserved abilities (Rees, 2005).

INTERNATIONAL CLASSIFICATION OF FUNCTIONING, DISABILITY AND HEALTH

The ICF is a biopsychosocial model of disability (WHO, 2001). It highlights how functioning and disability at the person level are created through dynamic interaction between a person's health conditions and contextual factors (see Fig 10.1).

The ICF 'is about *all people*' (WHO, 2001, p. 7, italics original). A patient's functioning 'is seen as associated with, and not merely a consequence of, a health condition' (Stucki et al., 2005, p. 349). *Functioning* is 'an umbrella term for body functions, body structures, activities and participation' (WHO, 2001, pp. 212–13). *Disability* is 'an umbrella term for impairments, activity limitations and participation restrictions' (WHO, 2001, p. 213). Of most importance in rehabilitation is *functional performance* which is what an individual can do in their 'societal context' which includes 'all aspects of their physical, social and attitudinal world' (WHO, 2001, p. 15). The components of ICF are defined in Table 10.2.

The ICF is advocated as a framework for acute care (Muller, Grill, et al., 2011; Muller, Stier-Jarmer, Quittan, Stucki, & Grill, 2011) and post-acute rehabilitation (Muller, Stier-Jarmer, et al., 2011; Stucki et al., 2007). It facilitates the selection of rehabilitation interventions that address the full impact of a health condition on a person's life (Kearney & Pryor, 2004). That is, rehabilitation interventions target:

- impairments of body structures and functions
- activity limitations
- participation restrictions

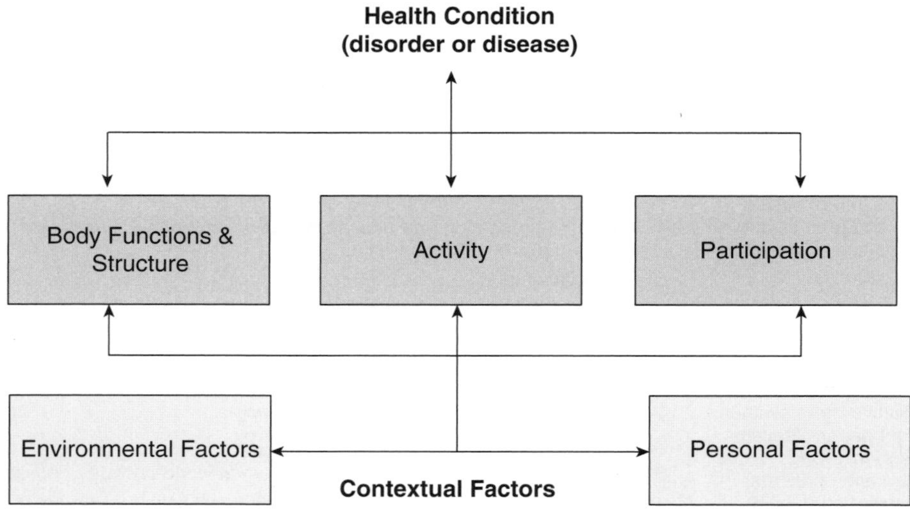

FIGURE 10.1 Interactions between the components of ICF. *Note*: From World Health Organization. (2001). *International Classification of Functioning, Disability and Health*. Geneva: WHO.

TABLE 10.2

Components of ICF. *Note*: From World Health Organization. (2001). *International Classification of Functioning, Disability and Health.* Geneva: WHO.

'In the context of health:

Body functions are the physiological functions of body systems (including psychological functions).

Body structures are anatomical parts of the body such as organs, limbs and their components.

Impairments are problems in body function or structure such as a significant deviation or loss.

Activity is the execution of a task or action by an individual.

Participation is involvement in a life situation.

Activity limitations are difficulties an individual may have in executing activities.

Participation restrictions are problems an individual may experience in involvement in life situations.

Environmental factors make up the physical, social and attitudinal environment in which people live and conduct their lives' (p. 10).

'**Personal factors** are the particular background of an individual's life and living, and comprise features of the individual that are not part of a health condition or health states' (p. 17).

- environmental factors
- personal factors.

This supports the move away from an impairment-oriented approach to a functional or task-oriented approach (Wade & deJong, 2000). While ICF is a useful framework for rehabilitation, the use of goals and teamwork are critical elements in the delivery of effective rehabilitation services. The ICF facilitates teamwork by providing a common language for all disciplines (WHO, 2001).

THE USE OF GOALS

As explained by Wade (2009, p. 291), most human behaviour is goal-directed regardless of how 'nebulous or unconsidered the behaviour may be'. The use of goals has become a hallmark of rehabilitation, and is recommended within clinical guidelines (e.g. National Stroke Foundation, 2010) and models of care (e.g. NSW Health, 2011). Current literature certainly discusses the challenges in regard to the robustness of evidence about the relationship between goals and health outcomes (Playford et al., 2009; Scobbie, Dixon & Wyke 2011); however there is consensus that goal setting is a core component of rehabilitation.

The setting of goals is said to facilitate self-determination and engagement in the activities of rehabilitation. Goal setting is widely supported as a pragmatic approach that fits with the problem solving and educational processes of rehabilitation (Wade, 1999). As described by Playford et al. (2009), goals may not necessarily have to be achievable but may reflect a person's ambitions; this is integral to person-centredness (McCance, Slater, & McCormack, 2008). Wade's (2009) caution that goals should not be used to predict outcomes of rehabilitation, but rather that goals should be identified to guide rehabilitation interventions, is worth remembering.

Long-term goals

The long-term goal of most patients is to return to their pre-injury or pre-illness life (Hafsteinsdottir & Grypdonck, 1997). Regardless of whether this is possible, this goal identifies what is important to a person and provides the rationale for the interventions of healthcare professionals. In relation to ICF (WHO, 2001), pre-injury or pre-illness life is often understood in terms of a person's participation in meaningful life situations (Cicerone, 2004); for example, recreational athlete, book lover, parent, farmer, gardener or house builder. To facilitate the setting of participation goals, Wade (1999) advocates using the 'Life Goals Questionnaire', on which a patient rates the importance of various aspects of their life.

Re-establishment of a 'person's sense of control over his or her body and life' (Ozer, 1999, p. 43) is an essential first step in rehabilitation. As Faull and Hills (2006, p. 729) note, 'the development of a resilient, intrinsic, spiritually based self' is central to rehabilitation outcomes. Ellis-Hill (2011) explains that this re-establishment is a process and recognises the role of nurses in the journey, as the often protracted transition to a new normal begins in hospital. Effective goal setting can assist in this process. Firstly, goals can help patients to move from pre-contemplation to action (van den Broek, 2005). Secondly, goals can be a powerful mechanism for enhancing patient ownership of, and engagement in, their rehabilitation (Levack et al., 2006). Thirdly, goals can be a reference point for evaluating rehabilitation outcomes (Scobbie et al., 2011).

Short-term goals

The conversion of a person's long-term participation goals into short-term goals that healthcare professionals can contribute to requires negotiation. We are reminded by Donnelly et al. (2005) and Levack et al. (2010) that depending on whose perspective is being considered (be it the person who is the patient, their family or clinicians), what are identified as problems in need of rehabilitation can differ. Discussion with and education of patients and families about the use of goals in rehabilitation is an essential first step in developing a shared understanding (Bowen, Yeates, & Palmer, 2010). Demystifying the goal-setting process enables patients to re-establish decisional autonomy over their situation (Cardol, DeJong, & Ward, 2002). Mutual goal-setting should also ensure that the needs of both service users and service providers are best served, rather than rehabilitation being viewed as 'a product to be dispensed' (Stewart & Bhagwanjee, 1999, p. 339) 'by one party to another' (Clapton & Kendall, 2002, p. 990). Clinicians need to consider the values and preferences of patients and families, their own clinical judgment, the time and resources required to work towards stated goals and the consequences of pursuing that goal (Levack, 2009).

Short-term goals are most useful when articulated as S(specific) M(measurable) A(agreed) R(relevant) T(time-limited) goals. The relevance of SMART goals is highlighted by Hill (1999), who herself has experienced traumatic brain injury; she notes that rehabilitation needs to assist injured persons to 're-orient or rebuild their life using a new set of "maps" with which to navigate life' (p. 839). SMART goals can contribute to the creation of these new maps.

In the short term, rehabilitation outcomes are evaluated by way of achievement of SMART goals. Healthcare professionals, however, need to be mindful that patients often evaluate their progress in relation to their pre-injury or pre-illness lifestyle and satisfaction with their reconstructed personal identity, not the small steps along the way (Ellis-Hill, 2011). As a discipline, nursing is ideally situated to ensure that the benefits of rehabilitation are available to all consumers of healthcare.

NURSING AND REHABILITATION

Rehabilitation is central to nursing practice across the continuum of care, regardless of a person's age, diagnosis or setting (Pryor, 2002). The overarching goal of rehabilitation, namely maximising human potential, is synonymous with the goal of nursing. Dittmar

TABLE 10.3

Four rehabilitative nursing functions. *Note*: From Kirkevold (1997).

Interpretive function	Nurses help patients and families make sense of what has happened to them, what is happening to them and what may happen in the future.
Consoling function	Nurses develop trusting relationships with patients and family members and provide emotional support.
Conserving function	Nurses are involved in maintaining normal bodily functions with a heavy emphasis on prevention and physical protection.
Integrative function	Nurses help patients integrate new learning, in relation to their activities of daily living, into their daily lives.

(1989, p. 2) describes rehabilitation as 'an approach, a philosophy, an attitude and a process', which can be woven into nursing practice regardless of the clinical setting. Hickey (2009a, p. 216) reinforces this point in noting the 'principles of rehabilitation are an integral component of independent nursing practice'. Rehabilitation is increasingly recognised for its interdisciplinary nature (Johnson et al., 2009) and should not be viewed as the exclusive domain of allied health.

Kirkevold's (1997) description of four nursing functions is one way to understand nursing's rehabilitation role. These functions, while derived from a Norwegian study of stroke nursing, are relevant to rehabilitative nursing practice regardless of diagnosis or setting (see Table 10.3).

The findings from other studies of rehabilitation and healthcare complement Kirkevold's work. Four particular aspects of this body of research are relevant to the practice of all nurses. Firstly, adopting a rehabilitative approach requires nurses to 'focus on a person's ability in order to see possibilities rather than focusing on disabilities' and to adopt 'a wellness model of care' (Pryor & Smith, 2002, p. 253). These are essential components for the person with an impairment in the reconstruction of their identity (Levack, Kayes & Fadyl, 2010) and could also be described as a humanised approach to care which encourages active participation in rehabilitation and healthcare (St-Germain, Boivin, & Fougeyrollas, 2011; Todres, Galvin, & Holloway, 2009).

Secondly, viewing 'every nurse–patient interaction as a teaching/learning opportunity' (Pryor & Smith, 2002, p. 253) ensures nurses assess patient readiness, ability and potential to be coached to self-care. This often starts with teaching patients about rehabilitation and about how the rehabilitation roles of patients and nurses differ from their acute care roles (Pryor, 2005). Kautz (2011) illustrates the sometimes subtle way in which nurses weave these teaching opportunities into everyday interactions and as identified in various studies (Long, Kneafsey, Ryan, & Berry, 2002; Pryor & Smith, 2002) occurs continually over a 24-hour period, which is unique to nursing.

Thirdly, like Kirkevold (1997) who reports that nurses create an atmosphere of positivity and optimism for each client, Pryor (2000) refers to a *rehabilitative milieu* that is contributed to by all people and activities on the unit. In a study of five inpatient rehabilitation units, Pryor (2010) reports nurses allowing time for patients to work at their own pace, keeping patients' spirits up by creating a light-hearted atmosphere, protecting patients from embarrassment and making hospitalisation more home-like to be important nursing contributions to the creation of this unique rehabilitation ward atmosphere. Tyrrell, Levack, Ritchie and Keeling, (2012) found that partnerships are formed between nurses, patients and families and in so doing nurses facilitate self-determination and motivation, the ultimate aim being for patients to regain control over their own lives.

Fourthly, there is agreement within the literature that coordination of each individual patient's rehabilitation is a nursing responsibility (Kautz, 2011; St-Germain et al., 2011). Long et al. (2002, p. 73) describe this responsibility as 'complex, including responsibilities for activities such as gathering, synthesising and disseminating information, liaison, referral, negotiation and discharge planning'. The introduction of a patient care coordinator was evaluated positively in an Australian study (Pryor, 2003), as have been similar initiatives elsewhere (e.g. Burton, 2000).

Three knowledge types, identified by Liaschenko and Fisher (1999) and discussed by Stein-Parbury (2009), are central to the effectiveness of nursing in supporting patients on their rehabilitation journey:

1 case knowledge (generalised and objective knowledge, such as anatomy and physiology, disease processes and pharmacology)
2 patient knowledge (knowledge of how a person is responding to their clinical situation)
3 person knowledge (understanding each person as unique, knowing their personal and private biography and understanding how actions make sense for that person).

While all three types of knowledge are essential, person knowledge is of particular importance for rehabilitation. It is through knowing a person that relevant, person-specific goals and motivators can be identified (Levack et al., 2010). Getting to know the patient, as a person, also communicates to their family and friends that they are valued by health-care workers as a person, not just a patient (Youngson, 2012).

The following factors are necessary if nurses are to get to know their patients: '(i) mutual trust and rapport; (ii) a positive nurse–patient attitude; (iii) sustained nurse–patient contact; and (iv) meaningful interaction' (Henderson, 1997, p. 112). Relationships built

CASE STUDY 10.1 Part 1

Matthew is a 30-year-old sheep farmer, who lives with his wife of 1 year in western NSW. His wife works part time at the local bank in the nearest town, approximately 20 kilometres away. Matthew is the eldest of six children, three of whom live locally and two in other parts of the state. Matthew's parents have retired from farming and now live in town. He is active in his local community, where he is a member of the Lions Club and the local branch of the National Farmers' Federation.

Matthew was involved in an accident on his property. While mustering sheep, his quad bike rolled over, trapping him for several hours. Matthew sustained a spinal cord injury and a traumatic brain injury, with a Glasgow Coma Scale score of 8/15 at the scene. Matthew was taken by road ambulance to the local hospital for medical stabilisation and from there transferred via air ambulance to a tertiary referral facility in Sydney for specialist care. His injuries included a left frontotemporal cerebral contusion and a T8 burst fracture resulting in T7 paraplegia.

Following an acute inpatient stay of 28 days, including 14 days with post-traumatic amnesia, Matthew was ready for transfer to a specialist inpatient rehabilitation centre. Matthew remained an inpatient at the rehabilitation centre for a period of 16 weeks, spending time in both a brain injury rehabilitation unit (BIU) (4 weeks) and a spinal injury rehabilitation unit (SIU) (12 weeks). Following discharge Matthew returned home to live with his wife on their farm, with support from family and friends.

upon these factors facilitate the negotiation of mutually agreed goals and the coaching of patients to take that next step on their journey towards self-care and independence.

In the remainder of this chapter, rehabilitation as a personal journey following injury or illness and as an intervention is illuminated through discussion of Matthew's story.

BRAIN INJURY — WHAT IS IT?

The human brain is a complex organ made up of approximately 100 billion cells (Hickey & Kanusky, 2009) and it controls everything we do. 'Acquired brain injury (ABI) is a collective term used to describe brain injury which may be as a result of traumatic or non-traumatic events' (O'Reilly & Pryor, 2002, p. 34). Brain injury is commonly classified as traumatic (TBI) or non-traumatic. A blow to the head or a motor vehicle accident where a person's head moves forwards and/or backwards too quickly injures the brain and is described as a TBI. Non-traumatic brain injury is caused by lack of oxygen to the brain as a result of an internal incident, such as infection or stroke.

Following brain injury a person does not simply emerge from coma and revert back to their pre-injury self. There is sometimes a period referred to as post-traumatic amnesia (PTA), when a person has difficulty in areas such as recalling personal information (e.g. age and date of birth), orientation to the environment and formation of new memories (Brain Injury Association of Queensland, 2006). During this time the person may be agitated, restless, confused, disoriented and, if mobile, may wander.

Along with the Glasgow Coma Scale, duration of PTA is a prognostic tool. If PTA lasts for more than 1 week, cognitive impairment is likely. However, as O'Brien, Nicholson, Johnson and Gravell (2002, p. 3) note, 'definitions of severe, moderate and mild head injury are not always based upon the same criteria'. For Matthew, PTA lasted 14 days, which indicates that his brain injury was 'very severe' (Brain Injury Association of Queensland, 2006, p. 11; Hannay et al., 2004, p. 160) (see Table 10.4).

Although a person may emerge from PTA, impairments to bodily functions, such as walking, bladder and bowel elimination and temperature control, along with communication and information processing limitations may present lifelong challenges. Brain injury can also affect a person's emotions, memory, their ability to concentrate and result in challenging behaviours, which may range from physical aggression to inertia (Australian Institute of Health and Welfare, 2007; Turner-Stokes, Disler, Nair, & Wade, 2005). These

TABLE 10.4

Severity of brain injury. *Note:* Adapted from Brain Injury Association of Queensland (2006), and Hannay H J, Howieson D B, Loring D W, et al (2004) Neuropathology for neuropsychologists. In M D Lezak, D B Howieson, D W Loring *Neuropsychological assessment* (4th edn:157–285). New York: Oxford University Press.

BRAIN INJURY ASSOCIATION OF QUEENSLAND (2006)		HANNAY ET AL. (2004)	
PTA duration	**Severity**	**PTA duration**	**Severity**
		< 5 minutes	Very mild
< 5 minutes	Mild	5–60 minutes	Mild
1–24 hours	Moderate	1–24 hours	Moderate
1–7 days	Severe	1–7 days	Severe
> 7 days	Very severe	1–4 weeks	Very severe
		> 4 weeks	Extremely severe

are just some of the difficulties a person who has sustained a brain injury may experience. These are significant in their own right, but it is the combination of these changes that can make it challenging for a person to return to their pre-brain injury life (Brain Injury Association of Queensland, 2006; O'Reilly & Pryor, 2002).

SPINAL CORD INJURY — WHAT IS IT?

The spinal cord is a continuation of the medulla oblongata and extends from the atlas down to the first lumbar vertebrae to the S2 level of the spinal column (Hickey, 2009b). The spinal cord 'is the communication highway from the brain to organs and muscles' (Branche-Spelich, Reyes, & Miller, 2012, p. 269). It is the main pathway for transmitting information between the brain and the nerves that lead to muscles, skin, internal organs and glands (Department of Veterans Affairs, 2009). The spinal cord is surrounded by the spinal column. This flexible bony structure is made up of 33 vertebral bodies (7 cervical, 12 thoracic, 5 lumbar, 5 sacral and 3 coccygeal), separated by discs but held together by ligaments and supported by muscles (Branche-Spelich et al., 2012). There are 31 pairs of spinal nerves (8 cervical, 12 thoracic, 5 lumbar, 5 sacral and 1 coccygeal) that exit the spinal cord through openings in the vertebral column (Hickey & Kanusky, 2009).

Any external force to the spinal column can result in damage to the cord. 'Traumatic injury can be caused by displaced bone fragments, disc material or ligaments that cause pressure, bruises or tears into the spinal cord tissue' (Branche-Spelich et al., 2012, p. 269). Transport-related injuries and falls accounted for nearly three-quarters of traumatic spinal cord injuries in Australia in 2007–08 (Norton, 2010). Non-traumatic causes include infections, tumours, degenerative changes and embolic events (Branche-Spelich et al., 2012).

An injury to the spinal cord can disrupt movement, sensation and function below the level of injury (Department of Veterans Affairs, 2009). The extent of disability is dependent upon the level and completeness of injury to the spinal cord. The higher and more complete the level of injury, the greater the deficit will be in terms of impairments of bodily functions. An impairment scale developed by the American Spinal Injury Association (ASIA) is widely used to classify spinal cord injury by level and type (see Table 10.5). Level of injury

TABLE 10.5
ASIA Impairment Scale. *Note*: From American Spinal Injury Association (2011).

A = COMPLETE	No sensory or motor function is preserved in the sacral segments S4–S5.
B = SENSORY INCOMPLETE	Sensory but not motor function is preserved below the neurological level and includes the sacral segments S4–S5 (light touch, pin prick at S4–S5: or deep anal pressure (DAP)), AND no motor function is preserved more than three levels below the motor level on either side of the body.
C = MOTOR INCOMPLETE	Motor function is preserved below the neurological level, and more than half of key muscle functions below the single neurological level of injury (NLI) have a muscle grade less than 3 (Grades 0–2).
D = MOTOR INCOMPLETE	Motor function is preserved below the neurological level, and at least half (half or more) of key muscle functions below the NLI have a muscle grade ≥ 3.
E = NORMAL	If sensation and motor function as tested with the ISNCSCI are graded as normal in all segments, and the patient had prior deficits, then the AIS grade is E. Someone without an initial SCI does not receive an AIS grade.

TABLE 10.6
Matthew's impairments

LEFT FRONTOTEMPORAL CEREBRAL CONTUSION	Blunt trauma injury caused by the brain impacting on the bony inner surface of the skull (Hickey & Prator, 2009).
T8 BURST FRACTURE	Compression injury causing shattering of the vertebral body with fragments of vertebral body impinging on spinal cord (Hickey, 2009b).
THORACIC SPINAL CORD LESION	Causing spastic paraparesis, hyperreflexia, neurogenic bladder and bowel and sensory loss below T7 (Branche-Spelich et al., 2012; Hickey, 2009b).

explains 'the most caudal level where both sensory and motor functioning is preserved bilaterally' (Hoeman, Liszner, & Alverzo, 2008, p. 241). Using this scale the patient with a spinal cord injury thus receives a diagnosis inclusive of the level of injury and ASIA Impairment Scale (AIS); for example, C4 ASIA C.

The range of impairments experienced by a person with spinal cord injury may present numerous activity limitations and participation restrictions. In addition to the loss of movement and sensation, physical functional deficits often include bladder, bowel and sexual dysfunction. Spinal cord injury requires ongoing management of these impairments to prevent or manage related problems, such as skin breakdown, pain and spasticity. Spinal cord injury can impact on many aspects of a person's life; hence, the ability to work, study, socialise and participate in leisure activities may be altered. The psychological impact of spinal cord injury can also be great, with many people experiencing 'adverse social consequences, including high risk of divorce, social discrimination and poor employment' (Craig & Perry, 2008, p. 9) following injury. A summary of Matthew's impairments is provided in Table 10.6.

In the following sections of the chapter, rehabilitation in acute care, specialist inpatient rehabilitation and the community will be discussed. Matthew's story will be used to illuminate rehabilitation as an intervention in each of these settings, but more importantly as an ongoing personal journey.

ACUTE CARE — WHERE REHABILITATION BEGINS

In an instant, life as Matthew knew it changed as a consequence of trauma to his body. Participation in valued life roles, such as managing his farming property, interacting with his family and involvement in the rural community, were interrupted. The complexity of physical impairments and psychological adjustment to disability challenged Matthew and those around him (Dickson, O'Brien, Ward, Flowers, Allan & O'Carroll, 2012), as they embarked on a journey of reconstructing life roles and identities (Ellis-Hill et al., 2008). Based on a qualitative meta-analysis of the literature, Morse (1997) describes this journey as a five-stage process of responding to threats to integrity (see Table 10.7).

In all acute care settings (emergency, high dependency and the ward), nurses actively facilitate Matthew's recovery, his rehabilitation and the preservation of his integrity and dignity as a person. In ICF (WHO, 2001) terms, Matthew has significant impairments of body structures and functions, activity limitations and participation restrictions.

Throughout his post-injury journey, Matthew's goal is to return to his pre-injury life. This goal guides the efforts of the multi-professional healthcare team. As nurses spend the

TABLE 10.7

Five stages of responding to threats to integrity. *Note*: From Morse J (1997).

1. VIGILANCE	'The first changes in the onset of acute or chronic illness bring about a dis-ease, with the individuals suspecting that something is wrong' (p. 28).
2. DISRUPTION: ENDURING TO SURVIVE	'The major task of the critically ill is to hold on to life' (p. 31).
3. ENDURING TO LIVE: STRIVING TO REGAIN SELF	'Once the acute crisis has been resolved, the real work derived from illness or the injury must begin' (p. 31).
4. SUFFERING: STRIVING TO RESTORE SELF	The person 'begins to struggle with grief, mourning what has been lost and the altered future' (p. 32).
5. LEARNING TO LIVE WITH THE ALTERED SELF	'The person must get to know and to trust the altered body' (p. 33).

most time with patients, they have a unique opportunity to ensure that the relationship between each healthcare intervention and Matthew's long-term goal is clearly explained to Matthew and his family. This is an essential aspect of nursing's interpretive function, as is explaining to Matthew and his family the nature of Matthew's injuries and the processes and rationale for the various treatments. Understanding how the interventions of healthcare workers relate to a person's everyday life assists people integrate what is happening into their lives.

The consequences of injuries like Matthew's on family and friends are significant, with several authors describing how these reverberate throughout the entire family and social network (Dickson et al., 2012; Flemming, Sampson, Cornwell, Turner, & Griffin, 2012). Pratt and Baldry (2002, p. 291) describe this reverberation as follows:

> It is during this journey from intensive care to a rehabilitation unit or ward that a metamorphosis occurs — relatives become 'carers'. As such, certain expectations are made and roles placed upon them by professional staff and by others in their environment. Carers, meanwhile, will have little time to adjust to this new role and will perceive themselves in their pre-injury condition.

Therefore, Matthew and his family members are likely to be emotionally and physically compromised learners. They are unlikely to be self-directed learners, because at this time they commonly experience difficulty knowing what they need to learn (Pryor & Jannings, 2004). While education helps people to cope, we need to appreciate that not all learning takes place within an inpatient setting (Olinzock, 2004). Much of a person's learning will be about how imparted information is integrated in line with their own values, physical environments and personal contexts (Schipper, Widdrshoven, & Abma, 2011). Therefore, many patients and their family members benefit from written as well as verbal information (Mateer, Sira, & O'Connell, 2005).

While nurses address all the components of ICF in acute care settings, a major aspect of acute care is maintaining normal bodily functions. With a heavy emphasis on prevention and physical protection (the conserving function), nurses make a significant contribution to patient rehabilitation through 'the management and promotion of homeostasis' (McPherson, 2006, p. 788). Unfortunately, overlooking the maintenance of existing function, a central aspect of rehabilitation (Pryor, 1999), can result in iatrogenic complications, such as joint contractures and imposed dependence (Gignac & Cott, 1998).

TABLE 10.8
Example goals and how nurses conserve Matthew's function in acute care

SHORT-TERM GOALS	NURSING INTERVENTIONS
Conserve function and prevent complications of immobility, such as deep vein thrombosis, pressure injury, joint contractures, pneumonia, constipation.	Regular range of motion exercises for all joints. Regular inspection of pressure points. Use of pressure-relieving mattresses. Airway management. Ensure adequate nutritional and fluid intake. Management of bowel and bladder elimination. Early identification of potential complications. Timely reporting of unexpected changes.
Conserve function and prevent secondary injury due to pulmonary aspiration associated with seizures (Ghaj, 2000).	Monitoring cerebral perfusion and oxygenation status and responding appropriately to changes (Albano, Comandante, & Nolan, 2005). Protecting and maintaining airway during seizures. Detailed and timely reporting of all seizure activity.
Conserve function and prevent secondary spinal injury due to unstable fracture site that may cause further cord damage.	Immobilising the spine when moving and handling Matthew.
Conserve function and prevent secondary injury due to infection resulting from thoracic and iliac crest wound.	Monitoring for signs of infection. Implement, follow and regularly review wound management plan.
Conserve function and prevent secondary injury due to spinal shock, such as paralytic ileus and neurogenic bladder.	Management of intravenous line and fluids. Insertion and management of nasogastric tube. Monitor for vomiting and abdominal distension. Monitor oral intake, bowel sounds and flatus. Insertion and management of indwelling urinary catheter. Accurate observation and recording of fluid intake and output (Hickey, 2009b).

In the early acute stage, while Matthew is in a barbiturate-induced coma, he cannot actively contribute to maintaining homeostasis. Therefore, nurses provide wholly compensatory care, shifting to partially compensatory care then educative–supportive care (Orem, 1995) as Matthew's condition allows. Knowing when to adopt a hands-on (wholly or partially compensatory) or hands-off (educative–supportive) approach is a hallmark of rehabilitation nursing expertise (Pryor & Smith, 2002). Table 10.8 gives examples of how nurses conserve Matthew's function.

PRE-TRANSFER EDUCATION

Pre-transfer education about what rehabilitation is and how it differs from acute care is vital for patients and their families (Pryor & O'Connell, 2008). Unless previously exposed to rehabilitation, most people do not understand it (Miller, 2003); even nurses who have not worked in specialist rehabilitation services commonly possess little rehabilitation knowledge. Therefore, staff from the rehabilitation unit should deliver this education so that accurate information can be provided and questions answered. Whenever possible, pre-transfer education should include written information and a visit to the rehabilitation unit by patient and family. These measures enhance the likelihood of informed decision-making.

The importance of pre-transfer education is highlighted in several studies (Gibbon, 2004; Pryor & O'Connell, 2008) that found pre-transfer preparation of patients for rehabilitation to be inadequate. Inadequate preparation can be detrimental to patient progress, because patients need time to adjust their expectations of hospitalisation to enable them to fully access the benefits of speciality rehabilitation. Nurses are ideally situated to ensure that patients, their family and friends have timely access to accurate information.

SPECIALITY INPATIENT REHABILITATION

Inpatient rehabilitation differs significantly from acute care. In the rehabilitation unit, patients are encouraged to work hard and interact with other patients as the momentum of rehabilitation increases. Each patient has an individualised rehabilitation plan consisting of short-term goals that are linked to the patient's personal longer term goals. All goals are reviewed regularly.

While patients do the work of rehabilitation, each person's rehabilitation is guided and supported by a multi-professional team. The patient and family are central team members, with others including specialist rehabilitation nurses, specialist rehabilitation doctors, recreation therapists, physiotherapists, occupational therapists, speech pathologists, psychologists, social workers, dietitians, pharmacists and rehabilitation assistants, as well as cleaning, administration and catering staff.

All family, friends and staff have the potential to make a valuable contribution to patient rehabilitation, but optimal teamwork is a major challenge. The role of nursing overlaps with the roles of all the other disciplines, and 'integrated action is a pre-requisite for successful rehabilitation' (Gutenbrunner, Meyer, Melvin, & Stucki, 2011, p. 760). This means nurses, medical and allied health staff assessing, planning, intervening and evaluating together, dialoguing, valuing and respecting each other's contribution. The coordination of patient, family and staff effort is a primary nursing responsibility (Pryor, 2003; Pryor & Smith, 2002). Furthermore, as Low (2003) explains, nurses are well positioned to ascertain a person's suitability for working with allied health staff and whether such participation will be of benefit in light of the person's other medical and nursing needs at a given time. This is central to ensuring patients' health and functional goals are addressed (Pryor, 2005).

Transfer to an inpatient rehabilitation unit does not guarantee patient readiness for active participation in rehabilitation. Despite clinicians' best efforts to ease patients into rehabilitation, patients are not always ready for the demands of a specialty inpatient rehabilitation program. On the other hand, failure by the multi-professional team to understand the patient and family perspective following trauma may inhibit a model of rehabilitation which is truly person-centred (Ellis-Hill et al., 2008; Youngson, 2012). Anxiety, loneliness, boredom and restricted visitors can lead to a lack of patient motivation (Flemming et al., 2012). Frustration (Hafsteinsdottir & Grypdonck, 1997) and lack of confidence (Pryor, 2005) have also been recognised as factors that impact on patient engagement with rehabilitation activities, although rehabilitation nurses who understand their vital role have been found to enhance patient engagement (Pryor & Buzio, 2010).

Patients with cognitive deficits are one group that has particular needs. Neurorehabilitation often fails when patients are not aware they have a problem that would benefit from rehabilitation (van den Broek, 2005). In this pre-contemplation stage of the transtheoretical model of change (Prochaska et al., 1992), problem identification by the patient is a primary goal of rehabilitation.

Establishing routines

Structure and routines are essential elements in assisting a person with memory impairment, fatigue, adynamia and, at times, depression as a result of brain or spinal cord injury. Nurses work with patients to establish routines for personal activities of daily living. Of particular importance is the establishment of routines for urinary and faecal elimination as this will support patients to gain the most benefit from rehabilitation programs and function more independently in the community (Hoeman et al., 2008; Ylvisaker, Jacobs, & Feeney, 2003). Timetables are an effective tool for establishing routines; an example is provided later in the chapter.

Cuing systems

For persons who are cognitively impaired, routine is supported by the use of cuing systems. Cuing systems involve the use of an external alarm to notify someone that something needs to be done. They help patients with poor initiation and memory problems. Cuing systems require little insight or internal motivation and they allow the patient to work collaboratively with others to decide what actions are to be prompted (Mateer et al., 2005).

Goal setting

Goal setting starts by identifying the activities a patient likes to do and the person/s they like to do them with; within the context of inpatient rehabilitation these become long-term goals. In so doing, rehabilitation 'invest[s] in the person and recognise[s] his or her unique talents' (Rees, 2005, p. 279); it also gives the multi-professional team insights into the person who is the patient. See Box 10.1 for examples of Matthew's long-term rehabilitation goals.

To achieve these goals, rehabilitation planning starts by identifying Matthew's specific impairments, activity limitations and participation restrictions. Doing this with Matthew creates an opportunity to explain to Matthew what has happened to his body and to help him explore what this means for his life. Use of a key worker to facilitate goal setting can be invaluable. Table 10.9 contains examples of Matthew's impairments, activity limitations and participation restrictions in the first 8 weeks of his inpatient rehabilitation stay.

In preparing Matthew's rehabilitation plan, healthcare professionals negotiate short-term goals with him. These are the goals that Matthew can work with staff to achieve during

BOX 10.1
Examples of Matthew's long-term rehabilitation goals

Matthew wants:

- to return to mustering cattle on the farm
- to resume a sexual relationship with his wife
- to organise meetings for the Lions Club
- to cook BBQs for family and friends
- to participate in camp drafting events.[1]

[1]Campdrafting is a sport involving a horse and rider, and cattle. The rider selects one animal (cattle) from a group of 6 or 8 to round up. The object is for the horse rider to control and direct the cattle away from the group into another area and around a set route in a figure-of-eight fashion (Australian Campdraft Association, 2012). The time limit to complete a camp drafting course is approximately 40 seconds so this sport is fast and requires the rider to be a competent and proficient horse rider. It is therefore a physically demanding sport and also requires the rider to be alert and strategic in their actions (Australian Campdraft Association, 2010).

TABLE 10.9
Examples of Matthew's impairments, activity limitations and participation restrictions

IMPAIRMENTS	ACTIVITY LIMITATION AND PARTICIPATION RESTRICTION
Motor dysfunction below the level of spinal cord injury, including spasm	Unable to mobilise independently, therefore: • dependent on slide board to transfer • dependent on manual wheelchair for all indoor mobility • dependent on power wheelchair for outdoor mobility • dependent on assistance of one person to wash and dress lower body • dependent on shower commode for showering and bowel evacuation.
Impaired sensation below the level of spinal cord injury	Unable to recognise need to relieve pressure, therefore: • requires pressure-relieving cushion for long periods of sitting.
Neuropathic pain	Pain and hyper-vigilance when performing any physical task, therefore: • altered ability to participate in recreation and leisure activities.
Neurogenic bladder	Unable to spontaneously void, therefore: • dependent on catheterisation to manage urinary elimination.
Neurogenic bowel	Unable to spontaneously evacuate bowel, therefore: • dependent on aperients and bowel management routine to manage faecal elimination.
Sexual dysfunction	Difficulty maintaining an erection, therefore: • unable to have spontaneous sexual intercourse.
Cognitive impairment	Poor short-term memory, therefore: • unable to remember schedules • unable to sequence events requiring more than 3 steps. Impulsive behaviour, therefore: • difficulty communicating (e.g. turn taking) impacting on relationships with others • unable to self monitor socially appropriate sexual behaviour. Problem-solving difficulties, therefore: • requires support to think through day-to-day problems (e.g. constipation).
Mood disturbance	Socially withdrawn, therefore: • reluctant to participate in social situations and group activities.

his inpatient stay. They depict specific patient behaviours that can be measured to determine progress towards goal achievement. When setting short-term goals, it is important to include goals that focus on all aspects of functioning and disability, as detailed in ICF (WHO, 2001). See Table 10.10 for examples of short-term goals used to guide Matthew's return to cooking a BBQ for family and friends.

Presenting SMART goals over a period of time helps to illustrate the complex nature of what is involved for Matthew to achieve independence. Nursing is one of many disciplines that guide Matthew through a process of engagement and learning. Olinzock (2004) explains that throughout this process both patient and clinician are required to assume changing roles. Matthew moves from dependence to self initiation and finally to self direction. In line with Matthew's increasing self-determination, clinicians move from an authoritative to a consultative role (Olinzock, 2004).

TABLE 10.10
Examples of short-term goals used to guide Matthew's return to cooking a BBQ

TIMEFRAME	SMART SHORT-TERM GOALS
Weeks 1–4 (BIU)	Open bowels each morning as planned with nursing assistance. Find way around unit without asking directions. Independent and safe in manual wheelchair (MWC) indoors including corners. Make a phone call to wife once each day. Make own sandwich for lunch under supervision.
Weeks 5–8 (SIU)	Report type of stool to nursing staff with 100% accuracy. Fill in own bowel chart each day accurately. Empty urine drainage bag using flip-flow valve. Record fluid balance accurately with assistance. Independent and safe in MWC in grounds of rehabilitation centre. Make a phone call each day to wife and demonstrate turn taking in the conversation by asking how she is, what happened on the farm today and has she seen any of their friends. Send a text to a friend. Make sandwich lunch for self and wife using memory aid. Prepare shopping list for hot lunch using memory aid.
Weeks 9–12 (SIU)	Attend to bowel care with supervision (enema insertion, abdominal massage, digital stimulation). Use flow chart to problem solve bowel issues with prompts. Perform clean intermittent self catheterisation (CISC) under supervision of nurse. Independent and safe in MWC in local community including crossing roads, negotiating kerbs and using traffic lights. Demonstrate turn taking in group conversation by not interrupting and waiting for responses to questions. Write an e-mail to a friend demonstrating interest in and concern for others. Purchase items from local shop performing money transaction under supervision. Cook hot meal for lunch with supervision.
Weeks 12–16 (SIU)	Attend all aspects of bowel care independently. Perform CISC four times per day independently. Independent and safe in MWC in unfamiliar environments, including over uneven terrain and using public transport. Participate appropriately in conversation with family and friends. Plan a BBQ deciding date, food and people to invite. Prepare BBQ shopping list using memory aid. Invite people to BBQ using telephone, email or text. Plan and undertake trip to shopping centre using bus to purchase supplies independently. Cook a BBQ for friends with wife close by for support as needed.

Timetabling

In a speciality rehabilitation setting, the flow of a patient's day should resemble, as far as possible, that of their usual lifestyle. Patients actively participate in all aspects of their personal care, dress in day clothes and commonly eat meals in a dining room. A combination of individual and group sessions with various disciplines is common. Matthew's mutually agreed timetable for week 12 of his inpatient rehabilitation program is presented in Table 10.11. Note the progression from less to more independence in some self-care activities; for example, self administration of medications (SAM).

As each rehabilitation journey is unique, we must remember that although some patients appear to transition through these stages seamlessly, others may falter or vacillate. It may take some patients more time to regain the 'capacity to direct one's life' (Schipper et al., 2011, p. 527), given the catastrophic event and challenging process of integrating this into a new way of living (DeSanto-Madeya, 2006).

NURSING'S CONTRIBUTION TO MATTHEW'S REHABILITATION

Nursing interventions, like other rehabilitation interventions, need to focus on maintaining and restoring function, promoting health and preventing and minimising disability. As with all interventions, nurses assess, plan, implement and evaluate their intervention. While Johnson et al. (2009) highlight the centrality of patient education to nursing's role, Boldt et al. (2005) illuminate the fuller breadth of nursing's contribution to rehabilitation. Nursing staff in two neurological hospitals in Germany documented 118 different nursing interventions that were matched to the components of the ICF: 19 related to body functions, 19 to body structures, 13 to activities and participation, and 5 to environmental factors (Boldt et al., 2005).

Although not so widely studied, the role of personal factors in an individual's rehabilitation is an important consideration for nursing. Personal factors can be assets or liabilities; hence they can be enablers or barriers of rehabilitation. Nurses have a responsibility to assist patients to identify and use their personal strengths and assets. This is as central to recapturing the ability to self-care (Guidetti, Asaba, & Tham, 2009), as it is to 'the social process of adaptation' (Duggan, Albright, & Lequerica, 2008, p. 979). Table 10.12 lists examples of interventions that nurses could use to support Matthew to achieve his rehabilitation goals.

Part 2 of Case Study 10.1 provides an update on Matthew's progress during inpatient rehabilitation.

LIFE AFTER HOSPITALISATION: REHABILITATION BEGINS IN EARNEST

A seamless transition from the inpatient rehabilitation unit to the community is essential to maintain the momentum of rehabilitation for the person and their family. To facilitate this transition, rehabilitation inpatients commonly access the community with a treatment team member or they have overnight leave. However, the environment in which this occurs is usually well structured, contained and controlled.

Transition from an inpatient to community setting can involve new challenges for the patient, their family and friends, as well as those working with them. Commonly, a person leaving inpatient rehabilitation believes they can get on with their life and things will return to normal quite quickly after discharge. The impact of an injury is often felt most when the person returns home. Here the reality of the altered body and altered life is most apparent (O'Brien, Nicholson, Johnson, & Gravell, 2002).

Appointment of a case manager from a community spinal service can help with community re-integration. Case management is a 'collaborative process that assesses, plans, implements, coordinates, monitors and evaluates the options and services required to meet

TABLE 10.11
Matthew's timetable for week 12

TIME	MONDAY	TUESDAY	WEDNESDAY	THURSDAY	FRIDAY	SATURDAY	SUNDAY
06.00	CISC with nurse supervising	CISC with nurse supervising	CISC with nurse supervising	CISC with nurse supervising	Independent CISC	Independent CISC	Independent CISC
06.30	Sleep	Sleep	Sleep	Sleep	Sleep	Sleep	Sleep
07.30	Breakfast	Breakfast	Breakfast	Breakfast	Breakfast	Breakfast	Breakfast
08.00	Medication education	SAM with nurse supervising	SAM with nurse supervising	SAM with nurse supervising	Independent SAM	Independent SAM	Independent SAM
08.00	Bowel care supervised by nurse	Bowel care supervised by nurse	Bowel care supervised by nurse	Bowel care supervised by nurse	Independent bowel care using flowchart	Independent bowel care using flowchart	Independent bowel care using flowchart
08.30	Shower independently	Shower independently	Shower independently	Shower independently	Shower independently	Shower independently	Shower independently
09.00							
09.30	Free time or rest	Session in the gym with physio	Free time or rest	Free time or rest	Group community access trip on buses & ferry with RT	Free time or rest	Free time or rest
10.00	WC skills outside with RT		Communication group with SP	Email practice with SP		Independent exercises in gym	Independent exercises in gym
10.30							
11.00	Car transfer practice with OT	Counselling session with clin psych	Free time or rest	Session in the gym with physio		Coffee group supported by nurses	Free time or rest
11.30							
12.00	CISC with nurse supervising	CISC with nurse supervising	CISC with nurse supervising	Independent CISC	Independent CISC in community	Independent CISC	Independent CISC
12.30	Lunch	Lunch	Lunch	Cook hot meal for lunch with supervision from OT	Lunch in community	Lunch	Cook lunch for wife with support as required
13.00	Meeting with key-worker to discuss progress and new goals	Free time or rest	Free time pr rest		Group community access trip	Free time or rest	
13.30		Peer support with local spinal injuries support group	Cardio group with physiotherapy assistant	Goal planning meeting with whole team to confirm next set of goals and actions		Trip out with parents transferring independently into their car	

(continued next page...)

TABLE 10.11

Matthew's timetable for week 12 — cont'd

TIME	MONDAY	TUESDAY	WEDNESDAY	THURSDAY	FRIDAY	SATURDAY	SUNDAY
14.00	Medication education	SAM with nurse supervising	SAM with nurse supervising	SAM with nurse supervising	SAM in community	Independent SAM	Independent SAM
14.30	Hydrotherapy with physio	Return to work discussion with VT	Free time or rest	Free time or rest	Group community access trip	Out with parents	Free time or rest
15.00			WC skills outside with RT		Physiotherapy session in the gym		Sunday afternoon film club supported by nurses
15.30							
16.00	Free time or rest		Car transfer practice with OT		Free time or rest		
16.30							
17.00	CISC with nurse supervising	CISC with nurse supervising	CISC with nurse supervising	Independent CISC	Independent CISC	Independent CISC	Independent CISC
18.00	Dinner	Dinner	Dinner	Dinner	Dinner	Dinner	Dinner
19.00	Phone wife	Phone mate	Skype sister and nephews	Phone mum and dad	Phone wife	Phone wife	Skype brother and nieces
20.00	Medication education	SAM with nurse supervising	SAM with nurse supervising	SAM with nurse supervising	Independent SAM	Independent SAM	Independent SAM
20.15	Transfer to bed using slide board supervised by nurses	Transfer to bed using slide board supervised by nurses	Transfer to bed using slide board supervised by nurses	Transfer to bed using slide board independently	Transfer to bed using slide board independently	Transfer to bed using slide board independently	Transfer to bed using slide board independently
21.00							
22.00	CISC with nurse supervising	CISC with nurse supervising	CISC with nurse supervising	Independent CISC	Independent CISC	Independent CISC	Independent CISC
	Sleep	Sleep	Sleep	Sleep	Sleep	Sleep	Sleep
02.00	CISC with nurse supervising	CISC with nurse supervising	CISC with nurse supervising	Independent CISC	Independent CISC	Independent CISC	Independent CISC
	Sleep	Sleep	Sleep	Sleep	Sleep	Sleep	Sleep

Abbreviations: CISC = clean intermittent self catheterisation; SAM = self-administration of medications; physio = physiotherapist; RT = recreation therapist; OT = occupational therapist; clin psych = clinical psychologist; WC = wheelchair skills; SP = speech pathologist; VT = vocational therapist.

TABLE 10.12 Example nursing interventions

GOAL	EXAMPLE INTERVENTIONS
To promote self-management of urinary elimination	• Education of patient regarding bladder management. • Prepare and educate patient about bladder investigations. • Support patient to maintain record of input and output. • Support patient through trial of void. • Education regarding CISC. • Practise CISC under supervision. • Gauge readiness for independence in CISC. • Educate and encourage patient to set alarms on memory aid for CISC timing. • Document and co-ordinate team evaluation of urinary elimination. • Modify program as required. • Education of family as/if required.
To promote self-management of faecal elimination	• Obtain a pre-injury history regarding faecal elimination. • Education regarding bowel management (including methods, diet, fluids etc). • Education regarding bowel movement classifications (Bristol Stool Chart). • Education regarding enema administration, abdominal massage and digital stimulation. • Attend to bowel care under supervision, prompts and support. • Support to problem solve around bowel problems using flow chart. • Gauge readiness for independent bowel care. • Document and coordinate team evaluation of bowel management. • Education of family as/if required.
To promote self-management of skin	• Education regarding SCI and how this affects skin and pressure area management. • Education regarding techniques for pressure relief (devices, frequency). • Support patient to problem solve around potential or real problems using flow chart. • Support in decision making around pressure relieving devices — cushions, mattresses. • Advice regarding appropriate clothing. • Education of family as/if required.

CASE STUDY 10.1 Part 2

By the end of week 16 of inpatient rehabilitation Matthew is able to:

- transfer independently in the morning and at night using a slide board
- independently get off the floor onto a chair
- mobilise independently indoors and in some outdoor situations
- mobilise outdoors using a 4 wheel drive power chair
- independently perform CISC
- independently perform bowel care
- access, set up and prepare a BBQ.

While Matthew is independent with self catheterisation and managing his skin within an inpatient rehabilitation setting, transferring these skills to manage these issues while working on the farm may take some time as Matthew is still developing an understanding of issues he may experience when he goes home. This transition will benefit from consultation with a community spinal injuries rehabilitation service.

an individual's health needs using communication and available resources to promote quality, cost effective outcomes' (Snowden, 2001, p. 3). Case management has an element of advocacy as a case manager assists the person, their family and friends to identify solutions to activity limitations and participation restrictions (Snowden, 2001). As such, the case manager helps individuals structure their rehabilitation in ways that are meaningful to them.

In the community the rehabilitation process is much slower as the intensity of sessions with health professionals is reduced, or ceased as in Matthew's case given the distance from home to services. Increased self-reliance and the support of family and friends are crucial to goal achievement at this stage (Ylvisaker et al., 2003) as rehabilitation is integrated into daily life. Furthermore, community rehabilitation is more likely to be multi-agency and multi-sectorial in nature. Every person, agency and service that Matthew interacts with has the potential to enable his rehabilitation. Unfortunately, it is also true that these same interactions can become barriers. This means that each of us has a responsibility to ensure that in our personal as well as our professional lives we are socially inclusive by enabling human functioning and participation.

Part 3 of Case Study 10.1 presents an overview of Matthew's progress after his return home.

CASE STUDY 10.1 Part 3

Matthew hosted his first BBQ within 1 month of returning home; inviting his friends and family as planned prior to discharge from hospital. Approximately 1 month after returning home, Matthew started to resume some light work around the farm, assisted by his close mates and one of his brothers who lived nearby. Initially he worked for only 3 hours a day, mostly directing and delegating tasks to his helpers until he gained confidence using his power wheelchair and navigating the uneven terrain. He then began to attend to heavier jobs, such as fixing fences and replenishing the feed lots and over the course of a month began to take on more and more of the jobs around the farm. Family and friends were able to assist in the modification of some of the machinery he was required to use and Matthew also was less hesitant to ask for help if he needed it from a select group of friends.

Two months after returning home, Matthew resumed his role as secretary of the local Lions Club and utilised his memory aid to assist with the organisation and planning of meetings. He was proficient in the use of a laptop computer to record and circulate meeting notes via email. In response to Matthew's residual memory deficits/impairments, Matthew and his wife recognised the potential for misunderstandings and miscommunication. Together they decided to use a whiteboard at home to improve communication and to minimise the potential for friction between them.

Matthew continued with his daily exercise program at home to maintain the upper body strength required for mobility in a manual wheelchair and to run his farm. Following on from the sexuality counselling he had received while an impatient on the rehabilitation unit, Matthew was able to resume a full sexual relationship with his wife shortly after he returned home using Viagra to maintain an erection. Twelve months after returning home Matthew has now set a goal to set up an online rural and remote support group for young men with spinal cord injuries. This project is in its infancy, but Matthew is determined to see this goal through; this started his wife thinking about setting up a similar group for wives.

Reflective questions

1. What rehabilitation interventions could you incorporate into your nursing practice in acute care?
2. Interview allied health professionals from a range of disciplines where you work and find out about the scope of practice for each discipline. What aspects of nursing overlap with the scopes of practice of allied health disciplines?
3. If you were Matthew's brother, how could you support his rehabilitation?

Recommended readings

DeSanto-Madeya, S. (2006). The meaning of living with spinal cord injury 5 to 10 years after the injury. *Western Journal of Nursing Research*, *28*(3), 265–289.

Kautz, D. D. (2008). Inspiring hope in our rehabilitation patients, their families and ourselves. *Rehabilitation Nursing*, *33*, 148–153.

Kearney, P., & Pryor, J. (2004). The international classification of functioning, disability and health (ICF) and nursing. *Journal of Advanced Nursing*, *46*(2), 162–170.

Levack, W. M. M., Kayes, N. M., & Fadyl, J. K. (2010). Experience of recovery and outcome following traumatic brain inury: a metasynthesis of qualitative research. *Disability and Rehabilitation*, *32*(12), 986–999.

Sparkes, A. C., & Smith, B. (2003). Men, sport, spinal cord injury and narrative time. *Qualitative Research*, *3*(3), 295–320.

References

Albano, C., Comandante, L., & Nolan, S. (2005). Innovations in the management of cerebral injury. *Critical Care Nursing Quarterly*, *28*(2), 135–149.

American Spinal Injury Association. (2011). *International Standards for neurological classification of spinal cord injury*. Retrieved July 9, 2012, from http://www.asia-spinalinjury.org/publications/59544_sc_Exam_Sheet_r4.pdf

Australasian Rehabilitation Nurses Association. (2002). *Rehabilitation Nursing — Scope of Practice Position Paper* (2nd ed.). Retrieved January 24, 2013, from http://www.arna.com.au/position.html

Australian Campdraft Association. (2010). *General information rules and guidelines*. Retrieved July 12, 2012, from http://www.campdraft.com.au/Page/208

Australian Campdraft Association. (2012). *About campdrafting*. Retrieved July 12, 2012, from http://www.campdrafting.com.au/index.php?page=about-campdrafting

Australian Institute of Health and Welfare. (2007). *Disability in Australia: acquired brain injury*, (Bulletin no.55. Cat no. AUS 96). Canberra: Author.

Barnes, M. P., & Ward, A. B. (2000). *Textbook of rehabilitation medicine*. Oxford: Oxford University Press.

Boldt, C., Brach, M., Grill, E., et al. (2005). The ICF categories identified in nursing interventions and administered to neurological patients with post acute rehabilitation needs. *Disability & Rehabilitation*, *27*(7/8), 431–436.

Bowen, C., Yeates, G., & Palmer, S. (2010). *A relational rehabilitation approach: Thinking about relationships after brain injury*. London: Karnac Book Ltd.

Brain Injury Association of Queensland. (2006). *Acquired brain injury the facts. The practical guide to understanding and responding to acquired brain injury*. Queensland: Author.

Branche-Spelich, M., Reyes, I. A., & Miller, D. (2012). Spinal cord injury. In K. L. Mauk (Ed.), *Rehabilitation nursing: A contemporary approach to practice* (pp. 268–282). Sudbury, MA: Jones & Bartlett.

Burton, C. R. (2000). A description of the nursing role in stroke rehabilitation. *Journal of Advanced Nursing, 32*(1), 174–181.

Burton, C., & Gibbon, B. (2006). Expanding the role of the stroke nurse: a pragmatic clinical trial. *Journal of Advanced Nursing, 52*(6), 640–650.

Cameron, I. D. (2010). Models of rehabilitation — commonalities of interventions that work and of those that do not. *Disability & Rehabilitation, 32*(12), 1051–1058.

Cardol, M., DeJong, B., & Ward, D. (2002). On autonomy and participation rehabilitation. *Disability & Rehabilitation, 24*(18), 970–974.

Cicerone, K. D. (2004). Participation as an outcome of traumatic brain injury rehabilitation. *Journal of Trauma Rehabilitation, 19*(6), 494–501.

Clapton, J., & Kendall E. (2002). Autonomy and participation in rehabilitation: time for a new paradigm? *Disability & Rehabilitation, 24*(18), 987–991.

Cott, C. (2004). Client-centred rehabilitation: client perspectives. *Disability & Rehabilitation, 26*(24), 1411–1422.

Craig, A., & Perry, K. N. (2008). *Guidelines for health professionals on the psychosocial care of people with spinal cord injury*. Retrieved July 9, 2012, from http://www.aci.health.nsw.gov.au/__data/assets/pdf_file/0019/155233/sci_ps_guideweb.pdf

Department of Veterans Affairs. (2009). *VA and spinal cord injury*. Retrieved July 9, 2012, from http://www1.va.gov/opa/publications/factsheets/fs_spinal_cord_injury.pdf

DeSanto-Madeya, S. (2006). The meaning of living with spinal cord injury 5 to 10 years after the injury. *Western Journal of Nursing Research, 28*(3), 265–289.

Dickson, A., O'Brien, G., Ward, R., et al. (2012). Adjustment and coping in spousal caregivers following a traumatic spinal cord injury: An interpretive phenomenological analysis. *Journal of Health Psychology, 17*(2), 247–257.

Dittmar, S. (1989). Scope of rehabilitation. In S. Dittmar (Ed.), *Rehabilitation nursing: process and application*. St Louis: CV Mosby.

Donnelly, J. P., Donnelly, K., & Grohman, K. K. (2005). A multi-perspective concept mapping study of problems associated with traumatic brain injury. *Brain Injury, 19*(13), 1077–1085.

Duggan, C., Albright, K., & Lequerica, A. (2008). Using the ICF to code and analyse women's disability narratives. *Disability & Rehabilitation, 30*(12), 978–990.

Ellis-Hill, C. (2011). Identity and sense of self; the significance of personhood in rehabilitation. *Journal of the Australasian Rehabilitation Nurses Association, 14*(1), 6–13.

Ellis-Hill, C., Payne, S., & Ward, C. (2008). Using stroke to explore the life thread model: An alternative approach to understanding rehabilitation following acquired disability. *Disability & Rehabilitation, 30*(2), 150–159.

Faull K., & Hills, M. D. (2006). The role of the spiritual dimension of the self as the prime determinant of health. *Disability & Rehabilitation, 28*(11), 729–740.

Flemming, J., Sampson, J., Cornwell, P., et al. (2012). Brain injury rehabilitation: The lived experience of inpatients and their family caregivers. *Scandinavian Journal of Occupational Therapy, 19*, 184–193.

Ghaj, J. (2000). Traumatic brain injury. *The Lancet, 356*(9233), 923–929.

Gibbon, B. (2004). Service user involvement: The impact of stroke and the meaning of rehabilitation. *Journal of the Australasian Rehabilitation Nurses Association, 7*(2), 8–12.

Gignac, M. A., & Cott, C. (1998). A conceptual model of independence and dependence for adults with chronic physical illness and disability. *Social Science Medicine, 47*(6), 739–753.

Grill, E., Quittan, M., Fialka-Moser, V., et al. (2011). Brief ICF core sets for the acute hospital. *Journal of Rehabilitation Medicine, 43*, 123–130.

Guidetti, S., Asaba, E., & Tham, K. (2009). Meaning of context in recapturing self-care after stroke or spinal cord injury. *American Journal of Occupational Therapy*, *63*, 323–332.

Gutenbrunner, C., Meyer, T., Melvin, J., et al. (2011). Towards a conceptual description of physical and rehabilitation medicine. *Journal of Rehabilitation Medicine*, *43*, 760–764.

Habilitation Benefits Coalition. (2011). *Coverage of habilitation services and devices in the essential benefits package under the Affordable Care Act.* Retrieved July 11, 2012, from http://www.aapmr.org/advocacy/health-policy/federal-reform/Documents/Habilitation-White-Paper.pdf

Hafsteinsdottir, T. B., & Grypdonck, M. (1997). Being a stroke patient: A review of the literature. *Journal of Advanced Nursing*, *26*, 580–588.

Hammell, K. W. (2007). Experience of rehabilitation following spinal cord injury: a meta-synthesis of qualitative findings. *Spinal Cord*, *45*:260–274.

Hannay, H. J., Howieson, D. B., Loring, D. W., et al. (2004). Neuropathology for neuropsychologists. In M. D. Lezak, D. B. Howieson & D. W. Loring (Eds.), *Neuropsychological assessment* (4th ed., pp. 157–285). New York: Oxford University Press.

Henderson, S. (1997). Knowing the patient and the impact on patient participation: A grounded theory study. *International Journal of Nursing Practice*, *3*, 111–118.

Hickey, J. V. (2009a). Rehabilitation of neuroscience patients. In J. V. Hickey (Ed.), *The clinical practice of neurological and neurosurgical nursing* (6th ed., pp. 213–267). Philadelphia: Lippincott, Williams and Wilkins.

Hickey, J. V. (2009b). Vertebral and spinal cord injuries. In J. V. Hickey (Ed.), *The clinical practice of neurological and neurosurgical nursing* (6th ed., pp. 410–453). Philadelphia: Lippincott, Williams and Wilkins.

Hickey, J. V., & Kanusky, J. T. (2009). Overview of neuroanatomy and neurophysiology. In J. V. Hickey (Ed.), *The clinical practice of neurological and neurosurgical nursing* (6th ed., pp. 40–88). Philadelphia: Lippincott, Williams and Wilkins.

Hickey, J. V., & Prator, B. C. (2009). Craniocerebral injuries. In J. V. Hickey (Ed.), *The clinical practice of neurological and neurosurgical nursing* (6th ed., pp. 370–409). Philadelphia: Lippincott, Williams and Wilkins.

Hill, H. (1999). Traumatic brain injury: a view from the inside. *Brain Injury*, *13*(11), 839–844.

Hoeman, S. P., Liszner, K., & Alverzo, J. (2008). Functional mobility with activities of daily living. In S. P. Hoeman (Ed.), *Rehabilitation nursing: prevention, intervention & outcomes* (4th ed., pp. 200–257). St Louis: Mosby Elsevier.

Johnson, K., Bailey, J., Rundquist, J., et al. (2009). Classification of SCI rehabilitation treatments SCIRehab project series: The supplemental nursing taxonomy. *Journal of Spinal Cord Medicine*, *32*(3), 329–335.

Kautz, D. (2011). Great rehabilitation nurses combine art and science to create magic. *Rehabilitation Nursing*, *36*(1), 13–15.

Kearney, P., & Pryor, J. (2004). The international classification of functioning, disability and health (ICF) and nursing. *Journal of Advanced Nursing*, *46*(2), 162–170.

Kirkevold, M. (1997). The role of nursing in the rehabilitation of acute stroke patients: toward a unified theoretical perspective. *Advances in Nursing Science*, *19*(4), 55–64.

Levack, W. M. M. (2009). Ethics in goal planning for rehabilitation: a utilitarian perspective. *Clinical Rehabilitation*, *23*, 345–351.

Levack, W. M. M., Kayes, N. M., & Fadyl, J. K. (2010). Experience of recovery and outcome following traumatic brain injury: a metasynthesis of qualitative research. *Disability & Rehabilitation*, *32*(12), 986–999.

Levack, W., Taylor, K., Siegert, R., et al. (2006). Is goal planning in rehabilitation effective? A systematic review. *Clinical Rehabilitation*, *20*, 739–755.

Liaschenko, J., & Fisher, A. (1999). Theorising the knowledge that nurses use in the conduct of their work. *Scholarly Inquiry for nursing practice: An International Journal*, *13*(1), 29–41.

Long, A. F., Kneafsey, R., Ryan, J., et al. (2002). The role of the nurse within the multi-professional rehabilitation team. *Journal of Advanced Nursing, 37*(1), 70–78.

Low, G. (2003). Developing the nurse's role in rehabilitation. *Nursing Standard, 17*(45), 33–38.

Mastos, M., Miller, K., Eliasson, A. C., et al. (2007). Goal-directed training: linking theories of treatment to clinical practice for improved functional activities in daily life. *Clinical Rehabilitation, 21*, 47–55.

Mateer, C., Sira, C. S., & O'Connell, M. E. (2005). Putting humpty dumpty together again. The importance of integrating cognitive and emotional interventions. *Journal of Head Trauma Rehabilitation, 20*(1), 62–75.

McCance, T., Slater, P., & McCormack, B. (2008). Using the caring dimensions inventory as an indicator of person-centred nursing. *Journal of Clinical Nursing, 18*, 409–417.

McPherson, K. (2006). Rehabilitation nursing — A final frontier? *International Journal of Nursing Studies, 43*, 787–789.

McPherson, K., Brander, P., Taylor, W., et al. (2001). Living with arthritis — what is important? *Disability & Rehabilitation, 23*(16), 706–721.

Miller, E. (2003). Rehabilitation nursing in a consumer-driven world. *Rehabilitation Nursing, 28*(5), 139, 163.

Morse, J. (1997). Responding to threats to integrity of self. *Advances in Nursing Science, 19*(4), 21–36.

Muller, M., Grill, E., Stier-Jarmer, M., et al. (2011). Validation of the comprehensive ICF core set for patients receiving rehabilitation interventions in the acute care setting. *Journal of Rehabilitation Medicine, 43*, 92–101.

Muller, M., Stier-Jarmer, M., Quittan, M., et al. (2011). Validation of the comprehensive ICF core set for patients in early post-acute rehabilitation facilities. *Journal of Rehabilitation Medicine, 43*, 102–112.

National Stroke Foundation. (2010). *Clinical guidelines for stroke management 2010*. Melbourne: Author.

New South Wales Health. (2011). *Rehabilitation redesign project final report*. North Sydney: Author.

Norton, L. (2010). *Spinal cord injury, Australia 2007–08. Injury research and statistics series no. 52. Cat. No INJCAT 128*. Canberra: Australian Institute of Health and Welfare.

O'Brien, J., Nicholson, P., Johnson, R., et al. (2002). Introduction. In R. Gravell & R. Johnson (Eds.), *Head injury rehabilitation a community team perspective* (pp. 1–36). London: Whurr Publishers.

O'Reilly, K., & Pryor, J. (2002). Young people with brain injury in nursing homes: not the best option! *Australian Health Review, 25*(3), 34–39.

Olinzock, B. (2004). A model for assessing learning readiness for self direction of care in individuals with spinal cord injuries: A qualitative study. *SCI Nursing, 21*(2), 69–74.

Orem, D. E. (1995). *Nursing: Concepts of Practice* (5th ed.). Philadelphia: Elsevier.

Ozer, M. N. (1999). Patient participation in the management of stroke rehabilitation. *Topics in Stroke Rehabilitation, 6*(1), 43–59.

Pagulayan, K. F., Temkin, N. R., Machamer, J., et al. (2006). A longitudinal study of health-related quality of life after traumatic brain injury. *Archives of Physical Medicine and Rehabilitation, 87*, 611–618.

Plaisted, L. M. (1978). Rehabilitation nurse. In R. M. Goldenson (Ed.), *Disability and rehabilitation handbook* (pp. 291–309). New York: McGraw-Hill.

Playford, E. D., Siegert, R., Levack, W., et al. (2009). Areas of consensus and controversy about goal setting in rehabilitation: a conference report. *Clinical Rehabilitation, 23*, 334–344.

Pratt, C., & Baldry, K. (2002). Families and carers. In R. Gravell & R. Johnson (Eds.), *Head injury rehabilitation: a community team perspective* (pp. 291–309). London: Whurr Publishers.

Prochaska, J. O., DiClemente, C. C., & Norcross, J. (1992). In search of how people change. *American Psychologist, 47*(9), 1102–1114.

Pryor, J. (1999). Goals and focus. In J. Pryor (Ed.), *Rehabilitation — A vital nursing function* (pp. 79–96). Canberra: Royal College of Nursing.

Pryor, J. (2000). Creating a rehabilitative milieu. *Rehabilitation Nursing, 25*(4), 141–144.

Pryor, J. (2002). Rehabilitative nursing: A core nursing function across all settings. *Collegian, 9*(2), 11–15.

Pryor, J. (2003). Co-ordination of patient care in inpatient rehabilitation. *Clinical Rehabilitation, 17*, 341–346.

Pryor, J. (2005). *A grounded theory of nursing's contribution to inpatient rehabilitation (PhD thesis)*. Melbourne: Deakin University.

Pryor, J. (2010). Nurses creating a rehabilitative milieu. *Rehabilitation Nursing, 35*(3), 123–128.

Pryor, J. (2012). Guest editorial: The nature of nursing interventions in rehabilitation. *Journal of the Australasian Rehabilitation Nurses Association, 15*(1), 2–3.

Pryor, J., & Buzio, A. (2010). Enhancing inpatient rehabilitation through the engagement of patients and nurses. *Journal of Advanced Nursing, 66*(5), 978–987.

Pryor, J., & Dean, S. (2012). The person in context. In S. Dean, R. Seigert & W. Taylor (Eds.), *Interprofessional rehabilitation: a person centred approach* (pp. 135–165). Oxford: Wiley-Blackwell.

Pryor, J., & Jannings, W. (2004). Preparing patients to self manage faecal continence following spinal cord injury. *International Journal of Therapy and Rehabilitation, 11*(2), 79–82.

Pryor, J., & O'Connell, B. (2008). Incongruence between nurses' and patients' understandings and expectations of rehabilitation. *Journal of Clinical Nursing, 18*, 1766–1774.

Pryor, J., & Smith, C. (2002). A framework for the role of registered nurses in the specialty practice of rehabilitation nursing in Australia. *Journal of Advanced Nursing, 39*(2), 249–257.

Rees, R. J. (2005). *Interrupted lives: Rehabilitation and learning following brain injury*. Melbourne: IP Communications.

Rusk, H. A. (1960). Rehabilitation: The third phase of medicine. *Rhode Island Medical Journal, 43*, 385–387.

Schipper, K., Widdrshoven, G., & Abma, T. (2011). Citizenship and autonomy in acquired brain injury. *Nursing Ethics, 18*(4), 526–536.

Scobbie, L., Dixon, D., & Wyke, S. (2011). Goal setting and action planning in the rehabilitation setting: Development of a theoretically informed practice framework. *Clinical Rehabilitation, 25*, 468–482.

Smith, S. (2005). Response to: Theory development and a science of rehabilitation. In R. J. Siegert, K. M. McPherson & S. G. Dean, *Disability & Rehabilitation, 27*(24), 1509.

Snowden, F. (2001). *Case Manager's desk reference* (2nd ed.). Gaithersburg: Aspen Publishers.

Stein-Parbury, J. (2009). *Patient and person: interpersonal skills in nursing* (4th ed.). Philadelphia: Elsevier.

Stewart, R., & Bhagwanjee, A. (1999). Promoting group empowerment and self reliance through participatory research: a case study of people with physical disability. *Disability & Rehabilitation, 21*(7), 338–345.

St-Germain, D., Boivin, B., & Fougeyrollas, P. (2011). The caring-disability creation process model: a new way of combining 'care' in nursing and 'rehabilitation' for better quality of services and patient safety. *Disability & Rehabilitation, 33*(21–22), 2105–2113.

Stucki, G., Cieza, A., & Melvin, J. (2007). The International Classification of Functioning, Disability and Health: A unifying model for the conceptual description of the rehabilitation strategy. *Journal of Rehabilitation Medicine, 39*, 279–285.

Stucki G., Ustun B., & Melvin J. (2005). Applying the ICF for the acute hospital and early post-acute rehabilitation facilities. *Disability and Rehabilitation, 27*(7/8), 349–352.

Todres, L., Galvin, K., & Holloway, I. (2009). The humanization of healthcare: A value framework for qualitative research. *International Journal of Qualitative Studies on Health and Well-being, 4*, 68–77.

Turner-Stokes, L., Disler, P. B., Nair, A., et al. (2005). Multidisciplinary rehabilitation for acquired brain injury in adults of working age (review). *Cochrane Database of Systematic Reviews*, Issue 3. Art. No.: CD004170. DOI: 10.1002/14651858.CD004170.pub2

Tyrrell, E., Levack, W., Ritchie, L., et al. (2012). Nursing contribution to the rehabilitation of older patients: patient and family perspectives. *Journal of Advanced Nursing, 68*(11), 2466–2476.

United Nations. (2006). *World Programme of Action Concerning Disabled Persons*. United Nations, New York. Retrieved June 29, 2012, from http://www.un.org/esa/socdev/enable/diswpa01.htm

United Nations. (2012). *Habilitation and rehabilitation*. Retrieved July 11, 2012, from http://www.un.org/disabilities/default.asp?id=238

van den Broek, M. D. (2005). Why does neurorehabilitation fail? *Journal of Head Trauma Rehabilitation, 20*(5), 464–473.

Wade, D. (1999). Goal planning in stroke rehabilitation: How? *Topics in Stroke Rehabilitation, 6*(2), 16–36.

Wade, D. (2005). Describing rehabilitation interventions. *Clinical Rehabilitation, 19*, 811–818.

Wade, D. (2009). Goal setting in rehabilitation: an overview of what, why and how. *Clinical Rehabilitation, 23*, 291–295.

Wade, D., & deJong, B. (2000). Recent advances in rehabilitation. *British Medical Journal, 320*, 1385–1388.

Ward, A. B., Barnes, M. P., Stark, S. C., et al. (2009). *Oxford handbook of clinical rehabilitation* (2nd ed.). Oxford: Oxford University Press.

Williams, J., & Pryor, J. (2010). Rehabilitation and recovery processes. In J. Williams, L. Perry, & C. Watkins (Eds.), *Acute stroke nursing* (Chapter 11, pp. 241–262). Oxford: Wiley-Blackwell.

World Health Organization. (2001). *International Classification of Functioning, Disability and Health*. Geneva: WHO.

Ylvisaker, M., Jacobs, H., & Feeney, T. (2003). Positive supports for people who experience behavioural and cognitive disability after brain injury: A review. *Journal of Head Trauma Rehabilitation, 8*(1), 7–32.

Youngson, R. (2012). *Time to care: How to love your patients and your job*. New Zealand: Rebelheart Publishers.

CHAPTER 11

Annette James
Gilbert Blandin de Chalain

Impact of obesity on chronic illness and disability

Learning objectives

When you have completed this chapter you will be able to:

- understand the impact obesity has on the development of chronic illnesses and disability
- identify the key factors that contribute to an obese population
- describe the preventative mechanisms and main treatment protocols for managing obesity
- discuss the importance of a multidisciplinary approach in the overall management of obesity
- explore the relationship of urban planning to the challenges presented by obesity in the community.

Key words

multidisciplinary approach, nutrition, obesity, overweight, urban planning

INTRODUCTION

Obesity is defined as abnormal and excess accumulation of adipose tissue. The World Health Organization (WHO) describes obesity as a worldwide epidemic that has more than doubled since 1980. In 2008 more than 1.4 billion adults aged 20 and older were overweight or obese. The incidence of overweight and obesity in developed countries is increasing at an alarming rate and because overweight and obesity is associated with many chronic diseases, it has a dramatic effect on health costs in the present and will have in the future.

Lowering the incidence of obesity in the community requires a multidisciplinary approach involving educators, urban planners and nursing and health practitioners.

INCIDENCE IN AUSTRALIA

According to the Australian Bureau of Statistics (ABS, 2012), the number of people who are obese is rising rapidly, making obesity one of the fastest developing public health problems. Recent studies estimate that more than half of all Australian women (56.2%) and two-thirds of men (70.3%) are overweight or obese. Almost 64% of the adult population in Australia is overweight or obese, and this has more than doubled in the past 20 years; the prevalence is 2.5 times greater than it was in 1980. Importantly, childhood obesity in Australia is amongst the highest in the developed nations with 25.3% of Australian children now overweight or obese (ABS, 2012). The prevalence of overweight and obesity is higher among children of lower socioeconomic status (Hardy, King, Espinel, Cosgrove, & Bauman, 2010; O'Dea, 2003).

A study of 20 347 Australian men and women showed that for the period 1980–2000 obesity increased by 250%, with the rate of growth in obesity higher in women than in men (34% compared to 27%). The study correlated obesity with lower socioeconomic status, higher television viewing time and lower physical activity (Cameron, 2003).

CLINICAL MEASUREMENTS

The most convenient way to measure overweight and obesity is by body mass index (BMI, kg/m^2). A person is overweight if their BMI is between 25 and 29 and obese if their BMI is 30 or greater. Obesity is also classified according to the increased health risks associated with increasing BMI levels: class I (BMI 30–34.9), class II (BMI 35–39.9) and class III (BMI 40+) (WHO 2000). In clinical practice children are classified according to BMI-for-age growth charts (Baur, 2000).

Some practitioners use waist-to-hip ratios, as there is a greater risk of heart disease, diabetes, infertility, liver disease and cancers associated with central adipose tissue accumulation ('spare tyre'), and a single measurement can be used. Men with a waist circumference greater than 102 cm and women with a waist circumference greater than 88 cm are classified as obese (Baur, 2000). A waist circumference greater than 93 cm for men and 80 cm for women increases the risk of some lifestyle-related chronic diseases (Department of Health and Ageing [DOHA], 2010).

There are also a number of electronic devices that can be incorporated into weighing scales or hand-held devices that can determine total adipose tissue but these have to be corrected for height, gender and athletic ability.

The obesity class into which a person falls determines the type of therapy and lifestyle changes that can be suggested. A reduction in dietary energy intake and an increase in physical activity would be considered for all obese people, and aggressive methods of weight reduction using drugs or bariatric surgery for people with class II or class III obesity, particularly if they have other risk factors (Katzmarzyk & Mason, 2006).

EPIDEMIOLOGY AND CAUSES OF OBESITY

A study of hospital and medical practice records in 2003 found that of 14 preventable health risks examined, obesity was responsible for 7.5%, and physical inactivity 7% of the incidence of the major diseases in Australia (Australian Institute of Health and Welfare

[AIHW], 2011). The highest risk factor was smoking (7.8%).The study also showed that a strong upsurge in the number of people with diabetes is likely, mostly due to higher levels of obesity.

Other studies (AIHW, 2005, 2011) have shown that two-thirds of avoidable hospital admissions were due to chronic conditions (non-communicable disease), many from diabetes complications, heart and respiratory conditions caused by obesity. This places an economic burden on the health system as well as a stress on health workers, as obese patients are physically difficult to manage. The annual cost to the Australian community was estimated at $3 billion in 2007, so the cost-effectiveness and therapeutic benefits of management strategies must have a high priority.

Humans have evolved to consume food when it is available and store excess energy as adipose tissue while at the same time reducing physical activity, which maintains this store. Some individuals have 'thrifty genes', which are very efficient at conserving energy, but in Western society we do not experience the food scarcity that would reduce the energy stores. 'Dieting' in these individuals may be ineffective because of metabolic adaptation that conserves energy (Williams & Ness, 1991; Pijl, 2011).

Men are less likely to regard themselves as overweight or to feel that they need to lose weight than are women. Women are likely to be concerned about their weight, particularly if they are in higher socioeconomic groups or are high-profile individuals such as models or movie stars. Social class is also correlated with other health risk factors associated with obesity and heart disease, the incidence of drug taking, alcohol and tobacco abuse increasing in lower socioeconomic groups (Skurray & Ham, 1999; DOHA, 2010).

In recent years research studies have suggested that increased obesity incidence has occurred despite no apparent increase in food intake. This has been dubbed the 'American paradox'. A decrease in physical exercise was suggested to be the cause of this obesity (Philips, 2004). However, the International Obesity Taskforce (IOT, 2002) has shown that the total amount of food may have remained constant but there has been an increase in the intake of energy-dense foods and drinks, as well as an environment that limits opportunities for physical activity. Australian national nutrition surveys have shown that in Australia the increase in energy consumption in recent years has come not from dietary fat but from carbohydrate in the form of sucrose in processed foods (Stubbs & Lee, 2004; NHMRC, 2005).

A common myth is that obese people have a lower-than-normal metabolic rate. However, a comparison of populations in Europe, Australia and the USA has shown that the total daily energy expenditure of obese people is the same as that of normal-weight individuals. The mass of the population has increased so that population total energy expenditure has increased (IOT, 2002; Swinburn, Caterson, Seidell, & James, 2004).

Surveys investigating changes in physical activity over the period in which the incidence of obesity has increased have shown that the percentage of people undertaking 30 minutes of exercise per day decreased from 62% to 57% even though there is evidence that 45 to 60 minutes of exercise is needed on a daily basis to prevent weight gain on the present energy-rich diet (IOT, 2002). More recent studies in Australia and the USA have pinpointed the cause of obesity in children and young adults as an increase in consumption of soft drinks, with Australian data indicating a 240% increase over a 30-year period. Children who consumed the most soft drinks were obese and intervention studies showed that adults gained weight after ten weeks of normal consumption of soft drinks; another group who consumed artificially sweetened soft drinks lost weight. Soft drinks do not appease the appetite compared with solid energy-rich foods (Gill, Rangan, & Webb, 2006).

Other factors that have given rise to an 'obesogenic' environment are:

- increased consumption of high-kilojoule foods such as takeaway foods and soft drinks
- increased serving sizes of takeaway foods (e.g. small pizzas are not available in the larger franchise stores)
- families not eating together or eating in front of the TV without concentrating on how much they are consuming
- people feeling guilty if they leave food on the plate ('clean plate' syndrome)
- increased availability of machines that do the physical work in industry and the home, thus reducing exercise
- greater dependence on cars for travel
- decreased incidence of walking and cycling because of road safety and crime
- increased television viewing and participation in computer games
- increased number of desk jobs rather than manual labour
- high 'hidden' fat and sugar content of many convenience foods
- decreased provision of healthy lunches
- decreased cost of high-energy foods
- increased popularity of ready-made meals, at the expense of home-cooked meals, due to competing work and social priorities
- low quality and high prices of vegetables and fruit in urban areas
- high rates of advertising of foods, drinks and takeaway foods high in fat and sugar (Catford & Caterson, 2003; Stanton, 2006; Swinburn et al., 2011).

THE ASSOCIATED DISEASES OF OBESITY

Overweight and Obesity has become one of the greatest health challenges in the Western world. It causes so much unnecessary morbidity and premature mortality and yet it is our most preventable risk factor of ill health and chronic disability (O'Brien, Brown, & Dixon, 2005). Individual characteristics and health-related behaviours influence health in a positive way (protective factor) or negative way (risk factor) and include social, economic and environmental factors that are said to be 'determinants of health' (WHO, 2012). The AIHW (2011) reported that our four major risk factors for ill health are physical inactivity, overweight and obesity, tobacco smoking and alcohol consumption.

The term 'malnutrition' is more often associated with under-nourishment and hunger than with obesity. However, the world is now seeing a dramatic increase in other forms of malnutrition characterised by obesity and the long-term implications of dietary and lifestyle practices associated with chronic non-communicable disease (WHO, 2007).

> Overweight or obesity is linked to the rising incidence and burden of type 2 diabetes, cardiovascular disease, respiratory disease, musculoskeletal problems and some cancers. Overweight or obesity during childhood and adolescence also increases the risk of overweight or obesity in adulthood. (AIHW, 2012)

Notwithstanding genetic factors, overweight and obesity is caused by an energy imbalance. This imbalance of nutrient energy occurs when energy intake exceeds energy expenditure over a period of time. The AIHW (2012) found that good nutrition and levels of physical activity play an important role in the prevention of weight gain and weight loss. Good nutrition is a crucial preventative mechanism in the achievement of good health.

A positive energy balance (consuming more energy than you use) is relatively easy to achieve with our sedentary lifestyle and is largely due to over-consumption of energy-dense foods and foods high in fat and sugar (Swinburn et al., 2004). Alcohol consumption also contributes to weight gain, and excessive alcohol consumption is a major risk factor for morbidity and mortality in Australia. The AIHW (2012) estimated that the harm caused by excessive alcohol consumption accounted for 2% of the total burden of disease in 2003. Highly sweetened, high-strength ready-to-drink (RTD) alcopops deliberately mask the flavour of alcohol and encourage excess intake by making it easier to get drunk faster. The 2005 Australian Government survey of secondary schools students' use of alcohol showed that 47% of 12–17-year-old girls and 13% of boys had consumed pre-mixed spirits in the last week and that the number of RTDs on the market had increased substantially (DOHA, 2006).

A major consequence of our increasing overweight and obesity is the rising incidence of type 2 diabetes and the newly recognised metabolic syndrome. According to Zimmet, Alberti and Shaw (2006) the global incidence of people with diabetes was said to be 150 million and by 2025 this number will have risen to 300 million. This poses a massive health problem in both developed and developing countries. Mohan (2001) observed that, in developed countries, overweight, obesity and diabetes correlate with lower socioeconomic groups, whereas the reverse applies in developing countries.

While the incidence of type 2 diabetes differs throughout the world, it is due to environmental, genetic and behavioural factors. People of Indian, Pacific Islander or Australian Aboriginal heritage are at particularly high risk of developing type 2 diabetes (Virtual Endocrine Centre, 2007). Indigenous peoples around the world are said to suffer diabetes at two to five times the rate of non-indigenous people (Paradies, Montoya & Fullerton, 2007).

One hypothesis proposes that a 'thrifty gene' is responsible for this increased susceptibility of indigenous peoples to type 2 diabetes. This genetic trait is said to help indigenous peoples survive extended periods without food, as it is associated with increased metabolic efficiency of nutrients. Now, a time of relative plenty, this 'thrifty gene' increases susceptibility to diabetes when indigenous populations migrate, urbanise or lead more modern, affluent and sedentary lifestyles. The Menzies School of Health Research, however, suggests that the 'thrifty gene' is not responsible for the high rates of diabetes in indigenous peoples but that the high rates of diabetes are linked to aspects of the social environment:

> Although there is certainly a genetic component to diabetes that affects people throughout society, the idea that indigenous people have a 'thrifty gene' is dispelled by our research which shows that when it comes to diabetes, genes are no more important for indigenous people than for anyone else.
>
> Instead, it is aspects of the social environment that are responsible for the high rates of diabetes among indigenous people. Poor diet, reduced physical activity, stress, low birth weight and other factors associated with poverty all contribute to the high rate of diabetes among indigenous people …
>
> For indigenous people, diabetes will only be tackled by addressing poverty and social disadvantage (Menzies School of Health Research, 2007).

Since 1981 the incidence of type 2 diabetes has doubled in Australia and the total number of cases has increased three-fold. According to Shaw and Chisholm (2003), more than 7% of Australian adults now have diabetes. Additionally, a further 16% of Australian adults have glucose intolerance. As the prevalence of diabetes increases with age, due in some part to degenerative processes, it is estimated that currently 20% of those aged over 60 years have type 2 diabetes. Alarmingly, more and more younger people, even children, are now developing type 2 diabetes. The increased number of obese young people will mean increased incidence of type 2 diabetes mellitus in this age group (Virtual Endocrine Centre, 2007).

Type 2 diabetes mellitus, also known as 'non-insulin-dependent diabetes mellitus', is a complex metabolic disorder characterised by hyperglycaemia, a relative deficiency of insulin secretion, along with a reduced response of target tissues to insulin (insulin resistance). This, in turn, produces a deranged metabolism of carbohydrate, fats and proteins (Shaw & Chisholm, 2003) and is associated with a myriad of complications which affect the feet, eyes, kidneys and cardiovascular health (Baker IDI Heart and Diabetes Institute, 2012).

According to Shaw and Chisholm (2003), insulin resistance is associated with a variety of cardiovascular risk factors, including central adiposity, glucose intolerance, dyslipidaemia and hypertension. When this association was realised, the concept of the metabolic syndrome was born, defined by WHO as having two components:

1 at least one of type 2 diabetes, impaired glucose tolerance or insulin resistance
2 plus at least two of:
   - hypertension (BP ≥ 140/90 mmHg)
   - obesity (BMI ≥ 30 kg/m^2, or waist–hip ratio >0.90 for men, >0.85 for women)
   - hypertriglyceridaemia (≥1.7 mmol/L) or low-serum HDL level (<0.9 mmol/L for men, <1.0 mmol/L for women)
   - microalbuminuria (albumin creatinine ratio >2.5 mg/mmol for men, >3.5 mg/mmol for women) (Shaw & Chisholm, 2003).

   (BP = blood pressure, BMI = body mass index, HDL = high-density lipoprotein)

Early identification and diagnosis of metabolic syndrome, as a precursor to type 2 diabetes and as a risk indicator for cardiovascular disease, could have a marked impact on preventing the development of these diseases and the burgeoning obesity epidemic if crucial behavioural and lifestyles changes are enacted. Therein lies the complexity of the problem.

Shaw and Chisholm (2003) give the example of a 52-year-old male with metabolic syndrome. Diagnosis was based on impaired glucose tolerance, central obesity, hypertension and dyslipidaemia. To halt this pre-diabetic state he needed to reduce all these risk markers in his lifestyle. To achieve this change he consulted with a dietitian to help reduce calories and saturated fat in his diet and to change the amount of food he ate. He undertook a 30-minute exercise regimen every day by alternating a brisk walk, swimming laps or riding an exercise bike before breakfast. After 6 months, while his weight had only decreased by 3 kg, his waist circumference had decreased by 6 cm and he felt generally better and more energetic and was enthusiastic to continue the diet and exercise regimen. Shaw and Chisholm emphasise that this type of lifestyle change needs to be ongoing, as discontinuing the program would put him (because of metabolic syndrome indicators) at high risk of developing type 2 diabetes, hypertension and cardiovascular disease.

Heart failure prevalence is increasing as a result of the ageing of the Australian population and also as a result of the increasing prevalence of overweight, obesity and diabetes. The risk of developing heart failure in Western countries is now about 20%. Campbell (2003) says that while treatment of heart failure has seen many major advances in recent years it remains a major burden on the community. 'Burden' refers to the cost, care and disability associated with the cardiovascular diseases. Preventative approaches offer great benefits to the whole population. The prospect of reducing the incidence of heart failure, other cardiovascular diseases and diabetes through multi-tiered preventative strategies should be a major incentive for governments to fund this priority approach to healthcare (Campbell, 2003).

An interesting paradox in the alcohol debate is that low-to-moderate alcohol consumption has been found to have a protective effect against hypertension, ischaemic heart disease, stroke and gallstones for some subgroups of the population. The cardiovascular health benefit of low-to-moderate alcohol consumption relates mainly to men over 40 years of age and post-menopausal women (AIHW, 2007).

While diabetes and cardiovascular disease are potential major consequences of overweight and obesity, the chronic debilitating effects of overweight and obesity are often more insidious. The following three consequences highlight the complexity of the compounding effects of excess weight gain: obesity and the musculoskeletal system, obesity and reproductive health and obesity and depression.

To understand the effect of weight gain on the musculoskeletal system of the human body you need to imagine how it would feel if you added extra weight to your present condition. As an exercise you could try this: add a series of ever-increasing leaded weights to your ankles and go about your normal daily activities. As you increase the leaded weights you start to tire more quickly and your productivity reduces. Your legs may start to ache as a result of the added weight, as it becomes harder to carry the extra load around. Ultimately overweight or obesity is a burden that you carry around. This burden of weight gain adds stresses and strains to all systems in the body, as it overtaxes all anatomical and biochemical systems (Anandacoomarasamy, Caterson, Sambrook, Fransen, & March, 2008).

Over time, adding weight to the skeletal and articulation systems puts extra load on the spine and hips and particularly weight-bearing joints such as the knees. While normal degenerative changes often necessitate orthopaedic reconstructions and replacements, excess weight is often the main contributing factor to the rate of degeneration. Invasive surgery of any sort is fraught with risks and these risks are exacerbated with increasing levels of overweight and obesity. Within our elective surgery system we already have cases where surgery is delayed until an individual loses weight so as to enhance post-operative recovery and the operative intervention. If acceptable weight loss is not achieved then the individual may progressively become reliant on aids, such as walking sticks, to maintain mobility and independence (Anandacoomarasamy et al., 2008).

It is in everyone's interest to maintain a healthy weight range and thus reduce their own potential burden of chronic illness and disability.

A lesser-documented effect of overweight and obesity is on reproduction function and obstetric outcomes (Nankervis, Conn, & Knight, 2006). The ability to conceive spontaneously is reduced by obesity. Overweight and obese women are over-represented among sub-fertile groups and those presenting with menstrual irregularity and anovulation (Nankervis et al., 2006).

Pregnancy outcomes are also affected by overweight and obesity as risks to mother and baby are increased. These include increased risks of miscarriage, gestational diabetes, pregnancy-induced hypertension, pre-eclampsia, thromboembolism, haemorrhage, caesarean section, sleep apnoea, wound infection and anaesthetic complications (Dietl, 2005; Andreasen, Andersen, & Schantz, 2004).

Nankervis et al. (2006) confirm that congenital abnormalities, birth-related injuries and fetal death in utero are more common in the offspring of overweight and obese women. Babies are more likely to be macrosomic — large for gestational age — which complicates 10% of all births and increases risks of birth trauma and caesarean deliveries.

As overweight and obesity are occurring at a younger age, often increasing with time, and women are becoming pregnant later in life, the problems associated with reproductive health will escalate as the incidence of overweight and obesity increases (Nankervis et al., 2006).

Overwhelming evidence exists that overweight and obese people die earlier, suffer more damage to their body systems and functions and are not the jolly individuals they are thought to be. Depression in the very obese is now well documented. Obese children and adults experience widespread prejudice, teasing and discrimination. As a group, they are less productive, accounting in Australia for some 4 million days away from work annually (Colagiuri, 2007).

There are a number of possible reasons for the links between obesity, anxiety and depression. One reason might be that being obese is socially undesirable. Our culture is bombarded with the 'thin is beautiful' message and people not fitting that image may be seen as lazy or lacking in willpower, or having little regard for their health. Social undesirability might lead to greater anxiety and depression (Skilton, Moulin, Terra, & Bonnet, 2007). As obesity eventually causes ill health and disability, the obese individual may be at risk of anxiety and depression, as we know that people who suffer from physical ill health and disability are more prone to anxiety and depression (The International Association for the Study of Obesity [IASO], 2012).

Overweight and obese people are less physically active. While it's harder for them to be physically active and while lower physical activity might contribute to their obesity, we know that physical activity has an antidepressant effect. The irony is that physical activity tends to reduce depression (IASO, 2012).

There is no doubt that obesity has a genetic component, and genes have always played a role in obesity and yet obesity is on the rise in epidemic proportions. Colagiuri (2007) asks 'Why? What has changed? What have we done? Do we have too much food and too little exercise, or have we changed the compositions of the food we eat? Is it our sedentary "touch of a button" lifestyle, or is it our thoughtless urban design that reduces incidental physical activity? Perhaps it is television and e-games. Or let's just blame our parents.'

One thing we do know is that we need comprehensive public health strategies that are multi-tiered and intersectorial to encompass the environmental and social determinants of lifestyle. Caterson (1999) and Swinburn et al. (2011) believe we need to legislate for healthier environments and healthier communities, and we need education about healthy lifestyles throughout life, along with aggressive control of risk factors in high-risk individuals.

The solution to obesity is simple but it requires a long-term commitment to permanently change eating and exercise habits — and therein lies the problem, says Stanton (2006). Prevention is always the first choice when tackling obesity. However, individual commitment to lifestyle and behaviour change is difficult, as it is influenced by powerful commercial forces that promote eating and physical inactivity. To challenge the advertising of energy-dense foods during children's TV viewing time would take strong political will (Brown & Siahpush, 2007).

What should we do about obesity? One view, according to Caterson (1999), is that weight loss and control are individual responsibilities, and another is that morbid obesity is inevitable because of genes, inherent appetite drives and metabolic set points, which need pharmacological or surgical weight-control help.

Brown & Siahpush (2007) suggest that the options for tackling overweight and obesity are:

- prevention (the first choice)
- lifestyle change
- drug therapy
- bariatric surgery (the surgical treatment of obesity).

Caterson (1999) says the goals of any treatment should be to optimise health, not necessarily to normalise body weight. The benefits of weight loss, regardless of how it is achieved, in improving quality of life and preventing lifestyle-related diseases can only be a bonus to health and wellbeing.

Bariatric surgery is rapidly growing in Australia today as it is said to provide a solution to an insoluble problem and is relatively safe and less invasive than earlier procedures. Current procedures are laparoscopic adjustable gastric banding (LAGB), Roux-en-Y gastric bypass and biliopancreatic diversion. In Australia LAGB accounts for 90% of procedures. The acceptance of LAGB is possibly due to its minimal invasiveness, relative safety, adjustability, reversibility and overall effective results (Brown & Siapush, 2007). Its popularity may also satisfy those who are still looking for the 'magic pill' to enable them to lose weight without effort, and to keep it off. That 'magic pill' comes at a price, however. In 2006 LAGB surgery cost around $10,000, according to weight loss online (AIHW, 2007). You will be $3000 out of pocket if you are privately insured, or face long public health system waiting lists, if you qualify.

Drug therapy to treat obesity effectively is still in development. Caterson (1999) says that two drugs, Orlistat, a pancreatic lipase inhibitor, and Sibutramine, which has both noradrenergic and serotonergic effects acting on appetite and thermogenesis, have shown some degree of success at achieving weight loss, though neither has shown sufficient long-term efficacy and the safety is unknown (Brown & Siapush, 2007). Some new drugs in development are aimed at altering energy expenditure or central appetite control pathways (Caterson, 1999).

Lifestyle solutions require changes that are simple to prescribe — eat less and exercise more — yet the achieved outcomes show limited success as the increase in overweight and obesity continues (Brown & Siapush, 2007). However, the lifestyle message is critical to the success of any sustained weight loss and improved health outcomes. To avoid weight gain, energy expenditure should exceed energy intake over a period of time. This can be achieved by combining regular physical activity with a healthy, well-balanced diet, as is demonstrated in The Healthy Living Pyramid (see Figure 11.1).

In addition, you should eat no more that two indulgences or extra food serves each day (cakes, biscuits, soft drinks, alcohol) and drink plenty of water.

The IASO (2012) offers suggestions to achieve a healthy well-balanced diet and lifestyle (see Table 11.1). If we all followed these guidelines the chronic health issues associated with overweight and obesity could be prevented.

Modern lifestyles make it very easy for individuals to be inactive. The greatest improvements in health are achieved when sedentary behaviour becomes active behaviour. Table 11.2 lists some suggestions for increasing physical activity levels.

Prevention strategies need to be aimed at changing our environment to prevent obesity. Health education has not been enough to halt the increase in obesity; we now need to make macro-environmental changes. This involves governments, policies, planning, business and health professionals and must involve urban planning, transport, roads and food production and distribution. Workplaces and schools must be involved. We need to plan for and create healthy environments that encourage health for all (Caterson, 1999; Swinburn et al., 2011).

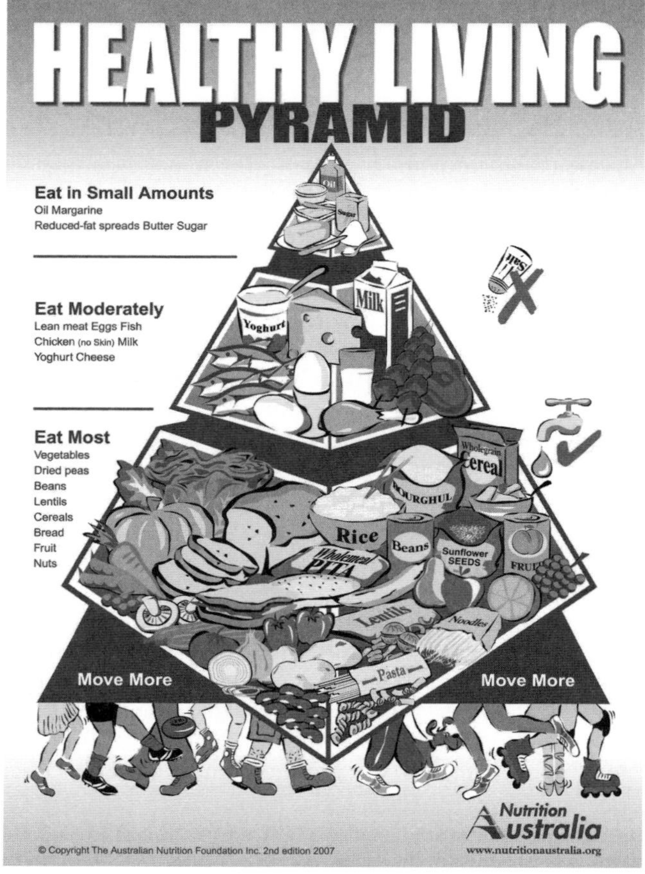

FIGURE 11.1 The Healthy Living Pyramid. Copyright Nutrition Australia.

URBAN PLANNING AND OBESITY

As our urban environments deteriorate, so does the physical and mental health of the people who live in them. However, it is suggested that these diseases can be moderated by the way that we design and construct our urban environments (Jackson & Kochtitzky, 2003).

Research indicates that the design, style and type of urban development can have a beneficial or an adverse impact on the health of the communities living within them (Rodriguez, Khattak & Everson, 2006). It has been suggested that the incidence of obesity can be effectively reduced under certain environmental conditions. That is, environments that encourage activity and human-powered movement seem to have a beneficial impact on the rate of obesity of those living within these environments. Furthermore, environments that provide easy access to nutritious food also seem to favour healthier communities and reduced rates of obesity. Bauman (2004) advises that 'the evidence appears consistent that those who participate in regular moderate-intensity activity and are not obese show protective benefits in terms of reduced risk of cardiovascular disease, diabetes

TABLE 11.1
Healthy eating suggestions

VARIETY	Include a wide variety of foods in your diet in moderate amounts.
ENERGY	Decrease the intake of foods high in energy to reduce the energy density of the diet.
FATS AND PROTEIN	Reduce the amount of fat in your diet. Eat a diet low in saturated fat. Choose low- or reduced-fat dairy. Select lean meats and try to limit fatty meats. Eat fish regularly. Limit takeaway foods. Limit high-fat, unhealthy snack foods.
CARBOHYDRATE	Increase the amount of carbohydrate in your diet. Choose mainly plant-based (or unrefined) foods, such as bread, cereals, whole grains, rice, pasta, vegetables, fruits and legumes. Increase intake of fruit and vegetables.
MEALS	Eat a nutritious breakfast, lunch and dinner. Do not skip meals. Avoid snacking regularly between meals. Ensure snacks are healthy and do not contribute to excess energy intake. Use healthy cooking methods. Become familiar with recommended portion sizes, and consider them when eating. Decrease portion sizes, especially of fast foods and takeaway foods.
BEVERAGES	Drink water rather than juice or soft drinks. Restrict alcohol intake; drink alcohol in moderation.
SHOPPING	Choose foods that are low in fat. Read food labels when you go shopping, to become familiar with products and to assist food choice, especially the fat and sugar content on the food label.

… and improved mental health and quality of life compared to those who are physically inactive and obese'. It is widely accepted that 'physical inactivity contributes to increased risk of many chronic diseases and conditions including obesity' (Ewing et al., 2003).

Rodriguez et al. (2006) argue that there is a strong connection between the built environment and inactivity and advise that there is 'accumulating evidence to suggest that people's decisions to walk or cycle are related to certain characteristics of the built environment'.

Therefore, if it is accepted that physical inactivity is a contributor to increases in the rate of obesity in the Australian population, the obvious means of addressing this problem would seem to be to encourage the population to be physically active. When considering this issue it is worth seeking an explanation for a reduction in physical activity. That is, why are we less active now than, say, 50 years ago? The answer to such a question is complex, but it is safe to suggest that our world has changed significantly in the last 50 years. Our lifestyles bear little relationship to those of 50 years ago. For instance, the ways in which we communicate, travel, commute and recreate are very different today. Our jobs and diets are vastly different from those of people who lived in 1950s Australia. We don't walk as

TABLE 11.2
Physical activity

SET YOURSELF SMALL, REALISTIC GOALS FOR YOUR ACTIVITY	Increase daily physical activity. Be active every day in as many ways as you can. Think of movement as an opportunity, not an inconvenience. Develop an exercise routine. Put together at least 30 minutes of moderate-intensity physical activity on most, preferably all, days. Enjoy some regular, vigorous activity for extra health and fitness. Participate in sports and active leisure activities. Choose activities you enjoy. Vary the type of activity you do. Be active with friends or a partner. Decrease inactive leisure. Increase incidental activity. Leave the car at home and walk whenever possible. Minimise the time you spend in front of a television, computer or other ways of not being active.

much or as far as we used to, and we don't expend as much energy at work as before. This has made it more difficult for us to control our weight. Technological and societal changes have contributed to a sedentary lifestyle, both at home and at work (Caterson, 1999).

Though the links between physical activity and health outcomes are well established, 74% of US adults do not get enough physical activity to meet public health recommendations (Ewing et al., 2003). As pointed out earlier in this chapter, Australia is in a similar position and 'unless we accept that the decades-long reliance on health promotion and intense media coverage of obesity has had virtually no effect', this unfortunate situation will continue (Zimmet & James, 2006).

Therefore, it is argued that it is pointless to long for the return of the active lifestyle of yesteryear and equally pointless to rely upon the general public to act on the advice provided through numerous education campaigns about the benefits of physical activity on general health and longevity.

The question that now arises is 'what type of activity needs to be encouraged if there is to be an improvement in community health and a reduction in the incidence of obesity?' It is interesting to note that studies point not to the need for increases in strenuous physical exercise as a means of tackling obesity in our community, but to the notion of 'incidental activity'. This simply means incorporating more activity in to our daily lives, coupled with the opportunity to do more if the individual chooses to (Caterson, 1999).

Modest increases in the level of physical activity could have significant health benefits, particularly for those who lead a mostly sedentary lifestyle (Frank, Andresen & Schmid, 2004).

Gebel et al. (2005) have summarised the elements of the built environment that may contribute to an increase in physical activity. It is suggested that there are several urban form characteristics (natural and built environment) that tend to be associated with physical activity:

- mixed land use and density
- footpaths, cycle ways and facilities for physical activity

- street connectivity and design
- transport infrastructure and systems, linking residential, commercial and business areas (Gebel et al., 2005).

Mixed land use and density

Land use refers to the way in which land is used in a locality, such as industrial, residential, business and retail uses. In many instances, planning and planners have gone to great lengths to separate these uses, as it was thought that it would be undesirable to allow some uses to be located in close proximity to others. For example, it may be undesirable to allow residential uses to be in close proximity to some industrial, business or retail activities. The result of this approach has been the separation of uses by significant distances. That is, this approach favours the establishment of lower density (fewer dwellings per unit area) residential neighbourhoods, remote from shopping and employment centres. This means that those who wish to access differing services, employment or shopping facilities are encouraged to do so via the use of a private motor vehicle. That is, the distance separating these land uses favours motor vehicular transport and not human-powered means of transport such as walking or cycling.

This development pattern is sometimes referred to as 'sprawl', or sprawling communities. Ewing et al. (2003) found that 'residents of sprawling counties were likely to walk less during leisure time, weigh more and have greater prevalence of hypertension than residents of compact counties' (Ewing et al., 2003).

Frank et al. (2004) found that land-use mix had the strongest association with obesity and found that 'each additional hour spent in a car per day was associated with a 6% increase in the likelihood of obesity. Conversely, each additional kilometre walked per day was associated with a 4.8% reduction in the likelihood of obesity' (Frank et al., 2004).

However, in instances where differing land uses are permitted in closer proximity or included together in a mix of land uses, the distance separating residential uses from goods and services is greatly reduced. This, when coupled with increases in density, has the effect of increasing neighbourhood 'walkability'. That is, these neighbourhoods are more conducive to walking and cycling as a means of transport to everyday goods and services.

Studies in the United States have found that residents living in older neighbourhoods (homes built before 1946) were more likely to walk longer distances with more frequency than those living in newer homes. This result was attributed to the greater likelihood of footpaths, dense interconnected streets and a mix of business and residential uses in older neighbourhoods (Frank et al., 2004).

In summary, with respect to land use mix and density, it is argued that allowing a mix of land uses in a locality, coupled with higher residential density, will most likely encourage higher levels of physical activity, such as walking and cycling.

Footpaths, cycle ways and facilities for physical activity

It seems obvious, but worth stating, that people are more likely to engage in some form of physical activity if facilities and infrastructure are provided. This does not have to be elaborate gymnasiums and sporting facilities because, as previously noted, only moderate increases in physical activity are recommended for significant improvements to general health and reductions in the likelihood of obesity.

The existence and design of footpaths and bicycle paths make walking and cycling as means of transport or recreation more attractive. Furthermore, parks and other recreational facilities provide residents with more opportunities to engage in physical activity. It is argued that public parks facilitate physical activity. On their own they provide places for people to walk or jog and in most cases they provide opportunity for organised sports and more vigorous activity. Studies in Australia have found that access to parks and large attractive open spaces are closely linked to walking. However, parks also provide a destination for people. A destination is thought to be advantageous as it provides the individual with a reason to walk (Cohen et al., 2007).

Street connectivity and design

Capon (2005) conducted an extensive review of the literature and found that greater levels of street connectivity decreased distances between trip origin and destination, and that this was likely to increase levels of walking and cycling. Furthermore, streets that are pedestrian- and bicycle-friendly saw increased foot and bicycle traffic.

Street layout and pattern affect connectivity. That is, older grid-style street patterns, with many intersecting streets, provide for more direct connection between point of origin and destination. Such neighbourhoods are considered to be more walkable and people living in them are more likely to walk for utilitarian purposes than those living in newer suburban environments.

Newer suburban environments tend to include curvilinear street patterns which increase distance between origin and destination. Such street patterns contain few intersections and seem to meander around a locality with few direct connections between point of origin and centre of activity.

Transport infrastructure and systems linking residential commercial and business areas

Higher urban density results in higher population in a smaller area and reduced distances between trip origin and destination. This type of urban environment tends to better support public transport. This is not only a benefit to the environment, as motor vehicle usage is reduced, but also encourages physical activity. Mason (2000) advocates 'active transport'. Active transport is transport that incorporates some form of physical activity. For instance, the use of public transport (e.g., rail, bus) generally requires that the commuter at least walk some distance to the train station or bus stop. Even if this distance is only moderate, the benefits to human health are significant.

PHYSICAL ENVIRONMENT AND PHYSICAL ACTIVITY

Having considered the brief summary above, it is argued that the built environment has a considerable impact on the level of physical activity and hence has an influence on the rate of obesity within our population.

Notwithstanding any of the above, Gebel et al. (2005) recommend caution when drawing the linkages between physical environment, physical activity and nutrition. That is, 'while there is an accumulating body of evidence on how physical environments affect physical activity, there is very little published or available research on influences of the environment on nutrition and obesity' (Gebel et al., 2005).

There is sufficient evidence to suggest that elements of the built environment contribute to an increase in physical activity and possibly improve and/or ensure access to nutritious food choices. This includes:

- providing for and encouraging land-use mix and increases in urban density
- ensuring that urban environments have adequate footpaths, cycle ways and facilities for physical activity

- designing and laying out streets so that they provide easy and logical connection between points of origin and destination
- making all possible efforts to provide a transport system that effectively links residential, commercial and business areas
- ensuring that provision is made for the inclusion of zoning and land uses that encourage access to fresh and nutritious food.

These elements and health-related benefits are summarised in Table 11.3.

This now leads to the next question: *Can the built environment be influenced so that the rate of obesity may be reduced?*

It is argued that the answer is definitely yes and that environmental planning has the ability, at least in theory, to influence the built environment so that the rate of obesity may be reduced. This is particularly true if it is accepted that environmental planning concerns itself with:

- ordering, influencing and controlling the use of land to sustain human life
- the provision of facilities and infrastructure to support the development and function of communities.

Furthermore, when the state-level legislation applying to environmental planning is reviewed it is clear that environmental planners at the state and local levels are provided with the power and means to influence and direct urban development at the state, local and neighbourhood levels. That is, environmental planners are provided with legislative powers to influence land use and urban design and are able to determine the type and mix of land use within a locality. For instance, environmental planners are able to make 'plans' that set aside land for public open space, areas where retail and business activities are to be located and even stipulate minimum/maximum residential densities.

Environmental planning is responsible for neighbourhood design and sets standards that apply to elements of the built environment, including:

- building design, location and/orientation
- street pattern
- footpath design
- urban landscaping
- public and private open space.

Setting standards such as these is a means of ensuring connectivity, safety and workability of residential neighbourhoods.

If access to fast food is considered to be an issue of concern, environmental planning could limit access to such foods by controlling the density and/or location of these establishments. For instance, it has been shown that when fast food restaurants are located in close proximity to schools, parents have difficulty controlling their children's exposure to them. If planning authorities were to accept that they have a responsibility to control the number and location of fast food outlets in the same manner that they already control the location of gambling establishments and licensed premises, then local planning authorities could draft and/or amend local planning laws to better control the location and density of fast food outlets (Ingleby, Prosser, & Waters, 2007).

Conversely, if access to fresh and nutritious food is to be a priority, local planning laws can be used to encourage the location of supermarkets in locations easily accessible to the local community and restrict the establishment of competing land uses in these locations.

TABLE 11.3

Elements of the built environment and health-related benefits. *Note*: From Gebel et al. (2005).

URBAN FORM CHARACTERISTIC	CONCEPT	KEY FEATURES	HEALTH-RELATED BENEFIT
Street network characteristics and design	Interconnectivity of roads	Grid-like pattern	Reduces distance between destinations, encouraging the use of active transport.
	Traffic-calming and other street design features	Street width, vehicular parking, kerb type; traffic management and control devices; street crossings, crossing aids, verge width, driveway crossovers, continuity; vehicular and cycle lane marking, sightings distance; density of street sign features.	Provides facilities that encourage cycling and walking and discourage driving.
	Separate integrated network of walking and cycling routes		Provides facilities that encourage walking and cycling.
Land-use mix	Food retail	Accessible supermarkets, plus local food stores.	Ensures a wide variety of nutritious food accessible at competitive prices.
	Food services	Limited density and number of fast food services around schools.	May reduce children's access to energy-dense food.
	Mix of residential, commercial and business uses	Different uses within a defined zone.	Increases opportunities for active transport.
	Public open space	Large public open spaces created/preserved close to residents, with pathway access, and good amenities.	Increases physical activity opportunities.
	Physical activity facilities	Swimming pools, basketball courts, gyms, football fields, tennis courts, playgrounds, bubblers etc.	Increases people's level of physical activity.
Housing Density	Density	Increased number of residential and commercial premises in an area.	Increases active transport, with reduced distances to destinations. Increases access to physical activity facilities.
Site design	Food production	Establishment of local community gardens, school gardens, home gardens and edible landscapes.	Provides cheap, fresh produce; potential educational, social and nutritional benefits.
	Breastfeeding	Establishment of public breastfeeding facilities.	Encourages breastfeeding, for longer, as recommended in dietary guidelines.
	Safety, aesthetics in local facilities and amenities.	Lighting; surveillance; maintenance and cleanliness of parks, gardens and streets; provision of public amenities and public transport facilities; building design, orientation and setback.	Influences perceived and actual safety and aesthetics; creates an environment that is conducive to active transport and physical activity.

TABLE 11.3
Elements of the built environment and health-related benefits — cont'd

URBAN FORM CHARACTERISTIC	CONCEPT	KEY FEATURES	HEALTH-RELATED BENEFIT
Transport planning	Access to food, retail	Footpaths, cycleway and public transport options to retail centres.	Improves access for food purchasing.
	Improved/ developed public transport systems and facilities	Bus shelters, cycling facilities near stops, pedestrian and cycle access to public transport.	Increases opportunities for active transport.

CASE STUDY 11.1

Over the last 30 years the fringe areas of the Sydney metropolitan area have experienced significant and sustained urban growth. Many would argue that the way in which this land was developed contributed to urban sprawl, bringing with it the many environmental and health-related problems noted in this chapter. However, while further urban growth is expected, the NSW Government in partnership with the private sector has sought to correct the planning mistakes of the past by encouraging plans that seek to guide development so that healthy and safe communities may evolve. Example of such a plan can be found on the Premier's Council for Active Living website accessed from http://www.pcal.nsw.gov.au/case_studies

There is a convergence of ideas that argues we must make meaningful lifestyle changes over the coming years that will allow us to protect our environment, improve our health and grow our economy and wealth in a sustainable way (Maberly, 2010).

However, environmental planners are not experts in human health and in this case it is imperative that health practitioners engage and challenge the planning process to ensure that human health outcomes are given the priority that they deserve.

CONCLUSION

The incidence of obesity in Australia is alarmingly high in both children and adults. Overweight and Obesity is increasing at an alarming rate each year due to a large number of factors. Obesity is of great concern as it can cause diabetes, cardiovascular and respiratory disease, musculoskeletal problems and some cancers. Obesity has links with genetics and ethnic background, and is more common in lower socioeconomic groups. Treatment of obesity can involve urban planning, reduced energy intake and increased physical activity; less preferable methods are drug therapy and bariatric surgery.

Reflective questions

1 Current evidence identifies that the majority of Western food habits and lifestyles are anything but healthy and the core of the problem is that we eat too much. Affluent lifestyles promote physical inactivity and the consumption of energy-dense, nutrient-poor foods. What needs to be done to turn the epidemic around?

2 The Australian guide to healthy eating recommends a daily intake of essential nutrients. Make an assessment of your daily dietary intake by recording the number of serves of food you consumed in the last 24 hours. A serve is roughly what fits into the palm of your hand. Compare your intake with the healthy eating guidelines. How many serves of vegetables, fruits and cereals/grains did you eat? Could you say that you eat a balanced diet? If not, what will you do about it?

3 Scenario: You have the opportunity to be part of a multidisciplinary team to design a new urban development on the outskirts of the city in which you live. As a health professional you are dedicated to improving the health of individuals and communities and reducing the incidence of preventable chronic disease. Best practice in obesity prevention requires attention to the content (what to do) and the process (how to do it). With this in mind explain what you would do and how you would do it. What urban design features would you want to see included? And what would be essential to create a healthy and safe community?

Recommended reading

Banks, G., Chairman, Productivity Commission, Health Policy Oration (2008). *Health costs and policy in an ageing Australia*. Canberra: Menzies Centre for Health Policy, John Curtin School of Medical Research, Australian National University. Retrieved from http://www.pc.gov.au/__data/assets/pdf_file/0011/81758/cs20080701-agedhealthpolicy.pdf

Barilla Center for Food & Nutrition. *Eating planet* (2012). Nutrition today: a challenge for mankind and for the planet. Retrieved from http://www.barillacfn.com/en/bcfn4you/il-libro/

Gwynn, J., Flood, V. M., D'Este, C. A., et al. (2012). Poor food and nutrient intake among Indigenous and non-Indigenous rural Australian children. *BMC Pediatrics*, 2012, 12:12 doi: 10.1186/1471-2431-12-12

Kent, J., Thompson, S. M., & Jalaludin, B. (2011). *Healthy built environments: A review of the literature*. Sydney: Healthy Built Environments Program, City Futures Research Centre, University of NSW. Retrieved from http://www.be.unsw.edu.au/sites/default/files/upload/pdf/cf/hbep/publications/attachments/HBEPLiteratureReview_FullDocument.pdf

Public Health Association of Australia. (2012). Future for food — healthy, sustainable, fair. Retrieved from http://www.phaa.net.au/documents/120214%20PHAA%20Report%202012_low%20res.pdf

References

Anandacoomarasamy, A., Caterson, I., Sambrook, P., et al. (2008). The impact of obesity on the musculoskeletal system. *International Journal of Obesity*, *32*, 211–222. Retrieved May 7, 2013, from http://www.nature.com/ijo/journal/v32/n2/pdf/0803715a.pdf.

Andreasen, K. R., Andersen, M. L., & Schantz, A. L. (2004). Obesity and Pregnancy. *Acta Obstetrica et Gynecologica Scandinavica*, *83*, 1022–1029. Retrieved July 10, 2013, from http://onlinelibrary.wiley.com/doi/10.1111/j.0001-6349.2004.00624.x/full

Australian Bureau of Statistics. (2012). Australian Health Survey: First Results. Retrieved May 7, 2013, from http://www.abs.gov.au/ausstats/abs@.nsf/Lookup/4364.0.55.001Chapter1002011-12

Australian Institute of Health and Welfare. (2005). *Obesity and workplace absenteeism among older Australians*. Canberra: Author.

Australian Institute of Health and Welfare. (2007). Retrieved June 1, 2007, from http://www.aihw.gov.au.

Australian Institute of Health and Welfare. (2011). *Key indicators of progress for chronic disease and associated determinants: data report*. Cat. no. PHE 142. Canberra: Author. Retrieved May 7, 2013, from http://www.aihw.gov.au/WorkArea/DownloadAsset.aspx?id=10737419243&libID=10737419242

Australian Institute of Health and Welfare. (2012). *Australia's health 2012. Australia's Health Series no.13*. Cat. no. AUS 156. Canberra: Author. Retrieved May 7, 2013, from http://www.aihw.gov.au/publication-detail/?id=10737422172&tab=2

Baker IDI Heart and Diabetes Institute. (2012). Diabetes: The silent pandemic and its impact on Australia. Retrieved May 7, 2013, from http://www.diabetesaustralia.com.au/Documents/DA/What's%20New/12.03.14%20Diabetes%20management%20booklet%20FINAL.pdf

Bauman, A. (2004). Physical activity and obesity — the connection with the built environment. In C. Johnson (Ed.), *Healthy environments – 11 essays* (pp. 57–68). Sydney: Government Architect's Publications.

Baur, L. (2000). How do we define or diagnose overweight and obesity in childhood? *Medical Journal of Australia*, *173*, S8–S9.

Brown, A., & Siahpush, M. (2007). Risk factors for overweight and obesity: results from the 2001 National Health Survey. *Public Health*, *121*(8), 603–613.

Cameron, A. (2003). Overweight and obesity in Australia: the 1999–2000 Australian diabetes, obesity and lifestyle study. *Journal of Australian Diabetes*, *178*(90), 427–432.

Campbell, D. J. (2003). Heart failure: How can we prevent the epidemic? *Medical Journal of Australia*, *179*(8), 422–425. Retrieved May 7, 2013, from http://www.mja.com.au/public/issues/179_08_201003/cam10108_fm.html

Capon, A. (2005). *Promoting nutrition, physical activity and obesity reduction through urban planning*. Sydney: Report prepared for NSW Centre for Overweight and Obesity.

Caterson, I. D. (1999). What should we do about overweight and obesity? *Medical Journal of Australia*, *171*(11), 599–600. Retrieved May 7, 2013, from http://www.mja.com.au/public/issues/171_11_061299/caterson/caterson.html

Catford, J. C., & Caterson, D. (2003). Snowballing obesity: Australians will get run over if they just sit there. *Medical Journal of Australia*, *179*(11/12), 577–579.

Cohen, D. A., McKenzie, T. L., Sehgal, A., et al. (2007). Contribution of Public Parks to Physical Activity. *American Journal of Public Health*, *97*(3), 509–514.

Colagiuri, R. (2007). The lion, the wardrobe and the witch hunt: An alternative take on obesity. *Medical Journal of Australia*, *186*(9), 476–477. Retrieved May 7, 2013, from http://www.mja.com.au/public/issues/186_09_070507/col11225_fm.html

Commonwealth Scientific and Industrial Research Organisation. (2005 ed.). A simple guide to healthy eating and weight control: CSIRO 12345 nutrition plan. Retrieved May 7, 2013, from http://www.csiro.au/proprietaryDocuments/12345_Plan.pdf

Department of Health and Ageing. (2006). Australian secondary school students' use of alcohol in 2005. Retrieved May 7, 2013, from http://www.nationaldrugstrategy.gov.au/internet/drugstrategy/publishing.nsf/Content/85D7B21B3E3A993ECA2572250007755F/$File/mono58.pdf

Department of Health and Ageing. (2010). Measure Up. Retrieved May 7, 2013, from http://www.health.gov.au/internet/abhi/publishing.nsf/Content/Weight%2C+waist+circumference+and+BMI-lp

Dietl, J. (2005). Maternal obesity and complications during pregnancy. *Journal of Perinatal Medicine*, *33*, 100–105. Retrieved May 7, 2013, from http://www.ncbi.nlm.nih.gov/sites/entrez

Ewing, R., Schmid, T., Killingsworth, R., et al. (2003). Relationship between urban sprawl and physical activity, obesity and morbidity. *American Journal of Health Promotion, 18*(1), 47–57.

Frank, L. D., Andresen, M. A., & Schmid, T. L. (2004). Obesity relationships with community design, physical activity, and time spent in cars. *American Journal of Preventative Medicine, 27*(2), 87–96.

Gebel, K., King, L., Bauman, A., et al. (2005). *Creating healthy environments: A review of links between the physical environment, physical activity and obesity*. Sydney: NSW Health Department and NSW Centre for Overweight and Obesity.

Gill, T. P., Rangan, A. M., & Webb, K. L. (2006). The weight of evidence suggests that soft drinks are a major issue in childhood and adolescent obesity. *Medical Journal of Australia, 184*(6), 263–264.

Hardy, L. L., King, L., Espinel, P., et al. (2010). *NSW schools physical activity and nutrition survey (SPANS) 2010: Short report*. Sydney: NSW Ministry of Health. Retrieved May 7, 2013, from www.health.nsw.gov.au/pubs/2011/pdf/spans_2010_summary.pdf

Ingleby, R., Prosser, L., & Waters, E. (2007). Fast food restaurants and obesity. *Australian Planner, 44*(2), 12–13.

International Obesity Taskforce. (2002). Obesity in Europe. The case for action. Retrieved May 7, 2013, from http://www.iotf.org/media/euobesity.pdf

Jackson, R. J., & Kochtitzky, C. (2003). *Creating a healthy environment: The impact of the built environment on public health*. Centers for Disease Control and Prevention Sprawl Watch, Clearinghouse Monograph Series.

Katzmarzyk, P. T., & Mason, C. (2006). Prevalence of class I, II and III obesity in Canada. *Canadian Medical Journal, 174*(2), 156–157.

Maberly, G. F. (2010). *Partnerships for health and wellbeing for Western Sydney Strategic Planning Session*. Centre for Health Innovation and Partnership (unpublished).

Mason, C. (2000). Transport and health: en route to a healthier Australia? *Medical Journal of Australia, 172*(5), 230–232.

Menzies School of Health Research. (2007). Media Release: Study shows that indigenous people are not genetically prone to diabetes. View from http://www.researchaustralia.com.au/files/MSHR_Studyshowsthatindigenouspeoplearenotgeneticallypronetodiabetes_16_04_07.pdf

Mohan, V., Shanthirani, S., Deepa, R., et al.(2001). Intra-urban differences in the prevalence of the metabolic syndrome in southern India — the Chennai urban population study. *Diabetic Medicine, 18*, 280–287. Retrieved May 7, 2013, from http://onlinelibrary.wiley.com/doi/10.1046/j.1464-5491.2001.00421.x/abstract

Nankervis, A. J., Conn, J. J., & Knight, R. L. (2006). Obesity and reproductive health. *Medical Journal of Australia, 184*(2), 51. Retrieved May 7, 2013, from https://www.mja.com.au/journal/2006/184/2/obesity-and-reproductive-health

National Health and Medical Research Council. (2005). Food for health: The Australian dietary guidelines. Retrieved May 7, 2013, from http://www.nhmrc.gov.au/_files_nhmrc/publications/attachments/n31.pdf

O'Brien, P. E., Brown, W. A., & Dixon, J. B. (2005). Obesity, weight loss and bariatric surgery. *Medical Journal of Australia, 183*(6), 310–314. Retrieved May 7, 2013, from http://www.mja.com.au/public/issues/183_06_190905/obr10369_fm.html

O'Dea, K. (2003). Difference in overweight and obesity among Australian schoolchildren. *Medical Journal of Australia, 179*, 63–65.

Paradies, Y., Montoya, M., & Fullerton, S. (2007). Racialized genetics and the study of complex diseases: the thrifty genotype revisited. *Perspectives in Biology and Medicine, 2*(50) (spring 2007), 203–227. Retrieved May 7, 2013, from https://bmw.curtin.edu.au/pubs/2009/Paradies_etal_2007.pdf

Phillips, G. (2004). Heart exercise. ABC Radio, 18 June 2004.

Pijl, H. (2011). Obesity: Evolution of a symptom of affluence. How food has shaped our existence. *The Netherlands Journal of Medicine*, April 2011, *69*(4).

Rodriguez, D. A., Khattak, A. J., & Everson, K. A. (2006). Can new urbanism encourage physical activity? *Journal of the American Planning Association*, *72*(1), 43–54.

Shaw, J. E., & Chisholm, D. J. (2003). Epidemiology and prevention of type 2 diabetes and the metabolic syndrome. *Medical Journal of Australia*, *179*(7), 379–383. Retrieved May 7, 2013, from http://www.mja.com.au/public/issues/179_07_061003/sha10375_fm.html

Skilton, M. R., Moulin, P., Terra, J.-L., et al. (2007). Associations between anxiety, depression, and the metabolic syndrome. *Biological Psychiatry*, *62*(11), 1251–1257.

Skurray, G. R., & Ham R. (1999). Drugs, alcohol and respiratory disease and social class in Sydney western metropolitan areas. *Australian Journal of Social Issues*, *27*(2), 144–149.

Stanton, R. (2006). Nutrition problems in an obesogenic environment. *Medical Journal of Australia*, *184*(2), 76–79. Retrieved May 7, 2013, from http://www.mja.com.au/public/issues/184_02_160106/sta10572_fm.html

Stubbs, C. O., & Lee, A. J. (2004). The obesity epidemic: both energy intake and physical activity contribute. *Medical Journal of Australia*, *181*(9), 489–491.

Swinburn, B. A., Caterson, I., Seidell, J. C., et al. (2004). Nutrition and the prevention of excess weight gain and obesity. *Public Health Nutrition*, *7*(1A), 123–146.

Swinburn, B. A., Sacks, G., Hall, K., et al. (2011). The global obesity pandemic: shaped by global drivers and local environments. *The Lancet*, *378*(9793), 804–814.

The International Association for the Study of Obesity (IASO). (2012). About obesity. Retrieved May 7, 2013, from http://www.iaso.org/resources/aboutobesity/

Virtual Endocrine Centre. (2007). Type 2 diabetes. Retrieved May 7, 2013, from http://www.virtualendocrinecentre.com/diseases.asp?did=826

Williams, G. C., & Ness, R. M. (1991). The dawn of Darwinian medicine. *Quarterly Reviews of Biology*, *66*, 1–22.

World Health Organization. (2000). *Obesity: Preventing and managing the global epidemic. WHO Technical Report Series 894*. Geneva: Author. Retrieved May 7, 2013, from http://whqlibdoc.who.int/trs/WHO_TRS_894.pdf

World Health Organization. (2007). The challenge of obesity in the WHO European Region and the strategies for response. Retrieved May 7, 2013, from http://www.euro.who.int/__data/assets/pdf_file/0010/74746/E90711.pdf

World Health Organization. (2012). Health impact assessment. Retrieved May 7, 2013, from http://www.who.int/hia/evidence/doh/en/

Zimmet, P. Z., & James, P. T. (2006). The unstoppable Australian obesity and diabetes juggernaut. What should politicians do? *Medical Journal of Australia*, *185*(4), 187–188.

Zimmet, P., Alberti, K., & Shaw, J. (2006). Metabolic syndrome — a new world-wide definition. A Consensus Statement from the International Diabetes Federation. *Diabetic Medicine: A Journal of the British Diabetic Association*, *23*(5), 469–480.

CHAPTER 12

Christine Haley
James Daley

Palliation in chronic illness

Learning objectives

When you have completed this chapter you will be able to:

- understand historical factors that led to the development of contemporary palliative care practices
- identify the philosophy and principles that underpin core palliative nursing care practices for life-limiting illnesses
- identify challenges that present as barriers to the holistic palliative care approach
- apply the core nursing skills required to provide appropriate palliative care
- identify the nurse's role in the multi-profession palliative care team.

Key words

palliative care, multidisciplinary team, quality of life, end of life, carers

INTRODUCTION

'Palliative care is provided for a person with an active, progressive advanced illness, who has little or no prospect of cure, and for whom the primary treatment goal is quality of life' (Palliative Care Australia [PCA], 2005). Ferrell and Coyle (2010, p. 3) define the goals of palliative care nursing as promoting quality of life across the illness trajectory through the relief of suffering, including care of the dying and bereavement follow-up. Broadening the scope of practice in palliative care is therefore necessary to enable care for all patients with life limiting illnesses. Standards of care for palliative care have been developed by the peak body, Palliative Care Australia (PCA). The underlying philosophy of their approach to palliative care is a positive open attitude towards death and dying (PCA, 2008).

This chapter will provide the student with a brief overview of the historical development of palliative care. Discussion will then focus on contemporary issues and challenges to providing care for patients with cancer and other life-limiting illnesses. The management of chronic illness is often complex and poly-symptomatic; individual planning is therefore a crucial component for successful nursing intervention. Two clinical case studies will be used to display examples of how philosophy and practice principles come together to guide care. These principles ensure a holistic patient-centred palliative approach is underpinned by core skills throughout the chronic illness trajectory. To be successful this approach requires a collaborative approach by a multi-professional team, which also includes doctors, allied healthcare disciplines, community support groups and increasingly complementary and alternative health practitioners. Each team member will be guided by the same underlying principles of care but will have a unique role to fulfil in an effort to meet the needs of the patient. The multi-professional team approach will be utilised in the case studies to show how key players can be incorporated into an effective plan of care.

In this technological age it is important that quality web-based information sites are recommended for further reading to inform and promote appropriate palliative care of advanced chronic illness. Informative internet sites include:

- Palliative Care Australia http://www.palliativecare.org.au/Home.aspx
- CareSearch Palliative care Knowledge network http://www.caresearch.com.au/caresearch/tabid/1477/Default.aspx
- Cancer Council of Australia http://www.cancer.org.au/aboutcancer/FAQ.htm#573
- Australian Institute of Health And Welfare http://www.aihw.gov.au/
- New Zealand Palliative Care http://www.health.govt.nz/our-work/life-stages/palliative-care

AN OVERVIEW OF HISTORICAL DEVELOPMENTS

Since the 1980s palliative care has become a subspecialty in medicine, nursing and allied health education programs. Up until the 20th century, palliative nursing care was the only option of care for the terminally ill. It was during the early part of the last century that palliation was lost to the biomedical preposition with aggressive measures to investigate disease and prolong life as long as possible (Macintosh & Zerwekh, 2006). Thus an obsession with cure or defeating disease processes prevailed while death was seen as failure of the healthcare system. Although the medical approach has improved the treatment of acute conditions, often a patient's family and carers were denied the truth regarding their poor prognosis, making them vulnerable to unnecessary aggressive and distressing interventions (Macintosh & Zerwekh, 2006).

The hospice movement of the last century was developed as a response to these concerns and nurses were often at the forefront in bringing about change. As Hiedrich (2007, p. 23) informs us, 'the overriding principle behind hospice was the notion that patients needed and deserved an alternative to an aggressive, cure orientated, hospital based system of care that generally failed to address the real issues of concerns to the dying'. In the early days of the hospice movement, palliative care was viewed as terminal care, this being the care given to a person in the last days to weeks of their life. It took place within the confines of the hospice, isolating death and dying in society. Death was no longer seen as a normal component to life. However with 'consumerism on the rise in healthcare, patients began to take more of a role in steering the cause of their care' (Macintosh & Zerwekh, 2006, p. 22). The right to make informed decisions was demanded by patients and family/friends especially in relation to the necessity of life-extending treatments that offered additional time, but limited the quality of life. The overwhelming impact on family and friends of the physical, psychological and social demands of caring for a loved one during the terminal stages of illness emerged as pivotal factors in redefining the palliative care movement.

Palliative care as we know it today is an evolving concept, defined and developed by the World Health Organization (WHO). (See Box 12.1.) This ensures that palliative care principles remain at the core of the treatment and that patients' individualised needs are central to the outcomes. Johnson (2005, p. 2) further defines the objectives drawn from the WHO definition as:

- to palliate physical symptoms
- to alleviate disease and maintain independence for as long and as comfortable as possible
- to alleviate isolation, anxiety and fear associated with advancing disease
- to provide as dignified a death as possible
- to support those who are bereaved.

The definition developed by the WHO in 2002 and principles drawn from it will be utilised to guide nursing practices and is displayed in Box 12.1.

BOX 12.1

World Health Organization's definition of palliative care Source: World Health Organization.

An approach that improves quality of life of patients and their family facing the problems associated with life threatening illness, through the prevention of suffering by early identification and impeccable assessment and treatment of pain and other problems, physical, psychological and spiritual. Appropriate palliative care:

- provides relief from pain and other distressing symptoms
- affirms life and regards dying as a normal process
- intends neither to hasten nor to postpone death
- integrates the psychology and spiritual aspects of patient care
- offers a support system to help patients live as actively as possible until death
- offers a support system to help the family cope during the patient's illness and their families, including bereavement counselling, if indicated
- uses a team approach to address the needs of patients and their families, including bereavement counselling if necessary
- will enhance quality of life, and may also positively influences the course of illness
- is applicable early in the course of the illness; in conjunction with other therapies that are intended to prolong life, such as chemotherapy or radiation therapy, and includes those investigations needed to better understand and manage distressing clinical complications.

A HEALTH PROMOTION APPROACH TO PALLIATIVE CARE

In recent years there has been a growing recognition of the fact that managing death and dying is not just a responsibility of health systems but of the community at large and although people generally die in hospitals they live out their lives in their communities not in a health service environment (Rumbold, Young, & Salu, 2007). This approach is based on a public health model of palliative care also known as health promoting palliative care. This is based on the public health concept of a population approach linking to the World Health Promotion guidelines 'the Ottawa Charter' (CareSearch, 2012). Kellehear (2010, p. 114) informs of the benefit of a health promotion framework for support of those living with life threatening illness, bereavement or carers for either enhances quality of life by strengthening a community's inherent capacity to support these people. Kellehear's previous work has been pivotal in developing a social model for palliative care practice and aligning primary healthcare concepts of health promotion to palliative care (Rumbold et al., 2007). Kellehear outlined the principles of a health-promoting model of palliative care as:

- building public policies that support dying, death, loss and grief
- creating supportive environments (in particular social supports)
- strengthening community action
- developing personal skills in these areas
- re-orientating the health system (Kellehear, 1999, p. 20).

The promotion of quality of life in the face of an incurable illness is firmly based on a caring, patient-centred approach which takes into account the person as a totality comprising physical, psychological, emotional and spiritual dimensions. It acknowledges the fact that people exist within a community, which greatly impacts on the delivery of care. Pivotal to the success of the palliative care process is recognition of the key role the carers have in the provision of care. This has been highlighted in the 2008 PCA position statement on End of Life and Carers.

- 'Dying is part of life. The care of people at the end of life, their families and carers is the responsibility of the whole community.
- Carers must be recognised as *both a key partner* in the care team *and a recipient of care* in accordance with the palliative care service provision model.
- Enabling people's preferences to receive quality care at the end of life in the setting of their choice is dependent upon ongoing physical, emotional, practical and spiritual support from individual carers and their communities as well as health professional support.
- The extent and quality of support provided to the carer and the person nearing the end of life is a key determinant of both of their experiences. The whole community should support them (PCA, 2008, p. 1).

It is acknowledged that palliative care practice and philosophy grew from the experience of managing advanced cancer (Walsh, Aktas, Hullihen, & Indura, 2011). Increasingly there has been recognition of the fact that palliative care must be a component in the management of life limiting chronic illnesses such as end-stage cardiac or pulmonary disease, advanced dementia, renal and liver failure and other neurological conditions (Maxwell, 2010). As in many other developed countries chronic illness in Australia and New Zealand continues to exact a high toll on the health of individuals. People are now living longer with increasing levels of morbidity associated with chronic illness. Chronic illnesses 'are estimated to make up the greatest burden of disease, mental problems and injury for the population as a whole' (Glover, Hetzel, & Tennan, 2004, p. 1).

LEVELS OF PALLIATIVE CARE INTERVENTION

When seeking to understand the various levels of palliative care provision it is useful to divide it into three dynamic categories or tiers: primary carer and informal community support; generalist health providers and formal community support services; and specialist palliative care services. All levels potentially form a network of care to support a patient as their illness inexorably progresses towards death. As the patient's illness progresses so will their need for care fluctuate. The complexity of the symptoms experienced and needs of the family/carers are critical factors in determining the need for services and support.

Palliative care can be conceptualised as being provided by four interlocking and mutually supporting elements which work across the spectrum of hospital and community settings: the primary carer; the specialist palliative care team; symptom control; and the settings of care. An understanding of how these components of care work towards providing care is integral to an understanding of palliative care as it is now practised in Australia and New Zealand.

The primary carer

The Australian Bureau of Statistics (ABS) in its profile of carers describes a primary carer as follows: 'A primary carer is the main provider of care to someone in the core activities of daily living such as dressing, eating or moving around the house' (ABS, 2008). They may also be supported by other informal carers. The role of the primary carer has become increasingly difficult as patients are now living longer with greater burdens of illness. Adding to the stress of caring is the fact that patients are now being discharged earlier from hospital with diminishing levels of community support. 'It has been estimated that carers provide 76% of all services to people needing help and support' (PCA, 2008, p. 2). Carer's roles include:

- Providing physical, psychological, emotional, spiritual support.
- Coordinating informal and formal care providers.
- Administering medications.
- Taking patient to various medical appointments (PCA, 2004).

As our population ages it is common that the primary carer is elderly with significant health issues of their own. The Carers Association of Australia in their publication *Warning: Caring is a health hazard* pointed out that up to 75% of carers of palliative patients have chronic health problems. As Nuzzo, McCorkle and Ercolano (2010, p. 897) have identified, 'the caregiver role has changed dramatically from promoting convalescence to providing high technology care and psychological support in the home'.

PCA's report on carers, *The hardest thing we have ever done* (2004, p. 14), outlines some important considerations when understanding the role of carers in palliative care.

- 50 to 70% of caregivers are spouses with two-thirds being wives and 20% daughters or daughters-in-laws, and half of them aged less than 60 years (Robbins, 1998; McIntyre, 1999).
- Caregivers experience ambivalence towards their role. Although 85% of family caregivers of cancer patients reported that they resented having to provide care (Barg et al., 1998).

- 97% acknowledged that caregiving was important, with 67% reporting getting enjoyment out of their role. Nevertheless, some caregivers may feel forced to take on roles they may not want to assume or for which they do not feel capable (Yates, 1999), or they may not be offered a choice regarding their role (Aranda & Pearson, 2001; PCA, 2004, p. 14).

Research has identified that carers themselves have many unmet needs and that caring places enormous physical, emotional and financial demands on the person assuming the role of primary carer and that the caregiving experience encompasses both positive and negative elements (Millberg & Strang, 2003). Studies have repeatedly shown that depression and anxiety is frequently experienced by care givers and that sleep deprivation is common, which adds to the burden of care (Given, Wyatt, & Given 2004).

Primary care providers

For patients with a relatively uncomplicated illness trajectory, care is most appropriately delivered by their primary care providers. These have been defined by PCA (2005, p. 29) as:

> general practitioners, community and hospital based doctors, nurses and allied health, staff of residential aged care facilities whose substantive work is not in palliative care. Primary care providers in the palliative context can also be other specialist care providers for example, oncologists, general physicians, and geriatricians.

Primary care providers have a pivotal role in the management and coordination of services to support the palliative patient and their carer. To be effective the primary provider needs to have an open and honest caring relationship with the patient and their carer, understand what their goals of treatment are, be confident in the management of symptoms commonly experienced by patients and be aware of the support networks that are available in their local community. It is also important that they know when to refer to specialist services when symptoms are or will become difficult to manage.

The specialist palliative care team

PCA (2005) define the specialist palliative care team as: 'providing care to those patients whose needs exceed the capacity and resources of the primary care provider. Referral to a specialist palliative care service will in most cases be through a primary care provider'. The specialist teams increasingly have a consultative role and work in collaboration with the primary health providers. Specialist palliative care services have achieved much in raising the profile of skill required for people at the end of life, particularly in pain and symptom management (Kralik, Van Loon, Alde, & Allen, 2011).

In the NSW Health Role Palliative Care Role Delineation Framework (2007) the specialist palliative care team's role is generally characterised by the following attributes:

- provides specialist palliative care for patients and their families where assessed needs exceed the resources and/or capability of primary care providers
- provides assessment and care consistent with the needs of the patient, caregiver and family and within available service capability and resources
- provides consultation and support to primary care service managing the care of people with life-limiting illness in community, acute care hospitals and residential aged care facilities
- provides ongoing care to patients with complex, unstable condition not restricted to physical symptoms but including psycho-emotional social and spiritual problems

- provides education to primary care providers (NSW Health Role Palliative Care Role Delineation Framework, 2007).

Symptom control

The relief of symptoms associated with advanced and progressive illness is one of the primary aims of palliative care and without optimal management of symptoms whether they are physical, emotional or existential the patient's quality of life quickly deteriorates. This in turn will also erode confidence in their ability to care and can very quickly feel overwhelmed by the responsibility of caring for someone who is in distress. If symptoms are not managed at home the situation can quickly escalate to a crisis which can culminate in the patient being taken to hospital for symptom management.

Good symptom control can only be achieved by a thorough holistic, patient-centred approach to assessment. Symptoms do not exist in a void unrelated to the whole person and their social context and good communication is the cornerstone on which the assessment process rests. A useful approach to clinical decision making in palliative care is called the WHY Framework (Currow & Clarke, 2006, p. 4). The framework is reproduced below.

Does this person have a life limiting illness?
An understanding of the natural course of the illness can help to make clearer the following questions.
Is today's new symptom:

- An expected manifestation of the illness?
- An unexpected manifestation of the illness?
- An exacerbation of a coexisting problem?
- Is it a totally new problem?

Is this person unwell today because of overall progression in a (maximally) treated disease?
OR
Is this person unwell today because of the effects of an acute problem with an easily reversible cause?

- Why has a change in condition occurred?
- What is the timeframe for the change?
- What else has changed in and around the same timeframe?

Can we do something about the problem?
Yes does not necessarily mean that we should start to treat. We need to consider:

- the underlying life-limiting illness and its current systemic manifestations (fatigue, weight loss, anorexia)
- whether the problem is likely to be reversible or not
- the whole person's wishes under these circumstances.

Where possible the best treatment for any symptom is still to treat the cause of the problem.
What can we reasonably do to maintain or improve comfort or function for this person?

Good symptom control is the responsibility of the whole team working with the patient and if symptoms are becoming unstable the primary care providers need to alert the case manager (usually the GP) to have medications adjusted or other interventions commenced. If the symptoms are proving difficult to manage a referral to the specialist palliative care team would be appropriate. Where there is any change made to the plan of care, particularly if there is any change made to medications it is important that the patient and carer are fully involved in the process and understand and agree with the changes.

Settings of care

Palliative care is the care provided to people with an advanced life-limiting illness with little or no prospect of cure. As discussed earlier the majority of the care for palliative patients is provided by the primary carer usually in the person's home in a community setting supported by primary care providers and supported by the specialist palliative care team when symptoms become difficult to manage. As the illness progresses the likelihood that the patient will require admitting to an acute inpatient facility becomes more likely. Reasons for admittance can be summarised as:

- receive treatment for an acute medical or surgical condition
- symptom control
- respite for carers
- to die.

Although a home is often the preferred place of death most people in fact die in hospital. A study in Victoria showed that 16% of patients in South Australia die at home and another study in Victoria showed that about 21% die at home (Hudson, 2003). In PCA's publication *The hardest thing that we have ever done* (2004) they summarise the factors that are usually present which enable a person to die at home as (PCA, 2004, p. 12):

- usually a man
- adequate financial resources
- having cancer or AIDS
- having a healthy full-time carer
- not living alone
- having personal needs which can be managed by carers
- expressing a desire to die at home.

THE NEEDS OF OLDER PEOPLE AT THE END OF LIFE

It comes as no surprise to say that we are living in a society in which the population is rapidly ageing and 'is characterised by an upwards shift in the age structure, so the proportion of younger people declines as the proportion of older people increases. The relative increase in the proportion of older people in the population will be accompanied by a sharply increasing number of older people. In 1999, 12% of the Australian population was aged over 65 years and 2% was over 80 years. It is predicted that by 2016, 16% will be over 65 years and 4% will be over 80 years (ABS, 2009).

Most people who now die are over 65 years of age and the prevalence of chronic illness and disability usually increases with age. About one quarter of all people aged 65 and over have a profound or severe core activity limitation, and chronic illnesses such as dementia, hypertension, asthma and diabetes are common conditions (Australian Institute of Health and Welfare [AIHW], 2007).

The Palliative Care Knowledge Network reports the AIHW's finding that, in June 2006, there were 2931 residential aged care services providing 164 008 places for people requiring care (CareSearch, 2012). The AIHW (2007) report:

> there has been a consistent trend of rising dependency levels among residents. In 2005/6 for 87% of residents the reason for separation from the residential aged care facilities (RACF) was due to death with 17% of those who died having stayed less than 3 months, 19% between 3 months and a year, 45% for 1 to 5 years and 20% for more than 5 years.

These statistics identify the need to take the current palliative approach in residential aged care to one that involves the aged care team and incorporates the embedding of palliative care skills in to resident care settings (Kralik et al., 2011).

CareSearch (2011) identify the key issues in providing palliative care in RACFs as:

- knowing when a resident's condition is palliative and making appropriate adjustments to the goals of care
- building stronger relationships between RACFs and specialised palliative care services
- raising awareness of general practitioners about the palliative approach
- that the skill mix in RACFs promotes a high level of care
- increased opportunities for education in the palliative approach for staff working in RACFs
- that RACFs have access to resources to support residents requiring palliative care.

PROVIDING CULTURALLY APPROPRIATE PALLIATIVE CARE FOR INDIGENOUS PEOPLE

The Indigenous peoples of Australia and New Zealand are not a homogenous group of people, and are comprised of a diverse group of people living in many different communities, sharing different values. Indigenous cultures do not exist within social vacuum and intersect in dynamic ways with non-Indigenous culture and community. Connections to traditional values are an individual choice and likewise there is much variability amongst Indigenous people particularly where there is mixed descent (PCA, 2004).

Indigenous peoples are more likely to die before they are old. The most recent estimates from the ABS show that an Indigenous male born in 2005–2007 was likely to live to 67.2 years, about 11.5 years less than a non-Indigenous male (who could expect to live to 78.7 years). An Indigenous female born in 2005–2007 was likely to live to 72.9 years, which is almost 10 years less than a non-Indigenous woman (82.6 years) (Australian Indigenous InfoNet, 2012).

The Māori experience is somewhat better, although still reflective of the Australian experience.

> Life expectancy at birth for non-Māori exceeded that of Māori by 8.6 years for males and by 7.9 years for females in 2005–07. For males, three-quarters of this difference is due to higher Māori death rates at ages 40–79 years. For females, three-quarters of this difference is due to higher Māori death rates at ages 50–84 years (Statistics New Zealand, 2012).

A very important principle that underlies practice of palliative care with Indigenous peoples is the principle of 'cultural safety': 'this is a practice which respects, supports and empowers the cultural identity and wellbeing of an individual. It is based on the palliative care practitioner understanding their own culture and the power relationships between the practitioner, the patient and/or their family and their community' (PCA, 2004). Berman and colleagues (2012) point out that it is not expected that nurses will fully understand Indigenous beliefs but there is an expectation of respect and individualised care. Despite the diversity there are some common themes which are strongly felt in Indigenous peoples which need to be acknowledged and respected.

Despite the diversity there are some important themes when working with Indigenous people that clinicians need to be aware of to maximise treatment choices:

- communicating in a way that is not clearly understood
- isolation of some groups from major treatment centres and the importance of 'country' and unwillingness to travel outside of 'country' for treatment
- the desire to die at home amongst family (McGrath, 2007)
- lack of trust of government agencies
- lack of compliance to medication regimens and safe storage issues in some areas
- the importance of kinship and the position of the patient within their community and its impact on treatment
- the importance of family and a broader concept of family which includes not only blood relatives but also significant others (McGrath, 2008).

Indigenous Australian advocates can help to overcome some of the above barriers to care — they could be an Aboriginal Health worker, an elder or a trusted community member (PCA, 2004).

PAEDIATRIC PALLIATIVE CARE

Paediatric palliative care is based on the same principles of adult palliative care, but also recognises the exceptional hardship which the death of a child has on the family of the child. Children's reactions to death are strongly influenced by their previous experiences and the family's attitude towards death (Haley, 2013, p. 950). Death in the paediatric sector is rarer than in adult populations. In developed nations the estimated number of children and young people likely to require palliative care services is 16 per 10 000 for the population aged between 0 and 19 years (including neonatal deaths). This figure is 15 per 10 000 excluding neonatal deaths (CareSearch, 2011).

Below is a list of some of the issues and concerns that need to be considered when working with children and their families.

- Family dynamics and willingness to engage with the team will have a profound impact on their willingness to accept palliative care (Summer, 2010).
- The child's age and level of understanding dictates the degree to which they are able to participate in the decision making around treatment options and discussions around death and dying.
- The child's siblings need to be involved in the process of care to the level that they feel comfortable and will require individualised support and education.
- Education and support may need to be directed towards the child's school and local activity groups in which the child is involved.
- Family members/friends pose a serious risk for complicated bereavement and will therefore need close follow-up after the death of the child.
- 'Parents struggle to cope with the diagnosis and learn the skills necessary to provide technical care and negotiate the care system for needed services and information' (Hellsten & Medellin, 2010).
- Barriers to pain control in children are similar to those in adults. They primarily relate to:
  - lack of assessment
  - incorrect attitudes or misconceptions by patients, their families or health providers about pain and its management
  - issues related to systems (Hellsten & Medellin, 2010).

Palliative care can be delivered at the same time as life-prolonging treatments are being pursued or can be the focus of treatment whose aims are based on symptom relief and quality of life. The stigma attached to the words palliative care can often be a real barrier to parents accepting a referral to the specialist palliative care team, as the word palliative is associated with death and giving up (Summer, 2010).

END OF LIFE CARE

A good natural death is really one of the principal aims of the palliative process, and particularly if the care has been good up until this point it is a tragedy of the greatest magnitude if the patient's death is difficult, not only for the dying but also for the family and those health professionals caring for them. It is essential that the team looking after the person recognise that the patient has entered the dying phase. This phase is unpredictable and can last days to sometimes weeks (although uncommon). As the patient gets closer to death they become increasingly weary, weak and sleepy, lose interest in getting out of bed, talking and receiving visitors, become less interested in what's going on around them (although they may rally for short periods of time) and often become confused and agitated (Furst & Doyle, 2004).

At this stage it is vitally important that the caring team communicate with the family and they are made aware of the deterioration in the patient's condition and the team sensitively discuss the plan of care with them. The family need to be able to express their concerns and have the rationale of care explained in a way that makes sense to them. This can be particularly important if some family members express a desire for the commencement of parenteral fluids or nutrition. All but the most necessary medication used to control symptoms can be ceased including anti-hypertensive and hyperglycaemic medication. If patients are having difficulty swallowing medication, most medications used in terminal care can be delivered subcutaneously via a syringe driver, which can deliver the medications continuously over 24 hours (*Therapeutic Guidelines Palliative Care*, 2005).

In some cases if symptoms prove too severe or difficult to manage a patient it may be necessary to sedate the patient to achieve an acceptable level of symptom relief. The key to this process and what distinguishes it from euthanasia is the goal, which is symptom relief and that the amount of medication used is proportional to the patient's needs for symptom relief and not intended to end his/her life. If palliative sedation is required it is important that the plan of care and its goals are communicated clearly to the family.

BEREAVEMENT AND GRIEF

Bereavement refers to the experience of the death of a significant person and the psychological and emotional adaptations those who had a close relationship with that person make in response to that death. Corless (2010) characterises bereavement as the process of 'adjusting to a world without the physical, psychological and social presence of the deceased'. Death is not the end for those that remain behind and it is very important that those charged with the care of a dying person maintain an awareness of the fact that the last days to weeks of a person's life remain locked in the memory of those left behind. How well the process was managed has a significant bearing on the quality of the bereavement of family and friends.

Grief is the term which describes the sadness that people experience after the death of a loved one. For most people's grief fluctuates in its intensity and doesn't require specialised counselling. For clinicians supporting a person or family who are grieving, listening compassionately and responding in a genuine manner is a powerful therapeutic intervention, particularly if the clinician knew the person and was involved in their care. As Tejada-Reyes (2000) points out, 'to provide this caring and reassuring approach, we often do not have to do much beyond sitting at the bedside or making and keeping a commitment to speak and be with the friend or family'. Cultural background profoundly affects how a person copes with the death of a significant person.

A small proportion of people will experience a complicated grief reaction which will require specialised interventions to help them manage their sadness. For this group of people it is appropriate to refer them to bereavement counsellors, or other psychological/psychiatric services. Many Palliative Care teams have bereavement counsellors or social workers with experience in working with grief. Bereavement groups are very useful for those that don't have enough social support or prefer talking about their sadness with those who have experienced similar loss.

The following two case studies will display the palliative care nursing approach. The first case study involves a young mother in declining health with a brain tumour situated in the community. The second case study refers to a patient with a life limiting heart condition in a residential care facility. After each case study a nursing response is provided based on the principles and practices of holistic patient-centred palliative care.

PALLIATIVE NURSING CARE RESPONSE (CASE STUDY 12.1)

It is not uncommon that after relapse a milestone is reached where patients receiving curative therapy for their cancers are faced with the realisations that cure is no longer possible. This decision is often made as a result of previous experiences. In Belinda's case, during

CASE STUDY 12.1

Belinda is a 36-year-old mother of two children who was employed as a part-time medical receptionist in a busy rural practice. Belinda's husband Tom owns his own business. Belinda was diagnosed with an inflammatory breast cancer and after extensive surgical intervention, radiotherapy and chemotherapy was progressing well. Nine months following the completion of her treatment Belinda developed pain in her hip. On investigation it was found that she had bony metastases.

Belinda was immediately referred back to her radiation oncologist and subsequently received radiation therapy to her pelvis. Following this she commenced second line chemotherapy. As a result of the chemotherapy Belinda experienced distressing side effects resulting in numerous hospital admissions.

During her treatment she developed a persistent headache followed rapidly by unsteadiness in her gait. After a CT scan of her body it was discovered that she had further brain and liver metastases. She was again reviewed by the radiation oncologist and received whole brain irradiation. This initially provided some relief but after some months her symptoms recurred. After medical consultation, discussion and deliberation Belinda decided that she would have no further chemotherapy and opted to remain at home utilising community support and naturopathy services for her palliative care needs.

her second line of chemotherapy she experienced overwhelming nausea and vomiting. These distressing symptoms resulted in crises which led to multiple admissions to hospital. After discussion with the medical oncologist and further deliberation involving the family and oncology nursing staff, Belinda realised that further treatment would not lead to a cure and potentially erode the quality of her life. Therefore she decided she would no longer have active treatment and has opted for palliative care. These decisions can be quite challenging for nursing staff involved in the care of an oncology patient and tests the multi-professional team's ability to stay focused on the patient's wishes.

In an effort to palliate Belinda's immediate symptoms (i.e. headache and unsteady gait) it was suggested that she be commenced on steroids to help reduce the intra-cranial pressure causing her symptoms. One of the roles of the nurse in this situation would be to reiterate the significant side effects associated with this treatment and ensure that Belinda understands the treatment and its rationale. As a result of the spread of her cancer to her bones Belinda began to experience moderate–severe aching pains. During the assessment process a pain management plan was discussed and it was recommended by the specialist palliative care nurse that Belinda be commenced on a combination of Paracetamol, non-steroidal anti-inflammatory and prn liquid morphine. In case Belinda experiences nausea with these medications it was also recommended that she be ordered prophylactic anti-nausea medications. At this stage a bowel management plan may be necessary to avoid constipation if regular use of opioids analgesia is used.

It must be stressed that at all levels of this debilitating disease, Belinda will have sexual, physical and emotional needs. Belinda is still relatively young and is in a long-term relationship with her husband. Both Belinda and her husband may require counselling to assist them to maintain some level of intimacy. White (2003, p. 247) informs us that 'the lack of assessment of sexuality is an issue for all palliative care staff, given that the importance of sexuality as an integral component of an individual's quality of life does not decrease in the palliative care phase'. The nurse will need to assess the importance Belinda places on her own personal body image and sexuality and be open to the appropriate communication skills required to allow Belinda to voice her feelings.

At this point Belinda was referred by the oncology nurses to the specialist palliative care team. Here it is important to clarify patient goals and assess symptom and supportive needs. By utilising therapeutic communication skills the patient and family and caregiver in consultation with the palliative team can reach a decision regarding their future care. Belinda's desire to remain as independent as possible can be facilitated by referral to the other members of the multi-professional team. The following individuals may be identified as being helpful in supporting Belinda to achieve her goals and meet these needs as they become evident during the palliative journey.

- **District and community nursing services** — Early referral to these services are vital to enable Belinda to realise her goal to remain at home with family. Home nurses are in a unique position to provide long-term care and a holistic approach. Nursing services provide essential nursing support that may include:
  - personal care
  - ongoing assessment of symptoms and recommendation for changes to management plan
  - monitoring medication requirements
  - liaising with other team members.
- **Medical practitioners** — the general practitioner's role in this community based scenario would be to support Belinda's decision to remain at home by ensuring that she receives the appropriate medical assessment for medication and

community support. The knowledge that the GP may have regarding Belinda's medical and social history will be invaluable for her future management.

- **Social worker** — Belinda's situation can create significant emotional and financial distress. Social workers can have an invaluable role in mobilising financial assistance (i.e. sickness benefits, carers' allowances and liaising with previous employers). At some point, Belinda's illness will most probably require some form of domiciliary support. They can also offer additional emotional support and counselling for her husband and children. Often where there is advanced cancers in younger people it must be acknowledged that it creates increased stress for family, carers and the healthcare team.
- **School counsellor** — in this situation would be an essential member of the team and can provide essential support for Belinda's children. This support may include the provision of academic assistances and specific counselling services for Belinda's children and their friends.
- **Cancer support services** — generic cancer support services offer a wide range of voluntary services and supportive networks. For example, body image **workshops,** Canteen, education pamphlets/DVDs and telephone counselling.
- **Mental health liaison team** — if depression and anxiety become a concern then referral to the mental health team would be appropriate. Medication and specific cognitive and behavioural therapies can promote wellness and improve quality of life in this situation.
- **Bereavement counsellor** — this form of counselling is focused on grief and offers bereavement support to surviving family, friends and carers.
- **Pastoral care** — the spiritual dimension of Belinda's journey will require significant consideration requiring support and guidance. Often patients who are experiencing religious death will express a desire to explore the spiritual aspect of their beliefs or reconnect with a religious group.
- **Dietitian** — in consultation with the patient assesses nutritional needs and develops a plan for maximising nutritional intake.
- **Occupational Therapist** — as Belinda has decided to die at home she will require specialised equipment and home medications as her illness progresses.
- **Complementary therapist** — Belinda's naturopath would be involved in helping to control a wide range of symptoms including homeopathic medicine. Belinda could also utilise the services of an aromatherapist for relaxation and pain control.

As a result of the support provided by the extended palliative care team and the mobilisation of community support networks, Belinda was able to maintain relative independence and autonomy at home. Over the period leading to her death Belinda was able to successfully adapt to her circumstances and participate in preparing family and friends.

PALLIATIVE CARE NURSING RESPONSE (CASE STUDY 12.2)

We highlighted earlier in this chapter the importance of palliative nursing care as a core generic skill in nursing practice for patients with life-limiting illnesses. However, it has been well discussed in recent literature that there is a reluctance to view the terminal stage of chronic heart failure as requiring palliative care. In fact, research suggest that the patient's

CASE STUDY 12.2

Peter is a 74-year-old retired factory worker who is estranged from immediate family. Fifteen years ago Peter's wife died suddenly and tragically. As a result Peter became depressed, his consumption of alcohol increased considerably. In conjunction with his drinking he smoked heavily and his nutritional intake became inadequate. Peter's health deteriorated and thirteen years ago he was diagnosed with chronic dilated cardiomyopathy.

He was commenced on a combination of Ace inhibitors, diuretics, Beta Blockers and Digoxin. His underlying depression was treated with medications and counselling and as a result he was able to make positive life style changes. His condition stabilised and for some time he maintained his health with the help of nursing and allied health support and medical supervision, which necessitated a number of medication adjustments. However the medications become less effective and symptoms increased. These included shortness of breath, oedema, fatigue and frequent chest pain.

Peter's health deteriorates significantly and requires an admission to hospital for acute shortness of breath. Once stabilised Peter was transferred to a local nursing home. Despite appropriate nursing and medical care Peter's cardiac condition continued to deteriorate and he has developed irreversible left-sided heart failure, which causes overwhelming pulmonary oedema. Peter now begins the palliative phase of his illness and has consented for nursing staff to contact family members.

experience of end-stage cardiac failure was similar to that of advanced cancer but palliation as a mode of care was not identified, and therefore patients dying of non-cancer diagnosis receive less coordinated palliative care than patients dying of cancer (Gott et al., 2007; Johnson & Houghton, 2006; Horne & Payne, 2004; Palmer & Howarth, 2005). This can be rectified by thorough and comprehensive patient-centred nursing assessment aimed at providing best care practices for patients nearing the end of life.

Appropriate and sensitive communication is the key to palliative care nursing practices. Although many nurses find it challenging to discuss death in the initial assessment, this is exactly where discussion on the outcome of Peter's treatment should be addressed. Patients in Peter's condition require the opportunity to discuss their feelings and emotions in preparation for death. This is part of the groundwork when one is working towards 'a good death' and is guided by the WHO (2002) principle of affirming life and regarding dying as a normal process. In attempting to discuss death with Peter the nurse must be aware of the impact of increasing hypoxia causing breathlessness and confusion resulting in difficulties in communication.

The generalist nurse can play a significant role in Peter's care. Physical symptoms associated with heart failure such as pain, breathlessness, weight loss (cardiac cachexia), nausea and vomiting, weakness and incontinence are common, and comparable with the physical symptoms of cancer. 'The morbidity and mortality rates of heart failure and cancer are often almost identical' (Palmer & Howard, 2005, p. 101). Nurses are quite aware of the important role they play in the basic physical need requirements and can provide skilled care in assisting Peter to maintain some functionality and ability to self-care. Oxygen, opioids and diuretic drug therapy all remain essential medical elements of Peter's care and therefore require vigilant monitoring for effectiveness with the aim to maintain comfort, not prolong death and enhance quality of life.

Peter's condition has clearly deteriorated where medical treatment with a curative intent would be inappropriate. That is not to suggest that palliation is not an active form of nursing treatment. Palliative care in this case study provides the necessary treatment to promote comfort levels and minimise suffering associated with his worsening chronic condition by:

- relieving distressing symptoms
- assist Peter to come to terms with end-of-life issues
- maintenance of a level of quality of life that is compliant with his personal wishes.

Often heart failure, like cancer, has a high level of unpredictability. Patients often experience sporadic improvements of health but heart failure is more likely than cancer to end in sudden death due to arrhythmias. The nurse must be aware of the anxiety as a result of the uncertainty of the situation and particularly the breathlessness. In this situation a long acting benzodiazepine in moderate doses can be helpful in ameliorating anxiety and helping to maximise respiratory function.

The instability of the situation can be addressed once the breathlessness has been stabilised and when appropriate the nurse can initiate dialogue making enquiries regarding his future care. It's timely then to consider, in consultation with medical practitioners and specialist palliative care nurses:

- contact with family and friends
- advance directives
- spiritual needs
- funeral arrangements
- living will.

As a consequence of holistic nursing care nurses can play a pivotal role in the coordination of the multidisciplinary health team approach in palliative care. As a result of the information gathered through ongoing assessment and monitoring, the nurse may find themselves as providing leadership and direction to other members of the multiprofessional team. This could also require the nurse to play an advocacy role assisting Peter to meet his end-of-life goals. The following individuals may be identified as being helpful in supporting Peter achieve his goals and meet his needs as they become evident.

- **Palliative care nurse specialist** — providing expert advice on symptom management, education to patient and staff. Liaising with generalist nursing and medical practitioners. If symptoms become very difficult to manage the palliative care nurse specialist can usually have access to a palliative doctor. The palliative care nurse specialist provides advice on the dying process and helps to ensure that appropriate medications are in place in case the situation deteriorates rapidly. This may include sedatives, adequate opioids titration and appropriate bowel management plan. Ensuring availability of prn medication to guide effective nursing interventions.
- **Medical practitioner** — general practitioners working as members of the multiprofessional team helping to provide medical intervention at an appropriate level, which is congruent with WHO principles of palliative medicine.
- **Social worker** — helping Peter with his financial and social needs. Liaison with social services and establishing contact with solicitors and funeral directors. Helping to liaise with family members and offer counselling and support for problematic or difficult family situations.

- **Mental health liaison team** — this community based team is available for patients experiencing emotional and psychological distress as a result of their condition. This may include the addition of antidepressant/anxiolytic medications and specific therapeutic interventions.
- **Bereavement counsellor** — offers bereavement support for the grieving process to surviving family, friends and carers.
- **Pastoral care** — spiritual leaders provide counselling for patients requiring spiritual guidance. Patients at this time are often re-evaluating the meaning and direction of their life.
- **Dietitian** — can provide patient consultation: with the patient assesses nutritional needs and develops a plan for maximising nutritional intake.
- **Physiotherapist** — can be helpful in providing additional support in teaching patient and nursing staff in assisting Peter to maximise his cardio-pulmonary function.
- **Occupational therapist** — can provide advice in minimising Peter's energy requirements. By assessing his physical capabilities and providing appropriate equipment.
- **Complementary therapist** — very useful in helping to control symptoms and maximising wellness using a range of therapeutic modalities including remedial massage, aromatherapy, acupuncture, music and diversional therapies.

In Peter's case study it was seen that even within a hospital setting, palliative care was able to be provided by a multiprofessional team approach. With thorough assessment and goal setting Peter was able to remain in control with the assistance of interventions that enhanced the quality of his life.

CONCLUSION

Caring is a core skill that underpins every nursing practice, and every nurse will be involved with a palliative care patient at some point in their career. It's vitally important for the wellbeing of those they are caring for that nurses understand what is expected of them. Palliative care is much more than the care offered in the terminal stages of an illness; it is now accepted as having a role in the management of all chronic life-limiting illnesses. Palliative care is holistic in its commitment to quality of life and embraces the challenge of death.

Reflective questions

1. Discuss the concept of the three levels of care provision for patients in palliative care.
2. If you were the primary nurse carer for a patient with end-stage lung disease what are the important considerations of care required to ensure comfort measures?
3. Identify the role of the generalist nurse as a member of a multi-professional team supporting a palliative care patient in the community.

Recommended readings

Abbott, J., O'Connor, M., & Payne, S. (2008). An Australian survey of palliative care and hospice bereavement services. *Australian Jourmal of Cancer Nursing*, *9*(2), 12–17.

Aoun, S. M., Breen, L. J., O'Connor, M., et al. (2012). A public health approach to bereavement support services in palliative care. *Australian and New Zealand Journal of Public Health*, *36*(1), 14–15.

Burns, C., Abernathy, A., Leblanc, C., et al. (2010). What is the role of friends when contributing care at the end of life? Findings from an Australian population study. *Psycho-Oncology*, *20*, 203–212.

Cancer Council Australia. (2012). *FAQ*. Retrieved July 26, 2012, from http://www.cancer.org.au/aboutcancer/FAQ.htm#573

Carers Association of Australia. (2000). *Warning: caring is a health hazard: Results of the 1999 National survey of carer health and wellbeing*. Retrieved August 6, 2012, from http://www.apa.org.au/upload/2004-5A_Hales.pdf

McKechnie, R., Macleod, R., & Jaye, C. (2011). The use of nurses in community palliative care. *Home Healthcare Nurse*, *29*(7), 408–415.

Rawlings, D., Hendry, K., Nyine, S., et al. (2011). Using palliative care assessment tools to influence and enhance clinical practice. *Home Healthcare Nurse*, *29*(3), 145–147.

Warner, R. (2009). Recovery from schizophrenia and the recovery model. *Current Opinion in Psychiatry*, *22*, 374–380.

References

Aranda, S., & Pearson, A. (2001). Caregiving in advanced cancer: lay decision making. *Journal of Palliative Care*, *17*(4), 270–276.

Australian Bureau of Statistics. (2008). *Who cares? 2.5 million Australians (media release)*. Retrieved August 2, 2012, from http://www.abs.gov.au/AUSSTATS/abs@.nsf/Latestproducts/4448.0Media%20Release12008?opendocument&tabname=Summary&prodno=4448.0&issue=2008&num=&view=

Australian Bureau of Statistics. (2009). *Future population growth and ageing*. Retrieved August 1, 2012, from http://www.abs.gov.au/AUSSTATS/abs@.nsf/Lookup/4102.0Main+Features10March%202009

Australian Indigenous InfoNet. (2012). *Summary of Australian Indigenous health*. Retrieved July 29, 2012, from http://www.healthinfonet.ecu.edu.au/

Australian Institute of Health and Welfare. (2007). *Older Australia at a glance* (4th ed.). Retrieved July 26, 2012, from http://www.aihw.gov.au/WorkArea/DownloadAsset.aspx?id=6442454209

Barg, F., Pasacreta, J., Nuamah, I., et al. (1998). A description of a psychoeducational intervention for family caregivers of cancer patients. *Journal of Family Nursing*, *44*, 394–413.

Berman, A., Snyder, S., Levitt-Jones, T., et al. (Eds.), (2012). *Kozier & Erb's fundamentals of nursing* (2nd Aust. ed.). Australia: Pearson Australia.

CareSearch. (2012). *Public health palliative care*. Retrieved August 6, 2012, from http://www.caresearch.com.au/caresearch/tabid/1477/Default.aspx

Corless, I. B. (2010). Bereavement. In R. Ferrell & N. Coyle (Eds.) *Oxford textbook of palliative nursing*. Oxford: Oxford University Press.

Currow, D., & Clarke, K. (2006). *Emergencies in palliative and supportive care*. Oxford: Oxford University Press.

Ferrell, R., & Coyle, N., (Eds.), (2010). *Oxford textbook of palliative nursing*. Oxford: Oxford University Press.

Furst, C. J., & Doyle, D. (2004). The terminal phase. In D. Doyle, G. Hanks, N. Cherny & K. Calman (Eds.), *Oxford textbook of palliative care* (3rd ed.). Oxford: Oxford University Press.

Given, B., Wyatt, G., & Given, C. (2004). Burden and depression among caregivers of patients with cancer at the end of life. *Oncology Nursing Forum, 31*(6), 1105–1115.

Glover, J., Hetzel, D., & Tennant, S. (2004). *The Socioeconomic gradient and chronic illness and associated risk factors in Australia and New Zealand Health Policy*. Retrieved August 6, 2012, from http://www.anzhealthpolicy.com/content/1/1/8

Gott, M., Barnes, S., Parker, C., et al. (2007). Dying trajectories in heart failure. *Palliative Medicine, 21*, 95–99.

Haley, C., (Ed.). (2013). *Pilliterri's child & family health nursing in Australia and New Zealand* (1st ed.). Australia: WoltersKluwer/Lippincott Williams & Wilkins.

Hellsten, M. B., Medellin, G. (2010). Symptom management in paediatric palliative care. In R. Ferrell & N. Coyle (Eds.), *Oxford textbook of palliative nursing*. Oxford: Oxford University Press.

Hiedrich, D. E. (2007). Palliative care & end of life care perspectives. In K. K. Kuebler, D. E. Heidrich & P. Esper (Eds.), *Palliative & end of life care, clinical practice guidelines* (2nd ed.). St Louis: Elsevier.

Horne, G., & Payne, S. (2004). Removing the boundaries: palliative care for patients with heart failure. *Palliative Medicine, 18*, 291–296.

Hudson, P. (2003). Home based support for palliative care families: Challenges and recommendations. *Medical Journal of Australia, 179*(6), 35.

Johnson, M. J., & Houghton, T. (2006). Palliative care for patients with heart failure: description of a service. *Palliative Medicine, 20*, 211–214.

Johnston, B. M. (2005). Introduction to palliative care: overview of nursing developments. In J. Lugton & R. McIntyre (Eds.), *Palliative care the nursing role* (2nd ed.). Edinburgh: Elsevier Churchill Livingstone.

Kellehear, A. (1999). *Health promoting palliative care* (p. 20). Melbourne: Oxford University Press.

Kellehear, A., & O'Connor, D. (2010). Policy and practice health — promoting palliative care: A practice example. *Critical Public Health, 18*(1), 111–115.

Kralik, D., Van Loon, A., Alde, P., et al. (Eds.), (2011). *Community Nursing in Australia: Context, Issues and Applications*. Australia: John Wiley & Sons.

Macintosh, E., & Zerwekh, J. (2006). Hospice and palliative care. In J. V. Zerwekh (Ed.), *Nursing care at the end of life, palliative care for patients and families*. Philadelphia: F.A. Davis.

Maxwell, T. (2010). Caring for those with chronic illness. In R. Ferrell & N. Coyle (Eds.), *Oxford textbook of palliative nursing*. Oxford: Oxford University Press.

McGrath, P. (2007). 'I don't want to be in that big city; this is my country here': research findings on Aboriginal peoples' preference to die at home. *Australian Journal Rural Health, 15*, 264–268.

McGrath, P. (2008). Family Caregiving for Aboriginal peoples during end of life: Findings from the Northern Territory. *Journal of Rural and Tropical Public Health, 7*, 1–10.

McIntyre, R. (1999). Support for family and carers. In J. Lugton & M. Kindlen (Eds.), *Palliative care: The nursing role*. Edinburgh: Churchill Livingstone.

Millberg, A., & Strang, P. (2003). Meaningfulness in palliative home care: An interview study of dying patients' next of kin. *Palliative Support Care, 203*(1), 171–180.

NSW Health Role Palliative Care Role Delineation Framework. (2007). *NSW Health Guideline, GL2007-22*. Retrieved August 6, 2012, from http://www.health.nsw.gov.au/policies/gl/2007/pdf/GL2007_022.pdf

Nuzzo, P., McCorkle, R., & Ercolano, E. (2010). Home care. In R. Ferrell & N. Coyle (Eds.), *Oxford textbook of palliative nursing*. Oxford: Oxford University Press.

Palliative Care Australia. (2004). *The hardest thing that we have ever done. The social impact for caring for a terminally ill person*. Retrieved August 12, 2012, from http://www.palliativecare.org.au/Portals/46/The%20hardest%20thing.pdf

Palliative Care Australia. (2005). *A guide to palliative care service development: A population based approach*. Retrieved July 26, 2012, from http://www.palliativecare.org.au/Portals/46/resources/PalliativeCareServiceDevelopment.pdf

Palliative Care Australia. (2008). *Carers and end of life. Position statement*. Retrieved August 12, 2012, from http://www.palliativecare.org.au/Portals/46/PCA%20Carers%20and%20End%20of%20Life%20Position%20Statement.pdf

Palmer, E., & Howarth, J. (2005). *Palliative care for the primary care team, issues for the primary care team*. London: Quay Books Division.

Robbins, M. (1998). *Evaluating palliative care: Establishing the evidence base*. Oxford: Oxford University Press.

Rumbold, B., Young, B., & Salu, S. (2007). From concept to care: Enabling community care through a health promoting palliative care approach. *Contemporary Nurse, 27*, 132–140.

Statistics New Zealand. (2012). *Population*. Retrieved July 26, 2012, from http://www.stats.govt.nz/browse_for_stats/population/births/new-zealand-life-tables-2005-07/chapter-2-national-trends-in-longevity-and-mortality.aspx

Summer, L. (2010). Paediatric hospice and palliative care. In R. Ferrell & N. Coyle (Eds.), *Oxford textbook of palliative nursing*. Oxford: Oxford University Press.

Tejeda-Reyes, I. (2000). Making death a meaningful transition. *Clinical Journal of Oncology Nursing, 6*(3), 173–174.

Therapeutic Guidelines Palliative Care, Version 2. (2005). Melbourne: Therapeutic Guidelines Ltd.

Walsh, D., Aktas, A., Hullihen, B., & Indura, R. (2011). What is palliative medicine? Motivation and skills. *American Journal of Hospice and Palliative Medicine, 28*(1), 52–58.

White, K. (2003). Sexuality and body image. In M. O'Connor & S. Aranda (Eds.), *Palliative care nursing: A guide to practice* (2nd ed., pp. 245–256). Melbourne: Ausmed.

World Health Organization. (2002). *Innovative care for chronic conditions: Building blocks for action; global report*. Geneva: Report No: ISBN 92 4 159 017 013. Retrieved August 22, 2012, from http://www.who.int/diabetes/publications/iccc_exec_summary_eng.pdf

Yates, P. (1999). Family coping: Issues and challenges for cancer nursing. *Cancer Nursing, 2*(1), 63–71.

CHAPTER 13

Louise O'Brien
Scott Fanker

Schizophrenia

Learning objectives

When you have completed this chapter you will be able to:

- describe the onset and course of schizophrenia
- identify the community beliefs about schizophrenia that lead to stigmatisation and self-stigmatisation
- discuss the concept of recovery in relation to schizophrenia
- identify the essential components of recovery-focused services for people with schizophrenia
- consider the role of the nurse in the recovery process for a person with schizophrenia.

Key words

psychosocial education, recovery, schizophrenia, stigmatisation, therapeutic alliance

INTRODUCTION

Schizophrenia is a severe mental illness that can affect every facet of a person's life. In the past schizophrenia was viewed as an inevitably deteriorating disorder marked by declining ability to live and participate in the community. However, people who have had an acute episode of schizophrenia often recover from that episode and for people who do not fully recover, or go on to have further episodes, their life is not necessarily marked by deterioration. This chapter will discuss the causes and course of schizophrenia, and its impact on quality of life. A focus of this chapter is the effect of stigmatisation and self-stigmatisation, as well as a focus on the recovery process and what this means for the delivery of mental health services and the role of the nurse.

DESCRIPTION OF THE DISORDER

Schizophrenia is a severe mental illness marked by psychotic phenomena such as hallucinations and delusions. The person has difficulty identifying reality, thinking, communicating, managing emotional responses and making judgments to the extent that the person's ability to function is impaired. Although the prevalence of schizophrenia varies, prevalence studies indicate that about seven individuals per 1000 population are affected (McGrath, Saha, Chant, & Welham, 2008). The onset of the illness is usually between 15 and 25 years of age.

SYMPTOMS OF SCHIZOPHRENIA

The symptoms of schizophrenia include:

- *Hallucinations:* hallucinations are the experience of hearing, seeing, smelling, sensing or tasting things not experienced by other people. Auditory hallucinations are the most common and may include the hearing of voices commenting on the person's behaviour, or hearing voices telling the person to act in particular ways.
- *Delusions:* people who are described as delusional hold beliefs that are not in keeping with the evidence, with strong conviction and against the beliefs of other members of the same culture. The person may believe that there is a conspiracy to harm them, with a lack of evidence that this is so, and when other members of the same community do not see such a threat. Delusions are unable to be shifted by reasoning or presenting evidence to the contrary.
- *Thought disturbances:* the person is described as suffering thought disturbance when they experience disruption to thoughts, such that they may feel that thoughts are being removed from their mind; that thoughts are being inserted into their mind; or that their thoughts are being broadcast aloud when they have not been spoken.
- *Disturbances in speech:* speech may not be understandable or speech patterns may not make links to what is happening or being discussed. Speech seems disconnected.

Other symptoms are sometimes described as negative symptoms and are marked by lack of energy, apathy, failure to initiate speech and responses to the environment that are inappropriate or blunted.

THE DIAGNOSIS OF SCHIZOPHRENIA

Schizophrenia is diagnosed in the presence of at least two of the following symptoms: hallucinations, delusions, disturbance of speech, disorganised behaviour, negative symptoms. In addition, the presence of these symptoms is accompanied by disruption to social and occupational functioning and the duration of the symptoms and dysfunction is at least six months, although if treated this may be shorter. Other disorders, such as mood disorders, substance abuse and physical illness, need to have been ruled out (American Psychiatric Association, 2000).

WHAT CAUSES SCHIZOPHRENIA

Schizophrenia appears to be caused by the interaction of a number of factors (Warner, 2004). Factors that have been implicated in vulnerability to develop schizophrenia in the individual include genetic predisposition, exposure to intrauterine infections, birth trauma, head injury in childhood and communication patterns in the family. In addition, environmental stress, such as change in role or relationships or drug use, is believed to interact with the vulnerability to precipitate the psychotic episode. A number of protective factors may mitigate the impact of the vulnerability and environmental stress (Treatment Protocol Project, 1997). People with good pre-morbid functioning in a number of areas such as relationships and employment tend to have better outcomes (Warner, 2004).

THE COURSE OF SCHIZOPHRENIA

The prodromal phase

Before the onset of acute symptoms (delusions and hallucinations, speech and thought disturbance) the person may have a number of poorly defined signs indicating change from previous functioning, but these signs may be attributed to developmental problems (for instance, adolescent behaviours) or to changes in the environment (stress related to family, social relationships, school or work). The person may be noted to have a general loss of interest in activity, withdrawal from social relationships, work or school difficulties. The person may also develop beliefs and interests that are seen as odd (for instance in the occult), develop odd ritualistic behaviours or begin talking to themselves.

The active phase

The active phase describes the onset of psychotic features of hallucinations and delusions, accompanied by disturbances in thinking and behaving. The person may be highly anxious, frightened of the world around them or depressed. They may have difficulty thinking through the most mundane of tasks, but because this experience is so frightening they may have difficulty admitting that there is a problem. Delusions can be undermining of trust in others, even the closest of family and friends (McCann & Clark, 2004).

The residual phase

This phase is marked by a diminution of active symptoms. However, the extent to which active psychotic symptoms resolve is variable. The assault of the active psychotic phase may take considerable time to resolve. The person may be left with a number of symptoms that do not seem to be responsive to medication. These residual symptoms are sometimes termed 'negative' symptoms, as they are marked by a lack of energy, failure to be able to initiate interest and engagement with others and lack of motivation. It may be difficult to differentiate between the residual symptoms of the illness, the effects of medication and the effect of the trauma of the acute psychotic illness. People who have suffered an acute psychotic episode may see their future as unpredictable, have little confidence in the reliability of their own mind and continue to fear that the illness will return (McCann & Clark, 2004).

The recovery style of people who have suffered a psychotic illness varies. Three recovery styles have been identified: an integrative style, a sealing-over style and a mixed integrative and sealing-over style (Thompson, McGorry, & Harrigan, 2003). The integrative style is one that is marked by the ability to accept the psychotic illness as part of their life experience. This style requires a level of flexibility in thinking, accepting the psychosis as another life experience that need not be viewed negatively. The sealing-over style utilises encapsulation of the psychotic experience, viewing it as a negative disruption and avoiding thinking about the experience. Some people use a mix of the two styles. Thompson et al. (2003) found that recovery styles may change over time, moving from sealing-over to integration and vice versa. It is noted that people with a sealing-over style of recovery had significantly more debilitating psychotic illness. In addition, the style of recovery appeared to be related to insight and understanding of the illness. These issues have implications for education about illness and sensitivity about the timing and style of education. Sealing-over style of recovery may be self-protective against stigmatisation, discussed later in this chapter.

The length and severity of each phase of the illness is highly variable, as is the outcome. The WHO suggests that it can be expected that 25% will experience full recovery, 40% will suffer recurrent active episodes with some measure of disability between episodes, while 35% will remain chronically disabled (Treatment Protocol Project, 1997).

SCHIZOPHRENIA AND CHRONICITY

Chronicity has been associated with schizophrenia since Kraepelin, in 1896, classified a group of mental disorders as dementia praecox and predicted that the recovery rate for this disorder was between 2.6% and 4.1%. Bleuler, in the early 1900s, further developed the definition of the illnesses, labelled them 'the schizophrenias', identified primary and secondary symptoms and also suggested that people never fully recovered (Corin, 1990). The pervasiveness of these views on the thinking about schizophrenia has been evidenced in medical diagnostic manuals and textbooks (Harding, Zubin, & Strauss, 1987; McGorry, 1992).

This view of schizophrenia, as an inevitably chronic illness, has since been questioned in long-term follow-up studies and it has been suggested that the course of the illness is sensitive not only to biological vulnerability but also to social development, culture, social networks and stress and coping (Cavelti, Kvrgic, Kossowsky, & Vauth, 2012; Mueser et al., 2006). Coping with the effects of the illness is compounded by the fact that people with long-term mental health problems face additional difficulties in coping with social systems. People with chronic schizophrenia have lives that are often marked by stress and impoverishment. Problems relate to role transition, living arrangements and financial concerns, as well as loneliness and difficulty in negotiating satisfactory relationships. Even in the face of an unhelpful social context, people with long-term mental illness have been shown not to inevitably decline into a deteriorating condition.

EFFECT OF SCHIZOPHRENIA ON THE ACTIVITIES OF DAILY LIVING

Schizophrenia can have a huge impact on the activities of daily living and all parts of the person's life are likely to be affected by the experience of having a psychotic illness. The difficulty of living with a mental illness such as schizophrenia is one of dealing with ongoing symptoms, managing the problems of medication and other treatments and suffering alienation, isolation and loneliness. Relating to others is difficult in that although there may be a need for contact with people there may also be a fear of closeness and the problem of managing the stress that closeness might create.

The extent of difficulties related to activities of daily living depends not solely on the severity of the illness, nor on the residual symptoms but also on the extent of developmental delay caused by the onset of the illness. Young people who develop psychotic illness may not have well-developed social and practical skills for daily living prior to the onset of the illness. Poor judgment and disordered thinking patterns make daily decision-making difficult.

Thus, the person with schizophrenia may need support for, and education about, organising hygiene, clothing, shopping, cooking and house-cleaning, managing finances, developing social relationships and managing time. Employment may present a huge difficulty and many people with schizophrenia are unemployed even when they wish to work. When they do have employment they may need support related to the management of medication and work, and disclosure of their health status (Bennett, Sundram, Farhall, Fossey, Grigg, & Jeffs, 2012).

STIGMA AND SCHIZOPHRENIA

Stereotyping is a way of organising information about groups of people. It can be positive and can be a quick way of communicating about a particular group. Stigmas are stereotypes that hold negative connotations about a group. There are a number of negative stereotypes associated with mental illness and particularly with schizophrenia. Beliefs that mental illness is a lifelong, deteriorating disease, that people with mental illness are violent and that people with mental illness cannot live on their own, or hold a job, or be in a relationship pervade thinking about people with mental illness. These stereotypes are perpetuated by media reports that link mental illness with violence, fear, need for exclusion or need for patronising care (Corrigan, Larson, Sells, Niessen, & Watson, 2007; Owen, 2012). Stigma leads to discrimination such as in housing, employment, health services and relationships (Warner, 2004). The social messages inherent in the stigma are powerful and strongly linked with poor self-image, a lack of self-esteem and self-stigmatisation.

Vauth, Kleim, Wirtz and Corrigan (2007) found that even when recovery from overt psychotic symptoms was good, people with schizophrenia perceived high levels of stigmatisation and devaluation. The authors found that participants in their study used withdrawal and secrecy as ways to manage anticipated discrimination and that these ways of coping affected self-image and led to self-stigmatisation.

IMAGE OF SELF

The effect on the sense of self of a person who develops schizophrenia may be one of the most profound effects of the illness. The onset of the illness presents an experience that is inexplicable to the person. The experience of hallucinations, perceptions of the world that are no longer reliable, difficulties in thinking and making themselves understood by others have a significant effect. Most people react with helplessness as efforts to make sense of their experience fail (Bauml et al., 2006). Helplessness and hopelessness are the outcomes of self-concepts that are negative, expectations of poor outcome of the illness and a locus of control that is external to the person. Thus the person has low self-esteem, feels that the outcome of the illness is beyond their control and thinks that they can do nothing to influence the course of the illness (Hoffmann, Kupper, & Kunz, 2000).

The issue of stigmatisation of people with mental illness, and in particular schizophrenia, was discussed earlier in this chapter. However, an important aspect of stigmatisation is self-stigmatisation, or internalised stigma (Hanzawa, 2012) and how it affects self-image. Self-stigmatisation is 'the agreement with negative prejudices' (Vauth et al., 2007) that is internal and directed towards self. The stereotypes of society are accepted by the person and turned inwards. This results in social isolation, as the person withdraws due to both the need to maintain secrecy about the illness and the overwhelming shame about having the illness (Corrigan, 2012). Self-stigmatisation affects the person's sense of self-efficacy and empowerment and this in turn affects levels of depression and is indicative of poorer quality of life.

The person with schizophrenia is in a dilemma. Do they reject the idea of having a mental illness, called lacking insight, or accept that they have a mental illness with the resultant stigmatisation and self-stigmatisation that occurs? Davidson (2003) eloquently tells the story of Kyle, a young man with delusions that he was involved in the CIA, who was labelled treatment-resistant. Kyle's explanation for his resistance to treatment was that to accept treatment was to accept the label of schizophrenia: 'I had to be either a CIA agent or a mental patient. Which would you choose?' (p. 142). This is also a dilemma for mental health service providers. How can service providers encourage acceptance of mental illness when we know that the consequence of such acceptance is likely to be self-stigmatisation? Warner (2004) suggests that in the process of encouraging insight into the illness, services need to encourage the development of mastery, to encourage ways of having a sense of being in charge of the illness in order to combat the effects of self-stigmatisation. Similarly Sibitz, Unger, Woppman, Zidek and Amering (2011) identified that people with schizophrenia had the capacity to counteract the stigma of mental illness through stigma resistance. People who showed higher levels of stigma resistance had higher self-esteem, empowerment and better quality of life.

QUALITY OF LIFE

People with severe psychiatric illness, including schizophrenia, often rate their quality of life as low (Hewitt, 2007). Many people with schizophrenia have lives marked by impoverishment and loneliness. Housing options may be sub-standard or they may have drifted into a life of homelessness, accessing shelter where they can. Some live in boarding houses of varying comfort and quality. Others may live in group homes, hostels or supported independent accommodation. While many families provide support, which affects quality of life, this may not be the chosen option for the person with schizophrenia or their family.

In a study of people with psychotic illness, mainly schizophrenia, Eklund and Backstrom (2005) identified a number of factors of importance that affected quality of life for this group. These factors were sense of self, satisfaction with daily activities, psychopathology and satisfaction with medical care. In addition, issues of independent living and education affected quality of life. Greenberg, Knudsen and Aschbrenner (2006) identified that prosocial family interactions marked by warmth and praise led to increased life satisfaction for the adult child with schizophrenia. Vauth, Kleim, Wirtz and Corrigan (2007) identified that people with schizophrenia tended to develop an avoidant coping style to deal with anticipated stigma, and that this led to reduction in self-efficacy, eroded empowerment and reduced quality of life. Clearly, the quality of life of a person living with schizophrenia is multifactorial and challenges mental health services to consider beyond the biological illness model to consider how to provide services that increase quality of life and satisfaction with life.

RECOVERY

The traditional view of recovery from illness is concerned with the amelioration of symptoms and the use of medication and perhaps some psychosocial education to achieve this. This has been described as 'clinical recovery' (Cavelti et al., 2012, p. 19). However there has also been identified 'personal recovery' (Cavelti et al., 2012, p. 19) that relates to the development of ways to manage the threat to the person's sense of self and meaning of their place in the world. Thus recovery as a concept involves not only the provision of high-quality treatment that is evidence-based, but also the active involvement of clients and their families in a process that supports people to live satisfying lives with the chronic illness. To embrace the concept of recovery in relation to schizophrenia means to challenge services that provide messages of hopelessness and accuse clients of not being motivated, or being too 'chronic' to be able to have goals and aspirations. The mental health consumer movement has been active in the process of making the voices of people with mental illness heard and in raising awareness that an understanding of the subjective experience of mental illness is essential to recovery services (Australian Mental Health Consumer Network, 2007).

Patricia Deegan, who has undertaken her own recovery process from mental illness, describes recovery as '... a journey of the heart' (Deegan, 1996) and argues that recovery is based on the awareness that people who have been diagnosed with mental illness are firstly human beings who can act, change their situation, speak for themselves and become the experts in their own recovery process. Recovery is concerned with 'hope, social connection, personal responsibility, meaningful life activities, a positive identity, full life beyond illness and personal growth' (Mueser et al., 2006).

In stories of consumers' perspectives of recovery there is a strong emphasis on hope. The reflection to consumers with schizophrenia that it is an inevitably deteriorating illness, that they will need to take medication for the rest of their lives and that their dreams and aspirations are highly unlikely to be achieved causes consumers to believe that all their efforts will be futile (Deegan, 1996). Deegan suggests that the 'apathy, withdrawal, isolation and lack of motivation' are more than negative symptoms of schizophrenia, but represent a 'hardening of the heart' by the person as a way of surviving. To care about the loss of hopes and dreams is to lay oneself open to possibility, and the despair and hopelessness if the possibility did not eventuate. The greatest danger is if those people who are there to support and care reflect back that hopelessness and despair, and give up on hope of recovery because the person is seen as unmotivated to change (Deegan, 1996). Consumers describe the important aspects of recovery from mental illness as being hope, self-responsibility, education, self-advocacy and peer support (Mead & Copeland, 2000).

People with schizophrenia have also identified the incremental nature of the recovery process. In an ethnographic study (Jenkins & Carpenter-Song, 2005) participants saw improvements as gradual and marked by setbacks, but nevertheless identified optimism in improvement. The markers of improvement for these people were often not dramatic but related to being able to get out of bed, meet friends, take care of others and distract themselves from annoying voices. Participants in this study also emphasised the importance of a sense of self in relation to the illness that could stand outside the illness, and learn strategies to deal with symptoms.

Studies of the impact of hopelessness on outcomes for people with schizophrenia indicate that a sense of hopelessness predicts a poor rehabilitation outcome. Hopelessness was linked to self-concepts that were negative, low expectations of self and the future and a sense of being under control of external forces (Hoffmann et al., 2000). The acceptance of the messages of society, including healthcare professionals, clearly affects the rehabilitation possibilities for the individual. Conversely services that are recovery-oriented are marked by optimism, focus on choice, empowerment and interpersonal support and pay attention to vocational rehabilitation (Warner, 2009).

In order to develop therapeutic relationships, nurses and other clinicians need a clear understanding of those assumptions that underpin the way they view consumers. Confronting the assumptions of hopelessness, of the consumer as the passive recipient of treatment with which they must comply, of the consumer as motivated, apathetic and inevitably deteriorating into chronicity requires the clinician to examine the foundations of their practice. It requires a level of critical analysis of the services offered and the philosophy that underpins that service.

A recovery journey from schizophrenia needs the collaboration of the person, the family, health professionals and the support of other survivors from mental illness. Exacerbation of psychotic symptoms is not uncommon and can interrupt the recovery journey. Programs informed by recovery concepts have been developed and introduced in Australia, the United States and Britain and the concept of recovery has been adopted as the framework for mental health services (Rickwood, 2006). Most recovery-informed programs involve education of both clients and their families. The Illness Management and Recovery Program (Mueser et al., 2006) piloted in the US and Australia included psychosocial education about mental illness and treatments, cognitive-behaviour approaches to medication adherence, a relapse prevention plan, social skills training and coping skills training (p. S33). Importantly, the structured program commenced with an exploration of what recovery meant for the individual. Measures of recovery used five factors: personal confidence and hope, willingness to ask for help, goal and success orientation, positive reliance on others and not being dominated by symptoms. Importantly none of the factors used to measure recovery include the absence of symptoms or an emphasis on independence. Rather, measures reflected a belief that the important issues in recovery are learning to live with and manage the illness.

PRINCIPLES OF CARE

Models of care for people with schizophrenia usually include medication to treat psychotic symptoms and a range of psychosocial interventions depending on the needs of the person and their family. Comprehensive models of care that have been evaluated as effective include attention to medication needs, psychosocial education for the person and their family and a range of options in relation to social and vocational skills. The relationship between the key health professional and the person may be the most potent factor in success of treatment.

MEDICATION

Medication is often seen as the mainstay of treatment for schizophrenia, and for many people medication has proven to be valuable. The newer anti-psychotics have been shown to be effective and to have a lower side-effect profile than the older anti-psychotics (Keltner & Folks, 2005). However for many people weight gain is a problem (Vandyk & Baker, 2012). For some people medication may be life-saving and even the reduction of some psychotic symptoms may make a difference to their quality of life. Finding the right medication in the optimal dose is a collaborative effort between the treating team and the consumer (for comprehensive information on psychotropic drugs see Keltner & Folks, 2005).

There are two major groups of anti-psychotic drugs, both used in the treatment of schizophrenia: first generation antipsychotics (FGAs) and second generation antipsychotics (SGAs). Choice of medication is usually related to the likelihood of adverse side effects. Both FGAs and SGAs have demonstrated efficacy in reducing psychotic symptoms and are recommended treatment of both acute and longer term psychotic illnesses (Buchanan et al., 2010).

Examples of FGAs include chlorpromazine, thioridazine, fluphenazine, trifluoperazine and haloperidol. Examples of SGAs include amisulpride, aripiprazole, olanzapine, quetiapine and respiradol.

CASE STUDY 13.1 Part 1

Matthew is a 17-year-old who completed his final exams at high school 6 months ago. He had planned to study engineering at university but he had found it increasingly difficult to concentrate over the previous 6 months and he did not achieve the results he wanted. His family had expressed concern at changes in him but felt it may have been related to the stress of the exams, a break-up with his girl-friend and the death of his grandfather. His family had also noticed a gradual withdrawal from social occasions, and a tendency to spend much more time in his room. Six weeks ago he was admitted to the local mental health adolescent inpatient unit following a serious suicide attempt. He was found to have symptoms of a psychotic illness. He believed he was being followed, that thoughts were being removed from his brain and that his life and that of his family was in danger. He could not identify the source of the danger or the identity of his followers. His attempt on his own life was because he believed that his family would be spared if he was sacrificed. He has been discharged from hospital on medication and referred to the early psychosis mental health team.

Case study questions

1. Identify the vulnerability, stress and protective factors that Matthew might have.
2. As Matthew's community nurse, what do you think are the important principles of care at this time?
3. You attempt to educate Matthew about the illness but he is clearly distressed about the information and he does not keep his next appointment. What might be the reason for this and what might you do?

The major problem with the FGAs is adverse side effects such as movement disorders (muscle spasms, restless limbs and abnormal movements). Some of these can be managed with medication. The major problem with SGAs is their link with increased appetite, weight gain and the development of metabolic syndrome marked by diabetes and heart disease. Olanzapine has been particularly noted for its link with metabolic syndrome (Buchanan et al., 2010).

The evidence for medication treatment is strong. Early treatment with antipsychotic medication reduces psychotic symptoms. Identifying and titrating medication to achieve the least side effects with the greatest desired effect for the individual is a skilled process (Buchanan et al., 2010).

The argument has been made by some consumers of mental health services that while medications are a choice for reducing symptoms, they are not the only choice and medication compliance should not be seen as the only way that symptoms can be managed. Medication can go a considerable way to improving the recovery journey for some people. However, even with the advent of new antipsychotics, 25–50% of people with schizophrenia will continue to have ongoing psychotic symptoms at some level (Mueser et al., 2006). Jenkins and Carpenter-Song (2005) noted that while participants in their study all talked of medication as important to their recovery, many of their participants stressed that medication could not provide all the ingredients for recovery.

In a 15-year follow-up study of people with schizophrenia Harrow and Jobe (2007) found that there was a subgroup of people who did not immediately relapse when off medication and even showed signs of recovery. What characterised this group of people was good development prior to the illness, positive personality and attitude, lower level of vulnerability, greater resilience and other favourable prognostic factors. This study indicates that not all people who develop a schizophrenic illness need to use antipsychotic medication on an ongoing basis for the foreseeable future. However, many people with schizophrenia will be on medication and benefit from it and it is important that mental health services are developed in a way that ensures collaboration about medication.

PSYCHOSOCIAL EDUCATION

> ... It is a fundamental right of patients to receive a comprehensive explanation of their illness and to be given the chance of an informed involvement in the drafting of their treatment (Bauml et al., 2006).

Programs that emphasise psychosocial education have been shown to positively affect the course of the illness, and the life of the person with the illness. Consumers who participate in psycho-educational programs such as the Illness Management and Recovery Program (Mueser et al., 2006) report high satisfaction with the program, finding it helpful for managing symptoms and for progressing towards goals. They also indicated significant improvements in hope and goal orientation. This program involved a nine-week educational format with topics covering:

- recovery strategies
- practical facts about schizophrenia
- stress-vulnerability model and treatment strategies
- building social support
- using medications effectively
- drug and alcohol use
- reducing relapses
- coping with stress
- coping with problems and persistent symptoms
- getting your needs met in the mental health system (Mueser et al., 2006).

The topics of the Illness Management and Recovery Program are consistent with the essential elements of psychosocial education groups outlined by Bauml et al. (2006) as therapeutic interaction, clarification and enhancement of coping competence through 'briefing patients about their illness, problem-solving training, communication training and self-assertiveness training' (p. S3). Therapeutic interaction is the approach adopted by the clinician as a 'therapist orientation guide' (p. S6) who explains the process of the illness with empathic understanding of the impact it has on the individuals in the group. The group process encourages sharing of experiences, modelling problem-solving behaviours and conveying respect and esteem for the opinions and struggles of group members. The clarification process reflected in the psychosocial educational model encourages a process of mutual respect for knowledge: both knowledge of self-experience and professional knowledge about the illness. This process allows for mutual understanding to develop between and among therapists and group members. The element of enhancing coping competence recognises the importance of acknowledging loss and grief in the process of coming to terms with the illness and what it may mean. This process emphasises strengths and not limitations, explores how medication can best work for the group members and identifies crisis management plans. It also emphasises the members of the group as the experts in their own illness (Bauml et al., 2006).

FAMILY AND CARERS

The families of people with schizophrenia are clearly very important to the way the illness progresses. Many early studies of families explored the negative impact of families (Warner, 2004), seeking causal relationships between the family communication, particularly from mothers, and the generation or the course of the illness. Later studies identified high-expressed emotion (the number of negative, critical comments directed at the person with schizophrenia) as having a negative effect on the course of the illness. More recent studies have identified the positive effects of communication between family members, particularly mothers and their adult children with schizophrenia. Greenberg and colleagues (2006) found that people with schizophrenia reported higher quality of life when their mothers were demonstrably warm and made positive comments about them. The mothers who were warm and positive (described by the authors as pro-social) displayed three types of behaviour: they encouraged activities that emphasised the abilities of their adult child with schizophrenia, they made acknowledgement of small positive steps and they were less reactive to residual symptoms such as lack of energy and detachment (Greenberg et al., 2006 p. 1776). This study emphasised the importance of providing families with education and support when they have a family member with schizophrenia.

When the person with schizophrenia is also a parent, consideration needs to be given to the needs of all family members, including the children. When there are children in the household, mental health services need to make specific consideration for their need for age-appropriate education, support and care (Foster, O'Brien & Korhonen, 2012; O'Brien, Brady, & Gillies, 2011). The issue of stigmatisation of people with mental illness affects the children of parents with schizophrenia as well as their parents. People with schizophrenia who are also parents may need additional support to continue in their role (Fudge, Falkov, Kowalenko & Robinson, 2004).

Many people with schizophrenic illness live with their families and their families may be their major source of support and social communication. Family education about mental illness has been demonstrated to provide positive outcomes including the reduction of relapse rates, the improvement of recovery from symptoms and the enhancement of family and psychosocial outcomes (Murray-Swank & Dixon, 2004). A range of models of family psycho-education programs have been developed, such as one-day workshops (Pollio et al., 2006), programs running over six months (Magliano, Fiorillo, Malangone, De Rosa, & Maj, 2006) and 90-minute ongoing workshops provided on a monthly basis (Sherman, 2003). The aims of psycho-education programs are: to provide families with information about mental illness, including symptoms, treatments and services, early intervention and prevention of relapse; to give families the opportunity to ask questions; to encourage support from a group of peers; to reduce stigmatisation; and to increase communication between health services and families.

IMPLICATIONS FOR NURSING

Nursing plays an integral role in the healthcare of people recovering from schizophrenia. Nurses need to have a knowledge base that includes understanding about schizophrenia and its course and treatment, knowledge of human responses to psychotic experiences and knowledge of those interventions that will ameliorate distress in the person and their family. Nursing skills need to include the ability to form therapeutic relationships that are based on collaboration, and to maintain hope and engender hope in people with severe mental illness.

CASE STUDY 13.1 Part 2

Matthew had a second admission two years later. He was diagnosed with schizophrenia with paranoid features. He had become increasingly withdrawn, agitated and distressed. Police had found him in the middle of the night, in a local park, shouting and gesticulating wildly. He claimed that his room had been bugged, and that his computer was monitoring his movements. He claimed that there was a conspiracy to kill him because he had done something terrible. He could not elaborate on what he had done. The police recognised that he was either mentally ill or affected by drugs, and brought him to hospital. Since his first episode he had enrolled in computer courses at a local college, had joined a local church group and had started bush walking and cycling to get fit.

Matthew had continued to live with his parents who were supportive. However recent stressors included his siblings moving out of home, his parents going on holiday and he had contracted a flu-like virus that caused him to take time off from college. Unfortunately, during the time Matthew was relapsing into a psychotic illness, he had frightened his neighbours and fellow students by talking about the computers being bugged. He had been behaving strangely in church, looking agitated and frightened. Matthew was deeply embarrassed about having a mental illness and had not told his friends at college or his social or church group, as he feared the consequences.

Since his discharge, following his second admission, Matthew has been increasingly depressed and isolated. He has not returned to college, avoids contact with his neighbours and has not resumed social activity.

Case study questions

1. As Matthew's community nurse, what approach would you take?
2. Review the information on stigma, self-stigmatisation and stigma resistance and consider what support Matthew might need to approach the problem of what to tell people about his previous behaviour.
3. If you were one of Matthew's fellow students how would you respond to being told that he had a mental illness that sometimes caused him to distrust those around him? What information might be helpful?

CASE STUDY 13.2

Patricia is a 28-year-old woman who has had five admissions to an acute psychiatric unit in the last ten years. On her first admission she was diagnosed with depression following a suicide attempt. She has been subsequently diagnosed with a schizoaffective disorder and finally with schizophrenia. The exacerbations of her illnesses are usually acute and marked by hallucinations and delusions with strong religious content. These exacerbations usually follow an increase in stress. Despite her frequent admissions to hospital she has managed to complete a university degree in business management and to gain experience as an office manager in small business. She enjoys her work and her employer is aware of her mental illness.

CASE STUDY 13.2 — cont'd

Patricia has no family history of schizophrenia; however several family members have been treated for depression. She describes a fairly happy childhood until her adolescence when her father died suddenly and she, her two brothers and her mother had to move into her grandparents' home. She suffered disruption to her schooling and has recently disclosed that she was sexually assaulted by an uncle who visited the house. The assaults continued until she left home after her first admission to hospital. Patricia has had no counselling for childhood sexual assault. She complains of flashbacks to the assaults that intrude on her thinking and disrupt her sleep.

Patricia lives on her own in a small unit. She volunteers with a bush-care group who meet monthly, and she belongs to a book club. She has one friend whom she met in hospital, but has not kept contact with other friends as she does not want to tell them about her illness.

She takes medication to treat her depression and psychosis. She is currently on an atypical antipsychotic and an antidepressant although she admits she does not always take these medications as prescribed as she finds the side effects, of weight gain and tiredness, are limiting. She admits to adjusting her medication dosage at weekends as she feels she is brighter and more sociable when she does. She also admits that when she does this in a context of increased stress she is more likely to relapse.

Case study questions

1 As Patricia's community nurse how would you approach discussion about the management of her medication? What principles would you use to frame the discussion?
2 Patricia asks about what might have caused her illness. What issues are important to discuss?
3 What stressors may have contributed to her illness?

Nursing care needs to be informed by recovery principles of attention to the subjective experiences, and choice, optimism, empowerment and interpersonal support (Warner, 2009).The most important role that nurses can undertake is the establishment of a collaborative therapeutic alliance with both the person and their family. This relationship can underpin all subsequent treatments. The establishment of such a relationship may take time, but persistent, consistent interactions that seek to understand the person and their situation in a respectful way are powerful in reducing anxiety and instilling hope.

Assessment is an important part of the therapeutic process and is comprehensive and ongoing. In addition to assessment of mental state, including substance use assessment and risk assessment, nurses need to assess physical health, response to medication and psychosocial status.

People with schizophrenia have a higher rate of physical illness that is undetected (Leucht, Burkard, Henderson, Maj, & Sartorius, 2007). Nurses are in an ideal position to encourage regular health checks, to promote contact between a general practitioner and the person and to promote a healthy lifestyle.

Nurses need to advocate for services that are consumer-centred. There are many barriers within traditional mental health services to the development of consumer-centred services (Carroll, Manderscheid, Daniels, & Compagni, 2006). For mental health services to be

Reflective questions

1. Identify three messages you have picked up from media representations of people with schizophrenia and discuss these in light of studying the current chapter.
2. Consider how you would develop a recovery-focused plan with a person with schizophrenia.
3. Consider how you would develop an information package for a person with schizophrenia including websites, information sheets and other material.

focused on recovery, services also need to be strength-focused rather than deficit-focused (Watkins, 2007). Nurses are in a position to drive change in the way mental health services are delivered.

In both inpatient and community mental health settings nurses are in an ideal position to provide and advocate for a range of psycho-therapeutic interventions, including education about the illness, and the treatment, for the person and their family, either in formal groups or in informal discussions; problem-solving approaches to psychosocial problems; development of relapse recognition plans; encouragement to use medication constructively; provision of assertive community treatment; and identification of a range of resources that may be useful in maintaining and sustaining community tenure (Beebe, 2007).

Nurses are also in an ideal position to advocate for the provision of a range of vocational and living skills support services that are in turn appropriately supported by mental health services.

CONCLUSION

Schizophrenia is a serious mental illness; however, the stereotypes of deterioration, alienation from society and paternalistic care are not inevitable. Some people recover; some people have episodes with good functioning between episodes. Recovery-focused services are consumer-centred and strengths-based. Recovery-focused services do not give up hope that a person, even when they have symptoms that do not respond well to medication, can live a satisfying and productive life.

Recommended reading

Davidson, L. (2003). *Living outside mental illness: Qualitative studies of recovery in schizophrenia*. New York: New York University Press.

Kleim, B., & McLean, R. (2003). *Recovered, not cured: A journey through schizophrenia*. Sydney: Allen & Unwin.

Psychotropic Expert Group. (2008). *Therapeutic guidelines: Psychotropic (Version 6)*. Melbourne: Therapeutic Guidelines Limited.

Slade, M. (2009). *Personal recovery and mental illness: A guide for mental health professionals*. Cambridge: Cambridge University Press.

Warner, R. (2009). Recovery from schizophrenia and the recovery model. *Current Opinion in Psychiatry*, *22*, 374–380.

Additional resources

SANE Australia http://www.sane.org/information/factsheets-podcasts

Schizophrenia Fellowship http://www.sfnsw.org.au/

Resources for parents with schizophrenia and their families http://www.copmi.net.au

References

American Psychiatric Association. (2000). *Diagnostic and statistical manual of mental disorders: DSM-IV-TR*. Washington DC: American Psychiatric Association.

Australian Mental Health Consumer Network. (2007). Network News 3 November 2007. Retrieved November 22, 2012, from www.amhcn.org.au

Bauml, J., Frobose, T., Kraemer, S., et al. (2006). Psychoeducation: A basic psychotherapeutic intervention for patients with schizophrenia and their families. *Schizophrenia Bulletin, 32*, 1–9.

Beebe, L. H. (2007). Beyond the prescription pad. Psychosocial treatments for individuals with schizophrenia. *Journal of Psychosocial Nursing, 45*(3), 35–43.

Bennett, C., Sundram, S., Farhall, J., et al. (2012). Schizophrenia and related disorders. In G. Meadows, J. Farhall, E. Fossey, et al. (Eds.), *Mental health in Australia: Collaborative community practice* (3rd ed., Ch 28, pp. 741–788). Melbourne: OUP.

Buchanan, R. W., Kreyenbuhl, J., Kelly, D. L., et al. (2010). The 2009 Schizophrenia PORT Psychopharmaceutical treatment recommendations and summary statements. *Schizophrenia Bulletin, 36*(1), 71–93.

Carroll, C. D., Manderscheid, R. W., Daniels, A. S., et al. (2006). Convergence of service, policy, and science toward consumer-driven mental health care. *Journal of Mental Health Policy and Economics, 9*(4), 185–192.

Cavelti, M., Kvrgic, E. M., Kossowsky, J., et al. (2012). Assessing recovery from schizophrenia as an individual process: A review of self-report instruments. *European Psychiatry, 27*, 19–32.

Corin, E. (1990). Facts and meaning in psychiatry: An anthropological approach to the lifeworld of schizophrenics. *Culture, Medicine and Psychiatry, 14*, 153–158.

Corrigan, P. W. (2012). Research and the elimination of the stigma of mental illness. *British Journal of Psychiatry, 201*(1), 7–8.

Corrigan, P. W., Larson, J., Sells, M., et al. (2007). Will filmed presentation of education and contact diminish mental illness stigma? *Community Mental Health Journal, 43*(2), 171–181.

Davidson, L. (2003). *Living outside mental illness: Qualitative studies of recovery in schizophrenia*. New York: New York University Press.

Deegan, P. E. (1996). Recovery as a journey of the heart. *Psychiatric Rehabilitation Journal, 19*(3), 91–97.

Eklund, M., & Backstrom, M. (2005). A model of subjective quality of life for outpatients with schizophrenia and other psychoses. *Quality of Life Research, 14*, 1157–1168.

Foster, K., O'Brien, L., & Korhonen, T. (2012). Developing resilient children and families when parents have mental illness: A family focussed approach. *International Journal of Mental Health Nursing, 21*(1), 3–11.

Fudge, E., Falkov, A., Kowalenko, N., et al. (2004). Parenting is a mental health issue. *Australasian Psychiatry, 12*(2), 166–171.

Greenberg, J. S., Knudsen, K. J., & Aschbrenner, K. A. (2006). Prosocial family processes and the quality of life of persons with schizophrenia. *Psychiatric Services, 57*(12), 1771–1777.

Hanzawa, S., Nosaki, A., Yatabe, K., et al. (2012). Study of understanding the internalised stigma of schizophrenia in psychiatric nurses in Japan. *Psychiatry & Clinical Neurosciences, 66*(2), 113–120.

Harding, C. M., Zubin, J., & Strauss, J. S. (1987). Chronicity in schizophrenia: Fact, partial fact, or artifact? *Hospital and Community Psychiatry, 38*(5), 477–485.

Harrow, M., & Jobe, T. H. (2007). Factors involved in outcome and recovery in schizophrenia patients not on antipsychotic medications: a 15-year multifollow-up study. *Journal of Nervous and Mental Disease, 195*(5), 406–414.

Hewitt, J. (2007). Critical evaluation of the use of research tools in evaluating quality of life for people with schizophrenia. *International Journal of Mental Health Nursing, 16*, 2–14.

Hoffmann, H., Kupper, Z., & Kunz, B. (2000). Hopelessness and its impact on rehabilitation outcome in schizophrenia — an exploratory study. *Schizophrenia Research, 43*, 147–158.

Jenkins, J. H., & Carpenter-Song, E. (2005). The new paradigm of recovery from schizophrenia: cultural conundrums of improvement without cure. *Culture, Medicine and Psychiatry, 29*, 379–413.

Keltner, N. L., & Folks, D. G. (2005). *Psychotropic Drugs* (4th ed.). Missouri: Elsevier.

Leucht, S., Burkard, T., Henderson, J., et al. (2007). Physical illness and schizophrenia: A review of the literature. *Acta Psychiatrica Scandinavica, 116*, 317–333.

Magliano, L., Fiorillo, A., Malangone, C., et al. (2006). Patient functioning and family burden in a controlled, real-world trial of family psychoeducation for schizophrenia. *Psychiatric Services, 57*(12), 1784–1791.

McCann, T., & Clark, E. (2004). Embodiment of severe and enduring mental illness: finding a meaning in schizophrenia. *Issues in Mental Health Nursing, 25*, 783–798.

McGorry, P. D. (1992). The concept of recovery and secondary prevention in psychotic disorders. *Australian and New Zealand Journal of Psychiatry, 26*, 3–17.

McGrath, J., Saha, S., Chant, D., et al. (2008). Schizophrenia: A concise overview of incidence, prevalence, and mortality. *Epidemiologic Reviews, 30*, 67–76.

Mead, S., & Copeland, M. E. (2000). What recovery means to us: Consumers' Perspectives. *Community Mental Health Journal, 36*(3), 315–328.

Mueser, K. T., Piper, S., Penn, D. L., et al. (2006). The illness management and recovery program: rationale, development and preliminary findings. *Schizophrenia Bulletin, 32*, 32–43.

Murray-Swank, A. B., & Dixon, L. (2004). Family Psychoeducation as an evidence-based practice. *CNS Spectrums, 9*(12), 905–912.

O'Brien, L., Anand, M., Brady, P., et al. (2011). Children visiting parents in inpatient psychiatric facilities: Perspectives of parents, carers and children. *International Journal of Mental Health Nursing, 20*(2), 137–143.

Owen, P. R. (2012). Portrayals of schizophrenia by entertainment media: A content analysis of contemporary movies. *Psychiatric Services, 63*(7), 655–659.

Pollio, D. E., North, C. S., Reid, D. L., et al. (2006). Living with severe mental illness — what families and friends must know: evaluation of a one day psychoeducation workshop. *Social Work, 51*(1), 31–38.

Rickwood, D. (2006). *Pathways of recovery: 4As framework for preventing further episodes of mental illness.* Canberra: Commonwealth of Australia.

Sherman, M. D. (2003). The Support and Family Education (SAFE) program: Mental health facts for families. *Psychiatric Services, 54*(1), 35–37.

Sibitz, I., Unger, A., Woppman, A., et al. (2011). Stigma resistance in patients with schizophrenia. *Schizophrenia Bulletin, 37*(2), 316–323.

Thompson, K. N., McGorry, P. D., & Harrigan, S. M. (2003). Recovery style and outcome in first episode psychosis. *Schizophrenia Research, 62*, 31–36.

Treatment Protocol Project. (1997). *Management of mental disorders* (2nd ed.). Sydney: World Health Organization Collaborating Centre for Mental Health and Substance Abuse.

Vandyk, A. D., & Baker, C. (2012). Qualitative descriptive study exploring schizophrenia and the everyday effect of medication-induced weight gain. *International Journal of Mental Health Nursing, 21*(4), 349–357.

Vauth, R., Kleim, B., Wirtz, M., et al. (2007). Self-efficacy and empowerment as outcomes of self-stigmatizing and coping in schizophrenia. *Psychiatric Research, 150*(1), 71–80.

Warner, R. (2004). *Recovery from schizophrenia* (3rd ed.). New York: Brunner Routledge.

Warner, R. (2009). Recovery from schizophrenia and the recovery model. *Current Opinion in Psychiatry, 22*, 374–380.

Watkins, P. (2007). *Recovery: a guide for mental health practitioners*. Edinburgh: Elsevier.

CHAPTER

14

Scott Fanker
Louise O'Brien

Depression

Learning objectives

When you have completed this chapter you will be able to:

- identify the epidemiology, clinical features and assessment of depression
- understand potential pharmacological and psychotherapeutic treatment approaches
- identify nursing assessment and management implications of depression
- understand the potential disability impacts of depression
- apply knowledge to a clinical case study.

Key words

antidepressant, depression, dysthymic disorder, epidemiology of depression, major depression

INTRODUCTION

> In the course of life, there is sadness and pain and sorrow, all of which, in their right time and season are normal — unpleasant, but normal. Depression is an altogether different zone because it involves a complete absence: absence of affect, absence of feeling, absence of interest. The pain you feel in the course of major clinical depression is an attempt on nature's part (nature after all abhors a vacuum) to fill up an empty space. But for all intents and purposes, the deeply depressed are just the walking, waking dead (Wurtzel, 1994, p. 19).

Depression is a public health issue of global proportions. It is anticipated that some 300 million people worldwide suffer from depression (Commonwealth Department of

Health and Aged Care, 2001). Depression is associated with significant distress for individual sufferers and their families, and can lead to impairment in educational, social, family and employment functioning and outcomes. As would be expected for a common and serious illness, a significant proportion of health expenditure in Australia is devoted to the treatment of depression. Approximately 24% of service contacts with public-sector community mental health services relate to mood disorders, and there are approximately 22 170 admissions to public hospitals and 11 870 admissions to private hospitals for mood disorders each year (Australian Institute of Health and Wellbeing, 2006). The direct cost of treating depression each year is estimated to be in excess of $600 million. The true cost of depression for the community, which includes the indirect costs associated with the reduced productivity that accrues from a disabling condition, defies quantification. In Australia depression has been identified as a National Health Priority Area in an attempt to elevate depression to the same level of community consciousness and coordinated health policy response — in the form of prevention, assessment and treatment — as heart disease, diabetes and cancer (Commonwealth Department of Health and Aged Care, 2001).

Nurses working in a variety of settings are well placed to be able to play a role in the identification, assessment and management of depression. The fact that depression is disconcertingly prevalent means that nurses working in acute hospital, community, primary and aged care contexts will encounter individuals with clinically significant depression, and may be the first clinician to directly explore the likelihood of depression. Early identification and mobilisation of effective treatment responses is the single most likely means by which the disability of burden of depression for individuals, their families and carers and the community can be reduced. Treatment for depression can be highly effective, potentially reducing the distress of depression and its disabling impact on occupational, social, family and relationship functioning. While there is some evidence of a decrease in suicide-related deaths in the Australian context, it remains a grim reality that each year over 2300 Australians choose to end their lives by suicide, many or most of whom have been depressed or suffering from another mental disorder at the time of their death, with over three-quarters of suicide deaths occurring among men (Australian Bureau of Statistics [ABS], 2010). This is a statistic that underscores the importance and potential of nurses and clinicians from varying disciplines to have an understanding of the epidemiology, clinical features, assessment, treatment and management of the depressive disorders.

THE SCOPE OF THE PROBLEM: THE EPIDEMIOLOGY OF DEPRESSION

Over the past two to three decades there has been significant research interest in identifying and understanding the epidemiology of depression (and mood disorders). This activity has, in large part, been driven by improved methodological approaches (e.g. the use of standardised diagnostic interviews) for undertaking large-scale community surveys to assess incidence and prevalence at a population level. Population-based surveys of the prevalence of depression — undertaken as part of larger studies of the epidemiology of mental disorders — have been conducted and reported in the United States (Regier & Robins, 1991; Weissman et al., 1988; Kessler et al., 1994), New Zealand (Wells et al., 1989), Britain (Jenkins et al., 1997) and Australia (ABS, 1998; Andrews, Henderson, & Hall, 2001).

Early findings of the community prevalence of depression arose from the Epidemiological Catchment Area Study, in which a standardised diagnostic interview was undertaken with some 20,000 participants in the United States. Approximately one-third of participants reported periods of dysphoria of at least 2 weeks' duration at some point in their lifetime. The study estimated that 6.3% of the US population aged 18 years or over had experienced at least one clinically significant episode of depression (major depressive episode) during their lifetime (Regier & Robins, 1991). A second large-scale study, the National Co-morbidity Study, used a different survey instrument and identified the lifetime rate of major depressive episode to be 17.1% among the adult population (12.7% for adult males and 21.3% for adult females) (Kessler et al., 1994).

Depression is a global concern. Bromet et al. (2011) have recently reported cross-national data for the prevalence of major depressive episode (MDE) in 18 countries. The lifetime and 12-month prevalence rates for MDE in 10 high socioeconomic status countries were 14.6% and 5.5%, and 11.1% and 5.9% in 8 medium- to low-income countries.

In the Australian National Survey of Mental Health and Wellbeing a sample of approximately 778,000 adults were interviewed with a standardised diagnostic instrument (the Composite International Diagnostic Interview), which identified that in the 12-month period prior to interview 5.8% of the adult population had experienced an identifiable and clinically significant depressive disorder (major depressive episode) (ABS, 1998). In the Second National Survey of Mental Health and Wellbeing conducted in 2007, the 12-month prevalence of depressive episodes was 4.1% (ABS, 2008). A separate child and adolescent component of the study identified that 3% of children and young people (6–17 years) experienced a depressive disorder in the 12-month period preceding the survey (Sawyer et al., 2001).

The differences in reported lifetime rates of major depression between studies are likely to be attributable to two factors: methodological variance and/or recall bias. Some variance may be accounted for by the different methodological approaches between studies, for example the diagnostic interview instrument employed. Also, there is the possibility that participants' ability to accurately recall having experienced episodes of depression across their lifetime may play a role in explaining the reported difference in prevalence rates (Andrews et al., 1999). Considering data from multiple studies, Wilhelm et al. (2003) have identified in a survey which asked participants to rate depressive symptoms in the previous 1-month period that the current prevalence of major depression among adults aged 18 years or over is between 3% and 5%.

A consistent finding across studies of the epidemiology of depression is a strong female preponderance, with most studies identifying up to a twofold increase in prevalence among women (Kuehner, 2003). The causes of this apparent gender difference have been the focus of significant research interest. It has been proposed that the gender 'difference' may be an artefactual finding, possibly reflecting that women are more likely to recall episodes of depression over their lifetime than men, or that women might be more likely to reflect on or amplify their mood states than men, who employ distraction or denial as means of coping with dysphoria (Parker & Brotchie, 2004). Differential exposure and vulnerability to social or environmental stressors, for example sexual violence, has also been suggested, although not consistently demonstrated in research. Kessler and McLeod (1984) proposed a 'cost of caring hypothesis', suggesting that female gender roles around caring could increase women's exposure and sensitivity to life events in their social networks. Biological difference has also been considered, with pubescent changes in hormones being a focus of interest, given that the female preponderance for depression commences between the ages of 15 and 18 (Arnold, Costello, & Worthman, 1998). Parker and Brotchie (2004) have hypothesised that, since the female preponderance for depression also extends to anxiety, there may be a post-pubertal effect of sex hormones on limbic system hyperactivity that increases risk of both depressive and anxiety disorders.

IDENTIFYING THE DISABILITY IMPACTS OF DEPRESSION

In 1996, the World Health Organization (WHO) and the World Bank commissioned the Global Burden of Disease study (Murray & Lopez, 1996). The study represented the most comprehensive attempt to quantify and explicate the mortality and disability impacts (burden of disease) of all diseases, injuries and risk factors using robust methodological approaches. Disability was estimated by using the Disability Adjusted Life Year (DALY) measure, which expresses the years of life lost due to premature death and years lived with a disabling illness of specified duration and severity (Joyce & Mitchell, 2004). Mental illness contributed a significant proportion of DALY-measured disability, with 'uni-polar major depression' estimated by 2020 to contribute the second largest share of disability worldwide (Murray & Lopez, 1997a, 1997b). These burden of disease projections have recently been revised; depressive disorders are expected to continue to be the second largest contributor to disability worldwide after HIV/AIDS (Mathers & Loncar, 2011).

In the Australian context, mental disorders are estimated to account for 13% of the total burden of disease, measured using DALYs. In females, anxiety and depression are the leading cause of disease burden (10% of total burden), while in males anxiety and depression are the third leading cause of disease burden after ischaemic heart disease and type 2 diabetes (4.8% of total burden) (Begg et al., 2007).

There is some evidence that men may experience more disability impacts associated with depressive and anxiety disorders. It is possible that this difference may be attributable to men being less likely to disclose and/or seek help in respect of mental health disorders, limiting their access to effective treatments and supports (Scott, 2011).

DEPRESSION, THE WORKPLACE AND DISABILITY

In recent years there has been recognition that depression in the workplace is a significant issue. Work forms an important part of the life of most people. There is good evidence that work can be inherently health-promoting. Paid work obviously provides an income that allows at least the potential for individuals to live as healthy a life as possible; work, whether paid or otherwise, also provides meaning and purpose in the lives of many people.

A stable and rewarding workplace can impact in a positive way on a person's mental health. The opposite of this also holds true; a workplace that is unrewarding or involves stress associated with, for example, the nature of the work undertaken and/or the relationships with colleagues or superiors can be detrimental to an individual's mental health.

A recent Victorian study estimated that depression affects 1.54 million Australians who are participating in the workplace, and that the costs associated with this are approximately $8000 per person per year, or $12.6 billion in total. These costs comprise lost workplace productivity, absenteeism, employee turnover and replacement and mental health related treatment costs (LaMontagne, Sanderson, & Cocker, 2010; Veronese et al., 2012).

Employers increasingly understand that workplace depression is a major issue. There are examples of workplace programs designed to identify and refer employees who are depressed and/or strategies aimed at making workplaces mental health promoting by changing aspects of job demands or employee dynamics.

DEPRESSION AND MEDICAL ILLNESS

There are complex inter-relationships between depression and physical illnesses. Having a serious or chronic physical health condition is, in and of itself, a risk factor for developing a depressive disorder. There is also evidence that depression is a risk factor for the development of a physical illness and early mortality. Epidemiological studies have identified a higher prevalence of depression in people with a number of physical illnesses, including coronary heart disease, cerebrovascular accident, diabetes, cancer, Parkinson's disease, HIV/AIDS, hepatitis C, epilepsy, arthritis and osteoporosis compared with the general population (Clarke & Currie, 2009: American Psychiatric Association, 2010).

The relationship between heart disease and depression is complex; there is evidence that depression is an independent risk factor for the development of heart disease. Van de Kooy and colleagues undertook a meta-analysis of 28 published studies of the relationship between depression and cardiovascular disease, concluding that 'clinically diagnosed major depressive disorder was identified as the most important risk factor for developing cardiovascular disease' (Van de Kooy, van Hout, Marwijk, Marten, Stewhouwer, & Beekman, 2007). A number of potential psychosocial (increased prevalence of lifestyle and traditional cardiac risk factors; medication adherence) and biological (effects of stress on autonomic nervous system, endocrine, platelet and inflammatory systems) explanations for the association between depression and the onset of heart disease have been identified (Lichtman, Bigger, & Blumenthal, 2008). The risk of mortality increased among those who experience depression following a myocardial infarction (de Jonge et al., 2007). There is evidence that treatment outcome is poorer for those who experience co-morbid depression and physical illness (Iosifescu et al., 2003; Evans, & Charney, 2003).

It is hardly surprising that medical illnesses that are chronic, debilitating or painful can cause stress and predispose an individual to depression. While depression in the course of medical illness may be understandable, depression is never 'normal' and requires assessment and definitive treatment (American Psychiatric Association, 2010).

CLINICAL FEATURES OF DEPRESSION AND ASSESSMENT APPROACHES

Depressed, sad or dysphoric mood is a common and normal response to life's challenges and vicissitudes. There would be few people who could not relate to the experience of having felt sad in response to a loss of some kind; this level of normal range of emotion and emotional reactivity does not in and of itself constitute 'clinical' depression. Distinguishing circumstances where depressed mood is indicative of a depressive disorder requiring definitive treatment, as against an understandable and transient feeling state, is a key challenge for clinicians working in a variety of clinical settings.

Major (clinical) depression is distinguished from what might be understood to be 'normal' depression on the basis of the presence of certain symptoms and the severity, duration and persistence of these symptoms. There is no single or pathognomonic symptom that is necessary or sufficient for the diagnosis of major depression. Although pervasive feelings of lowered mood or sadness are frequent features of major depression, it is not clear that depressed mood per se is the core pathological change. It has been suggested that mood disturbance may be an epiphenomenon of a syndrome of core deficits in relation to energy, motivation and activation. This possibility is suggested by the fact that some individuals who report depressive symptoms of reduced energy and motivation, poor concentration, inability to feel pleasure, reduced appetite and sleep problems do not report feeling sad or depressed in their mood (Joyce, 2004).

There are two widely used international diagnostic classification systems for mental disorders: the *Diagnostic and statistical manual of mental disorders* (4th edn, text revision) (DSM-IV-TR) published by the American Psychiatric Association (American Psychiatric Association, 2000), and the *Classification of mental and behavioural disorders* (10th edn,

ICD 10), published by the WHO (1992). Both systems identify operationalised diagnostic criteria for each of the mental disorders, including depression and other disorders of mood.

For a diagnosis of major depressive episode to be made, DSM-IV-TR requires the presence of at least a 2-week period of depressed mood or loss of interest or pleasure in most activities. The depressed mood or loss of interest and pleasure must be present for much of nearly every day, on the basis of an individual's self-report or the observation of others. In children the predominant mood state can be one of irritability. In addition, at least four of the following behavioural, biological, psychomotor or psychological symptoms must be present:

- significant weight loss when not dieting (e.g. a change of more than 5% of body weight in a 1-month period), or decrease in appetite nearly every day. In children failure to reach expected weight gains is also relevant
- insomnia or hypersomnia nearly every day
- psychomotor agitation or retardation nearly every day
- fatigue or loss of energy nearly every day
- feelings of worthlessness or excessive or inappropriate feelings of guilt (which may reach delusional intensity) nearly every day (not merely self-reproach or guilt about being ill)
- diminished ability to concentrate, or indecisiveness, nearly every day (based on subjective account or the report of others)
- recurrent thoughts of death (not just fear of dying), recurrent suicidal ideation without a specific plan, or a suicide attempt, or a specific plan for committing suicide (adapted from American Psychiatric Association, 2000).

The average age of onset of a first episode of depression is in the late 20s. Depression can, however, occur at any age. Both childhood and late-life depression are relatively common, and are sometimes under-recognised by health professionals (Bostic, Rubin, Prince, & Schlozman, 2005).

In children depression can sometimes present quite differently from adults. Depressed preschool children may display behavioural problems, apathy, withdrawal, irritability, regression or complain of somatic concerns such as headache or stomach aches. School-aged children may display crying spells, sadness or irritability and complain of somatic problems (Martin, 2004; Bostic et al., 2005).

Depression in older people has been estimated to occur at a rate of approximately 2–5%, while in residential aged care settings such as hostels or nursing homes the rate is estimated to be much higher, at 6–18%. In older people one of the key challenges from an assessment point of view is disentangling and distinguishing symptoms of depression from symptoms related to grief and loss, dementia, Parkinson's or other medical disease or the effects of prescribed medication (ABS, 1998; Byrne, 2004).

Depression: chronicity and recurrence

The duration of an episode of major depression is variable, lasting from weeks to years in some cases. Left untreated, and assuming that a person has been kept safe, major depression can remit of its own accord in 6 to 9 months (American Psychiatric Association, 2010). The likelihood of recurrence after an episode of treated depression is approximately 40% within 1 year. Studies that have assessed long-term outcome at 25 years following an index episode have found high rates of persisting symptoms or recurrence (Brodaty et al., 2001;

Royal Australian and New Zealand College of Psychiatrists Clinical Practice Guidelines Team for Depression, 2004).

Taken together these findings underscore the potential level of disability that can accrue from recurrent episodes of major depression (major depressive disorder). Depression can contribute chronicity and disability in other circumstances: where a dysthymic disorder (a low-grade and chronic form of depression) is present; where full remission of symptoms in response to adequate treatment is elusive (treatment resistance); or where symptoms are persistent in nature (chronic depression).

Dysthymic disorder (or dysthymia)

Dysthymic disorder is a diagnostic category within the DSM-IV-TR that refers to a chronic low-grade depression of at least 2 years duration (American Psychiatric Association, 2000). It is possible for individuals with dysthymic disorder to have periods of acute exacerbation (where diagnostic criteria for a major depressive episode is met); this is often known as 'double depression', due to the combination of an acute severe depression being overlaid on a background of chronic depression of mild to moderate severity (Klein, Shankman, & Rose, 2006).

Treatment resistance

Approximately 30% of people with major depression will not respond to adequate antidepressant therapy within an expected time period, for example show signs of improvement within the first 4 weeks of treatment. Switching antidepressant agents and/or the addition of an augmentation agent are common means by which treatment resistance is managed. Augmentation agents are those where their addition to the antidepressant is thought to have a potentiating effect. Various augmentation strategies have been applied in practice, including lithium, triiodothyronine (T3), buspirone, pindolol, antipsychotic agents (first generation, and atypical agents), anticonvulsants, folates, oestrogens and psychostimulants. To date, methodologically rigorous trials of psychological treatment strategies for treatment-resistant depression have not been reported (Stimpson, Agrawal, & Lewis, 2002; Ros et al., 2005).

Chronic depression

Approximately 10% of individuals who are treated for a major depressive episode will remain depressed in 12 months, despite appropriate treatment, and another 10–20% will experience only a partial remission in their symptoms. Clinical approaches to the treatment of chronic depression include making changes in antidepressant regimens (dose adjustment or switching agents), considering the use of ECT or adding a psychotherapeutic approach to the package of treatment (Joyce & Mitchell, 2004; American Psychiatric Association, 2010).

RECURRENCE AND INTER-EPISODE FUNCTIONING

About half of those who experience a first episode of major depression will go on to experience at least one other episode. The course of recurrent major depressive disorder is highly variable in terms of both episode duration and the interval of time between episodes. Some people have recurrent episodes separated by periods of years, while others experience clusters of episodes. There is evidence that some people have increased frequency of episodes as they age.

CASE STUDY 14.1 Part 1

John Smith is a 44-year-old married man who works as a solicitor in one of the larger inner city law firms. He specialises in commercial litigation. John lives with his wife, Megan, and their two daughters, Aisling who is 7 years old and Amelia who has just turned 4.

For some months Megan has been concerned about John. She is concerned that John has been behaving out of character at home. Megan has discussed her concerns with her general practitioner, Dr Morris, who agreed that John's behaviour (as described) was cause for concern. Dr Morris offered to see John, even if only for the purpose of referring him to another clinician. John has never had a regular general practitioner himself, tending to go to medical centres only when absolutely necessary.

Over approximately a 6-month period John has become increasingly withdrawn and irritable at home, spending his evenings and weekends working in his study. John has always taken his work very seriously and worked long hours. Two years ago John was made a partner in the law firm, a promotion that was expected to allow him to spend less time working on weekends. While John has always worked long hours, he has always previously prioritised spending time with Megan and the children, especially on weekends. Of late John has shown less interest in the children, often appearing visibly irritated when one or both of the girls had asked him to spend time with them or help them with their homework. When Megan most recently raised John's withdrawn behaviour with him, reminding him that the promotion was expected to mean that he would be able to spend more time with his family, John snapped at her stating, 'You knew what you were signing on for when you married me.' When Megan raised the possibility that John see Dr Morris, John replied, 'I don't need to see a doctor. I'm busy, that's all; there is nothing wrong with me.'

John himself has noticed that he hasn't been himself, although his coping style has always been one of 'soldiering on' and he hasn't felt comfortable discussing his own concerns with Megan. John has been experiencing trouble concentrating and completing tasks at work, requiring him to work longer hours to get through his work. His work performance was recently raised with him at a recent performance review, where a senior partner (someone John has never got along with) told him that his performance wasn't at the level of a new partner. John felt embarrassed and humiliated by the performance review. Even a month down the track John finds himself thinking about the review for some part of each day, and how he has failed the firm, and failed himself for failing to meet his own expectations.

For the past 5 months, John has trouble sleeping. He falls to sleep easily enough, but wakes at approximately 2 a.m. each morning and is then unable to return to sleep.

John has lost weight (approximately 9 kgs) in the 6 months. He has had to buy new clothes for work. John can't explain his weight loss. He has stopped participating in the between-firm sporting activities and had expected to gain weight.

John has noticed that he now takes the lift at work because he becomes breathless if he takes the stairs. He also has regular headaches that are not always relieved by simple analgesia.

John feels that his relationship with Megan is under strain because of his workload. He's always aware of tension associated with him having lost interest in sex in recent months. John blames his loss of libido, headaches and work performance on the

CASE STUDY 14.1 Part 1 — cont'd

unrealistic expectations of the firm and the senior partner. Privately he wonders how much longer he can continue to work under these conditions.

One morning on his way to work John notices a beyondblue advertisement on the side of a government bus. John recalls that beyondblue, Australia's national depression initiative, was mentioned at a continuing professional development seminar on lawyers and workplace stress that he attended some months ago. When John arrives at his office he uses the internet to search the beyondblue website; he reads that some of the things that he has been experiencing in recent months could be symptoms of depression.

Case study questions

1. What are some of the symptoms that John has been experiencing that suggest that he may have a depressive disorder?
2. What other aspects of John's presentation and recent history should a nurse be concerned about?

While most people who have recurrent depression experience a return to their normal level of functioning between episodes, approximately 25–35% of people have persistent residual symptoms, or social and occupational impairment. Persisting inter-episode symptoms and impairment increases the risk of a subsequent episode of major depression. For this reason biopsychosocial treatments aimed at promoting a full return to baseline levels of function are an important aspect of the treatment of depression (American Psychiatric Association, 2010; Guico-Pabia, Fayyad, & Soares, 2012).

MAPPING THE TERRAIN: SOME ISSUES IN SUBTYPING AND CLASSIFYING DEPRESSIVE DISORDERS

Depression is a term used to describe states of mood that are part and parcel of human experience, being felt by nearly everyone at times of, say, grief, loss or life stress. Depression is also understood to refer to a serious and, in some cases, life-threatening illness that requires clinical assessment and treatment. At face value it is tempting to assume a link between feeling states that are commonplace but generally transient and what is understood to be 'clinical' depression — an essentially single phenomenon that is distinguished by severity and persistence.

The extent to which depression represents a single dimensional phenomenon, as against a range of discrete disorders with differing symptoms and, by extension, treatment characteristics, has been the focus of close to a century of debate. The identification of meaningful subtypes of depression — either clinically or in research — is a profitable exercise if subtypes are associated with differential response to treatment. In a clinical setting, for example, being able to identify the circumstances under which a psychological versus a biological treatment approach would be most appropriate, or being able to decide with some confidence which of a range of treatments would be most suitable, would have significant utility. Table 14.1 identifies the subtypes of depression that are detailed in the DSM-IV-TR (American Psychiatric Association, 2000).

TABLE 14.1

Severity and subtypes of depression. *Note*: Adapted from Royal Australian and New Zealand College of Psychiatrists Clinical Practice Guidelines Team for Depression (2004).

SEVERITY OF MAJOR DEPRESSION (MD)	
Episodes can be classified as mild, moderate or severe	
Mild	• Just meets or slightly exceeds minimum required diagnostic criteria in DSM-IV-TR. • Level of disability and impairment in functional capacity is mild, or able to be maintained with effort.
Moderate	• More than the minimum required DSM-IV-TR diagnostic criteria present. • Increased level of impairment of social and occupational functioning.
Severe	• Most DSM-IV-TR diagnostic criteria present. • Severe impairment in social and occupational functioning.
DSM-IV-TR subtypes of major depression	
Subtypes are distinguished on the basis of symptoms present or nature of onset (e.g. post-partum onset or seasonal pattern of onset).	
Melancholia	• Characterised by significant psychomotor abnormality (retardation or agitation); loss of pleasure in almost all activities; severe mood state. • Considered to be particularly responsive to biological treatments (e.g. antidepressants, ECT).
MD with psychotic features	• Characterised by the presence of delusion and/or hallucinations. • Content of psychotic symptoms usually mood-congruent. • Considered to be particularly responsive to biological treatments. • Treatment with antipsychotic agents often required in addition to antidepressant agents.
Atypical depression	• Characterised by reactivity of mood and two or more of the following: weight gain, increased appetite, hypersomnia, leaden paralysis i.e. heavy leaden feelings in arms or legs, longstanding pattern of sensitivity to interpersonal rejection that results in social or occupation impairment. • The essential features and clinical significance of atypical depression is subject to debate.
MD with post-partum onset	• Onset of depression occurs within 4 weeks of birth of infant.
MD with seasonal pattern	• Onset and remission of major depressive episodes coincides with particular times of the year (e.g. autumn or winter onset and spring remission).

Of the subtypes described in DSM-IV-TR, two (major depression with melancholic subtype/'melancholia', and major depression with psychotic features/'psychotic depression') are noteworthy. 'Melancholic' depression is characterised by the presence of significant mood disturbance, psychomotor retardation or agitation and profound inability to experience pleasure. Identifying melancholia is clinically relevant as there is evidence that melancholia is specifically responsive to biological treatments (antidepressant therapy or ECT). 'Psychotic' depression is characterised by the presence of delusions and/or hallucinations. Profound feelings of guilt and/or severe psychomotor disturbance are also frequently present. In terms of treatment, combined therapy with an antidepressant and antipsychotic agents and/or ECT, is often required. The severity of symptoms and risks associated with suicide or nutritional or hydration compromise in melancholic and psychotic depression can often be such that hospitalisation is necessary.

THE COMPLEX AND MULTI-STRANDED CAUSES OF DEPRESSION

Depression is a complex disorder, or set of disorders, for which the underlying causes are not fully understood. Current thinking in relation to the pathophysiology of many mental disorders, including depression, involves the likely interaction of biological, psychological and psychosocial factors (O'Brien & Fanker, 2006).

Biological factors

The possibility of biological factors playing a role in the aetiology of depression has been proposed since antiquity. Hippocrates postulated that 'melancholy' was caused by an excess of 'black bile' (Radden, 2000). Interest in attempting to identify biological foundations of depression gained momentum from the 1950s, when it was observed that iproniazid (an anti-tuberculin) led to a noticeable improvement in the mood of those undergoing treatment for tuberculosis. More or less contemporaneous observations were also made that reserpine (initially used as an anti-hypertensive agent) and chlorpromazine (initially developed as an anti-histamine) reduced symptoms of psychosis. Taken together these findings encouraged research into identifying biological aspects of mood and psychotic disorders, and drove what has become the modern era of psychopharmacology. From the 1960s onwards research directed at identifying biological substrates of and treatments for mental disorders has continued apace (O'Brien & Fanker, 2006).

Genetics: the role of heredity in depression

Depression tends to run in families, raising the possibility of there being a genetic contribution to the aetiology of depressive disorders. This tendency has been demonstrated in a number of well-designed family studies. The odds ratio of an immediate relative of a person with a history of major depression also being affected has been calculated to be 2.84 (95% CI; 2.31–3.49); in other words an almost threefold increase in risk (Sullivan, Neale, & Kendler, 2000). Two of the three adoption studies published to date provide support for a genetic role, where there is increased risk of being affected by depression even when offspring of those with major depression have been raised in adoptive families. Twin studies have shown that the rate at which monozygotic twins are concordant (both affected) for depression is approximately 50%, whereas for dizygotic twins concordance is between 10% and 25% (Sullivan, 2004).

Neurotransmission

Serotonin — a neurotransmitter that plays a role in the regulation of a number of biological functions, including sleep, appetite and libido — has been the focus of significant research interest in relation to its potential role in the pathophysiology of depressive disorders. Data from a number of studies have found an association between low serotonin levels and depression, and artificial drug-induced depletion of serotonin (e.g. by reserpine) has been observed to precipitate depression. A number of antidepressant agents (e.g. the selective serotonin reuptake inhibitors) increase levels of serotonin in the central nervous system (CNS), implying that reduced levels of CNS serotonin play a role in the pathogenesis of depression.

There are interrelationships between the serotonergic and noradrenergic neurotransmitter systems, and noradrenaline has also been a focus of interest for its potential role in depression. Noradrenaline has roles in regulating autonomic nervous system responses and in the regulation of arousal, and a number of processes involved in depression including mood and sleep. Studies investigating noradrenergic function have yielded equivocal findings, but remain a focus of interest due to some antidepressant agents having up-regulation effects on noradrenaline (Schweitzer & Tuckwell, 2004; O'Brien & Fanker, 2006).

Psychological and psychosocial factors

Psychosocial stress and life events

Three psychosocial threads have been examined in relation to their potential role in precipitating depression: persistent stress (e.g. enduring environmental and life stressors), life events (dramatic and sudden stressors such as grief and loss) and the availability of social support (the protective nature of having supportive social networks). There appears to be a relationship between life events and the development (or relapse) of depression (Paykel, 2004).

Personality factors

Personality style has also been considered as a factor that may increase an individual's vulnerability for the development of depression. It is possible that people with certain personality types may use internalising defence mechanisms (e.g. self-blame), and that these patterns of coping may increase vulnerability to psychological disturbances such as depression (O'Brien & Fanker, 2006).

APPROACHES TO THE TREATMENT AND MANAGEMENT OF DEPRESSION

Joyce (2004) identified the overall approach to the assessment and management of depression as involving the following principles:

1. ensuring comprehensive (diagnostic) assessment
2. assessing and ensuring safety
3. providing education to the person who is affected, and their family and carers
4. establishing a therapeutic relationship
5. providing support and care
6. providing advice and recommendations for treatment (e.g. evidence-based biological or psychotherapeutic interventions)
7. ongoing assessment of treatment response
8. promoting treatment adherence (e.g. through active assessment and management of treatment-emergent adverse effects)
9. evaluating and responding to associated impairments
10. preventing relapse.

Choice of treatment is usually driven by factors such as severity, depressive subtype, previous history of successful treatment and patient preference.

'Biological' approaches

Medication

The pharmacological treatment of depression has been a fertile area of research and practice since the late 1950s with the introduction of imipramine (a tri-cyclic antidepressant). Its clinical usage is now widespread. The efficacy of imipramine impelled what David Healy

CASE STUDY 14.1 Part 2

John doesn't want to consult Dr Morris. John doesn't feel comfortable discussing his situation with Dr Morris, who has treated Megan and the children for many years. John approaches Ben, the in-house nurse employed by the law firm. John has always had a friendly relationship with Ben because Ben plays in the between-firm soccer tournament.

John meets with Ben and describes his concerns and the contents of material from the beyondblue website that he had printed out. John has highlighted some of the contents of this material, made handwritten notes on the paperwork and made a list of questions for Ben.

Ben asks John if he has ever experienced an episode with similar experiences in the past. John tells Ben that he took a semester off law school due to 'not coping' with the demands of the course. Ben learns that this episode was associated with weight loss, poor concentration, loss of energy, ruminations of guilt and failure and insomnia. John tells Ben that he went backpacking through Thailand and Cambodia, but didn't seek any formal treatment at the time. John did not discuss his symptoms with anyone at the time, not even his best friend from childhood. John tells Ben that his view at the time was that he 'just had to pull myself together'.

John states that his mother, Lucy, has had treatment for 'bad nerves' on and off throughout her adulthood. John is unsure of the exact nature of Lucy's diagnosis, but he believes that she has 'seen counsellors' and 'taken pills'. He tells Ben that he believes that his mother's problems had impacted on her ability to be as good a mother as she could have.

Ben asks John if this episode feels the same or different to that he experienced while at university. John states that he believes that his current symptoms are 'ten times worse' than the previous episode. John states that 'nothing or no one' gives him any pleasure anymore. He describes his mood as 'dead' and he states that his mood is 'stuck' at this point for all of the past 7 months. John describes feeling that his whole body is slowed down. He tells Ben that he knows it might sound silly, but his limbs feel heavier than they once did making everything he did an effort.

Case study questions

1. What factors may have contributed to John's development of a depressive disorder?
2. Is John experiencing any symptoms suggestive of a depressive subtype? If so, which subtype?
3. What other questions should Ben ask John in relation to his recent experiences and symptoms as part of his initial assessment?

has termed the 'anti-depressant era', a period of significant activity in relation to identifying, trialling and introducing into clinical practice an array of antidepressant agents (Healy, 1997).

An antidepressant agent is usually indicated in circumstances where a major depressive episode has been established. Antidepressants would almost always be indicated in circumstances where melancholic or psychotic subtypes of depression are present (Bauer et al.,

2002). Selection of an antidepressant agent would usually be determined on the basis of the following factors:

- the likelihood that the agent will work (efficacy)
- the likelihood that a person will be able to tolerate any adverse effects
- aspects of the person's symptoms (e.g. choosing a sedating antidepressant if insomnia is an issue)
- avoiding certain agents if they are likely to affect medical issues (agents that may affect blood pressure).

Mann (2005) has provided a useful summary of the clinical use of antidepressant agents in the treatment of depressive disorders. Table 14.2 provides a summary of commonly used antidepressants, therapeutic dose ranges, relative safety in overdose and adverse effect profile.

Electroconvulsive therapy

First used clinically in 1938, electroconvulsive therapy (ECT) retains a role as an effective and relatively safe treatment for depression (Greenberg & Kellner, 2005). The availability of a range of effective antidepressant agents has tended to relegate the use of ECT to situations where rapid resolution of symptoms is required (e.g. the presence of a very severe mood state, high suicide risk, dehydration and/or nutritional compromise). ECT is also used in circumstances where treatment resistance, failure to respond to adequate trials of antidepressant agents or an inability to tolerate pharmacological approaches is an issue. ECT involves the induction of a generalised tonic-clonic seizure in an anaesthetised patient via electrical stimulation. The basis for the therapeutic efficacy of ECT is poorly understood, but is believed to relate to the action of the seizure rather than the electrical stimulus (UK ECT Review Group, 2003; American Psychiatric Association, 2010).

St John's Wort

The herb St John's Wort (*Hypericum perforatum*) has been the focus of interest in the past decade in both the popular media and the scientific literature on the basis of its purported antidepressant properties. There is some evidence that St John's Wort is superior to placebo in trials of its efficacy in the treatment of depression, although its comparative efficacy against conventional antidepressants has not been fully established. Until data emerges from well-designed randomised controlled studies of the efficacy of St John's Wort, its use as a stand-alone treatment for depression cannot be recommended. Having said this, there is evidence from community-based studies that St John's Wort is commonly used as a means of gaining relief from depression, and patients should be asked if they are taking any herbal or non-prescribed preparations in the assessment process (Jorm et al., 2004; Kessler et al., 2001). There is evidence that St John's Wort possesses enzyme-inducing properties, which means that it can interfere with the metabolism of a number of prescribed drugs and cause significant drug interactions (American Psychiatric Association, 2010).

Omega-3 fatty acids

The brain is a lipid-rich organ, and lipids are involved in the structure and function of all cell membranes in the brain, raising the possibility that omega-3 fatty acid supplementation could have a therapeutic effect and role. There is significant current interest in the potential role of omega-3 fatty acids in the treatment of a range of disorders, including cardiovascular and mental disorders. To date studies of the use of omega-3 fatty acids in the treatment of depression have involved omega-3 fatty acids being given as an adjunctive

TABLE 14.2

Commonly used antidepressants: doses, safety and adverse effect profile. Adapted from Mann J. (2005) The medical management of depression. *New England Journal of Medicine* 353:1819–1834 and Castle D & Bassett D (2010). *A primer of clinical psychiatry*. Sydney: Churchill Livingstone.

AGENT AND CLASS/ MECHANISM OF ACTION	STARTING DOSE	STANDARD DOSE (A)	LETHALITY IN OVERDOSE	ADVERSE EFFECTS						
	MG/DAY			INSOMNIA OR AGITATION	SEDATION	HYPO-TENSION	ANTI-CHOLINERGIC EFFECTS (B)	NAUSEA OR GI EFFECTS	SEXUAL DYSFUNCTION	WEIGHT GAIN
Selective serotonin reuptake inhibitors (SSRIs)										
Fluoxetine	20	20–40	Low	Moderate	None or mild	None or mild	None or mild	Moderate	Moderate	Mild or infrequent
Paroxetine	20	20–40	Low	Moderate	None or mild	None or mild	Mild	Moderate	Moderate	Mild or infrequent
Sertraline	50	50–150	Low	Moderate	None or mild	None or mild	None or mild	Moderate	Moderate	Mild or infrequent
Fluvoxamine	50	100–250	Low	Moderate	Mild	None or mild	None or mild	Moderate	Moderate	Mild or infrequent
Citalopram	20	20–40	Low	Moderate	None or mild	None or mild	None or mild	Moderate	Moderate	Mild or infrequent
Escitalopram	20	20–40	Low	Variable	Moderate	None or mild	None or mild	Moderate	Moderate	Mild or infrequent
Tricyclic agents										
Amitriptyline	25–50	100–300	High	None or mild	Moderate	Moderate	Severe	None or mild	Mild	Moderate
Dothiepin	25–50	100–300	High	None of mild	Moderate	Moderate	Moderate	None or mild	Mild	Moderate
Imipramine	25–50	100–300	High	Moderate	Mild	Moderate	Moderate	None or mild	Mild	Moderate

(continued next page...)

TABLE 14.2

Commonly used antidepressants: doses, safety and adverse effect profile — cont'd

AGENT AND CLASS/ MECHANISM OF ACTION	STARTING DOSE	STANDARD DOSE (A)	LETHALITY IN OVERDOSE	ADVERSE EFFECTS						
	MG/DAY			INSOMNIA OR AGITATION	SEDATION	HYPO-TENSION	ANTI-CHOLINERGIC EFFECTS (B)	NAUSEA OR GI EFFECTS	SEXUAL DYSFUNCTION	WEIGHT GAIN
Nortriptyline	25–50	75–200	High	Mild	Mild	Mild	Mild	None or mild	Mild	Mild
Clomipramine	25–50	100–250	High	Mild	Moderate	Moderate	Moderate	Mild	Mild	Moderate
Desipramine	25–50	100–300	High	Mild	None or mild	Moderate	Mild	None or mild	Mild	Mild
Mono-amine oxidase inhibitors										
Phenelzine (non-reversible)	15	30–90	High	Moderate	Mild	Moderate	Mild	Mild	Moderate	Mild
Moclobemide (reversible)	150	150–300	Low	Mild	None or mild	None or mild	Mild	Mild	None or mild	None or mild
Other agents										
Mianserin	30	60–120	Low	None or mild	Moderate	Mild	Mild	Never or mild	Never or mild	Mild
Mirtazapine	30	30–60	Low	None or mild	Severe	Mild	None or mild	Mild	Mild	Severe
Ventafaxine	37–75	75–225	Moderate	Moderate	None or mild	None or mild	None or mild	Moderate	Moderate	None or mild
Duloxetine	30	30–60	Low	Variable	Moderate	Low	None or mild	Frequent	None or mild	Low
Reboxetine	8	8–12	Low	Frequent	Low	Low	None or mild	Mild	None or mild	Low
Desvenlafaxine	50	50–200	Low	Low	Low	Low	Low	Low	Low	None or mild

[a]These doses reflect usual practice, and may vary depending on clinical circumstances.

[b]Anti-cholinergic side-effects include dry mouth, constipation, sweating, blurred vision and urinary retention.

therapy; for instance, combined with a conventional anti-depressant. The evidence of efficacy is currently difficult to interpret due to the small nature of the studies and methodological difference between studies, but the potential role of omega-3 fatty acids in the treatment of depression is interesting and warrants further consideration (American Psychiatric Association, 2010).

Psychotherapeutic approaches

A variety of psychotherapeutic (talking therapy) approaches to the treatment and management of depression have been proposed and used. Psychotherapy was the dominant approach until the 1950s, when effective antidepressant drugs first came into widespread use. Two approaches, cognitive behaviour therapy and interpersonal therapy, have been widely used and have empirical support for their effectiveness in depression (McKenzie, Carter, & Luty, 2004; American Psychiatric Association, 2010).

Cognitive behaviour therapy

Cognitive behaviour therapy (CBT) is a robust psychotherapeutic technique that is based around a model of depression causation that postulates that certain people are predisposed to depression due to them having certain patterns of thinking. These patterns of thinking, or 'cognitive schemata', are thought to involve negative or distorted ways of thinking about the self, present and future. Treatment is geared towards challenging and reversing these patterns of thinking. There is some evidence that CBT may be more efficacious for depression of mild to moderate severity and/or where the melancholic subtype is not present (Parker & Fletcher, 2007; American Psychiatric Association, 2010).

Interpersonal therapy

Interpersonal therapy (IPT) is a psychotherapy technique that focuses on losses, life transitions, social and other interpersonal skill-related aspects of the person. Therapy is directed towards addressing these issues through promoting mourning, understanding the link between experience and feeling states and the development of skills that promote supportive and functional interpersonal relationships. While there is some evidence from controlled studies supporting the superiority of IPT over placebo for the treatment of depression, further studies are required to fully establish efficacy (McKenzie et al., 2004). Again, IPT may not be effective in melancholic or psychotic depression or severe depression (Parker & Fletcher, 2007).

PRINCIPLES OF NURSING CARE

Rapport and meaning

Elizabeth Wurtzel's description of depression being akin to a state of 'walking, waking dead' gives a sense of how distressing and unpleasant the experience of being depressed can be. The establishment of a therapeutic relationship in which rapport and trust are established is a cornerstone of being able to provide helpful responses and interventions. Crowe and O'Malley (2004) have identified that assisting a person to understand and find meaning in their experience of depression is an important nursing role.

Providing education

One of the key roles that nurses can play in the treatment and management of depression is the provision of education to the person who is depressed and their family and carers. Education can explore issues around the nature of depression (e.g. that it is a common and treatable disorder), strategies for coping with the experience of depression and treatment.

Ongoing assessment

Nurses play an important role in the ongoing assessment of depression, because they are often well positioned to provide assessment on a 24-hour basis in the case of hospital settings, or over a significant ongoing time period in the case of community-based settings. Assessment should include consideration of changes (increases or decreases) in domains such as nutrition and hydration, interactiveness, mood, energy, motivation, concentration, ability to experience pleasure, suicide risk and patterns of depressive thinking.

Depressed thinking

Strategies for dealing with the negative thinking patterns that some depressed people have can involve helping the person to identify and evaluate alternative viewpoints about particular thoughts, feelings or actions. For example, it can be helpful to challenge a statement such as 'I am not getting any better; I will never be rid of this depression' with responses such as 'You have been able to sit with me today and talk about how you are feeling for longer than previous days; this is a sign of improvement'. It is helpful to respond in ways that acknowledge an individual's experience, while at the same time encouraging a more positive outlook; for example: 'I understand that you are still feeling depressed and that it is taking some time for you to feel improvement, but you have been able to spend more time out of your room today, you have eaten and have interacted with me. These are signs of improvement' (O'Brien & Fanker 2006).

Promoting sleep

Sleep disturbance is a frequent feature of mood disorder, including depression, and includes problems getting to sleep at night (initial insomnia), overnight wakefulness and inability to resume sleep (middle insomnia), or early morning wakening. Disrupted sleep can make navigating the daily tasks of living significantly more difficult and compound feelings of tiredness and fatigue, both of which can then have the effect of making the subjective experience of being depressed more unendurable. Some of the newer-generation antidepressant agents, especially the selective serotonin reuptake inhibitors (e.g. fluoxetine, paroxetine, sertraline, fluvoxamine and citalopram) and the selective serotonin noradrenaline reuptake inhibitor venlafaxine can also either induce or increase insomnia, especially during the first few weeks of treatment (Lam, 2006).

Strategies to promote adequate sleep are important foci of nursing care of the depressed person. Nursing advice and intervention can assist with promoting adequate sleep (O'Brien & Fanker, 2006; Crowe & O'Malley, 2004). For example, the nurse can:

- assist the person to establish a regular sleep routine, such as listening to relaxing music or having a warm bath prior to going to bed, and going to bed at the same time every night
- provide advice about the potential value of avoiding alcohol, caffeine and nicotine, especially in the late afternoon or evening, due to their stimulant effects
- encourage the introduction of regular exercise in the late afternoon
- assist the person to establish a comfortable environment that is conducive to sleeping, for example controlling the intrusion of noise and light
- provide advice about avoiding daytime napping, wherever possible, to increase the likelihood of feeling sleepy at night

- assist with teaching relaxation techniques such as progressive muscle relaxation
- suggest that the person get up at night and undertake an activity in another room (e.g. reading) rather than lying in bed tossing, turning and ruminating about their inability to sleep
- encourage the avoidance of stimulating activities while in bed, such as reading or watching television
- suggest the potential value of using soothing and relaxing stimuli, such as burning essential oils, massage or listening to meditative music.

Promoting activity and exercise

There has been significant research interest in recent years in relation to the potential antidepressant effect of exercise. A number of studies have demonstrated that exercise has been associated with decreased severity of depressive symptoms among people 'prescribed' exercise versus no-exercise control groups. It is possible that there are biological and psychosocial factors at play, as exercise can promote the release of neurotransmitters such as serotonin; there are also potentially positive psychosocial reinforcers that can be derived from exercise (e.g. social interaction, sense of achievement and mastery, promotion of sleep). Exercise can potentially distract people from negative thinking and reduce the feelings of tiredness and fatigue that can accompany depression. The effect sizes, or the size of the relationship between the variables of exercise and reduced depression scores in reported studies, to date have been relatively modest, with exercise perhaps best regarded as an adjunctive component of treatment as against a treatment in and of itself (Callaghan, 2004). The introduction of any exercise program needs to consider issues around a person's baseline level of fitness and exercise tolerance, and any concurrent medical problems that might have an influence on the appropriateness of introducing exercise.

Withdrawn behaviour

Withdrawn behaviour is common among people who are experiencing depression. Retreating into a withdrawn state is to some extent understandable given that depression often causes reduced energy, reduced motivation and fatigue. Depression also affects a person's willingness (or capacity) to interact with others, and the subjectively distressing and alienating experience of being depressed can promote a desire for aloneness. Crowe and O'Malley have described withdrawn behaviour as potentially reflecting a depressed person's '… desire for refuge, confinement, protection and escape' (2004, p. 272).

Nurses can use a range of strategies to assist patients who experience withdrawn behaviour during the course of an episode of depression. Identifying and understanding a person's subjective experience of the need to withdraw is an important starting point in determining helpful interventions, including the following.

- Acknowledge the person's need for aloneness, but reformulate activity and social interaction as important antidepressant strategies in and of themselves.
- Identify time to interact with a person on a one-to-one basis to encourage communication.
- Encourage the person to feel comfortable to be around other people, even if they feel initially unable to interact for any length of time.
- Use positive reinforcement or encouragement in response to a person's efforts to interact.

- Encourage a graded approach to activity and interaction with others; for example, starting with as little as 15 minutes of social contact and building up gradually as mood improves.

Encourage the use of passive stimulants (e.g. a radio), especially while a person might be experiencing the nadir of their depressed mood (Crowe & O'Malley, 2004; Shultz & Videbeck, 2009).

Suicidality

Assessing and responding to potential risk of suicide is a key component of the management of depression. Nurses who work with people who are suspected or known to be depressed should canvass the issues of suicide candidly during initial and ongoing assessments. Received notions that asking directly about suicide risk can 'put the idea in people's minds' and/or increase the likelihood of suicidal behaviour are myths; many people who are suicidal are relieved to be able to divulge their thoughts or plans in a supportive environment. Nursing strategies for managing suicidal risk and behaviour include:

- assess risk openly and on an ongoing basis, by asking questions related to thoughts, intentions or plans directed towards self-harm or suicide
- consider information from families, carers or friends who might have knowledge about risk not divulged by the person who is depressed or at risk
- give consideration to whether assessment by a specialist mental health clinician is warranted, in order to assess whether definitive treatment or a change in care environment (one-on-one nursing, admission to a mental health unit, detention under mental health legislation) is necessary
- frame suicidal behaviour as a symptom of overwhelming stress and/or an illness, and encourage the view that suicidal thinking can pass with support, safe care and the initiation of treatment
- employ strategies such as encouraging the person to focus on 'reasons for living', and encourage use of self-soothing and distracting techniques.

CASE STUDY 14.1 Part 3

Ben asks John a direct question in relation to whether he has had any thoughts of suicide. John avoids eye contact with Ben and appears to become visibly anxious and agitated. After a significant pause John states that he sometimes thinks that Megan and his daughters would be 'better off without him'. He goes on to state that he has investigated if his life insurance policy would pay a benefit to Megan in the event that he 'took the coward's way out'. When Ben explores this further with John, John admits to having had thoughts of suicide involving jumping from a height or driving his vehicle into a stationary object at speed.

Case study questions

1. What immediate steps should Ben take in relation to the disclosures that John has made to him?
2. What types of treatments, interventions or supports are likely to be appropriate for John given the symptoms that he has reported?

Reflective questions

1 In what settings should nurses consider asking their patients about depression and suicidality?
2 Depression is a significant public health issue. What are some of the potential public health responses that could be used to increase the recognition and treatment of depression?
3 What are some of the ways that workplaces can respond to the issue of workplace depression?

Self-soothing and pleasant events

Nurses can assist people to adopt self-soothing strategies that are designed to bring comfort or respite from depression, including relaxation, distracting strategies, identifying and facilitating pleasant events and use of aromatherapy or other complementary interventions.

CONCLUSION

Depression is a common, disabling and potentially life-threatening illness. Over the past three decades there have been steady improvements in the body of knowledge in relation to the effective treatment of depressive disorders. Nurses working in a variety of clinical settings have potential roles in the assessment, identification and management of depression. Early identification and management is the single best means by which the disabling effects of depression can be prevented, at both the individual and the community levels.

Recommended reading

American Psychiatric Association. (2000). *Diagnostic and statistical manual of mental disorders* (4th ed., text revision). Washington, DC: American Psychiatric Association.

Castle, D., & Bassett, D. (2010). *A primer of clinical psychiatry*. Sydney: Churchill Livingstone.

Crowe, M., & O'Malley, J. (2004). Mental health nursing care for individuals experiencing mood disorders. In P. Joyce & P. Mitchell (Eds.), *Mood disorders: Recognition and treatment* (Chapter 22, pp. 270–282). Sydney: University of NSW Press.

Parker, G. (2003). *Dealing with depression. A commonsense guide to mood disorders*. Sydney: Allen & Unwin.

Stahl, S. (2008). *Stahl's essential psychopharmacology. Neuroscientific basis and practical applications*. Cambridge: Cambridge University Press.

References

American Psychiatric Association. (2000). *Diagnostic and statistical manual of mental disorders* (4th ed., text revision). Washington: American Psychiatric Association.

American Psychiatric Association. (2010). *Practice guideline for the treatment of patients with major depressive disorder* (3rd ed.). Published October 2010. Retrieved October 29, 2010, from www.psychiatryonline.com/pracguide/pracguidetopic_7.aspx.

Andrews, G., Anstey, K., Brodaty, H., et al. (1999). Recall of depressive episode 25 years previously. *Psychological Medicine, 29*, 787–791.

Andrews, G., Henderson, S., & Hall, W. (2001). Prevalence, co-morbidity, disability and service utilisation: overview of the Australian National Mental Health Survey. *British Journal of Psychiatry, 178*, 145–153.

Arnold, A., Costello, E., & Worthman, C. (1998). Puberty and depression: the roles of age, pubertal status and pubertal timing. *Psychological Medicine, 29*, 1043–1053.

Australian Bureau of Statistics. (1998). *Mental health and wellbeing: Profile of adults.* ABS Catalogue No 4326.0. Author.

Australian Bureau of Statistics. (2008). *National survey of mental health and wellbeing.* ABS Catalogue No 4326.0. Canberra: Author.

Australian Bureau of Statistics. (2010). *Suicides, Australia, 2010.* ABS Catalogue No 3309.0. Canberra: Author.

Australian Institute of Health and Wellbeing. (2006). *Australia's health.* AIHW Catalogue No Aus 73. Canberra: Author.

Bauer, M., Whybrow, P., Angst, J., et al. (2002). WFSBP Taskforce on Treatment Guidelines for Unipolar Depressive Disorders, World Federation of Societies of Biological Psychiatry. Guidelines for biological treatment of unipolar depressive disorders, Part 1: Acute and continuation treatment of major depressive disorder. *World Journal of Biological Psychiatry, 3*(1), 5–43.

Begg, S., Vos, T., Barker, B., et al. (2007). *The burden of disease and injury in Australia.* PHE 82. Canberra: Australian Institute of Health and Wellbeing.

Bostic, J., Rubin, D., Prince, J., et al. (2005). Treatment of depression in children and adolescents. *Journal of Psychiatric Practice, 11*(3), 141–154.

Brodaty, H., Lupscombe, G., Peisah, C., et al. (2001). A 25-year longitudinal, comparison study of the outcome of depression. *Psychological Medicine, 31*, 1347–1359.

Bromet, E., Andrade, L., Hwang, I., et al. (2011). Cross-national epidemiology of DSM-IV major depressive disorder. *BMC Medicine, 9*, 90–96.

Byrne, G. (2004). Depression in older people. In P. Joyce & P. Mitchell (Eds.), *Mood disorders: Recognition and treatment* (Chapter 33, pp. 410–420). Sydney: University of NSW Press.

Callaghan, P. (2004). Exercise: A neglected intervention in mental health care. *Journal of Psychiatric and Mental Health Nursing, 11*, 476–483.

Castle, D., & Bassett, D. (2010). *A primer of clinical psychiatry*. Sydney: Churchill Livingstone.

Clarke, D., & Currie, K. (2009). Depression, anxiety and their relationship with chronic diseases: A review of the epidemiology, risk and treatment evidence. *Medical Journal of Australia, 190*(6), s54–s60.

Commonwealth Department of Health and Aged Care. (2001). *National action plan for depression. Mental Health and Special Projects Branch*. Canberra: Author.

Crowe, M., & O'Malley, J. (2004). Mental health nursing care for individuals experiencing mood disorders. In P. Joyce & P. Mitchell (Eds.), *Mood disorders: Recognition and treatment* (Chapter 22, pp. 270–282). Sydney: University of NSW Press.

de Jonge, P., Honig, A., & van Melle, J. (2007). Non-response to treatment for depression following myocardial infarction: Association with subsequent cardiac events. *American Journal of Psychiatry, 164*, 1371–1378.

Evans, D., & Charney, D. (2003). Mood disorders and medical illness: A major public health problem. *Biological Psychiatry, 54*, 177–180.

Greenberg, R., & Kellner, C. (2005). Electroconvulsive therapy. A selected review. *American Journal of Geriatric Psychiatry, 13*(4), 268–281.

Guico-Pabia, C., Fayyad, R., & Soares, C. (2012). Assessing the relationship between functional impairment/recovery and depression: A pooled analysis. *International Clinical Psychopharmacology, 27*, 1–7.

Healy, D. (1997). *The antidepressant era*. Cambridge, MA: Harvard University Press.

Iosifescu, D., Nierenberg, A., & Alpert, J., et al. (2003). The impact of medical comorbidity on acute treatment in major depressive disorder. *American Journal of Psychiatry, 160*, 2122–2127.

Jenkins, R., Bebbington, P., & Brugha, O., et al. (1997). The national psychiatric morbidity surveys of Great Britain — Strategy and methods. *Psychological Medicine, 27*, 765–774.

Jorm, A., Griffiths, K., & Christensen, H., et al. (2004). Actions taken to cope with depression at different levels of severity: A community survey. *Psychological Medicine, 34*, 293–299.

Joyce, P. (2004). The assessment and classification of depression. In P. Joyce & P. Mitchell (Eds.), *Mood disorders: Recognition and treatment* (Chapter 3, pp. 25–36). Sydney: University of NSW Press.

Joyce, P., & Mitchell, P. (Eds.), (2004). *Mood disorders: Recognition and treatment*. Sydney: University of NSW Press.

Joyce, P., & Mitchell, P. (2004). Mood disorders and the global burden of disease. In P. Joyce & P. Mitchell (Eds.), *Mood disorders: Recognition and treatment* (Chapter 40, pp. 496–500). Sydney: University of NSW Press.

Kessler, R., McConagle, K., Zhao, S., et al. (1994). Lifetime and 12-month prevalence of DSM-III-R psychiatric disorders in the United States. *Archives of General Psychiatry, 51*, 911–918.

Kessler, R., & McLeod, J. (1984). Sex differences in vulnerability to undesirable life events. *American Sociology Review, 49*, 620–631.

Kessler, R., Soukup, J., Davis, R., et al. (2001). The use of complementary and alternative therapies to treat anxiety and depression in the United States. *American Journal of Psychiatry, 158*, 289–294.

Klein, D., Shankman, S., & Rose, S. (2006). Ten-year prospective follow-up study of the naturalistic course of dysthymic disorder and double depression. *American Journal of Psychiatry, 163*(5), 872–880.

Kuehner, C. (2003). Gender difference in unipolar depression: An update of epidemiological findings and possible explanations. *Acta Psychiatrica Scandinavica, 108*, 163–174.

Lam, R. (2006). Sleep disturbances and depression: A challenge for antidepressants. *International Clinical Psychopharmacology, 21*(Suppl 1), 25–29.

LaMontagne, A., Sanderson, K., & Cocker, F. (2010). *Estimating the economic benefits of eliminating job strain as a risk factor for depression*. Carlton, Australia: VicHealth. Retrieved October 10, 2012, from www.vichealth.vic.gov.au/jobstrain

Lichtman, J., Bigger, T., & Blumenthal, J. (2008). Depression and coronary heart disease: Recommendations for screening, referral, and treatment. A science advisory from the American Heart Association Prevention Committee of the Council on Cardiovascular Nursing, Council on Clinical Cardiology, Council on Epidemiology and Prevention, and Interdisciplinary Council on Quality of Care and Outcomes Research. *Circulation, 118*, 1768–1775.

Mann, J. (2005). The medical management of depression. *New England Journal of Medicine, 353*, 1819–1834.

Martin, G. (2004). Childhood depression. In P. Joyce & P. Mitchell (Eds.), *Mood disorders: Recognition and treatment* (Chapter 28, pp. 349–357). Sydney: University of NSW Press.

Mathers, C., & Loncar, D. (2011). Projections of global mortality and burden of disease from 2002 to 2030. *PLOS Medicine, 3*(11), 2011–2030.

McKenzie, J., Carter, J., & Luty, S. (2004). Psychological therapies for depression. In P. Joyce & P. Mitchell (Eds.), *Mood disorders: Recognition and treatment* (Chapter 20, pp. 250–261). Sydney: University of NSW Press.

Murray, C., & Lopez, A. (Eds.), (1996). *The global burden of disease: A comprehensive assessment of mortality and disability from diseases, injuries and risk factors in 1990 and 2020*. Cambridge, MA: Harvard University Press on Behalf of the World Health Organization and the World Bank.

Murray, C., & Lopez, A. (1997a). Global mortality, disability, and the contribution of risk factors: Global burden of disease study. *Lancet, 349*, 1436–1442.

Murray, C., & Lopez, A. (1997b). Alternative projections of mortality and disability by cause 1990–2020: Global burden of disease study. *Lancet, 349*, 1498–1504.

O'Brien, L., & Fanker, S. (2006). Mental health breakdown. In E. Chang, J. Daly & D. Elliott (Eds.), *Pathophysiology applied to nursing* (Chapter 16, pp. 425–447). Sydney: Elsevier.

Parker, G., & Brotchie, H. (2004). From diathesis to diamorphism. The biology of gender differences in depression. *Journal of Nervous and Mental Disease, 192*(3), 210–216.

Parker, G., & Fletcher, K. (2007). Treating depression with the evidence-based psychotherapies: a critique of the evidence. *Acta Psychiatrica Scandinavica, 115*(5), 352–359.

Paykel, E. (2004). Psychosocial stress and depression. In P. Joyce & P. Mitchell (Eds.), *Mood disorders: Recognition and treatment* (Chapter 9, pp. 98–109). Sydney: University of NSW Press.

Radden, J. (Ed.), (2000). *The nature of melancholy. From Aristotle to Kristeva*. Oxford: Oxford University Press.

Regier, D., & Robins, L. (1991). Introduction. In L. Robins & E. Regier (Eds.), *Psychiatric disorders in America* (pp. 1–10). New York: Free Press.

Ros, S., Aguera L., de la Gandara, J., et al. (2005). Potentiation strategies for treatment-resistant depression. *Acta Psychiatrica Scandinavica, 112*(Suppl 428), 14–24.

Royal Australian and New Zealand College of Psychiatrists Clinical Practice Guidelines Team for Depression. (2004). Australian and New Zealand clinical practice guidelines for the treatment of depression. *Australian & New Zealand Journal of Psychiatry, 38*, 389–407.

Sawyer, M., Arney, F., Baghurst, P. A., et al. (2001). *The Mental Health of Young People in Australia.* Canberra: Mental Health and Special Projects Branch, Commonwealth Department of Health and Aged Care.

Schweitzer, I., & Tuckwell, V. (2004). The Neurobiology of Depression. In P. Joyce & P. Mitchell (Eds.), *Mood Disorders. Recognition and treatment.* Sydney: University of NSW Press.

Scott, K. (2011). Sex differences in the disability associated with mental disorders. *Current Opinion in Psychiatry, 24*, 331–335.

Shultz, J., & Videbeck, S. (2009). *Lippincott's manual of psychiatric nursing care plans* (8th ed.). Philadelphia: Lippincott Williams & Wilkins.

Stimpson, N., Agrawal, N., & Lewis, G. (2002). Randomised controlled trials investigating pharmacological and psychological interventions for treatment-resistant depression. *British Journal of Psychiatry, 181*, 284–294.

Sullivan, P. (2004). The genetic epidemiology of major depression. In P. Joyce & P. Mitchell (Eds.), *Mood disorders: Recognition and treatment* (Chapter 7, pp. 75–84). Sydney: University of NSW Press.

Sullivan, P., Neale, M., & Kendler, R. (2000). Genetic epidemiology of major depression: Review and meta-analysis. *American Journal of Psychiatry, 157*, 1552–1562.

UK ECT Review Group. (2003). Efficacy and safety of electroconvulsive therapy in depressive disorders: A systematic review and meta-analysis. *Lancet, 361*, 799–808.

Van de Kooy, K., van Hout, H., Marwijk, H., et al. (2007). Depression and the risk for cardiovascular diseases: Systematic review and meta-analysis. *International Journal of Geriatric Psychiatry, 22*(7), 613–626.

Veronese, A., Ayoso-Mateos, J., Cabello, M., et al. (2012). Work disability and depressive disorders. *American Journal of Physical and Medical Rehabilitation, 91*(Suppl 2), 62–68.

Weissman, M. M., Leaf, P. J., Tischler, G. L., et al. (1988). Affective disorders in five United States communities. *Psychological Medicine, 18*(1), 141–153.

Wells, H., Bushnell, J., Hornblow, A., et al. (1989). Christchurch psychiatric follow-up study. Part 1: Methodology and lifetime prevalence for specific psychiatric disorders. *Australian and New Zealand Journal of Psychiatry, 23*, 315–326.

Wilhelm, K., Mitchell, P., & Slade, T., et al. (2003). Prevalence and correlates of DSM-IV major depression in an Australian national survey. *Journal of Affective Disorders*, *75*(2), 155–162.

World Health Organization. (1992). *Classification of mental and behavioural disorders (ICD-10)*. Geneva: Author.

Wurtzel, E. (1994). *Prozac nation. Young and depressed in America. A memoir*. London: Quartet Books.

CHAPTER

15

Esther Chang
Amanda Johnson
Karen Hancock

Advanced dementia

Learning objectives

When you have completed this chapter you will be able to:

- comprehend the pathophysiology of a person who has dementia
- adopt a holistic approach in managing the symptoms and behaviours of a person with advanced dementia
- identify the potential challenges and implications for nursing a person with advanced dementia
- recognise communication skills are essential in the provision of nursing care to a person with advanced dementia and their family
- appreciate the importance of family carers as an integral feature in planning care for the person with advanced dementia.

Key words

advanced dementia, Alzheimer's, carers, communication, family, symptom management

INTRODUCTION

Worldwide there is much evidence to suggest that recognising dementia as a chronic disease through awareness, early diagnosis, good management and research is paramount to providing effective care (Alzheimer's Australia, 2011a). Dementia is becoming an increasingly burdensome health issue in both Australia and New Zealand. It is associated with a number of diseases characterised by impairment of brain function inclusive of memory, understanding and reasoning (Australian Institute of Health and Welfare [AIHW], 2012). This group of diseases leads to a progressive, incurable decline in cognitive abilities and normal daily functioning which severely limits quality of life (AIHW, 2012). Dementia is also acknowledged as the leading cause of disability in older Australians (Access Economics, 2009). Latest estimates reveal 266 574 people currently have dementia in Australia (Deloitte Access Economics, 2011) with 44 000 in New Zealand (Alzheimer's Association of New Zealand, nd). Projections in Australia for 2030 show an increase in people affected by dementia to be 553 285 and 942 624 by 2050 (Deloitte Access Economics, 2011). Similarly, by 2050 it is projected more than 147 000 New Zealanders will be diagnosed with dementia (Alzheimer's Association of New Zealand, nd). Dementia is frequently linked to advancing age, affecting less than 1% the population under 65 years of age and 1 in 4 people aged 85 years or older (AIHW, 2012). The Australian projections support the prediction that in two decades health and residential aged care spending will constitute the third highest source of spending (Access Economics, 2009). Further, by 2023 dementia will become one of the fastest growing sources of major disease burden overtaking coronary heart disease (Access Economics, 2009). In acknowledging these projections the Australian government has recognised, for the first time, dementia as a national health priority. Alzheimer's disease is the most common form of dementia that people experience affecting up to 50–75% of the population. This is followed by vascular dementia as the second most frequent type. Dementia with Lewy bodies and frontotemporal lobe dementia makes up a smaller percentage overall (AIHW, 2012). In New Zealand, in 2007 there were over 32 000 people with dementia. In 2011, 48 182 New Zealanders had dementia — 1.1% of the New Zealand population. This has increased over 18% in 3 years, from 40 746 people in 2008 (Alzheimer's Association of New Zealand, 2013).

As a disease, dementia is now ranked as the third leading cause of death in Australia (Australian Bureau of Statistics [ABS], 2010) and the fourth leading cause of death among the population aged 65 years and over in New Zealand (Alzheimer's Association of New Zealand, 2013). The number of deaths directly attributed to dementia in 2010 represented 6.3% of all Australian deaths overall, demonstrating a 3.4% increase since 2001, almost doubling during this time period and expected to continue to rise with the projections previously detailed (ABS, 2010). It is highly probable that a similar pattern of increase will be reflected in the New Zealand population in worldwide trends (World Health Organization [WHO], 2012). Symptoms of advanced dementia frequently resemble those of a person dying from advanced cancer (Alzheimer's Association of Australia, 2011b; Chang et al., 2009). This scenario suggests people with dementia would significantly benefit from the interventions traditionally directed to cancer-related end-of-life care (Mitchell, Teno, & Kiely, 2009; van der Steen, 2010); however palliative care interventions are infrequently accorded to this group of people so their needs are likely to be unmet (Chang et al., 2009; Chang & Walter, 2010). Further exacerbation of this lack of palliative care intervention may also be attributed to the person with advanced dementia possessing impaired communication (Johnson et al., 2009). As a result of this and the disease itself, the symptoms of dementia are likely to present as a challenge for family and professional carers.

ADOPTING A HOLISTIC APPROACH

The pathology of dementia means that many challenges and disruptions occur along the illness trajectory, manifesting as a multitude of symptoms across cognitive, functional, behavioural and psychological areas (Maher & Hemming, 2005; Grand, Caspar, & MacDonald, 2011). Because of the extensive needs of individuals with dementia, they often require care beyond traditional medical practice (Grand, Caspar, & MacDonald, 2011). The person becomes increasingly reliant on caregivers to provide his/her entire essential physical, psychological and social needs (Long, 2009). The challenge faced by nurses is to provide high-quality care that addresses all these facets. Hughes (2010) reported that people with dementia are less likely to have their pain and spiritual and religious needs addressed than those without dementia. Dementia can rob a person of their personhood (Long, 2009, p. 21). It is important to treat the person as an individual (Grand et al., 2011). This leads to a care environment in which the nurse's practice is complex and multi-layered, as a direct consequence of dementia pathology. The basic principle of care is to meet the needs of the person by managing their total symptom experience rather than responding to discrete segments; for example, attending to a person's emotional status while also assessing their pain (Maher & Hemming, 2005).

The illness trajectory of dementia is frequently slow and insidious, with family often acting as the primary caregivers for substantial periods of time. Ultimately, for the majority of people with dementia, a move to institutional care in a residential aged care facility (RACF) is required (WHO, 2012). The long involvement of family carers is unique to this client group; nurses, as part of their holistic approach and principle of care, must include the family in their caregiving. Recognising how family are feeling has a direct impact on the person with dementia (Nugent, 2005) and may further contribute to their anxiety, depression, wandering and other displays of behaviour. It is through the relationships the nurse has with the person and their family and the actions the nurse demonstrates in providing holistic care that healing occurs. Healing in this context means seeing the person as a whole, attending to all dimensions of care, giving meaning to their life, offering hope to the family and showing compassion, respect and patience. It is from this understanding that nurses can make a difference to the lives of the person affected by dementia and their family. Holistic nursing therefore delivers nursing care that addresses the person's physical, intellectual, emotional and spiritual dimensions. The person and their family's needs are considered as an interrelated entity of these dimensions (Taylor, 2009). If holistic nursing is not undertaken, significant levels of distress and suffering may be experienced by the person and their family (Maher & Hemming, 2005).

When nurses believe and demonstrate through their actions that they view a person as a whole human being embracing the interconnectedness of mind, body and spirit, evidence of a holistic approach to the delivery of nursing care is present (Erickson, 2007; Nugent, 2005). Erickson sees a person's wholeness as the dynamic interaction of the mind, body and spirit components within the person, between and among others and with the universe (2007, p. 140). For a healthy state to exist, balance and harmony in all aspects of the person's life — physical, social, emotional, cognitive and spiritual — must be present, irrespective of the presence or absence of physical disease (Erickson, 2007). This implies that in the presence of disease, a person has the potential to achieve a state of wellbeing if their needs are addressed holistically and the person remains in a relational context with other people (Erickson, 2007). In these circumstances, the person seeks, in partnership with the nurse, to ameliorate the imbalance and disharmony present through the alleviation of suffering, promotion of comfort, finding inner peace, assisting with healing and preventing illness and injury (Erickson, 2007; Mariano, 2007). Practising in this way demonstrates a shift in care from being disease-oriented to embracing the needs of the person and their family (Erickson, 2007; O'Brien, King, & Gates, 2007).

The following principles underpin holistic nursing: understanding the person as a unique human being who possesses a connectedness with everyone and everything; recognising the need for healing in states of illness where cure is not possible but where management of symptoms will lead to the alleviation of suffering; promoting comfort and restoration of balance and harmony; engaging in care practices that embrace both the science and the art of nursing; performing nursing care in relationship with the person and their family based on the values of compassion, respect, trust and authenticity; and participating in self-care activities to promote healing and personal development of self (Mariano, 2007; Nugent, 2005).

When a holistic approach to care is adopted, the journey taken by both the nurse and the patient is of a healing nature. This journey is predicated on the notion that healing is reflective of the following: having a presence; intent; unconditional acceptance; love and compassion (Erickson, 2007, pp. 154–9). Healing leads to the attainment of wellbeing in the presence of disease for the patient and, for the nurse, provides an energy source derived from the balance and harmony achieved that nurtures the nurse to continue caregiving. Understanding where the person and their family are at is the beginning point of the journey for the nurse, the person with dementia and their family members (Mariano, 2007).

Assessment of the person and their family's needs, at this point, offers the opportunity to identify and discuss care options across the illness trajectory in the context of the person's preferences (Mariano, 2007). Understanding the personal characteristics of the individual allows for the tailoring of interventions to support the person's deficits, to maximise their strengths and to identify the coping mechanisms of the person and their family (Kolanowski & Whall, 2000, p. 74) in the management of end-of-life issues.

Holistic nursing therefore offers nurses a means of practice that responds to the whole person by addressing their physical, psychological, social, spiritual and cultural needs as a collective entity rather than directing care to discrete segments of a disease (Erickson, 2007; Maher & Hemming, 2005; Nugent, 2005). For example, a person with dementia may scream or lash out as a result of feelings of anxiety, fear or depression due to their incapacity to express themselves and not as a consequence of dementia pathology (Kolanowski & Whall, 2000, p. 69). Alternatively, in the presence of non-assessed or misdiagnosed fatigue, thirst, hunger and/or pain, a person with dementia may respond by wandering, physical aggression and disruptive vocalisations (Kolanowski & Whall, 2000, p. 70) or exacerbations of these behaviours in response to an unmet physiological need.

Nurses who engage in a holistic nursing approach use a repertoire of actions that demonstrate their commitment to the concept of holism, including touch, massage, eye contact, moderated and empathic voice, comfort measures, aromatherapies, exercise, music, active listening, creation of trusting relationships, an approach that is non-confrontational and calm and the sensitive eliciting of information (Erickson, 2007; Maher and Hemming, 2005; Nugent, 2005; Kolanowski & Whall, 2000).

The case studies in this chapter show how holistic nursing care can be considered in practice. They show the interrelationship that exists between a person's mind, body and spirit and their care needs.

In Case Study 15.2 Anthony Harrison doesn't recognise his children any more. In this situation the nurse can use holistic nursing care to support both the individual and their family in their experiences of loss.

These two case studies highlight the complexity of providing holistic care and involving the family in the care of the person, viewing the person as a whole and understanding the significance of the interconnectedness between the components of mind, body and spirit, in order to meet the person's and their family's needs.

ADVANCED DEMENTIA AND THE EXPERIENCE OF PAIN

Pain is a subjective experience as illustrated in the definition by McCaffrey (1968), which is still commonly used today: 'Pain is whatever the experiencing person says it is, existing

CASE STUDY 15.1

Mary Jane is a 68-year-old woman who was diagnosed with vascular dementia 10 months ago. She had been living with her husband who is also her caregiver. They have no children. Five months ago Mary Jane was admitted to the RACF because of her behavioural problems. Her husband was increasingly concerned about her wandering, aggressive manner and the potential risk of harm. Other co-morbidities included heart disease, anxiety and depression and a past history of right mastectomy 10 years ago.

The staff in the RACF identified that Mary Jane was in the advanced stage of dementia. She had a Mini-Mental State Examination (MMSE) score of 12; she walked with the assistance of one nurse and was at a high risk of falling if she tried to ambulate independently. Mary Jane has recently displayed frequent episodes of extreme agitation. She regularly calls out loudly, bangs things like plates against the wall, is resistant to care and often becomes more physically aggressive to staff when they provide care. She previously attended resident activities run by the diversional therapist, but this has stopped because the other residents complained that she was too disruptive and noisy.

Mary Jane is receiving regular antipsychotic medication and sixth-hourly paracetamol for pain. When Mary Jane appears to have pain, the care staff initiates non-pharmacological pain interventions known to settle her, such as spending some time with her, distracting her to reduce her distress and agitation. She will sometimes settle without medication. Mary Jane's husband, a retired accountant, comes to visit her every day. She is less agitated when he is there.

From a holistic nursing perspective, the nurse would communicate with Mary Jane's husband in the planning of care and decision making to manage Mary Jane's symptoms.

Case study questions

1. What are the key elements of care for Mary Jane?
2. What are the key elements of building a trusting relationship with Mary Jane and her husband so that they feel valued?
3. How do you provide holistic care for Mary Jane?

whenever he or she says it does'. The challenge for the nurse, then, is how to assess and manage pain in people with advanced dementia who cannot usually communicate verbally how they feel due to the disease processes involved. It is commonly believed that people with dementia have decreased ability to experience pain; however, this conviction may be due to the pain tools used that rely on verbal report (Smigorski & Leszek, 2010). Pain is under-recognised and under-treated in advanced dementia (Jordan et al., 2011). A paper on bioethical issues in dementia by the Nuffield Council on Bioethics (2009) reported that research shows people with dementia receive poor end-of-life care, in particular poor pain control. It also found that older hospitalised people with dementia are less likely to receive palliative care than those who do not have dementia. Impairment in communicative ability, self-report in particular, has been recognised as the primary reason for inadequate pain management in this group (Sheu et al., 2011). Another challenge is that people with

CASE STUDY 15.2

Anthony Harrison is an 84-year-old man. He was diagnosed with Alzheimer dementia 6 years ago and has a history of diabetes and cardiovascular disease. Anthony was admitted to an RACF 3 years ago because his wife could no longer care for him at home. He required assistance to transfer from bed to chair, and assistance with all his activities of daily living. He was a large man who was difficult for his wife to lift.

Anthony's notes reveal that he is chair fast, requiring two nurses to transfer him using a Pelican belt or similar equipment. He is now incontinent of both urine and faeces if not taken to the toilet regularly and incontinent overnight. He can communicate a little, but his vocabulary is very restricted. He requires staff assistance to feed him a normal diet. Anthony was unable to complete any of the MMSE questions; his MMSE was therefore assessed as being zero.

Staff members have identified that Anthony's condition is deteriorating. He has lost weight and is becoming increasingly frail. Anthony is taking regular Celestone, Clamaxyl Duo, Chlorvescent and analgesics intermittently (PRN) if staff note that he appears to be in pain on movement. He no longer recognises his wife or children during their visits. This distresses his children a great deal, as they want him to share their lives, and those of their small children. He has no advance directive, no evidence that any discussion about prognosis or end-of-life care has been undertaken, nor goals of care stated.

From a holistic nursing perspective, the nurse would communicate with his wife in the planning of care and decision making of advance directives for Anthony.

Case study questions

1. What are the key elements for advanced care planning for Anthony?
2. How do you involve the family in the care of Anthony?
3. What are some of the issues raised when discussing end-of-life care?

dementia do not follow a linear trajectory towards death, and as a result pain management can be variable (Aupperle, MacPhee, & Strozeski, 2004). In addition, an observable behaviour symptom (e.g. agitation) may be symptomatic of conditions other than pain, highlighting the complexities in symptom management in people with advanced dementia. There is also a common belief that being a neurological disorder, central nervous system experience of pain in dementia is reduced (Reynolds, Hanson, DeVellis, Henderson, & Steinhauser, 2008). However, significant pain is a common experience in advanced dementia (Aminoff & Adunsky, 2004; Black et al., 2006; Feldt, Warne & Ryden, 1998; Ferrell et al., 1995; Gove et al., 2010; Kupper & Hughes, 2011; McClean, 2000; Parmelee, 1996; Smigorski & Leszek, 2010; Won et al., 2004; Young, 2001). As stated in the Australian Guidelines for a Palliative Approach in Residential Aged Care (Australian Department of Health and Ageing, 2006, p. 62), 'One of the most difficult aspects for the aged care team who is caring for the resident with advanced dementia is assessing whether they are experiencing pain'. Clinical experience of the authors supports this finding, with many Australian aged care nursing clinicians stating that the ability to not only assess but also address pain issues for the cognitively impaired resident remains a constant issue of concern as clinicians struggle to function within a system not designed or educated to cope with this challenge.

The literature indicates that people with dementia are at high risk for unrecognised, untreated or under-treated pain (Black et al., 2006; Evans, 2002; Reynolds et al., 2008; Shega, Hougham, Stocking, Cox-Hayley, & Sachs, 2006; Snow & Shuster, 2006). Apart from the challenges in assessment described above, this situation may be partly due to a common perception among many in our community, as well as trained health professionals, that individuals with dementia do not experience pain because of their impaired cognitive state (Boller et al., 2002) and their inability to verbalise and self-report their pain. This is not a logical assumption, because although communication deficits and motivational and complex thinking impairments may blunt pain behaviour, they do not necessarily alter pain perception (Schuster, 2000). Even towards the end of life such individuals continue to interact with their environment and are not in a vegetative state (Boller et al., 2002; Volicer & Hurley, 1998).

The majority of people with advanced dementia are over the age of 65 (WHO, 2012), and as such are likely to have underlying medical conditions that can cause pain (McClean, 2000). In advanced dementia, pain is frequently the result of constipation or diarrhoea, lodged food particles, contractures, decubitus ulcers or urosepsis (Smith, 1998). Other possible causes of pain include sore gums, broken teeth and cavities, headaches, back pain, osteoarthritis, hip fractures, skin rash, sore throat and cold (Rabins, Lyketsos, & Steele, 2006). A US study on nursing homes found that there was a lack of good quality palliative care, with distressing symptoms and burdensome interventions being more common in people at the end stage of dementia, unless their relatives were well informed (Cervo et al., 2009). For people with advanced dementia, pain may be expressed in terms of irritability, increased confusion or resistance to care. Nursing staff are in an ideal position to be able to notice changes in function or behaviour that may be signs of pain, as they are so closely involved in the care of the person that only they may be able to interpret the meaning of the symptoms. They also have an ethical and legal obligation to make all attempts to ensure the comfort and pain management of their patients, especially for those who are unable to express their pain verbally (Kerr & Chenoweth, 2003).

ASSESSING PAIN IN PEOPLE WITH ADVANCED DEMENTIA

An expert-based consensus statement of pain assessment in older adults recommended that adequate assessment is vital in providing a basis for clinical decision making and optimal care (Hadjistravropoulos et al., 2007; Herr et al., 2011). One of the main reasons that pain management in patients who are older and cognitively impaired is inadequate is that there is a lack of or inappropriate assessment (Hadjistravropoulos et al., 2007; Smigorski & Leszek, 2010). A systematic approach is required, using all members of the caring team within the facility, including family members.

Experts recommend that best practice for this population is to utilise behavioural observation-based assessment, due to difficulties with recall, interpretation of sensations and verbal expression in dementia (AGS Panel on Persistent Pain in Older Persons, 2002; American Medical Directors Association, 2005; Australian Department of Health and Ageing, 2006). Thus nursing staff base their decisions on an objective assessment of pain relief needs rather than simply relying on subjective impressions. An attempt should always be made to obtain a self-report of pain from the person with advanced dementia before changing to behavioural observation (Snow & Shuster, 2006) because 'any reports of pain from the cognitively impaired resident should be accepted as just as valid and reliable as those of residents who can communicate' (Australian Pain Society, 2005). Kerr and Chenoweth (2003) recommend the following interviewing skills when assessing pain in people with cognitive impairment: ask simple and specific questions about how the person is feeling (e.g. 'Do you have an ache?'); speak calmly and at a pace the person can comprehend; adopt a caring and patient manner; maintain eye contact and keep checking that the person understands the question; and use a safe, quiet environment. However, the nurse should also remember that, if the person's self-report of pain is negative, and pain discomfort behaviours are present, pain is likely (Snow & Shuster, 2006). A family carer report is also recommended if one is available, as they are familiar with the person's usual demeanour (Kerr & Chenoweth, 2003).

Other components of pain assessment apart from behavioural observation include physical assessment and a comprehensive review of the history of the person with dementia. Physical touch appears to be lacking when reviewing how pain is assessed in the resident with dementia. Health professionals and carers tend to base their decisions on verbal response rather than physical examination of the body and the reactions of the person with advanced dementia. Clinical examination of the individual, using a simple physical assessment that includes movement of the limbs while observing the person with dementia, will provide evidence of pain even in a person at the end stage of dementia, who may grimace, moan or resist being moved. The findings, when taken together with the results from using a pain assessment tool, the nurse's clinical judgment and the opinions of other care staff and family members, will provide evidence on which to base pain interventions.

The medical history should also be reviewed, especially in relation to factors and conditions known to be associated with pain. Additionally, it is useful to know the history of the pain being experienced itself. Useful questions include: 'When did the pain start?'; 'What aggravates the pain?'; 'What relieves the pain?' and 'Is there a certain time of the day when the pain is present?' While a resident with advanced dementia may not be able to recall and respond to these questions, family members and other members of the care team may be able to assist.

Potential behavioural indicators of pain

The American Geriatrics Society identified six main types of pain behaviours and indicators, based on a literature review (AGS Panel on Persistent Pain in Older Persons, 2002). These are listed in Table 15.1 with specific examples of observable behaviours. However, it

TABLE 15.1
Pain behaviours/indicators

PAIN BEHAVIOUR/INDICATOR	EXAMPLE
Facial expressions	Slight frown, sad, frightened face, grimacing, wrinkled forehead, closed or tightened eyes, any distorted expression, rapid blinking.
Verbalisations, vocalisations	Sighing, moaning, groaning, grunting, chanting, calling out, noisy breathing, asking for help.
Body movements	Rigid, tense body posture, guarding, fidgeting, increased pacing, rocking, restricted movement, gait or mobility changes.
Changes in interpersonal interactions	Aggressive, combative, resisting care, decreased social interactions, socially inappropriate, disruptive, withdrawn, verbally abusive.
Changes in activity patterns or routines	Refusing food, appetite change, increase in rest periods or sleep, changes in rest pattern, sudden cessation of common routines, increased wandering.
Mental status changes	Crying or tears, increased confusion, irritability or distress.

is important to take into account the influence of culture on the expression of pain, so not all cues listed will apply (Kerr & Chenoweth, 2003).

Tools for assessment of pain for advanced dementia

People with advanced dementia unable to self-report their pain are particularly at risk for under-recognised or under-treated pain, and the symptoms of dementia can be exacerbated by the pain experience. For example, the person may be more irritable, aggressive, depressed or withdrawn, with changed appetite or sleep. Recognition of these non-verbal behaviours as a potential sign of discomfort needs to be systematically addressed, with the use of appropriate pain assessment tools. Herr, Bjoro and Decker (2006) conducted a critical review of existing tools issued for pain assessment in non-verbal older adults with dementia. The tools they identified as meeting criteria are listed in Table 15.2. All the tools require the rater to observe the person and rate the behaviours in terms of their presence, intensity or frequency (Snow & Shuster, 2006). Although existing tools are still in the early stages of development and testing, particularly in terms of established validity (Herr et al., 2006), the advantage of these tools is that their use raises the nurse's awareness of the need to assess the patient for pain, and they provide an objective assessment that can augment the nurse's subjective judgment. One must always remember that a tool is only as good as the assessor and cannot take away the clinical judgment of the health professional or carer. Bearing this in mind, how, then, does the nurse ensure that all residents with possible pain are assessed? Adopting a systematic approach to pain assessment and management is the

TABLE 15.2
Pain assessment

PAIN ASSESSMENT TOOL	AUTHORS
Abbey Pain Scale (Abbey)	Abbey et al. (2004)
Assessment of Discomfort in Dementia (ADD) protocol*	Kovach et al. (1999)
Checklist of non-verbal pain indicators (CNPI)	Feldt (1998)
Certified Nursing Assistant Pain Assessment Tool (CPAT)	Cervo et al. (2009)
Discomfort of Dementia of the Alzheimer's Type (DS-DAT)	Hurley et al. (1992)
The Doloplus 2	Lefebvre-Chapiro & the Doloplus Group (2001)
The Face, Legs, Activity, Cry, and Consolability Pain Assessment Tool (the FLACC)	Merkel et al. (1997)
Mahoney Pain Scale	Mahoney & Peters (2008)
Noncommunicative Patient's Pain Assessment Instrument (NOPPAIN)	Snow et al. (2004)
Pain Assessment Checklist for Seniors with Limited Ability to Communicate (PACSLAC)	Fuchs-Lacelle and Hadjistravropoulos (2004)
Pain Assessment for the Dementing Elderly (PADE)	Villanueva et al. (2003)
Pain Assessment in Advanced Dementia (PAINAD)	Warden et al. (2003)
Pain Assessment In Noncommunicative Elderly (PAINE)	Cohen-Mansfield & Lipson (2008)

*Since this review the authors of the ADD have refined the protocol to develop the Serial Trial Intervention, which has been positively evaluated using a randomised controlled trial (Kovach et al., 2006b).

best practice (Kerr & Chenoweth, 2003; Kovach et al., 2006a, 2006b, 2006c; Snow & Shuster, 2006).

Systematic approach to assessment of pain

One example of a systematic approach for this population is the Serial Trial Intervention (STI) developed by nurses (Kovach et al., 2006c) to systematically assess and treat the unmet needs of people with dementia. This approach is a refinement of the Assessment of Discomfort in Dementia (ADD) protocol that has previously been found to be effective in improving pain assessment and management in nursing home residents with dementia (Kovach et al., 1999; Pieper, Achterberg, Francke, van der Steen, Scherder, & Kovach, 2011). The STI identifies the cause of discomfort behaviours and then treats the causes, such as pain, that lead to discomfort behaviours, and has been evaluated in a randomised controlled trial. The study of 114 nursing home residents with moderate or severe dementia found that those who received the STI had significantly lower levels of discomfort, were more likely to return to their baseline levels, received a broader scope of physical affective assessment and received more pharmacological comfort treatments than those in the control group (Kovach et al., 2006b). An application of this approach to the cases in this chapter will be given below.

APPLYING A SYSTEMATIC APPROACH TO THE ASSESSMENT OF PAIN

Current best practice guidelines set out by the Australian Government are that pain management should be conducted using a comprehensive assessment of the resident's pain and evidence-based analgesic decision making (Australian Department of Health and Ageing, 2006).

Table15.2 shows behavioural measures of pain assessment derived from a review (Herr, Bjoro, & Decker, 2006). Measures satisfied criteria of being:

1 based on behavioural indicators of pain
2 developed for assessment of pain in non-verbal older adults with severe dementia or evaluated for use with non-verbal older adults
3 available in English
4 psychometrically evaluated.

A position statement with clinical practice recommendations set out by Herr et al. (2011) poses the following hierarchy of pain assessment techniques for dementia, based on findings by Pasero and McCaffery (2011) and Hadjistravropoulos et al. (2007):

1 Obtain self-report. Self-report of pain is often possible in mild to moderate cognitive impairment, but ability to self-report decreases as dementia progresses.
2 Search for potential causes of pain. Consider common chronic pain aetiologies: Musculoskeletal and neurological disorders are the most common causes of pain in adults.
3 Observe patient behaviour. Observe facial expressions, verbalisations/vocalisations, body movements, changes in interactions, changes in activity patterns or routines and mental status. Behavioural observation should occur during activity whenever possible.

In the cases of Mary Jane and Anthony, any one of the behaviours listed in Table 15.1 could alert the nurse to the possibility that they may be experiencing pain. Mary Jane is reportedly agitated, and is frequently resistive to care and physically aggressive. Both of them have heart disease, disabling conditions known to cause pain and lower quality of life (Cunningham, 2006; Frondini, LanFranchi, Minardi, & Cucinotta, 2007). Recent research (Leonard, Tinetti, Allore, & Drickamer, 2006) indicates that aggressive cognitively impaired people are significantly more likely than a non-aggressive cognitively impaired person to have two or more pain-related diagnoses, including strokes, contractures and decubitus ulcers. However, Mary Jane's disruptive behaviours could also reflect other problems, such as depression, boredom or over- or under-stimulation (Snow & Shuster, 2006).

Using a systematic approach to managing Mary Jane and Anthony's symptoms, the nurse would respond to the behavioural symptoms by implementing multiple levels of assessment and treatment, tailored to the individual person (Kovach et al., 2006a). Detailed explanation of this approach can be found in Kovach et al. (2006a) and Snow and Shuster (2006).

1 Conduct a physical need assessment focusing on conditions associated with discomfort. In Mary Jane's or Anthony's case, there could be behavioural indications of specific locations of discomfort, so the nurse could physically move Mary Jane's and Anthony's limbs and watch for verbal and non-verbal cues that might indicate pain, such as grimacing; or when Mary Jane is taken for a walk while assessing her movement.
2 Examine environment and activity pacing (alternating in excessive periods of stimulation and rest) to identify potential causes of behaviour and treat accordingly if assessment positive. For Mary Jane and Anthony this would involve checking that sources of environmental stress, such as the chair used by Anthony, are eliminated or reduced to a minimum. Mary Jane and Anthony both require combinations of meaningful human interaction and rest, even if they appear not to be responding. This is an important step to help identify whether a particular symptom (e.g. agitation) is due to pain or other reasons, such as lack of meaningful human interaction or stimulation.
3 Initiate an analgesic regimen trial when indicated by physical examination. This would also be started if no clear potential cause of discomfort can be identified and non-pharmacological interventions to increase comfort have been unsuccessful. This should be carefully monitored and regularly reassessed. In Mary Jane's case, paracetamol was ineffective in controlling the pain. Although the pain was reduced after staff spent considerable time distracting her, this form of management is time-consuming, increases environmental stress and adds to the strain of caring (Kovach et al., 2006c). It does not assist with the underlying cause of the pain. Regular analgesic regimens will assist here. Anthony is also only being given analgesia 'as required'. With his history of diabetes and cardiovascular disease, he should be commenced on an 'around the clock' treatment regimen, commencing with paracetamol. The fact that Mary Jane was not given a stronger pain reliever than paracetamol is reflective of common under-treatment of pain that occurs in this population (Black et al., 2006; Evans, 2002; Shega et al., 2006; Snow & Shuster, 2006). However, the situation does appear to be improving, with a Swedish study (Haasum, Fastbom, Fratiglioni, Kåreholt, & Johnell, 2011) finding that people with dementia were more likely than those without dementia in a residential setting to receive analgesia. Perhaps awareness is increasing in medical and allied health staff on pain management in dementia. Adopting a palliative approach to the care of people with dementia (Australian Department of Health and Ageing, 2006) in the case of Mary Jane means that a strong analgesic may be appropriate in the absence of effective pain relief following simple analgesia. Although nurses do not have a prescribing role, they have a crucial role in

decisions about assessment, medication regimens and management procedures as well as reviewing practice and outcomes (Cunningham, 2006).

4 Non-pharmacological intervention trial: this occurs when indicated by Step 2 (examination of environment and activity pacing). Examples that could be applied to Mary Jane and Anthony include reduced or increased environmental/sensory stimulation, soothing and supportive verbal communication and/or touch, physical exercise/movement/massage and music therapy (Snow & Shuster, 2006). Best practice guidelines recommend that these treatments be used to complement analgesia, and may decrease the amount of analgesia required (AGS Panel on Persistent Pain in Older Persons, 2002; American Medical Directors Association, 2005). Review the use of complementary therapies such as aromatherapy and relaxation techniques.
5 If behaviour continues, consult with other disciplines or practitioners.
6 Using this approach requires persistence in terms of regular assessment, management and reassessment.

PRINCIPLES OF COMMUNICATION WITH FAMILY CARERS

When planning care for a person with advanced dementia the health and wellbeing of family members who act as primary carers (family carers) need to be assessed, monitored and referral made for interventions if indicated. Family carers provide physical care and emotional support to the person with dementia throughout the illness trajectory, frequently undertaking this responsibility even before a diagnosis is made (Wackerbath & Johnson, 2002). The care they provide is time-consuming, sometimes unpleasant, emotionally and physically stressful and falls outside the bounds of normal family relationships (Yap, Seow, Henderson, & Goh, 2005). For these reasons, the health and quality of life of the family carer may be adversely affected by their caring role. Dementia family carers may also be required to initiate, supervise and sometimes evaluate the effectiveness of medications (Brodaty & Green, 2002) and act as the substitute decision maker, providing consent for complex healthcare decisions for the person with dementia who no longer has the capacity to either consent to, or refuse, treatment.

Potential impact on family carers

Family carers can experience negative health outcomes as a result of their caring role. Carers of people with dementia have poorer physical and psychological health, life expectancy, quality of life and economic security (WHO 2012). Many are older people themselves who may have their own health problems and the round the clock care they need to give can be physically and mentally exhausting (Gove et al., 2010). Family carer grief associated with dementia may be a major factor in stress and burn-out, which if unaddressed can precipitate earlier admission of the person with dementia to a RACF (Brodaty, Green, & Koschera, 2003). The negative impacts of caring are found across geographic regions, cultures and healthcare delivery systems, and have an impact more on women carers than men carers (Torti et al., 2004; WHO, 2012). Despite experiencing the caring role as burdensome, however, many family carers report great satisfaction from their involvement in care (Andren & Elmstahl, 2005).

Assessment of family carers

Assessment of role strain potentially affecting the health of the family carer is an important dimension of nursing work. Validated tools are available to assist the assessment, such as the Caregiver Strain Index (Robinson, 1983), widely utilised in Australia (Australian Government Department of Veteran's Affairs). In New Zealand, the Caregiver Assessment Tools (Guberman et al., 2000) are recommended, although they require adapting for use with Māori and Pacific Islander people (New Zealand Guidelines Group, 2003). Assessment for depression is also necessary. One simple way for a nurse to screen a family carer for depression (Arroll et al., 2005) is to ask the family carer to answer 'yes' or 'no' to two questions: 'During the past month have you often been bothered by feeling down, depressed or hopeless?' and 'During the past month have you been bothered by little interest or pleasure in doing things?' These questions assess whether two core symptoms of depression are present. A 'yes' response to these questions may indicate the family carer is depressed. One further question, 'Is this something with which you would like help?', with three possible responses — 'yes', 'no' or 'yes but not today' — will assist the nurse to determine whether the family carer wants assistance. If indicated, the family carer can be referred to their usual medical practitioner for further investigation and treatment.

Consideration must also be given to the assessment of the family carer's previous grief and loss experiences in order to provide appropriate support. Less educated family carers with lower incomes who are experiencing more depressive symptoms are more likely to experience complicated grief reactions after the death of the person with dementia (Hebert, Dang, & Schulz, 2006). Family carers therefore may require referral to a counsellor, social worker, pastoral care worker or other spiritual adviser for additional support. Many family carers adjust rapidly following the death of the person with dementia. This adjustment has been attributed to remarkable resilience, possibly due to the prolonged period of caring before death, giving rise to a sense of relief following their loved one's demise (Schulz et al., 2003).

During the assessment process it is necessary to establish which family carer is the legal substitute decision maker for the person with dementia, able to give consent for medical and dental treatments. Legal requirements vary within Australia, and differ also to New Zealand, so the nurse needs to enquire locally about the legal standard for consent. Failure to identify the correct person may result in medico–legal difficulties and family conflict when the person with dementia is unable to make their own decisions (Peisah, Brodaty, & Quadrio, 2006). Disputes about treatment, or the absence of a legal substitute decision maker, require intervention from a legal authority such as a guardianship board or similar to make decisions in the best interests of the person with dementia. Mary Jane's husband (Case Study 15.1) appears to be the substitute decision maker for his wife. If he does not have legal authority to consent to treatments being given or withheld, then his decisions about his wife's care can be challenged.

Interventions to assist family carers

Anthony Harrison's wife (Case Study 15.2) was exhausted by her caring role, and as Anthony's medical condition deteriorated, her quality of life and wellbeing were also being eroded, to the point that her children implored her to admit Anthony to a RACF, which she did. What could be done to assist Anthony's wife and other family carers? Effective interventions across the dementia trajectory that have been shown to help family carers, and may delay admission of the person with dementia to a RACF, include giving the family carers information about the course of dementia and what to expect; giving them long-term social support, in the form of counselling and support groups; and improving their problem-solving skills so they can handle new situations as they arise (Mittelman, 2005; Mittelman, Haley, Clay, & Roth, 2006; WHO, 2012). Teaching them to think in a more clinical manner about their role — that is, more objectively — may also help (Hepburn et al., 2005). Interventions for family carers are more successful if the person with dementia is also involved (Brodaty et al., 2003). A home care program in India (Dias et al., 2008) found that providing information to carers on dementia, guidance on behaviour management, a single psychiatric assessment and psychotropic medication if needed effectively reduced caregiver strain and improved their mental health.

Encouraging the family carer to take a break from their caregiving duties is also beneficial, by providing respite care, which may be available on a daily basis in the home, or a day care centre; or for longer periods of a few weeks to months at a time, in a RACF, depending on the area in which the person with dementia is living (Brodaty et al., 2003; Mittelman, 2005; Mittelman et al., 2006). While Anthony Harrison (Case Study 15.2) lived at home, his wife may have required encouragement to use her respite time to undertake some physical activity, such as a walk, to relieve stress and maintain her own physical health and to attend her own medical and dental appointments as necessary. Now that he has been admitted to a RACF, the staff should encourage her to continue with these activities, as well as encouraging her to eat a healthy diet, get as much sleep as possible and maintain contact with her social circle whenever she can to reduce social isolation. Not all family carers use available support services, either because they don't think they need them or because they are not aware of their availability. Nurses in all care sites can assist family carers by making sure the family carer receives information and referral to available support services in their area (Brodaty et al., 2005).

In terms of caregiver interventions, it is important to conduct a comprehensive assessment of the needs, strengths, weaknesses and available resources to guide the selection of the intervention (WHO, 2012).

THE FAMILY CARER ROLE IN PLANNING CARE FOR THE PERSON WITH DEMENTIA

An advance directive (also called 'advance healthcare directive' or 'living will') may be either a document or an oral statement that gives instructions in advance of a health-related event, either consenting to, or refusing, certain treatments if the affected person does not have the capacity to make their own decisions. The legal requirements for making an advance directive differ in each state and territory of Australia, and in New Zealand, so nurses need to enquire about their local laws in relation to directives.

In both Australia and New Zealand the making of an advance directive is a relatively new concept; nurses working with people with advanced dementia may find that there is no formal advance directive available when caring for people with dementia and decisions fall to the family carer or other appointed guardian legally responsible for that person. For many carers of people with dementia, not knowing the right decision and being afraid of doing the wrong thing is a major source of stress (Hughes, 2010). Having an advance directive can help ease this stress.

The solution to the lack of a directive is to engage the family carer in a series of conversations about the likely future healthcare needs of the person with dementia, and together reach consensus about a future plan of care that optimises the quality of life and wellbeing of the person with dementia, and utilises a palliative approach to treat symptoms as they arise. Family carers may feel unprepared to make difficult end-of-life decisions and lack adequate information about the dementia trajectory (Sampson, Jones, & Thune-Boyle, 2010), which is why the focus should be on giving them accurate, honest information during a number of encounters. Research evidence remains scant. One study (Koopmans, van der Sterren, & van der Steen, 2007) revealed that the majority (85%) of people with dementia die before the very end stage of dementia is reached; and death, regardless of

Reflective questions

1. How can adopting a holistic approach to nursing practice be relevant for a person with advanced dementia?
2. What are some potential behavioural symptoms displayed by Mary Jane and Anthony that could be signalling that they are experiencing pain?
3. What are some non-pharmacology therapies that could be used in conjunction with medication to relieve Mary Jane and Anthony's pain?

when it occurs, is most commonly associated with cachexia/dehydration (35.2%), cardiovascular disorders (20.9%) and acute pulmonary diseases such as pneumonia (20.1%), so decisions about future treatment or palliation of the symptoms associated with these causes of death needs to form part of the plan of care. In the study by Koopmans et al. (2007), approximately 9% of people with dementia died of an unknown, acute cause. Nurses therefore also need to help family carers understand that death may occur due to other conditions that may be unpredictable.

An Australian study found that families of dementia patients who had died and who had advance directives demonstrated less stress, anxiety and depression than those who did not (Detering et al., 2010).Thus, despite the reluctance of carers to write plans (Sampson et al., 2010), advance care planning appears to be effective in ensuring quality patient care as well as the wellbeing of carers.

CONCLUSION

Advanced dementia brings numerous somatic, affective and behavioural symptoms, impairments and co-morbidities. Diagnosing and managing pain, and other symptoms, in people with advanced dementia is often made difficult by the communicative difficulties of the person with dementia. Pain and other symptoms may exacerbate the behavioural symptoms of dementia and the uncertain illness trajectory of advanced dementia. Nursing staff, because they are closely involved in the care of the person with dementia, often detect and interpret changes in behaviour that may signal pain. Furthermore, they have a pivotal role in managing the medication regimen of such patients. Adopting a systematic and holistic approach to assessment and management of pain and other symptoms in advanced dementia means that patients are more likely to receive appropriate treatment. These challenges can also point to the need for professional development and training needs for carers. Advance care directives expressing the resident's prospective care preferences would give clinicians clearer guidelines for responding to the patient, and would assist in negotiating care decisions with family members.

Acknowledgment: Sally Easterbrook, Megan Luhr and Kathleen Harrison in the first edition.

Recommended reading

Bidewell, J. & Chang, E. (2011). Managing dementia agitation in residential aged care. *Dementia, 10*(3), 299–315.

Chang, E. M., Daly, J., Johnson, A., et al. (2009). Challenges of care in advance dementia. *International Journal of Nursing Practice, 15*(1), 41–47.

Chang, E., Easterbrook, S., Hancock, K., et al. (2010). Evaluation of an information booklet for family and caregivers of people with dementia: An Australian perspective. *Nursing & Health Sciences, 12*(1), 45–51.

Chang, E., & Johnson, A. (2012). Challenges in advanced dementia. In E. Chang & A. Johnson (Eds.), *Contemporary and innovative practice in palliative care*. Croatia: InTech Open Science.

Johnson, A., Chang, E., Daly, J., et al. (2009). The communication challenges faced in adopting a palliative care approach in advance dementia. *International Journal of Nursing Practice, 15*(5), 467–474.

References

Abbey, J., Piller, N., Bellis, D. E., et al. (2004). The Abbey pain Scale: a 1-minute numerical indicator for people with end-stage dementia. *International Journal of Palliative Care, 10*(1), 6–13.

Access Economics. (2009). Keeping dementia front of mind: Incidence and prevalence 2009–2050. Retrieved August 6, 2012, from http://www.fightdementia.org.au/access-economics-reports.aspx

AGS Panel on Persistent Pain in Older Persons. (2002). The management of persistent pain in older persons. *Journal of the American Geriatrics Society, 50*, S205–S224.

Alzheimer's Association of Australia. (2011a). National strategies to address dementia. Retrieved August 6, 2012, from http://www.fightdementia.org.au/alzheimers-australia-reports.aspx

Alzheimer's Association of Australia. (2011b). Planning for the end of life for people with dementia. Retrieved August 6, 2012, from http://www.fightdementia.org.au/alzheimers-australia-reports.aspx

Alzheimer's Association of New Zealand. (2013). Reports and statistics. Retrieved May 9, 2013, from http://www.alzheimers.org.nz/information/reports-statistics

American Medical Directors Association. (2005). *Clinical practice guideline: Pain management in the long-term care setting*. Columbia, MD: Author.

Aminoff, B., & Adunsky, A. (2004). Dying dementia patients: Too much suffering, too little palliation. *American Journal of Alzheimer's Disease and Other Dementias, 19*(4), 243–247.

Andren, S., & Elmstahl, S. (2005). Family caregivers' subjective experiences of satisfaction in dementia care: aspects of burden, subjective health and sense of coherence. *Scandinavian Journal of Caring Sciences, 19*(2), 157–168.

Arroll, B., Goodyear-Smith, F., Kerse, N., et al. (2005). Effect of the addition of a 'help' question to two screening questions on specificity for diagnosis of depression in general practice: diagnostic validity study. *British Medical Journal, 331*, 884–886A.

Aupperle, P. M., MacPhee, E. R., & Strozeski, J. E. (2004). Hospice use for the patient with advanced Alzheimer's Disease: The role of the geriatric psychiatrist. *American Journal of Alzheimer's Disease and Other Dementias, 19*, 94–104.

Australia Bureau of Statistics. (2010). Causes of death, Australia, 2010. Retrieved August 6, 2012, from http://www.abs.gov.au/ausstats.

Australian Department of Health and Ageing. (2006). *Guidelines for a palliative approach in residential aged care (enhanced version)*. Canberra: Author.

Australian Institute of Health and Welfare. (2012). Australia's health 2012. Retrieved August 6, 2012, from http://www.aihw.org.au

Australian Pain Society (2005). Pain in residential aged care facilities. Management strategies. Retrieved December 23, 2005, from http://www.apsoc.org.au

Black, B. S., Finucane, T., Baker, A., et al. (2006). Health problems and correlates of pain in nursing home residents with advanced dementia. *Alzheimer's Disease and Associated Disorders, 20*(4), 283–290.

Boller, F., Verny, M., Hugonot-Diener, L., et al. (2002). Clinical features and assessment of severe dementia. A review. *European Journal of Neurology, 9*(2), 125–136.

Brodaty, H., & Green, A. (2002). Defining the role of the caregiver in Alzheimer's disease treatment. *Drugs & Aging, 19*(12), 891–898.

Brodaty, H., Green, A., & Koschera, A. (2003). Meta-analysis of psychosocial interventions for caregivers of people with dementia. *Journal of the American Geriatrics Society, 51*(5), 657–664.

Brodaty, H., Thomson, C., Thompson, C., et al. (2005). Why caregivers of people with dementia and memory loss don't use services. *International Journal of Geriatric Psychiatry, 20*(6), 537–546.

Cervo, F., Bruckenthal, P., Chen, J., et al. (2009). Pain assessment in nursing home residents with dementia: Psychometric properties and clinical utility of the CNA pain assessment tool (CPAT). *Journal of the American Medical Directors Association, 10*(7), 505–510.

Chang, A. & Walter, L. C. (2010). Recognizing dementia s a terminal illness in nursing home residents. *Archives of Internal Medicine, 170*(13), 1107–1109.

Chang, E. M., Daly, J., Johnson, A., et al. (2009). Challenges for professional care of advanced dementia. *International Journal of Nursing Practice, 15*(1), 41–47.

Cohen-Mansfield, J., & Lipson, S. (2008). The utility of pain assessment for analgesic use in persons with dementia. *Pain, 134*(1–2), 16–23.

Cunningham, C. (2006). Managing pain in patients with dementia in hospital. *Nursing Standard, 46*, 54–58.

Deloitte Access Economics. (2011). Dementia across Australia: 2011–2050. Retrieved August 6, 2012, from http://www.fightdementia.org.au/access-economics-reports.aspx

Detering, K., Hancock, A., Reade, M. C., et al. (2010). The impact of advance care planning on the end of life care in elderly patients: randomized controlled trial. *British Medical Journal, 340*, 847.

Dias, A., Dewey, M. E., D'Souza, J., et al. (2008). The Effectiveness of a Home Care Program for Supporting Caregivers of Persons with Dementia in Developing Countries: A Randomised Controlled Trial from Goa, India. *PLoS ONE, 3*(6), e2333. Published online June 4, 2008. http://www.plosone.org/article/info%3Adoi%2F10.1371%2Fjournal.pone.0002333

Erickson, H. L. (2007). Philosophy and theory of holism. *Nursing Clinics of North America, 42*(2), 139–163.

Evans, B. D. (2002). Improving palliative care in the nursing home: from a dementia perspective. *Journal of Hospice and Palliative Nursing, 4*(2), 91–102.

Feldt, K. S., Warne, M. A., & Ryden, M. B. (1998). Examining pain in aggressive cognitively impaired older adults. *Journal of Gerontological Nursing, 24*(11), 14–22.

Ferrell, B. A. (1995). Pain evaluation and management in the nursing home. *Annals of Internal Medicine, 123*, 681–687.

Frondini, C., LanFranchi, G., Minardi, M., et al. (2007). Affective, behavior and cognitive disorders in the elderly with chronic musculoskeletal pain: the impact on an aging population. *Archives of Gerontology and Geriatrics, 44*(Suppl 1), 167–171.

Fuchs-Lacelle, S., Hadjistravropoulos, T. (2004). Development and preliminary validation of the pain assessment checklist for seniors with limited ability to communicate (PASLAC). *Pain Management in Nursing, 5*, 37–49.

Gove, D., Sparr, S., Dos Santos Bernardo, A., et al. (2010). Recommendations on end-of-life care for people with dementia. *The Journal of Nutrition, Health and Aging, 14*(2), 136–139.

Grand, J., Caspar, S., & MacDonald, S. (2011). Clinical features and multidisciplinary approaches to dementia care. *Journal of Multidisciplinary Healthcare, 4*, 125–147.

Guberman, N., Keefe, J., Fancey, P., et al. (2000). CARE tool and caregiver risk screen. University Institute of Social Gerontology, Centre de recherché sur les services communautaires (CLSC). René Cassin. Retrieved June 1, 2007, from http://www.msvu.ca

Haasum, Y., Fastbom, J., Fratiglioni, L., et al. (2011). Pain Treatment in Elderly Persons With and Without Dementia: A Population-Based Study of Institutionalized and Home-Dwelling Elderly. *Drugs & Aging, 28*(4), 283–293.

Hadjistravropoulos, T., Herr, K., Turk, D., et al. (2007). An interdisciplinary expert consensus statement on assessment of pain in older persons. *Clinical Journal of Pain, 23*(1), S1–S43.

Hebert, R., Dang, Q., & Schulz, R. (2006). Preparedness for the death of a loved one and mental health in bereaved caregivers of patients with dementia: findings from the REACH study. *Journal of Palliative Medicine, 9*(3), 683–693.

Hepburn, K. W., Lewis, M., Narayan, S., et al. (2005). Partners in caregiving: A psychoeducation program affecting dementia family caregivers' distress and caregiving outlook. *Clinical Gerontologist, 29*(1), 53–69.

Herr, K., Coyne, P., McCaffery, M., et al. (2011). Pain assessment in the patient unable to self-report: Position statement with clinical practice recommendations. *Pain Management Nursing, 12*(4), 230–250.

Herr, K., Bjoro, K., & Decker, S. (2006). Tools for assessment of pain in nonverbal older adults with dementia: A state-of-the-science review. *Journal of Pain and Symptom Management, 31*(2), 170–192.

Hughes, J. (2010). Ethical issues and decision-making in dementia care. Presentation to National Press Club of Australia, June 2010.

Hurley, A. C., Volicer, B. J., Hanrahan, P. A., et al. (1992). Assessment of discomfort in advanced Alzheimer patients. *Research in Nursing and Health, 15*, 369–377.

Johnson, A., Chang, E., Daly, J., et al. (2009). The communication challenges faced in adopting a palliative care approach in advance dementia. *International Journal of Nursing Practice, 15*(5), 467–474.

Jordan, A., Hughes, J., Pakresi, M., et al. (2011). The utility of PAINAID in assessing pain in a UK population with severe dementia. *International Journal of Geriatric Psychiatry, 26*(2), 118–263.

Kerr, S., & Chenoweth, L. (2003). Pain management. In R. Hudson (Ed.), *Dementia nursing: A guide to practice* (pp. 162–173). Melbourne: Ausmed Publications.

Kolanowski, A. M., & Whall, A. L. (2000). Toward holistic-theory based intervention for dementia behavior. *Holistic Nursing Practice, 14*(2), 67–76.

Koopmans, R. T., van der Sterren, K. J., & van der Steen, J. T. (2007). The 'natural' endpoint of dementia: death from cachexia or dehydration following palliative care? *International Journal of Geriatric Psychiatry, 22*, 350–355.

Kovach, C. R., Cashin, J. R., & Sauer, L. (2006a). Deconstruction of a complex tailored intervention to assess and treat discomfort of people with advanced dementia. *Journal of Advanced Nursing, 55*(6), 678–688.

Kovach, C. R., Logan, B., Noonan, P. E., et al. (2006b). Effects of the serial trial intervention on discomfort and behavior in demented nursing home residents. *American Journal of Alzheimer's Disease and Other Dementias, 21*(3), 147–155.

Kovach, C. R., Noonan, P. E., Schildt, A. M., et al. (2006c). The serial trial intervention: An innovative approach of meeting needs of individuals with dementia. *Journal of Gerontological Nursing, 32*(4), 18–25.

Kovach, C., Weissman, D., Groffie, J., et al. (1999). Assessment and treatment of discomfort for people with late stage dementia. *Journal of Pain and Symptom Management, 18*, 412–419.

Kupper, A. L., & Hughes, J. (2011). The challenges of providing palliative care for older people with dementia. *Current Oncology Reports, 13*, 295–301.

Lefebvre-Chapiro, S., The Doloplus Group (2001). The Doloplus–2 scale — evaluating pain in the elderly. *European Journal of Palliative Care, 8*, 191–194.

Leonard, R., Tinetti, M., Allore, H., et al. (2006). Potentially Modifiable Resident Characteristics That Are Associated With Physical or Verbal Aggression Among Nursing Home Residents With Dementia. *Archives of Internal Medicine, 166*, 1295–1300.

Long, C. (2009). Palliative care for advanced dementia: Approaches that work. *Journal of Gerontological Nursing, 35*(11), 19–24.

Maher, D., & Hemming, L. (2005). Understanding patient and family: holistic assessment in palliative care. *British Journal of Community Nursing, 10*(7), 318–322.

Mahoney, A., & Peters, L. (2008). The Mahoney pain scale: examining pain and agitation in advanced dementia. *American Journal of Alzheimer's Disease and other Dementias, 23*, 250–261.

Mariano, C. (2007). Holistic nursing as a specialty: Holistic nursing — scope and standards for practice. *Nursing Clinics of North America, 42*(2), 165–188.

McCaffrey, M. (1968). *Nursing practice theories related to cognition, bodily pain, and man-environment interactions.* Los Angeles: UCLA Student's Store.

McClean, W. (2000). *Practice guide for pain management for people with dementia in institutional care.* Stirling: The Dementia Services Development Centre, University of Stirling.

Merkel, S. I., Voepel-Lewis, T., Shayevitz, J. R., et al. (1997). Practice applications of research. The FLACC: a behavioural scale for postoperative pain in young children. *Pediatric Nursing, 23*, 293–297.

Mitchell, S. L., Teno, J. M., & Kiely, D. K. (2009). The clinical course of advanced dementia. *New England Journal of Medicine, 361*(16), 1529–1538.

Mittelman, M. (2005). Taking care of the caregivers. *Current Opinion in Psychiatry, 18*(6), 633–639.

Mittelman, M. S., Haley, W. E., Clay, O. J., et al. (2006). Improving caregiver well-being delays nursing home placement of patients with Alzheimer disease. *Neurology, 67*(9), 1592–1599.

New Zealand Guidelines Group. (2003). Assessment processes for older people. Retrieved May 9, 2013, from http://www.health.govt.nz/publication/assessment-processes-older-people-summary

Nuffield Council on Bioethics. (2009). Dementia: Ethical Issues. Nuffield Council on Ethics. Retrieved August 7, 2012, from www.nuffieldbioethics.org/sites/default/files/Nuffield%20Dementia%20report%20Oct%2009.pdf

Nugent, J. (2005). *A passion for caring book 5. Applying holistic skills in dementia care.* Adelaide: NurseLink Australia.

O'Brien-King, M., & Gates, M. F. (2007). Teaching holistic nursing: The legacy of Nightingale. *Nursing Clinics of North America, 42*(2), 309–333.

Parmelee, P. A. (1996). Pain in cognitively impaired older persons. *Clinical Geriatric Medicine, 12*, 473–487.

Pasero, C., & McCaffery, M. (2011). *Pain assessment and pharmacological management.* St Louis: Mosby.

Peisah, C., Brodaty, H., & Quadrio, C. (2006). Family conflict in dementia: prodigal sons and black sheep. *International Journal of Geriatric Psychiatry, 21*(5), 485–492.

Pieper, M., Achterberg, W., Francke, A., et al. (2011). The implementation of the serial trial intervention for pain and challenging behavior in advanced dementia patients (STA OP!) a cluster randomized trial. Retrieved May 9, 2013, from http://www.biomedcentral.com/1471-2318/11/12

Rabins, P. V., Lyketsos, C. G., & Steele, C. D. (2006). *Practical dementia care* (2nd ed.). New York: Oxford University Press.

Reynolds, K. S., Hanson, L. C., DeVellis, R. F., et al. (2008). Disparities in pain management between cognitively intact and cognitively impaired nursing home residents. *J Pain Symptom Manage, 35*, 388–396.

Robinson, B. C. (1983). Validation of a caregiver strain index. *Journal of Gerontology, 38*(3), 344–348.

Sampson, E., Jones, L., & Thune-Boyle, I. (2010). Palliative assessment and advance care planning in severe dementia: An exploratory randomized controlled trial of a complex intervention. *Palliative Medicine, 25*(3), 197–209.

Schulz, R., Mendelsohn, A. B., Haley, W. E., et al. (2003). End-of-life care and the effects of bereavement on family caregivers of persons with dementia. *The New England Journal of Medicine, 349*(20), 1936–1942.

Shega, J. W., Hougham, G. W., Stocking, C. B., et al. (2006). Management of non-cancer pain in community-dwelling persons with dementia. *Journal of the American Geriatrics Society, 54*(12), 1892–1897.

Sheu, E., Versloot, J., Nader, R., et al. (2011). Pain in the elderly: Validity of facial expression components of observational measures. *Clinical Journal of Pain, 27*(7), 593–601.

Shuster, J. L., Jr. (2000). Palliative care for advanced dementia. *Clinics in Geriatric Medicine, 16*(2), 373–386.

Smigorski, K., & Leszek, J. (2010). Pain experience and expression in patients with dementia, health management. Retrieved May 9, 2013, from: http://www.intechopen.com/books/health-management/the-experience-and-expression-of-pain-in-patients-with-dementia

Smith, S. J. (1998). Providing palliative care for the terminal Alzheimer patient. In L. Volicer & A. Hurley (Eds.), *Hospice care for patients with advanced progressive dementia* (pp. 247–256). New York: Springer Publishing.

Snow, A. L., & Shuster, J. L., Jr. (2006). Assessment and treatment of persistent pain in persons with cognitive and communicative impairment. *Journal of Clinical Psychology, 62*(11), 1379–1387.

Snow, A. L., Weber, J. B., O'Malley, K. J., et al. (2004). NOPAIN: a nursing assistant-administered pain assessment instrument for use in dementia. *Dementia Geriatric and Cognitive Disorders, 17*, 240–244.

Taylor, D. (2009). *Living with medicines for dementia — patient and carer perspectives.* University of Bath, UK: Pharmacy Practice Research Trust.

Torti, F. M. J., Gwyther, L. P., Reed, S. D., et al. (2004). A multinational review of recent trends and reports in dementia caregiver burden. *Alzheimer Disease & Associated Disorders, 18*(2), 99–109.

van der Steen, J. (2010). Dying with dementia: What we know after more than a decade of research. *Journal of Alzhiemer's Disease, 22*, 37–55.

Villanueva, M. R., Smith, T. L., Erickson, J. S., et al. (2003). Pain assessment for the dementing elderly: reliability and validity of a new measure. *Journal of the American Medical Directors Association, Jan/Feb*, 1–8.

Volicer, L., & Hurley, A. (1998). *Hospice care for patients with advanced progressive dementia.* New York: Springer Publishing.

Wackerbarth, S., & Johnson, M. (2002). Essential information and support needs of family caregivers. *Patient Education & Counseling, 47*(2), 95–100.

Warden, V., Hurley, A. C., & Volicer, L. (2003). Development and psychometric evaluation of the pain assessment in advanced dementia scale. *Journal of the American Medical Directors Association, 4*(1), 9–15.

Won, A. B., Lapane, K. L., Vallow, S., et al. (2004). Persistent non-malignant pain and analgesic prescribing patterns in elderly nursing home residents. *Journal of the American Geriatrics Society, 52*, 867–874.

World Health Organization. (2012). *Dementia: A public health priority*. Geneva: Author.

Yap, L. K. P., Seow, C. C. D., Henderson, L. M., et al. (2005). Family caregivers and caregiving in dementia. *Reviews in Clinical Gerontology, 15*(3–4), 263–271.

Young, D. M. (2001). *Pain in institutionalised elders with chronic dementia (PhD dissertation).* Iowa City: University of Iowa.

CHAPTER 16

Andrew Scanlon

Stroke (cerebrovascular accident)

Learning objectives

When you have completed this chapter you will be able to:

- identify known risk factors for stroke
- understand the mechanism for stroke (both ischaemic and haemorrhagic)
- understand the difference in acute care treatment between ischaemic and haemorrhagic stroke
- understand the aims of primary and secondary stroke prevention
- establish rehabilitation goal in light of deficits related to the stroke.

Key words

acute stroke care, haemorrhagic stroke, ischaemic stroke, risk factors, stroke rehabilitation

INTRODUCTION

Stroke, also known as cerebrovascular accident (CVA) or brain attack, is a debilitating condition and an enormous personal and financial burden for not only the sufferer and their loved ones but also society as whole. Its onset is often sudden and without warning, leaving long-lasting effects from which the individual may never fully recover. Despite the insidious nature of stroke its modifiable risk factors are well known and so too are its long-term ramifications.

This chapter discusses stroke incidence, signs and symptoms, pre-hospital care, diagnosis, types, acute care and rehabilitation issues that may arise during the trajectory of care. Two case studies will also be presented to demonstrate care priorities for two very different types of stroke.

STROKE

Most recent data (2008–2010) shows that in Australia there are 41 977 acute stroke presentations each year (Australian Institute of Health and Welfare [AIHW], 2012), of which approximately 11 204 result in death, accounting for nearly 7.8% of all deaths in Australia (Australian Bureau of Statistics [ABS], 2012). Globally, there are about 6.2 million acute stroke presentations each year and stroke is the second leading cause of death in the developed world (World Health Organization, World Heart Federation, & World Stroke Organization, 2011). In 2003, it was estimated that over 346 700 Australians experienced a stroke at some time during their lives, with 146 400 suffering from some form of disability as a direct result (AIHW, 2006). The cost of stroke and other cerebrovascular diseases amounted to $896 million in 2000–01 (1.8% of total health system expenditure), of which aged care homes accounted for 50% and hospitals 40% (National Health Priority Action Council [NHPAC], 2006). In New Zealand, over 8000 people each year will have a stroke, one third will die within the first year after the event and at least 70% will have a long-term disability and at least three-quarters of this number will die or be disabled (Feigin et al., 2006).

As a consequence, stroke prevention is an international priority, as there are many identified risk factors that can be modified or targeted to save countless lives as well as lifelong expense.

Stroke can occur in two main ways, either through a sudden blockage of cerebral arterial blood flow, such as found in ischaemic stroke (80% of cases), or through the rupturing of cerebral arteries in haemorrhagic stroke such as intracerebral haemorrhage (15%), or subarachnoid haemorrhage (5%) (Donnan, Fisher, Macleod & Davis, 2008). This abrupt cessation or alteration in cerebral arterial blood flow directly affects the part of the brain the artery feeds, leading to loss of function, which is directly related to the signs and symptoms exhibited by the patient. The physical manifestation of stroke (signs and symptoms) can be transient or permanent, depending on the extent of brain cell death, patients' existing co-morbidities, how early it is diagnosed, type of stroke, treatment options available, complications from the stroke and rehabilitation options available.

RISK FACTORS AND PRIMARY PREVENTION

Risk factors for stroke are similar to those for other common chronic diseases, especially those involving the cardiovascular system. These can include physiological, social and behavioural determinants. These factors can influence one another, further compounding the devastating effects of stroke. Understanding the following risk factors and actively preventing them (if possible) is considered to be primary prevention.

Social factors

Potential risk factors or vulnerability towards conditions can be avoidable but, due to personal circumstances, may be extremely difficult to overcome and can be seen as (personally) unmodifiable. Social determinants have been and will continue to be used to determine an individual's predisposition to conditions such as stroke. Numerous factors associated with the socially disadvantaged such as level of education, informed health decisions and access to healthcare all contribute to overall risk (Scanlon & Lee, 2007).

Age (the elderly)

With advancing age also comes the increased risk of debilitating conditions such as stroke (Iadecola, Park, & Capone, 2009). The incidence of mortality and ongoing severity morbidity associated with stroke also increases with age (Lloyd-Jones et al., 2010).

The National Health and Hospitals Reform Commission commissioned the Australian Institute of Health and Welfare to undertake projections of Australian healthcare expenditure. The resulting publication released in 2008 was to determine health expenditure from 2003 to 2033. In relation to stroke it projected that although the number of strokes was going to rise over time due to an ageing and growing population to 55.9%, the age-standardised incidence rate of stroke will decline (40.4% and 40.6% for males and females, respectively) (Goss, 2008).

Ethnicity

There is evidence that racial background is associated with biological predisposition and/or social determinants towards developing certain conditions. In the United States, those of African-American or Hispanic descent (Lloyd-Jones et al., 2010) are more likely to suffer a stroke than the general population. In Australia, Aboriginal and Torres Strait Islander peoples are more than twice as likely to suffer a stroke than the general population (AIHW, 2008). This may also be related to modifiable determinants of health compounding these risks. In the New Zealand population Māori/Pacific and Asian/other people are at higher risk of ischaemic stroke but there similar rates of subarachnoid haemorrhage across all ethnic groups (Feigin et al., 2006).

Heredity

Positive family history of conditions has well been established as an indicator for risk. Through ongoing genetic research numerous genes have been identified as known risk factors for both ischaemic and haemorrhagic stroke (Nahed et al., 2007). Unfortunately, the availability of genetic testing and awareness of this particular risk are not widespread. Education is required about the positive outcomes of pre-emptive screening and possible modifiable risk factors.

Sex

Gender differences are common for most cardiovascular conditions. Men are more likely than women to have a stroke below the age of 65 but after the age of 75 women are at higher risk (Towfighi, Saver, Engelhardt, & Ovbiagele, 2007). The reason for this may be related to the failure of many men to have regular check-ups or act on early warning signs and symptoms of conditions such as stroke (Scanlon & Lee, 2007). In the age group above 75 women have a tendency to experience more strokes and have worse outcomes (quality of life, depression, disability) than men; the exact reason behind this is not well understood (Gargano & Reeves, 2007).

Transient ischaemic attack

A transient ischaemic attack (TIA) mimics stroke symptoms and is sometimes called a 'mini stroke'. The symptoms last less than 24 hours and spontaneously resolve. If left untreated, however, a transient ischaemic attack can further develop into embolic stroke. The causes of TIAs are predominantly clots or embolisms that can originate from atherosclerotic plaque or thrombosis from elsewhere in the body. Transient ischaemic attack must be actively and aggressively treated because of this increased risk of stroke (Lloyd-Jones et al., 2010). The risk of stroke after TIA is approximately 5% at 7 days and 10–15% at 90 days (Giles & Rothwell, 2007, 2009).

High blood pressure

There are numerous complications that occur as a result of hypertension, none more serious than the associated vascular changes such as loss of smooth motor function (Iadecola et al., 2009). These changes can weaken (thus rupture) or degrade (through constant vasoconstriction to maintain the hypertensive state) the cerebral vasculature to such an extent that stroke is inevitable. Lowering blood pressure is an effective method for reducing the risk of stroke and subsequent stroke (Lakhan & Sapko, 2009).

High blood cholesterol

Hypercholesterolaemia is of particular concern due to changes to the vascular system, including profound changes that take place in the cerebral vascular system. Its direct effects on the cerebral vascular system and stroke, however, are currently widely debated as to whether there is a correlation or not. Regardless of this, the indirect effects can be attributed to the damage caused to the arteries supplying the heart, causing cardiac dysfunction, which may in turn lead to ischaemic stroke through embolisation (Prinz & Endres, 2011).

Carotid stenosis

The increased incidence of clot formation (and thus thrombosis and embolism) associated with stenosis of the carotid arteries also increases the potential for stroke (Altaf et al., 2007). This stenosis may also be attributed to the atherosclerotic changes associated with hypercholesterolaemia, as mentioned previously, leading to emboli lodging in (usually) the middle cerebral artery.

Atrial fibrillation

This heart condition has a tendency to produce emboli secondary to turbulent blood flow in the atria. These in turn are 'flicked off' towards the path of least resistance (aorta — carotid arteries — cerebral arterial circulation) until they can travel no further, lodging in an arterial vessel and causing stroke. Those suffering with atrial fibrillation have an increased risk of more severe stroke (Wang et al., 2003). Patients with this condition require anti-coagulation to decrease this very real complication.

Diabetes

Apart from the well-documented effects that diabetes has on all vital functions of the body, its effects on the vascular system in particular not only substantially increase the risk of stroke but also complicate patient outcomes (Giorda et al., 2007; Yakubovich & Gerstein, 2011). If left untreated hyperglycaemia can further complicate recovery, as it is linked to associated brain oedema as well as infarct expansion within 24 hours of initial stroke (Baird et al., 2003). Oedema related to the infarcted brain tissue expands within the limited space of the cranial vault and causes adjacent brain cells also to become damaged and even temporarily or permanently cease functioning.

Tobacco smoking

Tobacco smoking is a well-known risk factor for all cardiovascular disease, including stroke (Scanlon, 2006). Nicotine, apart from being highly addictive, is also a known poison. The effects of smoking tobacco cause a rise in blood pressure, increase in heart rate and vasoconstriction of all arteries. Each of these on its own could cause stroke; together the likelihood is increased. Smokers' risk for stroke is approximately double that of non-smokers (Lloyd-Jones et al., 2010).

Alcohol consumption

Evidence for the relationship between alcohol use and stroke can be seen as conflicting as the effects of alcohol can be both beneficial and detrimental. The anticoagulation effect of moderate alcohol use is beneficial for ischaemic stroke, lessening the potential for clot or thrombosis formation (Goldstein & Hankey, 2006). However, the overall risk increases exponentially with heavy alcohol use (Reynolds et al., 2003) as the increased anticoagulation effect of alcohol use also increases the risk of haemorrhagic stroke.

Obesity

There are clear links between obesity and any number of chronic conditions, and stroke is no different. The risk of ischaemic stroke — in particular stroke caused by atherosclerosis — is increased by 10 to 20% with obesity (Chen, Bai, Yeh, Chiu, & Pan, 2006). Obesity puts the individual at risk of hypertension and diabetes, both known risk factors of stroke, and further increases their potential. Studies have also shown that regular exercise can also reduce the chance of stroke (Gallanagh, Quinn, Alexander, & Walters, 2011).

Other factors

Hormone replacement therapy and the contraceptive pill are associated with an increase of stroke incidence. However, they are not seen as priorities in assessing and preventing stroke (Lloyd-Jones et al., 2010).

Stroke prevention clinics

In response to the overwhelming evidence of known risk factors, some healthcare facilities run clinics whose specific purpose is to prevent stroke. Of note is Austin Health's stroke prevention clinic. This clinic is run by the stroke team, who review patients identified as having any or a combination of the above established risk factors. During the consultation the patient is reviewed and appropriate early referral made to a specialised member of the multidisciplinary team, be it a dietitian, cardiologist, smoking cessation specialist, etc. The aim of the clinic is to reduce the incidence but also the potential severity of morbidity associated with stroke and provide a means of primary prevention of stroke.

PRE-HOSPITAL CARE

Of paramount importance for stroke survival is appropriate and timely pre-admission or hospital care. Worldwide, guidelines support this rapid response to presenting symptoms in order to achieve better patient outcomes (Hachinski et al., 2010; National Stroke Foundation, 2010). Symptoms associated with stroke should never be ignored, as any delay in diagnosis and treatment can further exacerbate the sufferer's condition and lead to preventable complications, including death.

Signs and symptoms of stroke

Abrupt cessation of stroke or alteration in blood flow is directly attributed to a sudden loss of function demonstrated by common signs and symptoms. These can include:

- weakness, numbness or paralysis of the face, arm or leg on either or both sides of the body

- difficulty speaking or understanding
- dizziness, loss of balance or an unexplained fall
- loss of vision, or sudden blurred or decreased vision on one or both eyes
- headache, usually severe and sudden in onset, or unexplained change in the pattern of headaches
- difficulty swallowing (National Stroke Foundation, 2010).

Stroke symptoms typically last more than 24 hours or result in the death of the sufferer (not to be confused with TIAs, which last less than 24 hours). The National Stroke Foundation has developed a public media campaign to increase awareness around stroke and what to do. The campaign (which started in 2006) is aimed at presenting the symptoms of stroke simply, allowing for assessment that could be performed by anyone, thus increasing the likelihood of rapid assessment and appropriate treatment (National Stroke Foundation, 2012a). The campaign is based on the acronym FAST:

- **F**acial weakness — can the person smile? Has their mouth or eye drooped?
- **A**rm weakness — can the person raise both arms?
- **S**peech difficulty — can the person speak clearly and understand what you say?
- **T**ime to act fast — seek medical attention immediately (National Stroke Foundation, 2012b).

This process allows the assessor to decide on the appropriate action for their patient or loved one as quickly as possible, as there is a very small window of opportunity in which to seek treatment to reverse or lessen the potentially devastating and fatal side-effects of stroke.

DIAGNOSIS

Once clinical signs and symptoms of stroke are present the sufferer has a very limited amount of time to receive treatment to obtain maximum benefit. This timeframe has been conservatively estimated at 2 hours (Adams et al., 2007). On presenting to the emergency department, rapid assessment and diagnosis should be performed to rule out all possibilities. Signs and symptoms of stroke do mimic other possible life threatening conditions and differential diagnosis to stroke can include, but is not limited to, traumatic brain injury, migraine, hypoglycaemia, seizure, brain tumour and systemic infection. The first and most definitive diagnostic test is the computed tomography (CT) scan. A CT scan can at least differentiate very quickly between ischaemic and haemorrhagic stroke, as well as other possible diagnoses such as brain tumour or trauma. Haemorrhagic strokes often have telltale signs of acute blood characterised white appearance or hyperdense regions anywhere within the cerebrospinal fluid pathways (the ventricles, gyri and sulci etc.), whereas ischaemic stroke areas of infarction may appear dark or hypodense within normal structures of the brain (Wardlaw et al., 2004). Sometimes, however, ischaemic stroke may not be evident on a CT scan for up to 48 hours after initial symptoms are present (Frizzell, 2005). At this point treatment for stroke diverges. If a CT scan rules out haemorrhagic stroke or other differential diagnosis then appropriate treatment is commenced. If it confirms haemorrhagic stroke then further investigation is necessary to determine the source of the bleed. This is usually performed by angiography, which can be done by CT scan or magnetic resonance imaging (MRI) scans but most commonly is done with fluoroscopy digital subtraction. Angiography of the cerebral arteries allows visualisation of abnormalities such as aneurysms or arteriovenous malformations.

TYPES OF STROKE

Ischaemic stroke

Ischaemic strokes account for the vast majority of all strokes; between 80 and 85% (Therapeutic Guidelines Limited, 2011). Its presentation is similar to haemorrhagic but its treatment is very different due to the nature of the cerebral blood flow disruption. The three main types of ischaemic stroke are thrombotic, lacunar and embolic.

Thrombotic stroke is usually a result of atherosclerosis weakening the cerebral artery wall to such an extent that a thrombus forms and eventually blocks the artery. This type of stroke accounts for roughly 30% of all stokes and predominantly affects large vessels of the brain (Therapeutic Guidelines Limited, 2011).

Lacunar stroke accounts for about 15% of all strokes and is regarded as a subtype of the thrombotic stroke (Therapeutic Guidelines Limited, 2011). The reason for this is that it develops in a similar way to thrombotic stroke, but on smaller vessels usually in and around the brain stem.

Embolic stroke occurs as a result of an embolism travelling into the cerebral circulation and eventually becoming lodged in the capillary bed, leading to loss of blood flow and cell death. These emboli frequently come from the heart due to atrial fibrillation, artificial heart valves or myocardial infarction. They can also occur due to other cardiovascular disorders such as deep vein thrombosis or through surgery or trauma that frees particles of adipose tissue or air bubbles. This type of stroke accounts for approximately 20% of all strokes (Therapeutic Guidelines Limited, 2011).

There are also strokes that can occur from rare conditions such as dissection, venous infarction, vasculopathies and these make up approximately 5% of all strokes. There are also strokes which develop from unknown causes which make up about 15% of all strokes (Therapeutic Guidelines Limited, 2011).

Haemorrhagic stroke

Haemorrhagic stroke accounts for approximately 15–20% of all strokes and over 50% of the mortality related to all strokes (Therapeutic Guidelines Limited, 2011). Its devastating effects require at times both medical and neurosurgical intervention. This type of stroke includes both intracerebral haemorrhage (10% of all strokes) and subarachnoid haemorrhage (SAH) (5% of all strokes) (Therapeutic Guidelines Limited, 2011). Both types of haemorrhagic stroke occur due to ruptured blood vessels. This can be attributed to trauma but more commonly it is weakened cerebral vessels as a result of atherosclerotic changes, hypertension, congenital malformations and a mixture of previous causes or can also be idiopathic.

SAH affects approximately 6.5 people per 100 000 throughout Australia and New Zealand every year (Brophy et al., 2000) with devastating effects. Usually SAH is caused by a weakened blood vessel which may be berry-like in shape, have an appearance of a general weakening of one particular area (fusiform) or by arteriovenous malformation (AVM). An AVM affects cerebral vasculature in such as way that it is both arterial and venous in nature. This 'mixed' circulation causes the vessels to develop into multiple fistula-like formations that also drastically weaken them, particularly to increases of pressure. Once ruptured there is an increased risk of re-bleed shortly after the initial event as well as cerebral vasospasm (which can induce an ischaemic stroke up to 28 days post initial SAH), hydrocephalus and hyponatraemia associated with the initial and any subsequent bleeds (Diringer, 2009).

ACUTE STROKE CARE

Once the stroke has been defined as being ischaemic or haemorrhagic, ongoing treatment is determined. The two types of stroke require very different approaches to care as there are contraindications for some treatment modalities in both. Despite the differences in approach, however, there is clear evidence in both cases for the need for specialist stroke care, usually in the form of a dedicated stroke unit within a large public hospital. These units are characterised by a focus on rapid, thorough assessment and early management, utilising a multidisciplinary team (Adams et al., 2007; Hachinski et al., 2010; National Stroke Foundation, 2010). Well-established evidence supports the existence of these units, which have been shown to improve overall patient outcomes (Lakhan & Sapko, 2009) by reducing associated mortality by approximately 20%; in comparison with less organised services these specialised units also have reduced rates of morbidity (Lakhan & Sapko, 2009; Therapeutic Guidelines Limited, 2011).

Ischaemic stroke care

The principles of ischaemic stroke care are to reduce and try to re-establish cerebral health; prevent any further formation of clots, cerebral oedema, increase cerebral perfusion, control for pain and protect from further damage the area of the body that now has the resultant neurological deficit.

Acute treatment for ischaemic stroke requires initial dissolving of the clot (thrombosis or embolism) in the acute stage, commonly referred to as thrombolytic or 'clot buster' therapy, but this must be administered within a very short period after onset of symptoms Intravenous alteplase (t-PA) has been shown to improve long-term outcomes in both morbidity and mortality for selected patients (van der Worp & van Gijn, 2007). The criteria for determining who is eligible for t-PA are as follows:

- ischaemic stroke confirmed (by CT or MRI scan)
- onset of symptoms is within the previous three hours
- no major changes of early ischaemia (on CT or MRI scan)
- no other contraindication for thrombolytic therapy:
  - bleeding disorder
  - recent peptic ulceration
  - serious medical condition
  - recent surgery
- the availability of a specialised stroke unit or high dependency unit care
- aggressive treatment of hypertension
  - close monitoring of blood pressure
- neurological assessment
  - close monitoring for at least 24 hours post-infusion. (National Stroke Foundation, 2010; Therapeutic Guidelines Limited, 2011)

The use of aspirin within 48 hours of ischaemic stroke has been shown to reduce mortality/morbidity to approximately one death or recurrent stroke per 100 people in the first few weeks (Therapeutic Guidelines Limited, 2011). Aspirin works by inhibiting thromboxanes, which are substances that influence platelet aggregation and thus clot formation. However, aspirin cannot be used in conjunction with thrombolytic therapies.

Secondary prevention

Follow-up therapy has shown to decrease the likelihood of future strokes. It is termed secondary prevention, while primary prevention is used to prevent initial stroke.

Secondary prevention usually involves (Davis & Donnan, 2012; Therapeutic Guidelines Limited, 2011):

- anti-platelet therapy
  - aspirin or clopidogrel
- anti-hypertension therapy, if hypertension is evident
- anti-coagulation, if atrial fibrillation is diagnosed
- smoking cessation
- treatment of hypercholesterolaemia
- carotid endarterectomy, for carotid stenosis.

Haemorrhagic stroke care

The principles of haemorrhagic stroke care are to correct the site of rupture (if possible), reduce any associated intracranial pressure and cerebral oedema, manage the unconscious patient, maintain airways and breathing and reduce pain from headache.

Once the stroke is identified as haemorrhagic stroke consultation is sought by the patient's parent unit (usually a medical or dedicated stroke unit) for neurosurgical services for intervention. If a clearly defined cause is apparent though diagnosis investigation, be it an aneurysm or AVM, then corrective surgery, such as clipping on endovascular coiling of the damaged vessel, is an option. If there is no clear reason for the haemorrhage, further investigation is warranted. Regardless of the outcome of the investigations, aggressive blood pressure lowering must be initiated to reduce haematoma expansion (Bederson et al., 2009; Therapeutic Guidelines Limited, 2011). However, if the bleed is large, a craniectomy and evacuation of the clot, or drainage of bloodstained cerebrospinal fluid (which may cause hydrocephalus) through the insertion of an external ventricular drain, may need to be performed to relieve pressure on the already damaged brain. Those suffering from an SAH of aneurysmal origin are at an increased risk of cerebral vasospasm, which may cause further stroke. Cerebral vasospasm should be aggressively treated and once an aneurysm is stabilised hypertensive and hypervolumic therapy should be commenced to improve perfusion and dilation of cerebral vessels (Therapeutic Guidelines Limited, 2011).

REHABILITATION

Approximately 25% to 30% of stroke patients are candidates for comprehensive inpatient rehabilitation (Good, Bettermann, & Reichwein, 2011). Stroke rehabilitation is individual to each patient and is dependent on a number of factors including the type of stroke (ischaemic or haemorrhagic), pre-existing co-morbidities and/or risk factors and initiation of appropriate treatment and complications immediately after the stroke. However, there are some common problems that are universal to stroke rehabilitation.

- Movement:
  - limb spasticity or contracture
  - loss of motor strength or sensation
  - loss of balance

- dysphagia
- DVT prevention
- pressure sore prevention.
- Cognition:
  - changes in attention span or memory
  - agnosia or apraxia
  - aphasia
  - mood changes
  - depression
  - incontinence.

Therefore, rehabilitation and discharge planning should be directed at achieving maximum level of function to undertake the activities of daily living, drive, return to work, pursue leisure activities and lead a sexual life (National Stroke Foundation, 2010). It may be that maximal recovery will not be achieved because of a lack of services available in some areas of Australia and internationally (Hachinski et al., 2010) and so the nurse has a responsibility to ensure that the patient has been put in touch with as many services as possible prior to discharge.

Apart from ongoing physical therapy, the patient will also need ongoing services in relation to respite care, outpatient visits to speech and occupational therapy and perhaps assistance with home duties or cooking (Good et al., 2011). The nurse discharging the patient will have an important role in facilitating the forging of these links to ensure ongoing care is delivered and so make the transition to home successful.

Brain repair and recovery after stroke involves a process of axonal sprouting in connected cortical neurons and in basic terms occurs when neural connections take over lost functions secondary to stroke (Benowitz & Carmichael, 2010; Carmichael, 2010). As a result a reorganisation of motor, sensory, language and other cognitive operations within the brain can occur (Benowitz & Carmichael, 2010). This is possibly further facilitated by skill learning through rehabilitation exercises.

Physical repair and functional recovery commonly occurs in the weeks and months after stroke (Benowitz & Carmichael, 2010). The extent of this recovery will be initially determined by the resolution of the ischaemic area surrounding the infarction and the ability of the brain to reorganise in such a way that new areas of the brain can perform functions originally performed by the now damaged area.

Better results seem to correlate with early and frequent practice of simple skills that stimulate the use of the affected muscle groups (Krakauer, 2006). Indeed, Krakauer referred to research that demonstrates that recovery is maximised when the skills that are designed to be practised can be varied in some way (e.g. reaching for a glass and reaching for a toothbrush) and so enabling memory about more general applications of the skill that then can be applied to activities of daily living. Further, success may be achieved if the practice sessions are punctuated with rest periods that are more frequent and longer as time goes on, allowing motor memory of these activities to be formed.

The recovery phase is characterised by a reduction in cerebral oedema and an increased activation of the neuronal network (Rijntjes, 2006). There is an initial increased neuronal activity of the unaffected side which, when this level of activity has peaked, is then followed by increased neuronal activity of the affected side (Rijntjes, 2006). This activity seems to be at the basis of reorganisation. Reorganisation of the brain involves areas of the brain performing functions they did not previously perform (Krakauer, 2006).

Thus recovery is the result of several factors: spontaneous recovery of areas that were previously swollen but not damaged; focused rehabilitation activities to facilitate motor learning; and compensation, which is the use of alternative muscle groups to achieve the same end; for example, using the right hand instead of the left to pick something up. For motor recovery, for example, the stroke sufferer needs to learn the sequence of movements along with velocity, which is achieved by using visual and proprioceptive cues (Krakauer, 2006).

The result is to reduce the level of physical impairment through the minimisation of cerebral damage. In addition, the rehabilitation process assists the sufferer to overcome the consequences of any residual physical impairment through reorganisation or motor learning.

The nurse's role in rehabilitation comprises numerous functions and brings a distinctive holistic perspective to the patient care process (Miller et al., 2010). As the Australian Nurse and Midwifery Council (ANMC) competency standard for the RN describes, a RN:

> ... provides evidence-based nursing ... includes promotion and maintenance of health and prevention of illness for individual/s with physical or mental illness ... as well as alleviation of pain and suffering at the end stage of life.
>
> ... assesses, plans, implements and evaluates nursing care in collaboration with individual/s and the multidisciplinary healthcare team so as to achieve goals and health outcomes ...
>
> ... provides care in a range of settings that may include acute, community, residential and extended care settings ... modifies practice according to the model/s of care delivery.
>
> ... [assumes] a leadership role in the coordination of nursing and healthcare within and across different care contexts to facilitate optimal health outcomes ... contributes to quality healthcare through lifelong learning and professional development of herself/himself and others, research data generation, clinical supervision and development of policy and clinical practice guidelines ... (Australian Nursing and Midwifery Council, 2006; Nursing and Midwifery Board of Australia, 2010).

As members of the interdisciplinary rehabilitation team, registered nurses are responsible for identifying, developing and then implementing treatment plans to address therapy goals for stroke survivors. This is in addition to their role in the management of co-morbid existing conditions (that were present) prior to, complicated by or directly attributed to the stroke (Miller et al., 2010).

CASE STUDY 16.1 Ischaemic Stroke

Barbara presented with left-sided weakness involving her face and upper and lower limbs, and dysarthria after going to the toilet to use her bowels. Barbara is a 68-year-old female with a past history of hypertension, hypercholesterolaemia, paroxysmal atrial fibrillation and type 2 diabetes mellitus.

Non-contrast scans of the brain followed by a CT perfusion of the brain demonstrate no evidence of acute intracranial haemorrhage, but a chronic lacunar infarct is seen as well as a possible left posterior cerebral artery infarct. As she met all the criteria for thrombolysis therapy (t-PA) she was administered within 2 hours of onset of symptoms.

Barbara's dysarthria improved within 2 hours of thrombolysis, however she had ongoing problems with balance and coordination but not strength. She was admitted to rehabilitation and was discharged after 14 days. She had outpatient follow-up organised for the stroke prevention clinic to plan secondary prevention measures.

CASE STUDY 16.2 Haemorrhagic Stroke

Tri is a 49-year-old man of Vietnamese origin who was brought in by ambulance from home to a major metropolitan hospital after being found by his wife collapsed on the floor next to a pool of vomit at 2330 hours. Tri has a past history of hypertension, hypercholesterolaemia, is an ex intravenous drug user and is hepatitis C positive. At the time of referral, his Glasgow Coma Scale (GCS) score was 6 with both pupils at about 2–3 mm, with minimal reaction. He was hypertensive at about 270 mmHg systolic. After initial assessment, he was intubated and a CT scan and CT angiogram showed extensive intraventricular haemorrhage arising from a possibly ruptured anterior communication artery aneurysm.

After a discussion with Tri's wife, it was decided to perform bi-frontal EVDs to try and reduce the pressure and drain off the intraventricular blood. On day two he experienced a tonic clonic seizure and was commenced on anticonvulsant therapy. On day seven he deteriorated neurologically and underwent digital subtraction angiography and injection of nimodipine intra-arterially as he developed cerebral vasospasm. On day 9 he had a tracheotomy tube inserted as he was unable to maintain his own airway. On day 12 he became febrile from an unknown source and was commenced on vancomycin and ceftriaxone empirically. On day 21 he was transferred to the ward as he clinically improved to GCS 10. On day 24 he neurologically deteriorated and a MET call was initiated. It was then it was decided that he was for palliative care. This was discussed at length with the family at which time it was pointed out there would be no functional gains and they were given a poor prognosis on his survival. The family agreed for him to be transferred to the palliative care unit. All invasive therapies were ceased and he was commenced on a Graseby pump of methadone and midazolam. He was transferred to the palliative care unit 2 days after and died at day 40 post initial presentation.

Reflective questions

1. List three nursing interventions and their rationales that you as a nurse can initiate to lessen the effects of stroke.
2. Name the types of stroke and the usual treatment options available for them.
3. In acute clinical practice what are the main secondary preventions which you can implement for your patients post stroke?

CONCLUSION

The statistics on stroke and its associated mortality and morbidity are alarming. As a consequence, stroke prevention, early diagnosis and appropriate treatment and rehabilitation are understandably national priorities, attracting significant government funding and expert clinician input into best practice. As nurses it is our moral duty to provide best-practice care to patients, as well as appropriate information and ongoing education about their condition to them and their loved ones, along with information about reasonable steps that can be taken to alleviate possible complications.

Acknowledgments: thanks to James Kevin, for his contribution to the original chapter as well as Bronwyn Coulton, nurse practitioner candidate, for her contribution to ischaemic stroke case study.

Recommended reading

Bederson, J. B., Connolly, E. S., Jr., Batjer, H. H., et al. (2009). Guidelines for the management of aneurysmal subarachnoid haemorrhage: a statement for healthcare professionals from a special writing group of the Stroke Council, American Heart Association. *Stroke*, *40*(3), 994–1025.

Gallanagh, S., Quinn, T. J., Alexander, J., et al. (2011). Physical activity in the prevention and treatment of stroke. *ISRN Neurology, 2011*, 953818.

Miller, E. L., Murray, L., Richards, L., et al. (2010). Comprehensive overview of nursing and interdisciplinary rehabilitation care of the stroke patient. *Stroke*, *41*(10), 2402–2448.

National Stroke Foundation. (2010). Clinical guidelines for stroke management 2010. Available from http://www.strokefoundation.com.au/pages/Default.aspx?PageID=192&id=1

Summers, D., Leonard, A., Wentworth, D., et al. (2009). Comprehensive overview of nursing and interdisciplinary care of the acute ischemic stroke patient: a scientific statement from the American Heart Association (guideline review). *Stroke; A Journal of Cerebral Circulation*, *40*(8), 2911–2944.

References

Adams, H. P., Jr., del Zoppo, G., Alberts, M. J., et al. (2007). Guidelines for the early management of adults with ischemic stroke: A guideline from the American Heart Association/American Stroke Association Stroke Council, Clinical Cardiology Council, Cardiovascular Radiology and Intervention Council, and the Atherosclerotic Peripheral Vascular Disease and Quality of Care Outcomes in Research Interdisciplinary Working Groups: the American Academy of Neurology affirms the value of this guideline as an educational tool for neurologists [practice guideline]. *Stroke*, *38*(5), 1655–1711.

Altaf, N., MacSweeney, S. T., Gladman, J., et al. (2007). Carotid intraplaque hemorrhage predicts recurrent symptoms in patients with high-grade carotid stenosis. *Stroke*, *38*(5), 1633–1635. PubMed PMID: 17379827.

Australian Bureau of Statistics. (2012). Causes of death, Australia 2010. Retrieved 12 June, 2012, from http://www.abs.gov.au/AUSSTATS/abs@.nsf/ProductsbyReleaseDate/9E7B7AFA9DF69E20CA2571F60017A972?OpenDocument

Australian Institute of Health and Welfare. (2006). *Chronic diseases and associated risk factors in Australia, 2006*. Cat no PHE 81. Canberra: Author.

Australian Institute of Health and Welfare. (2008). *Cardiovascular disease and its associated risk factors in Aboriginal and Torres Strait Islander peoples 2004–2005*. Canberra: Author.

Australian Institute of Health and Welfare. (2012). Separation statistics by principal diagnosis in ICD-10-AM, Australia, 2008–09 to 2009–2010. Retrieved June 30, 2012, from http://www.aihw.gov.au/hospitals-data-cube/?id=10737419429

Australian Nursing and Midwifery Council. (2006). *National competency standards for the Registered Nurse*. Dickson: Author.

Baird, T. A., Parsons, M. W., Phanh, T., et al. (2003). Persistent post-stroke hyperglycemia is independently associated with infarct expansion and worse clinical outcome. *Stroke*, *34*(9), 2208–2214. PubMed PMID: 12893952.

Bederson, J. B., Connolly, E. S., Jr., Batjer, H. H., et al. (2009). Guidelines for the management of aneurysmal subarachnoid hemorrhage: a statement for healthcare professionals from a special writing group of the Stroke Council, American Heart Association. *Stroke*, *40*(3), 994–1025.

Benowitz, L. I., & Carmichael, S. T. (2010). Promoting axonal rewiring to improve outcome after stroke. [Research Support, N.I.H., Extramural Research Support, Non-U.S. Gov't Research Support, U.S. Gov't, P.H.S.] *JAMA*, *290*(8), 1049–1056.

Brophy, B. P., Riddell, J., Mee, E., et al. (2000). Epidemiology of aneurysmal subarachnoid hemorrhage in Australia and New Zealand: incidence and case fatality from the Australasian Cooperative Research on Subarachnoid Hemorrhage Study (ACROSS). *Stroke*, *31*, 1843–1850.

Carmichael, S. T. (2010). Targets for neural repair therapies after stroke. [Research Support, N.I.H., Extramural Research Support, Non-U.S. Gov't Review.] *Stroke*, *41*(10 Suppl), S124–S126.

Chen, H. J., Bai, C. H., Yeh, W. T., et al. (2006). Influence of metabolic syndrome and general obesity on the risk of ischemic stroke. [Research Support, Non-U.S. Gov't.] *Stroke*, *37*(4), 1060–1064.

Davis, S. M., & Donnan, G. A. (2012). Clinical practice. Secondary prevention after ischemic stroke or transient ischemic attack. [Review.] *The New England Journal of Medicine*, *366*(20), 1914–1922.

Diringer, M. N. (2009). Management of aneurysmal subarachnoid hemorrhage. *Critical Care Medicine*, *37*(2), 432.

Donnan, G. A., Fisher, M., Macleod, M., et al. (2008). Stroke. [Review.] *Lancet*, *371*(9624), 1612–1623.

Feigin, V., Carter, K., Hackett, M., et al. (2006). Ethnic disparities in incidence of stroke subtypes: Auckland regional community stroke study, 2002–2003. [Research Support, Non-U.S. Gov't.] *Lancet Neurology*, *5*(2), 130–139.

Frizzell, J. P. (2005). Acute stroke: pathophysiology, diagnosis, and treatment. [Review.] *AACN Clinical Issues*, *16*(4), 421–440; quiz 597–598.

Gallanagh, S., Quinn, T. J., Alexander, J., et al. (2011). Physical activity in the prevention and treatment of stroke. *ISRN Neurology*, *2011*, 953818.

Gargano, J. W., & Reeves, M. J. (2007). Sex differences in stroke recovery and stroke-specific quality of life: results from a statewide stroke registry. [Research Support, Non-U.S. Gov't Research Support, U.S. Gov't, P.H.S.] *Stroke; A Journal of Cerebral Circulation*, *38*(9), 2541–2548.

Giles, M. F., & Rothwell, P. M. (2007). Risk of stroke early after transient ischaemic attack: a systematic review and meta-analysis. [Research Support, Non-U.S. Gov't Review.] *Lancet Neurology*, *6*(12), 1063–1072.

Giles, M. F., & Rothwell, P. M. (2009). Transient ischaemic attack: clinical relevance, risk prediction and urgency of secondary prevention. [Review.] *Current Opinion in Neurology*, *22*(1), 46–53.

Giorda, C. B., Avogaro, A., Maggini, M., et al. (2007). Incidence and risk factors for stroke in type 2 diabetic patients: the DAI study. [Multicenter Study.] *Stroke*, *38*(4), 1154–1160.

Goldstein, L. B., & Hankey, G. J. (2006). Advances in primary stroke prevention. [Research Support, N.I.H., Extramural Research Support, Non-U.S. Gov't Research Support, U.S. Gov't, Non-P.H.S. Review.] *Stroke*, *37*(2), 317–319.

Good, D. C., Bettermann, K., & Reichwein, R. K. (2011). Stroke rehabilitation. *CONTINUUM: Lifelong Learning in Neurology*, *17*(3 Neurorehabilitation), 545–567.

Goss, J. (2008). Projection of Australian health care expenditure by disease, 2003 to 2033. *Health and Welfare Expenditure Series*, Number 36.

Hachinski, V., Donnan, G. A., Gorelick, P. B., et al. (2010). Stroke: working toward a prioritized world agenda. [Review.] *Stroke*, *41*(6), 1084–1099.

Iadecola, C., Park, L., & Capone, C. (2009). Threats to the mind: aging, amyloid, and hypertension. *Stroke*, *40*(Suppl. 3), S40–S44.

Krakauer, J. W. (2006). Motor learning: its relevance to stroke recovery and neurorehabilitation. *Current Opinion in Neurology*, *19*(1), 84–90.

Lakhan, S. E., & Sapko, M. T. (2009). Blood pressure lowering treatment for preventing stroke recurrence: a systematic review and meta-analysis. *International Archives of Medicine*, *2*(1), 30.

Lloyd-Jones, D., Adams, R. J., Brown, T. M., et al. (2010). Heart disease and stroke statistics — 2010 update. *Circulation, 121*(7), e46–e215.

Miller, E. L., Murray, L., Richards, L., et al. (2010). Comprehensive overview of nursing and interdisciplinary rehabilitation care of the stroke patient. *Stroke, 41*(10), 2402–2448.

Nahed, B. V., Bydon, M., Ozturk, A. K., et al. (2007). Genetics of intracranial aneurysms. *Neurosurgery, 60*(2), 213–225; discussion 225–216.

National Health Priority Action Council. (2006). *National service improvement: Framework for heart, stroke and vascular disease.* Canberra: Australian Government Department of Health & Ageing.

National Stroke Foundation. (2010). Clinical guidelines for stroke management 2010. Retrieved May 8, 2013, from http://www.strokefoundation.com.au/pages/Default.aspx?PageID=192&id=1

National Stroke Foundation. (2012a). Signs of stroke — FAST. *FAST.* Retrieved July 25, 2012, from http://strokefoundation.com.au/event/signs-of-stroke-fast-3/

National Stroke Foundation. (2012b). Signs of Stroke — FAST. *FAST.* Retrieved May 27, 2012, from http://strokefoundation.com.au/what-is-a-stroke/signs-of-stroke/

Nursing and Midwifery Board of Australia. (2010). Recency of practice registration standard. *Codes and Guidelines.* Retrieved May 1, 2011, from http://www.nursingmidwiferyboard.gov.au/documents/default.aspx?record=WD10%2f142&dbid=AP&chksum=BFUtVLcmL7kAJIZY06vrrg%3d%3d

Prinz, V., & Endres, M. (2011). Statins and stroke: prevention and beyond. [Research Support, Non-U.S. Gov't Review.] *Current Opinion in Neurology, 24*(1), 75–80.

Reynolds, K., Lewis, B., Nolen, J. D., et al. (2003). Alcohol consumption and risk of stroke: a meta-analysis. [Erratum appears in *JAMA.* 2003 Jun 4, *289*(21), 2798.] [Meta-Analysis Research Support, U.S. Gov't, P.H.S.] *JAMA: The Journal of the American Medical Association, 289*(5), 579–2588.

Rijntjes, M. (2006). Mechanisms of recovery in stroke patients with hemiparesis or aphasia: new insights, old questions and the meaning of therapies. *Current Opinion in Neurology, 19*(1), 76–83.

Scanlon, A. (2006). Nursing and the 5As guideline to smoking cessation interventions. *Australian Nursing Journal*, Oct, *14*(5), 25–28.

Scanlon, A., & Lee, G. (2007). The use of the term 'vulnerability' in acute care. Why does it differ and what does it mean? *Australian Journal of Advanced Nursing, 24*(3), 54–59.

Therapeutic Guidelines Limited. (2011). *Stroke, Therapeutic Guidelines: Neurology, version 4, 2011 (Vol. 2007).* West Melbourne: Therapeutic Guidelines Limited.

Towfighi, A., Saver, J. L., Engelhardt, R., et al. (2007). A midlife stroke surge among women in the United States. [Comparative Study.] *Neurology, 69*(20), 1898–1904.

van der Worp, H., B., & van Gijn, J. (2007). Acute Ischemic Stroke. *New England Journal of Medicine, 357*(21), 2203–2204.

Wang, T. J., Massaro, J. M., Levy, D., et al. (2003). A risk score for predicting stroke or death in individuals with new-onset atrial fibrillation in the community: the Framingham Heart Study. [Research Support, Non-U.S. Gov't Review]. *Neurobiology of Disease, 37*(2), 259–266.

Wardlaw, J. M., Keir, S. L., Seymour, J., et al. (2004). What is the best imaging strategy for acute stroke? [Comparative Study Review.] *Health Technology Assessment (Winchester, England), 8*(1), iii.

World Health Organization, World Heart Federation, & World Stroke Organization. (2011). *Global Atlas on cardiovascular disease prevention and control.* S. Mendis, P. Puska, & B. Norrving (Eds.). Geneva: World Health Organization.

Yakubovich, N., & Gerstein, H. C. (2011). Serious cardiovascular outcomes in diabetes: the role of hypoglycemia. [Research Support, Non-U.S. Gov't Review.] *Circulation, 123*(3), 342–348.

CHAPTER 17

Robin Ray
Anne Kavanagh
(with contributions from Laraine McAnally)

Parkinson's disease, multiple sclerosis and motor neuron disease

Learning objectives

When you have completed this chapter you will be able to:

- describe the symptoms of Parkinson's disease (PD), multiple sclerosis (MS) and motor neuron disease (MND) and some of the treatments used to manage these diseases
- discuss the possible impact each disease may have on the person living with PD, MS or MND
- discuss the possible challenges faced by family and/or friends in providing in-home care for people living with PD, MS or MND
- explain the importance of assessing the individual needs and providing an interdisciplinary approach to supportive care
- discuss relevant strategies that would enable people and their carers to live well with neurodegeneration.

Key words

degenerative, mobility, interdisciplinary team, neurological, supportive care

INTRODUCTION

The three neurological diseases featured in this chapter — Parkinson's disease (PD), multiple sclerosis (MS) and motor neuron disease (MND) — are all progressive disorders of motor function, with sensory function also affected in MS. Additionally, each disease has specific non-motor symptoms. Study of these three neurological diseases reveals that they have some initial symptoms in common, especially those associated with movement, highlighting the need for careful diagnosis. Following a stressful and sometimes frustrating period of hypothesising and indecision, symptomatic people and their families are confronted with a devastating, often life-limiting diagnosis.

Progressive neurological diseases present unique lifestyle challenges for the person and their carers living in the community. Every case is different and each person has their own cultural and social understanding of illness, its impact and the eventual end-of-life process. People with the disease and their carers become very knowledgeable about disease management. This expertise must be recognised and valued by nurses and other members of the healthcare team (Forbes, While, & Taylor, 2007; Heisters, 2007). In this chapter, case studies have been provided to develop nurses' insight into the individual manner in which each disease may affect a person's life, their family and their relationships with the community.

Providing care for people with any of these neurological diseases is very challenging, not only because of the complex and sometimes confronting symptomatology, but also the variable presentation of motor and non-motor signs in each person. An interdisciplinary approach to care is recognised as the preferred model, with nursing as a key discipline coordinating and providing care, facilitating advanced care planning, giving advice, support and education and monitoring the effect of medication. Effective care will only occur if nurses are prepared to work with other members of an interdisciplinary team and family carers to continually assess individual needs and collaboratively plan relevant supportive care, including timely access to community resources and end-of-life care.

PARKINSON'S DISEASE

In 1817, after the publication of his 'Essay on a shaking palsy', James Parkinson gave his name to the condition we now know as Parkinson's disease. PD is a chronic, degenerative neurological disorder, the second most common neurodegenerative condition after Alzheimer's disease (Australian Bureau of Statistics [ABS], 2010). At the time of diagnosis, there is an estimated loss of around 60% of dopamine-producing cells in the substantia nigra of the mid-brain, causing a loss of dopamine in the brain (Przedborski, 2007). Dopamine is an important neurotransmitter in the basal ganglia, a collection of very specialised brain cells at the base of the brain that are responsible for the modulation of movement. Loss of dopaminergic neurons has been found in other parts of the body, for instance in the gut, causing gastrointestinal dysfunction (Anderson et al., 2007), and in the olfactory tract, causing partial loss of smell (Micieli, Tosi, Marcheselli, & Cavallini, 2003).

Despite extensive research, the cause of PD remains unknown. However, there are recognised risk factors such as ageing, exposure to certain pesticides, head trauma, gender (more males than females), anaemia in women and genetics; while coffee consumption has been reported as a protective factor (Przedborski, 2007; Savica, Grossardt, Bower, Ahlskog, & Rocca, in press). PD is sporadic in more than 90% of cases, with no known familial or genetic risk factors (Przedborski, 2007). However, five genes have been identified for PD in a small percentage of people (Tan & Skipper, 2007). Although PD is seen in all age groups its incidence increases with age. The 17% increase in diagnoses of PD over the last 5 years — 54 700 to 64 000 (Deloitte Access Economics, 2011) or 1 : 350 Australians, and 8000 to 10 000 or 1 : 500 New Zealanders (Parkinsonism Society of New Zealand, 2012) — reflects the increasing percentage of the population in the older age groups. The median age at diagnosis is 59 years while the median age of death is 83.3 years with more males dying of PD than females (ABS, 2010).

Applying the United Kingdom Parkinson's Disease Society Brain Bank diagnostic criteria, Parkinson's disease is suspected when the person presents with bradykinesia — indicative of Parkinsonism and one of the following: muscular rigidity, resting tremor or postural instability. Stroke, head injury and encephalitis need to be excluded and other supporting criteria met before a diagnosis can be established (Hughes, Daniel, Kilford, & Lees, 1992). While PD has varied symptomatology, it usually presents asymmetrically. The signs of PD are divided into motor and non-motor.

Motor:

- the classical triad of (resting) tremor, rigidity (muscular stiffness) and akinesia (slowness and difficulty in initiating movement)
- flexion on the trunk, gait difficulties with shuffling and freezing and reduced arm swing
- akinesia results in difficulty turning in bed, small handwriting and a soft voice, which is difficult to understand (see secretary's comments regarding Bill in Case Study 17.1).

Non–motor:

- autonomic symptoms — postural hypotension, abnormal sweating
- urinary and bowel dysfunction, sexual difficulties
- cognitive decline, depression and anxiety
- sleep disturbances, fatigue
- loss of smell (anosmia)
- sensory phenomena, including pain not responsive to analgesia if caused by a lack of levodopa.

When functional disability affects quality of life, medications such as levodopa are used to treat dopamine deficiency, with no effect on the degenerative course of this disease. However, clinical trials are currently being conducted into the use of neuroprotective substances such as antioxidants to slow the progression of PD (Mythri & Bharath, 2012).

As PD progresses people find that the medication effects wear off between doses, signalling further degeneration. Since the 1980s deep brain stimulation (DBS) has been used to improve the advanced PD symptoms that respond to levodopa medication effects, but has no benefit for non-motor symptoms such as cognitive decline. Stimulation of the subthalamic nucleus has been found to improve a range of PD symptoms such as tremor, gait,

CASE STUDY 17.1

Bill was born in Wagga Wagga, NSW in 1944, while his father was serving in the Air Force during World War II. After the war, they returned to Coolangatta where Bill spent long periods surfing and swimming. He attended the local school then boarding school at 12 years of age. Bill worked with the Justice Department and the Courts for 13 years. During this time he married Jenny and they had three children. With further study Bill became a solicitor and then a partner in a commercial law firm after just 3 years. Throughout his working life, Bill had several changes of employment while continuing community involvement, especially volunteering with Surf Lifesaving.

CASE STUDY 17.1 — cont'd

Bill had been fairly fit, normotensive and generally well, but always overweight. He worked long hours, but by mid 2000s he realised he was producing less and not coping. He had a series of visits to a psychologist who identified issues which Bill thought were beyond resolution and causing depression. Bill's depression wasn't going away and he also noticed that stress in the legal practice and in the family was contributing to his problems with organisational skills. His wife Jenny was having difficulty understanding his speech. Handwriting was becoming more of a chore and harder to read. Bill's secretary confirmed the deterioration in handwriting and dictation voice levels. In 2009, a psychiatrist prescribed Lexapro 100 mg daily (currently 150 mg) and also Lumin (10 mg per day) and gave Bill some research material on Parkinson's disease (PD). The research pointed to other aspects of his condition that had not been noted, but were certainly present. Bill thought he might be a future candidate for PD, but his GP did not think he could diagnose PD at the time because Bill's gait was not consistent with that diagnosis (refer to the UK PD Society Brain Bank diagnostic criteria). Bill's own research identified a number of seemingly innocent habits that correlated with PD symptoms.

Bill's GP referred him to a specialist doctor dealing with PD. The doctor diagnosed PD and prescribed 3 Kinson tablets (levodopa 100 mg, carbidopa [anhydrous] 25 mg) which eased the symptoms. This dose has been bolstered over the intervening time to 4.5 Kinson tablets per day, Comtan (entacapone) 600 mg daily and Symmetrel 100 mg daily. With medication, Bill's right hand tremors have improved, while his left hand weakness and fine motor skills are gradually worsening. He can write legibly if he concentrates and his organisational skills have improved slightly. Speech therapy has enhanced his voice projection, but slurring of words and stammering is happening more often. His eyesight is weakening, yet he still hears well. Mobility challenges are increasing: Bill favours bending forward, has a shuffle gait, 'sticky feet', leans to the right and is experiencing balance problems particularly near water, which have led to a couple of recent falls. He has little control over a continuous heel/toe motion in right leg while sitting, unless asleep. He often exhibits a face mask expression resulting from rigidity of facial muscles. Bill finds that he is sleeping more and experiencing hallucinations and illusions. He wonders if this might be a side effect of the drugs he is taking.

Swimming sessions, no matter how strenuous, set Bill up for the day and make him feel better overall. He finds physical and spiritual fulfilment from tai chi exercises; particularly posture and balance enhancement. Bill loves fishing but tackle tasks are almost impossible due to left hand weakness and lack of fine motor skills. Additionally, he is disinclined to interrupt his mates to do these tasks for him. The motion of the boat in even the calmest of conditions causes extreme discomfort across the lower back and stomach (core muscles), so unfortunately fishing is likely to fade out of his life.

Consistent with his self-management approach, Bill is keen to learn more about PD while continuing his regimen of exercise and medication. He is researching deep brain stimulation (DBS) and considering his options. Meanwhile, Bill heads up the Parkinson's Support Group in a regional city and was a key player in organising a recent symposium on DBS.

rigidity, bradykinesia and improve sleep (Rodriguez-Proz, Matsubara, Clavero, Guridi, & Obeso, 2009). The positive effects of DBS are evident in this patient anecdote. Garry described how 'continual shakes and legs that felt like concrete' were alleviated by DBS enabling him to relax for the first time in 10 years. He now travels to the capital city to have 6 monthly appointments to adjust the controls. Currently, Garry is free from shakes and aches, except when he gets anxious or expects his body to do too much. Despite these improvements, DBS has little effect on speech and can induce paraesthesia (Fasano, Daniele, & Albanese, 2012). Not all people living with PD will benefit from DBS.

Altered mobility and fatigue

Fatigue is a common but not well-understood symptom of PD. However, it does not affect all people with PD and is not always directly related to function or stage of disease (Friedman et al., 2007). Sleep disturbances, the high incidence of depression and some PD medications can result in daytime tiredness. Therefore, it is important to monitor and treat, where possible, these extraneous factors. Fatigue has to be considered, as well as 'on' and 'off' states, when planning the daily routine.

People with PD have different levels of motor function depending on whether they are in the 'off' or 'on' states. The 'off' state describes the patient when the signs and symptoms of PD are most obvious, while the 'on' state describes the best the person can achieve with PD medications. The same patient who requires full care in feeding, showering and transferring may be able to manage their care independently or with assistance in the 'on' state, after their medications take effect. Speech is an exception as a positive medication impact on functional speech intelligibility has not been established (Sapir, Ramig, & Fox, 2008). Difficulty with gait, posture and balance means that mobility is often compromised, and showering, toileting and ambulating require careful assessment by a physiotherapist and an occupational therapist (OT) where available. Measures can then be put in place to accommodate the individual mobility limitations and the person can achieve a measure of independence within safety limits. As the disease progresses, balance often deteriorates and falls are common. Walking aids may be required after review from the physiotherapist. To enable the person to realise their daily goals, their routine needs to be planned around the 'on' time.

Dopamine replacement, in the form of levodopa combined with a dopa decarboxylase inhibitor to prevent the peripheral side effects of levodopa (such as Sinemet, Madopar or Kinson), remains the first-line treatment for PD. At the onset of PD this medication often returns the person close to a normal baseline, but with disease progression many people find that the 'on' time shortens, leading to motor fluctuations complicated by chorea-like involuntary movements called 'dyskinesias'. It is important to differentiate tremor from dyskinesia to ensure that correct treatment options are considered. Other PD drug therapies include synthetic dopamine agonists (pramipexole; pergolide; bromocriptine; cabergoline; and apomorphine), which act on the dopamine receptor sites with a similar but weaker action, except for apomorphine. Apomorphine, a by-product of morphine without opiate activity, is an injectable dopamine agonist that has a comparable effect to levodopa. It can be used as an injection to rescue the person from 'off ' states or as an infusion for management of symptomatology. Postural hypotension is common with this group of medications and they are more likely to cause hallucinations in susceptible patients (refer to Case Study 17.1). Obsessional behaviours such as hyper-sexuality, excessive eating and excessive gambling are recognised as side effects of levodopa and dopamine agonist therapy in susceptible patients (Avanzi et al., 2006).

The COMT inhibitor (entacapone) prevents the rapid uptake of levodopa, thus allowing a longer effect time. A combination drug (levodopa/carbidopa/entacapone) is also available. Anti-cholinergic drugs (benzhexol, benztropin, biperidin) are rarely used because of their many side effects and limited benefit. Amantidine has a mild benefit in motor symptoms and is more useful in controlling dyskinesias.

It is crucial that PD medications, in particular levodopa, are given on time, as delay may cause much discomfort as well as a reduction in the level of function. Dietary protein can interfere with the absorption of medications. Thus medications should be given at least 30 minutes before food, wherever possible. Timing of the effect of medication is important and can be measured with PD diaries, where motor fluctuations and dyskinesias (which are a side effect of long-term dopamine replacement), as well as 'on' and 'off' states, can be documented.

PD medications should not be stopped or drastically reduced abruptly, as this can lead to a rare but life-threatening condition called neuroleptic malignant syndrome (Ward, 2005). This syndrome is associated with worsening of Parkinsonian signs, altered mental state, hyperpyrexia, tachycardia, raised serum CK, renal insufficiency and a high mortality. Also there are many medications, including certain anti-emetics and phenothiazine medications, that may cause acute and severe exacerbation of PD and should be avoided.

It is accepted that people with PD have difficulty in motor sequencing. The use of external cues is very helpful to foster independence, especially with mobility, although swallowing or speech problems also respond to cues. Cues can be given by the nurse or carer or, where possible, instigated by the patient. Some useful cues, which initiate recovery from freezing of gait, include counting aloud, stepping over a laser line, humming a march tune or pretending to climb a stair. Getting out of bed can be broken down into motor segments and cues can be used to get the patient through the entire sequence of movements.

Body image

Many changes occur with PD that can lead to an altered body image. A stooped posture, slowness in movement and gait disturbance ages the person. Drooling, reduced facial expression, unblinking eyes, slowness in thought (bradyphrenia) and voice disturbances not only lead to a loss of personal dignity, but also interfere with communication and the person may appear of low intellect. Social isolation for both the person with PD and the carer can ensue. People with PD may resent their wishes, feelings and opinions being interpreted and reported by others and may often feel shunned by previous friends as the condition progresses (Habermann, 2000).

There are many complementary therapies available for people with PD to treat non-motor symptoms and improve body image and quality of life. Natural therapies, herbs and over-the-counter medications have been used for constipation, urinary frequency and urgency, postural hypotension, sexual difficulties, depression, anxiety and dementia. However, preparations should be checked by the pharmacist to ensure they do not interfere with PD medications or aggravate PD symptoms.

Quality of life

Quality of life means different things to different individuals and is adversely affected in PD for a variety of reasons. Motor symptoms have an effect on areas such as role change, independence, working, driving and physical comfort. Yet, studies show non-motor symptoms such as pain and sexual limitations are more troublesome and have a negative impact on quality of life (Mott, Dixon, Bird, & Kendrick, 2004; Mott, Kenrick, Dixon, & Bird, 2005). The incidence of depression in up to 50% of cases is much higher than in other chronic neurological conditions (Ravina et al., 2007). Psychiatric complications can reduce quality of life in patients and family and require careful monitoring and expert intervention.

Social interaction diminishes as the disease progresses, not only because of body image changes but also because of communication difficulties. Communication is a basic human need and nurses need to be aware that establishing an effective means of communication is paramount to developing a rapport with people with PD. When faced with people who have soft monotonic voices, rapid and/or slurred speech and reduced facial expression, it is important to listen to content rather than delivery of speech to gauge needs, mood and cognitive function. Ensuring a face-to-face position, making eye contact and using cues to encourage people to speak key words loudly, and with the use of a pacing board if prescribed, are helpful and enable the personal expression of needs. For people unable to speak communication boards paired with a pointing device are useful. Recent technological advances have brought many innovations so that speech generating devices can be individualised and operated via specialised switches even when fine hand motor control is severely impaired. Regardless of how a person with PD communicates, it is essential to allow them ample time to express themselves and check that you have understood their intended message.

Family and carers

As with the majority of chronic conditions, Parkinson's disease is a family affair. The dynamics, relationships and traditional roles in the family may change and resentment, guilt and grieving can become major problems if changes are not addressed. Social support is important and counselling outside the family is often helpful to resolve these issues.

A well-informed family is more able to assist the person with PD to engage in advance care planning and make decisions about their care, as well as solve many of the day-to-day quality-of-life issues. While direct caregiving may be exhausting in later stages of PD, the family also carries the burden of the condition vicariously as observers of the toll that PD is taking on their loved one. Support for carers needs to include monitoring of health particularly of older spousal carers, and opportunities for respite to avoid burn-out (Abendroth, Lutz, & Young, 2012).

MULTIPLE SCLEROSIS

Multiple sclerosis (MS) is a demyelinating disease affecting the nerve fibres in the white matter of the brain, the spinal cord and the optic nerve (Porth, 2005). Myelin forms around the axon as an insulator that interprets and conducts the message along the fibre tract. A process of acute inflammation causes demyelination to occur. In some instances the body remyelinates the axon and function returns. In other situations the myelin is lost and scarring or sclerosis occurs, slowing or impairing the transmission of the nerve impulse (De Souza & Bates, 2004) and increasing axon vulnerability to environmental influences (Kipp, Amor, Krauth, & Beyer, 2012). The size and distribution of the sclerotic plaques dictate the locations and types of symptoms experienced.

Geographical variations in incidence have led to several hypotheses about causal factors, including climatic influences, environmental exposure and ethnically based genetic differences (Taylor et al., 2010; Wallin & Kurtzke, 2003). However the initial trigger for demyelination is unclear (Lassmann, 2005). Studies suggest that the immune response generated in young adults with viral infections such as measles, mumps, rubella and Epstein-Barr induces demyelination, but no definitive link has been established (Compston & Coles, 2008).

The revised McDonald criteria consisting of a year of disease progression and two of the following: positive brain magnetic resonance imaging (MRI) with visually evoked potential (measurement of sensory, visual and auditory nerve conduction), positive spinal cord MRI or positive cerebrospinal fluid, is used to establish a diagnosis of MS (Polman et al., 2005). This combination of testing is required because abnormalities in one test, for example the presence of lesions on MRI, are inconclusive and could be the result of other disease processes (Frankel, 2007).

Various presentations of MS are classified into four categories.

1 Relapsing remitting MS: this is the most common form (attributed to 85% of MS cases), characterised by episodic attacks of neurological symptoms, commonly sensory disturbance that may not be accompanied by clinical signs. Symptoms are usually experienced in one or more limbs, with optical, cerebellar and vestibular disturbances, pain depression, sleep disturbances and accompanying fatigue (Newland, Fearing, Riley & Neath, 2012). Between attacks the person recovers partial or complete neurological function. Arona's condition (see Case Study 17.2) exemplifies one of 16 forms of relapsing remitting MS.
2 Primary progressive MS: about 10% of older people with MS live with primary progressive MS. This form begins with vague symptoms that develop into gait deficits, sometimes confused with the ageing process. Neurological damage continues to occur without remyelination, resulting in a steady increase in the level of disability. Antibodies that attack central nervous system antigens are thought to prevent remyelination in this form of MS (Pender, 2004).
3 Secondary progressive MS: This begins in a similar manner to relapsing remitting MS, but develops a more constant progressive path with only minor occasional remissions and plateaus (Chelune, Stott, & Pinkston, 2008).
4 Progressive relapsing MS: in this form the disease progression is continuous, with acute attacks occurring at intervals, accompanied by minor recovery (Frankel, 2007).

Listed as the most common chronic neurological disease in adults worldwide, the incidence of MS is increasing by 7% per year (MS Research Australia, 2012). Prevalence figures estimate that 21 000 Australians and 4000 New Zealanders live with MS. However,

CASE STUDY 17.2

Arona was 26 years old, single and enjoying life as a secondary science teacher when she had her first attack of MS. She experienced reduced sensation in the skin across the entire left side of her body. Her general practitioner referred her to a neurologist, who undertook a range of tests including CAT (computed axial tomography, now referred to as CT) scans, visual evoke response tests to test optic nerve transmission and lumbar punctures. A stressful time of repeated testing occurred before a diagnosis of relapsing remitting MS was finally made 18 months later.

At the age of 27, Arona was told she should never work full-time, never get married or have children. She should just sit around and wait for all the bad things to happen! Arona felt that her social life had ceased — 'I was a "lemon", no guy would want to know me!'.

After changing neurologists and taking some control of her destiny, Arona began living her life to the full. She taught for nearly 30 years, got married and later divorced, and had a son, who is now 23 years old and working in engineering customer support.

CASE STUDY 17.2 — cont'd

Over the years, MS has attacked her left side again and again, leaving a lasting left-sided weakness. During these attacks, Arona lost the sight in her left eye, the use of her left arm, and developed cerebellar ataxia, which upset her balance and coordination. These symptoms created movement problems that Arona described as 'walking in thick mud', as well as restrictions on her ability to undertake self-care and other life activities. Arona was in her mid-forties when Betaferon became part of the pharmaceutical benefits scheme, making the antiviral, immunoregulatory drug affordable. Arona injected herself every second day, lessening the effects of MS attacks.

Arona was inspired by the work of an Australian doctor, Professor George Jelinek, who was also living with MS. In his book *Taking control of multiple sclerosis*, he proposed that changing the fats in diet would rebuild the cell membrane phospholipid bi-layer and thus increase its resistance to MS. As a result, Arona became a fish-eating vegan who avoided chemical additives such as preservatives in food. Her attacks are now less severe. She still has problems with balance and occasional vertigo and her movement is very affected by hot temperatures and humidity: 'I'm like a Raggedy Anne doll or someone who is drunk'.

At about the young age of 49 years, Arona noticed a gradual deterioration in her cognitive capacity to process information and problem-solve, as well as increased fatigue levels. These symptoms affected her ability to continue school teaching. Two years later, after extensive neurological testing, Arona retired for medical reasons.

In 2005, Arona was hospitalised to treat a large, red lump in her thigh, which was eventually diagnosed as fat cell necrosis. As very few MS patients are hospitalised, the doctors and nursing staff knew very little about MS and its treatment. Arona recounted: 'I had my Betaferon with me, and explained what it was and how it was used. No one seemed to connect the lump in my leg with my injections, except my GP. The infectious diseases specialist pumped me full of intravenous drugs, even Vancomycin. I went in with three allergies, and came out after 4 weeks with six allergies and a cannulation phobia!'

The hospital kitchen even had difficulty meeting Arona's dietary restrictions, which made it very hard for Arona to continue to manage MS while in hospital.

Thirty-one years on from diagnosis, Arona continues to manage her MS with Rebif injections three times a week, a fish-eating vegan diet, a modified gym program to relax and tone (mostly done on machines; her 28th program since leaving teaching), transdermal natural progesterone and a positive outlook. There are several theories about the specific action of progesterone, but evidence supports the role of progesterone in regulating 'myelination during development and myelin repair' (Kipp et al., 2012, p. 11).

Reflecting on living with MS, Arona says:

> I'm not about to give up and go quietly. MS has had an effect of serious proportions on my life, but there are worse things that could happen. I consider myself lucky — I do not look disabled — it is the invisible companion I live with and nurture, rather than rejecting. Information and education, strategies for dealing with situations, being able to help others cope with serious illness — there are many positives to all that has happened. My wonderful neurologist supports all my complementary approaches. I know more than most doctors about my condition, and they allow me to guide them. I respect this greatly.

incidence in the Māori population is significantly less than for those of European descent, suggesting a similar protective factor to that found in Asians and Pacific islanders (Taylor et al., 2010). MS occurs two to three times more often in women than men, and women are a greater risk for transmitting familial MS (15 times greater in first-degree relative) to their children (Frosch, Anthony, & De Girolami, 2010). While the disease trajectory is hard to predict, younger women who recover well after attacks have more favourable outcomes than men (Frankel, 2007).

Altered mobility and fatigue

Fatigue is a common symptom for people with MS. Its debilitating effects, not evident to others, are often taken for laziness. The constant tiredness is difficult to assess and quantify, making it hard to balance life, work, activity and rest (Benito-Leon et al., 2007). During the course of daily living, MS symptoms may be exacerbated by intense periods of physical and/or emotional stress, such as work schedules or personal problems. Yet, controlled exercise improves muscle tone, assists bladder and bowel function, reduces fatigue and promotes a positive outlook.

Living with MS has physical and emotional implications for many aspects of daily life, including making provision for regular immunoregulatory antiviral injections. Work demands and life activities have to be programmed to include a few hours of quiet and rest after the injection has been given to assist with the management of side effects such as influenza-like symptoms and short-term fatigue. Loss of sensation may induce numbness in the affected parts of the body that can result in the person being unaware of injury. For example, loss of sensation in the face resembles the feeling generated by dental injections. The person may unknowingly bite their tongue or cheek and not feel pain. Likewise, hands or limbs may not detect heat from stoves, fires or steam from a kettle resulting in burns. People living with MS should be educated to avoid physical heat and stay cool in the summer. An increase in body temperature brought on by hot baths, hot weather or infection slows nerve conduction and creates mobility and coordination problems.

As well as being frustrating and socially challenging, tremors may reduce the person's ability to undertake tasks requiring fine motor skills. Neurological disturbances that alter the intent of voluntary movements and unpredictable loss of balance can result in falls, bruising and ligament damage as well as loss of confidence and self-esteem. Muscle spasm may cause pain that is effectively treated with Baclofen. Unresolved spasms may result in contractures that restrict the range of movement of affected joints. However, spasms may also be useful in areas of weakness when they create the stability needed to mobilise (Frankel, 2007). Short-term use of walking aids may be appropriate, but use needs to be monitored by a physiotherapist to ensure other muscle groups, particularly the upper limbs, are not compromised. Likewise, physiotherapy may improve muscle strength, tone and posture, but fatigue must be avoided (De Souza & Bates, 2004).

Body image

Preserving positive body image is contingent on seeing the whole person who is living with MS and not the disabling condition. Listening to people's needs and encouraging them to make an effort with personal appearance diverts attention from the disability focus and enhances self-esteem. However, the process of the illness affects body image and needs to be addressed in a sensitive manner. For example, localised tissue reactions to drugs such as Betaferon often leave people with unsightly, persistent red blotches. Emphasising the role these medications play in staying well will encourage people to balance the blotchy image with the health benefit.

Maintaining hydration and muscle tone and avoiding infection are important keys to bladder control. However, bladder control may be difficult to maintain during attacks and as the disease progresses. Frequency, urgency and the fear of incontinence are important body image issues (Christopherson, Moore, Foley, & Warren, 2006). Loss of bladder control may require a range of interventions from incontinence supports to intermittent or continuous catheterisation. Progressive forms of MS may result in the need for long-term catheterisation, sometimes in the form of suprapubic catheterisation. Body image is affected by visualisation of a catheter, the impediment to sexual activity and concern about the care needed to prevent infection. Effective management of the bowel, including treatment for constipation, managing the fear of incontinence and untimely flatus are also important for preserving body image (Christopherson et al., 2006). Neural disturbances may block the feeling of fullness in the bowel that signals the need for defecation. Regular eating patterns and a diet that includes fibre and a high fluid intake, together with a regimen of suppository insertion, can be used to re-establish regular bowel movement (Iggulden, 2006).

Loss of sensation and motor function arising from the nature of the disease, drug therapy or psychological issues can affect the person's sex life. Sexual issues such as impotence, loss of libido, reduced lubrication and loss of sensation may result in slow arousal and decreased satisfaction. Partners need to be patient and explore a variety of alternative techniques to achieve the sexual expression of love. Counselling, medication and assistive devices may also be helpful (Frankel, 2007).

Quality of life

Quality of life is closely associated with personal empowerment. Being willing to be involved in care decision making and setting their own priorities enables people living with MS to take control in the management of the disease. At several points in Arona's story (Case Study 17.2), she identifies times when she took control, reflecting her positive attitude to disease management.

The unpredictable nature of the disease and the limitations on work, leisure and life roles can result in anxiety and depression for those living with MS. Symptoms may change through the day and the timing of attacks cannot be predetermined (Frankel, 2007). Frustration, inadequacy and uselessness are common feelings that contribute to the increased incidence of depression among people with MS. Therefore, staying positive and fighting depressive moods through involvement in a range of activities and modified exercise (as per Arona's example) are important for maintaining quality of life.

Variations in quality of life can be correlated with the type and severity of symptoms being experienced at that time and the perceived level of social support (Reade, White, White, & Russell, 2012). Effective communication is essential for social interaction in everyday life. Slurred speech, usually found in more progressive forms of MS, makes communication difficult and may be mistaken by others for cognitive impairment or drunkenness, particularly when ataxia is also present. Although not considered a primary clinical feature of MS, difficulty with swallowing (dysphagia) has been reported in up to 43% of people with MS and is a leading cause of morbidity and mortality due to complications associated with dehydration, malnutrition and aspiration pneumonia (Abraham & Yun, 2002). Assessment by a speech pathologist is recommended in cases where speech and swallowing difficulties persist.

Visual disturbances may create reductions in visual acuity or double vision, making employment tasks and lifestyle activities such as driving difficult to perform. Deficiencies in short-term memory, conceptual function and problem solving can occur (De Sousa & Kalman, 2002).

Cognitive function is affected in about 60% of cases. While the research about stimulating more effective cognitive function is inconclusive, compensatory strategies such as routines, lists, diaries, visualisation techniques and avoiding detailed interactions in noisy, distracting environments have all been found to be useful in promoting cognitive function (Frankel, 2007).

The community understanding of MS is limited and people with MS are often anxious about being labelled with the stigma of chronic illness or disability. People living with MS have been refused employment or 'forced' out of work as a productivity liability. Disclosure of their MS status might be avoided for fear of jeopardising relationships, the potential for employment or roles in community groups. Nurses can play an important role in community education and advocacy to enhance opportunities and acceptance of MS in the community.

Family and carers

As with other chronic illnesses, living with MS affects family life in a number of ways, including roles, relationships, finances and general family organisation. The family carers' adaptive abilities will depend on family relationships prior to diagnosis, the attitudes to illness and rehabilitation, the effectiveness of their coping and stress management strategies and the availability of social support. Families have to accommodate the person's need for rest and the effects of symptoms during an attack, and generally rearrange their lives to provide care when needed. Many people living with relapsing remitting MS do not require intensive hands-on care. Instead they need love, understanding and support. However, in progressive forms of MS or during a severe attack people need varying degrees of assistance with activities of daily living, mobility, bowel and bladder management and in some cases catheter care and cognitive function as well as psychological support.

Family members also need to contend with their own responses to physical and emotional losses, including lifestyle restrictions, relationships and effective communication. Fear of future disease implications and end of life may also add to family stress. As with family carers in most situations, feelings of uselessness and guilt are common when family members are no longer able to provide care. Therefore, families are also people living with MS who need supportive care at various times during the illness trajectory (Hubbard, McLachlan, Forbat, & Munday, 2012).

MOTOR NEURON DISEASE

Motor neuron disease (MND) is a collective term that encompasses a number of neurodegenerative disorders including amyotrophic lateral sclerosis, primary lateral sclerosis and progressive bulbar palsy (Borasio, Rogers, & Voltz, 2004). Degeneration occurs in the upper motor neurons of the cerebral cortex, the anterior horn cells of the spinal cord and the motor nuclei of the brain stem (lower motor neurons) and results in multiple failures in nerve impulse transmission. Functional changes are first observed in the distal tracts of nerves and progress backwards until the parent nerve cell dies (Porth, 2005). Features of frontotemporal lobe dementia such as behaviour changes and some higher order cognitive processes occur in a significant number of cases (Hodges, 2011). Yet, the sensory system and intellect remain intact and the person is keenly aware of the degeneration of their body. Another complicating factor of this disease is that it mostly affects people aged between 40 and 60 years with a mean age onset of 55 years; an era of life when people are usually moving from direct parenting to living their own life, preparing for retirement and/or caring for elderly parents.

Some controversy exists in the literature about the rise in incidence of MND, but most authors agree that the prevalence of MND is increasing (Talbot, 2007). It is estimated that at any one time 1400 Australians and 300 New Zealanders are living with MND (MND Association of New Zealand, 2012; Motor Neuron Disease Association Australia, 2012). These figures indicate that MND is not a common condition, yet it is the most common degenerative disorder of the motor-neuronal system in adults (Borasio et al., 2004).

People living with MND present with a history of muscle weakness in one or more of the following areas: limbs, speech, swallowing or respiration. Problematically, the course of this disease is not consistent across cases and progressive muscle weakness, shrinkage and muscle fibre atrophy can occur at varying rates in different parts of the body. Four distinct phenotypes of MND have been developed in an attempt to categorise variations in presentation and disease progression: global, flail arm, flail leg and primary lateral sclerosis (Talman, Forbes, & Mathers, 2009). The global and flail phenotypes are the most common and are usually associated with a life expectancy of three to 5 years from diagnosis to death. The additional presence of bulbar symptoms such as dysphagia and dysarthria compounds functional loss and shortens life expectancy due to compromised respiratory function. Pain arising from stress on joints associated with muscle decline, muscle spasm and cramping as well as skin pressure pain is common across all phenotypes (Oliver & Borasio, 2004). Regular fasciculations or twitching of a single muscle group is an indicative feature of MND (Vucic & Kiernan, 2007).

- People with global symptoms experience muscle weakness and wasting throughout the body, particularly in the legs, feet, hands, arms, neck and head.
- Flail arm and flail leg phenotypes present with increasing flaccidity of arms or legs, quickly limiting the person's ability to manipulate even the lightest of objects or mobilise within their environment.
- Degeneration in primary lateral sclerosis (PLS) occurs in the upper neurons and manifests as hyperreflexes and spasticity. These people are more prone to atypical laughing or crying — referred to as emotional lability. Life expectancy in PLS is usually longer, sometimes up to 10 or 12 years (Kiernan, Talman, Henderson, & Harris, 2006).

Extensive research is being undertaken to establish the cause of MND. Most cases are thought to be sporadic, but approximately 5–10% of cases are familial in origin. Twenty percent of familial cases are associated with any of 100 mutations of the SOD1 gene (Battistini et al., 2005). Recent research has identified a new genetic aberration C9ORF72 in 46% of familial and 21% of sporadic cases in the Finnish population, but not in Asian populations (Renton et al., 2011).

The neuroprotective drug Riluzole extends life by months, but needs to be prescribed early to be most effective (The EFNS Task Force on Diagnosis Management of Amyotrophic Lateral Sclerosis et al., 2012). Life can also be extended through the use of assisted ventilation and gastrostomy feeding (Bourke et al., 2006; Forbes et al., 2004). Thus, from diagnosis, an interdisciplinary palliative approach is the most effective way to provide care and promote quality of life for people living with MND. Additionally, advance care planning (ACP) needs to begin soon after diagnosis to facilitate conversations about symptom management and preparations for end-of-life care (Oliver, 2007; Ray, Brown, & Street, 2012). As part of the interdisciplinary team, nurses provide supportive care including ACP, family education to sustain in-home care, institutional respite and acute care when patients need new treatments such as respiratory support, percutaneous endoscopic gastrostomy (PEG) placement or care related to co-morbidities.

CASE STUDY 17.3

At 37, Trigger was married to Lola, had a 6-year-old daughter, Sally, and was running a metal polishing business. He enjoyed competitive sports, raced motorbikes in Super Motard competitions and organised and played professional Pool (ranked 64th out of the top 500 players nationally), 7 days a week. He began to notice a problem with his hands losing strength. He was unable to touch his third and fourth fingers to his thumb. As his livelihood and sport relied on good hand function he consulted an OT who specialised in hands. A painful nerve conduction test that took 6 months to organise returned a normal result. He persisted with prescribed hand strengthening exercises for 6 months, hoping for some improvement. However, during a Pool competition he was unable to hold up his left thumb to guide his pool cue resulting in his national rank slipping to 124.

A few more months later Trigger's speech began to slur and he had coughing fits with a mildly painful burning sensation in his throat when drinking water. He consulted an ear, nose and throat specialist who noticed tongue fasciculations and said he may have MND. Trigger thought 'Good! Now they can fix me'. He had never heard of MND before. Within weeks he saw a neurologist who repeated the nerve conduction tests plus electromyography (EMG) on his skeletal muscles causing severe muscle spasm. Twenty-two months after he first noticed his hand weakness the neurologist confirmed that Trigger had MND and told him that there was no cure, that his motor function would continue to rapidly deteriorate and that it was terminal. He was devastated by the diagnosis and found it difficult to talk about his condition and symptoms without dissolving into tears, further distressing himself, Lola and Sally. Health professionals described him as emotionally labile. Trigger resisted the idea of anti-depressive medication, but after he began to take them his distress reduced a little and he was able to better engage in decisions about his care and support.

Not long after his diagnosis of MND Trigger began to experience cramping in both lower legs and noticed that walking seemed to ease the discomfort. A physiotherapist developed a suitable leg stretching regimen that kept his legs functioning well enough to stand independently for a while, and then later with the aid of a four wheeled walker. Laryngeal spasms began to cause him some anxiety as he felt that he was choking. A speech pathologist explained what was happening in his throat and taught him some swallowing techniques that improved his confidence in swallowing safely and comfortably.

Trigger bought a house from the proceedings of an income protection insurance policy. The financial security this would provide to his family as his condition progressed was important to him. It also meant that he could continue to oversee the running of his business which provided income as well as enjoyable social interactions with his colleagues. Lola was able to continue working in her part time job knowing that Trigger was not always alone at home during the day. Home ownership also made it easier to adopt OT recommendations for home modifications including ramps and the conversion of the shower.

As his mobility continued to decline continence became a concern because Trigger couldn't get to the toilet quickly with his four-wheel walker. The soiling caused him and Lola great distress and was an affront to his dignity. The situation became critical when he fell backwards one night when trying to access the toilet. The limb weakness made it impossible for him to control his fall. The result was a 9 cm gash in his scalp

CASE STUDY 17.3 — cont'd

that required an ambulance trip and five staples. That incident plus a previous fall that had resulted in a wrist fracture, displaced collar bone and torn intercostal muscle led to a decision to move his bed and computer, which had become an important source of recreation, to a room large enough to also accommodate a commode, four-wheel walker and the manual wheelchair he used for community outings. Trigger's continence concerns eased once he had easier and safer access within his new space.

Trigger's new central location within the home increased opportunities to request attention from Lola. While she was happy to care for him and understood his unrelenting and at times unreasonable demands, the increasing claim on her physical and emotional resources was draining. Lola enlisted the help of Sally, now 11, when she was willing to help take care of her father, but the frequent frustrated exchanges between Sally and Trigger over expectations left Lola reluctant to ask for Sally's help too often.

Five years after the first symptoms of MND Trigger's speech is slow and slurred but he communicates well enough with familiar people without the need for an alternative system. He requires assistance at mealtimes as he can't lift drinks or cutlery to his mouth, but he maintains adequate swallowing function, enjoying his favourite soft foods. Trigger has decided to have a PEG inserted but not until his swallowing ceases to be functional. After initially rejecting the idea of a powered wheelchair, believing it to be an admission of defeat that would hasten his death, a trial of use has shown him the benefits of easier and independent access to both his home and the community as well as more opportunities to engage in activities with Sally.

Trigger is a proactive and independent problem solver in his own care. This provides him with a sense of control over his condition despite the relentless deterioration in physical function. While he has received regular input from a specialised multidisciplinary team, it is Lola who provides consistent care and support. She has managed all of his increasing daily needs with occasional assistance from close family members. In the future, when Trigger requires more assistance with activities such as showering and dressing, Lola knows that she can call on the Palliative Care Community Nursing services for help so that he can remain living at home, where he chooses to be.

Altered mobility and fatigue

Mobility is altered to varying degrees depending on which neural tracts are affected by MND. Global symptoms may begin with muscle cramping, stumbling or falling unexpectedly as the legs and/or feet muscles deteriorate. Loss of balance and difficulty holding objects or lifting anything also herald changes in the person's level of mobility and ability to undertake the activities of daily living. Splinting may be useful and prolong capability, but carers quickly have to assume responsibility for tasks such as doing up buttons, zips and shoe laces, turning pages, operating remote controls, showering, dressing, shaving, feeding and turning door knobs. In fact, anything that requires the hand to have strength and grip.

Early introduction of mobility aids is recommended to enhance independence and reduce the load on the degenerating muscles. Large pieces of equipment such as hoists and electric wheelchairs with high back support present particular problems because they are hard to hide in a family home. The image of these mobility aids indicates the extent of the disease progression to anyone who visits, forcing what might have been private knowledge into a more public arena. Health professionals need to be aware that mobility aids may threaten the person's self-image and compel them to confront the next stage of degeneration. Sensitivity to the emotional as well as the physical needs of the person and their family is important when discussing additional mobility supports. Nevertheless, OT and physiotherapy assessments need to be commenced soon after diagnosis and continue at regular intervals as new losses become evident.

People living with MND experience increasing fatigue as their muscle tissue, including their intercostal muscles, diminishes. Fatigue increases through the day as fewer muscles are available to achieve the required work load. Small studies suggest that certain forms of exercise provide short-term improvements in function (Dalbello-Haas, Florence & Krivickas, 2008), but activities need to be timed for periods when the person is most rested to prevent fatigue. Weakened respiratory muscles lead to chronic hypoventilation, making less oxygen available to the tissues. Non-invasive ventilation (NIV) via a mask improves oxygenation, relieves fatigue and improves the person's quality of life (The EFNS Task Force on Diagnosis Management of Amyotrophic Lateral Sclerosis et al., 2012). However, while NIV can increase life expectancy, continuing body degeneration increases family carer burden.

Body image

In MND, body image is threatened by the relentless physical degeneration. Muscle wasting and weight loss are increasingly evident, particularly around the shoulders, trunk and sometimes the face. Losing the ability to participate in expected family routines and to undertake the personal activities of daily living such as showering, dressing, toileting and eating not only alters personal roles and boundaries, but also threaten body image. Family members can do little more than watch as their relative wastes away and becomes more dependent. Body image is further jeopardised for people with bulbar symptoms. When swallowing becomes a problem, quantities of saliva that are normally swallowed each day dribble uncontrollably from the mouth. Drooling and the need to be assisted with eating or PEG feeding is not consistent with social interaction. Children of people with MND could become embarrassed by the changed appearance and apparent loss of body control of their parent and cease having friends visit. This restricts opportunities to stay connected with social support systems and reduces quality of life for the person and their family.

Quality of life

As illustrated in Trigger's story (Case Study 17.3), quality of life for people living with MND is focused on effective symptom control, maintenance of personhood including independence and social relationships (Oliver, 2007). Early assessment, the establishment of a safe living environment and the well-timed introduction of functional devices that enable people to remain independent as long as possible improve quality of life for the person and family carers. The person with MND feels more in control of their life and the family carer is able to continue employment and other life activities for longer periods.

Symptom management in MND includes pain control, respiratory support, dysphagia management, drooling control, enhanced communication and, for some, management of emotional lability and cognitive changes. Pain resulting from strain on joints responds to anti-inflammatory medication, muscle relaxants such as Baclofen are useful for spasms from upper neuron damage, while skin pressure pain is relieved by repositioning and opioid medication (Oliver, 2007). Swallowing problems are managed initially by modified cups, postural changes, fluid thickening and food modification. Later, if the person agrees to active treatment, a gastrostomy is performed. Anticholinergic drugs or injecting the parotid glands with botulinum toxin can reduce saliva (The EFNS Task Force on Diagnosis Management of Amyotrophic Lateral Sclerosis et al., 2012). However, these drugs can also result in the development of tenacious saliva that is hard to swallow. Natural products such as dark grape juice, papaya enzyme and horse radish with garlic capsules have also been found to be helpful in managing saliva.

Quality of life through social relationships depends on effective communication. In Trigger's case he was able to maintain verbal communication with familiar people despite slurred speech. The loss of the ability to communicate restricts social relationships to those who can engage socially without needing verbal participation. This is especially important, as the majority of people with MND develop dysarthria and many will progress to anarthia during the course of the disease. There are a variety of communication devices available and the explosion in smart phone technology has increased accessibility and affordability for most affected people. However, their success is dependent on the rate of degenerative progression and the willingness of the person and others to adapt to that style of communication. For example, iPad applications require some hand control, computer programs can be voice, foot or laser activated, lightWRITERS use synthesised voice to verbalise typed words, while Etran boards rely on eye movements to spell out words. Despite these devices, communication can be hard work and social relationships decline, especially in the younger age groups (Ray & Street, 2005).

Family and carers

In Australia, most people with MND (as in Trigger's case) are cared for in the home by family members and many die at home. Access to community resources is sporadic and depends on availability of services and eligibility criteria. In recent years people with MND have become eligible for palliative care services, but the uncertainty of the disease trajectory and resource limitations makes it difficult for services to be instituted in a timely manner. Care in degenerative illness is constant as the person becomes less mobile and unable to carry out personal tasks. This means that family members, usually a partner or child, have to provide care 24 hours each day of the week. Family carers experience many situations that cause them to redefine themselves and their relationship with the person living with MND. The consistent and sometimes ambiguous losses caused by the effects of the disease, change roles and reconstruct the future. Details of some of the challenges faced by family carers, including the lack of social support, are evident in the recommended additional readings for this chapter. While family carers need and value the support of community resources, these resources should be integrated and structured so that family privacy and personal space in the family home are respected and preserved as much as possible. Coordination of services is essential to reduce the traffic through the home. Providing time to support family carers rather than just meeting the physical needs of the person with MND is vital for the maintenance of effective in-home care.

Education for the person and family living with PD, MS or MND

The management of PD, MS and MND is a shared function involving the person, their family or other carers and health professionals. It is important that those who care for the person with PD, MS or MND understand the complexities of the condition, the motor and non-motor aspects and the importance of the relevant medications and treatment options. It is easier to understand the motor and sensory problems, but the non-motor problems such as constipation, anxiety, depression, sexual difficulties and social withdrawal can prove to be more insidious and chip away at quality of life. However, many carers are well informed about the disease in general and the particulars in relation to their loved one by the time they need the care of nurses (Hubbard et al., 2012). Educational information needs to be incremental, relevant to achieving immediate care, address specific problems and be inclusive of planning for future care needs through ACP conversations. These conversations require advanced communication skills and sensitivity concerning the difficulty some may experience in confronting the reality of living with degenerative illness. Therefore, nurses need to be cognisant of the person or their family's existing knowledge, look for opportunities presented by changes in health status and recognise cues indicating readiness to engage in education and future planning.

Topics that might be useful include:

- effective ways to assist with activities of daily living (ADL) and manage care requirements to prevent injury
- repositioning techniques to relieve pressure and strain and to promote breathing
- communication techniques and devices, assisted coughing
- effective use of medications and complementary therapies to promote quality of life
- use and maintenance of interventions such as PEG, NIV devices, mobility aids
- effective cueing strategies
- available community services and resources to support in-home care
- strategies for identifying and mobilising social support networks
- importance of talking about the impact of the disease on relationships, lifestyle, ACP and preparations for end of life
- strategies for managing the losses and emotional burden of caregiving
- carer health and wellbeing, including plans for personal time and resources for respite
- access to the resources of relevant associations:
  - Australia (http://www.parkinsons.org.au/)
  - The Parkinson's Society of New Zealand (http://www.parkinsons.org.nz/)
  - MS Society (http://www.msnz.org.nz/) (http://www.msaustralia.org.au/)
  - MND Association (http://www.mndaust.asn.au/) (http://www.mnda.org.nz/).

While members of the interdisciplinary team may initiate some of these topics, nurses are often required to revise, support and consolidate knowledge and skills, and facilitate advanced care planning especially in rural and regional areas.

CONCLUSION

The degenerative disabling nature of PD, MS and MND creates multiple physical, emotional and lifestyle challenges for people and their families. Changes in the level of mobility and capacity to self-care as well as alterations in body image and self-concept change the nature of roles and relationships and affect quality of life. Support and encouragement that enables people to plan ahead and take control of disease management is integral to promoting a positive approach. Through understanding of the distinctive features of each disease and the available interventions nurses along with the interdisciplinary team will be equipped to provide focused support for people and their families living with PD, MS and MND.

Reflective questions

1. Timely interventions are important for maintaining quality of life and enabling people to live at home. Describe the likely patient care needs and the corresponding interdisciplinary team members that could be involved in facilitating effective in-home care across each disease trajectory.
2. Discuss the place and importance of supportive care for family carers of people living with PD, MS and MND.
3. Describe the challenges and enablers for facilitating advanced care planning among people living with PD, MS and MND.

Acknowledgments: the authors wish to thank the people living with PD, MS and MND for their willingness to share stories of their journey with each disease so that others may learn and improve their ability to provide supportive care.

Recommended reading

Abendroth, M., Lutz, B. J., & Young, M. E. (2012). Family caregivers' decision process to institutionalize persons with Parkinson's disease: A grounded theory study. *International Journal of Nursing Studies, 49*(4), 445–454. doi: 10.1016/j.ijnurstu.2011.10.003

Aoun, S., McConigley, R., Abernethy, A., et al. (2010). Caregivers of people with neurodegenerative diseases: profile and unmet needs from a population-based survey in South Australia. *Journal of Palliative Medicine, 13*(6), 653–661. doi: 10.1089/jpm.2009.0318

Forbes, A., While, A., & Taylor, M. (2007). What people with multiple sclerosis perceive to be important to meeting their needs. *Journal of Advanced Nursing, 58*(1), 11–22.

Ray, R. A., & Street A. F. (2007). Nonfinite loss and emotional labour: family caregivers' experiences of living with motor neurone disease. *Journal of Clinical Nursing, 16*(3a), 35–43.

Reade, J. W., White, M. B., White, C. P., et al. (2012). What would you say? Expressing the difficulties of living with multiple sclerosis. *Journal of Neuroscience Nursing, 44*(1), 54–63.

References

Abendroth, M., Lutz, B. J., & Young, M. E. (2012). Family caregivers' decision process to institutionalize persons with Parkinson's disease: A grounded theory study. *International Journal of Nursing Studies, 49*(4), 445–454. doi: 10.1016/j.ijnurstu.2011.10.003

Abraham, S. S., & Yun, P. T., (2002). Laryngopharyngeal dismotility in multiple sclerosis. *Dysphagia, 16*, 69–74.

Anderson, G., Noorian, A. R., Taylor, G., et al. (2007). Loss of enteric dopaminergic neurons and associated changes in colon motility in an MPTP mouse model of Parkinson's disease. *Experimental Neurology, 207*(1), 4–12. doi: 10.1016/j.expneurol.2007.05.010

Australian Bureau of Statistics. (2010). *Causes of Death, Australia, 2010. ABS diseases of the nervous system (G00–G99)*. Canberra: Author.

Avanzi, M., Baratti, M., Cabrini, S., et al. (2006). Prevalence of pathological gambling in patients with Parkinson's disease. *Movement Disorders, 21*(12), 2068–2072. doi: 10.1002/mds.21072

Battistini, S., Giannini, F., Greco, G., et al. (2005). SOD1 mutations in amyotrophic lateral sclerosis. *Journal of Neurology, 252*(7), 782–788. 10.1007/s00415–005–0742–y

Benito-Leon, J., Martinez-Martin, P., Frades, B., et al. (2007). Impact of fatigue in multiple sclerosis: the Fatigue Impact Scale for Daily Use (D-FIS). *Multiple Sclerosis, 13*(5), 645.

Borasio, G. D., Rogers, A., & Voltz, R. (2004). Palliative medicine in non-malignant neurological disorders. In D. Doyle, G. Hanks, N. I. Cherny, et al. (Eds.), *Oxford textbook of palliative medicine* (3rd ed., pp. 925–934). Oxford: Oxford University Press.

Bourke, S. C., Tomlinson, M., Williams, T. L., et al. (2006). Effects of non-invasive ventilation on survival and quality of life in patients with amyotrophic lateral sclerosis: a randomised controlled trial. *Lancet Neurol, 5*, 140–147.

Chelune, G., Stott, H., & Pinkston, J. (2008). Multiple Sclerosis. In J. E. Morgan & J. H. Ricker (Eds.), *Textbook of clinical neuropsychology* (pp. 599–615). New York: Taylor & Francis.

Christopherson, J. M., Moore, K., Foley, F. W., et al. (2006). A comparison of written materials vs. materials and counselling for women with sexual dysfunction and multiple sclerosis. *Journal of Clinical Nursing, 15*(6), 742–750.

Compston, A., & Coles, A. (2008). Multiple sclerosis. *The Lancet, 372*(9648), 1502–1517. doi: 10.1016/s0140–6736(08)61620–7

Dalbello-Haas, V., Florence, J., & Krivickas, L. (2008). Therapeutic exercise for people with amyotrophic lateral sclerosis or motor neuron disease. *Cochrane Database of Systematic Reviews, 16*(2), CD005229.

De Sousa, E. A., & Kalman, A. R. H. (2002). Cognitive impairments in multiple sclerosis: a review. *American Journal of Alzheimer's Disease and Other Dementias, 17*(1), 23–29.

De Souza, L., & Bates, D. (2004). Multiple Sclerosis. In M. Stokes (Ed.), *Physical management in neurological rehabilitation* (pp. 177–201). Edinburgh: Elsevier Mosby.

Deloitte Access Economics. (2011). *Living with Parkinson's Disease — update.* Barton: Deloitte Access Economics.

Fasano, A., Daniele, A., & Albanese, A. (2012). Treatment of motor and non-motor features of Parkinson's disease with deep brain stimulation. *The Lancet Neurology, 11*(5), 429–442. doi: 10.1016/s1474–4422(12)70049–2

Forbes, A., While, A., & Taylor, M. (2007). What people with multiple sclerosis perceive to be important to meeting their needs. *Journal of Advanced Nursing, 58*(1), 11–22.

Forbes, R. B., Colville, S., & Swingler, R. J. (2004). Frequency, timing and outcome of gastrostomy tubes for amyotrophic lateral sclerosis/motor neurone disease. A record linkage study from the Scottish Motor Neurone Disease Register. *Journal of Neurology, 251*(7), 813–817.

Frankel, D. I. (2007). Multiple Sclerosis. In D. A. Umphred, G. U. Burton, R. T. Lazaro, et al. (Eds.), *Neurological rehabilitation* (pp. 709–731). Philadelphia: Mosby Elsevier.

Friedman, J. H., Brown, R. G., Comella, C., Working Group on Fatigue in Parkinson's Disease, et al. (2007). Fatigue in Parkinson's disease: A review. *Movement Disorder, 22*(3), 297–308.

Frosch, M. P., Anthony, D. C., & De Girolami, U. (2010). The central nervous system. In V. Kumar, A. K. Abbas, N. Fausto, et al. (Eds.), *Robbins and Coltran: Pathologic basis of disease* (pp. 1279–1344). Philadelphia: Saunders Elsevier.

Habermann, B. (2000). Spousal perspective of Parkinson's disease in middle life. *Journal of Advanced Nursing, 31*(6), 1409–1415.

Heisters, D. (2007). Caring for a resident with Parkinson's disease. *Nursing & Residential Care, 9*(9), 116–118.

Hodges, J. R. (2011). *The clinical spectrum of cognitive changes in MND.* Paper presented at the 22nd International Symposium on ALS/MND, Sydney.

Hubbard, G., McLachlan, K., Forbat, L., et al. (2012). Recognition by family members that relatives with neurodegenerative disease are likely to die within a year: A meta-ethnography. *Palliative Medicine, 26*(2), 108–122. doi: 10.1177/0269216311402712

Hughes, A. J., Daniel, S. E., Kilford, L., et al. (1992). Accuracy of clinical diagnosis of idiopathic Parkinson's disease: a clinico-pathological study of 100 cases. *Journal of Neurology, Neurosurgery and Psychiatry, 55*, 181–184.

Iggulden, H. (2006). *Care of the neurological patient*. Oxford: Blackwell Publishing.

Kiernan, M. C., Talman, P., Henderson, R. D., et al. (2006). Establishment of an Australian motor neurone disease registry. *Medical Journal of Australia, 184*(7), 367–368.

Kipp, M., Amor, S., Krauth, R., et al. (2012). Multiple sclerosis: Neuroprotective alliance of estrogen–progesterone and gender. *Frontiers in Neuroendocrinology, 33*(1), 1–16. doi: 10.1016/j.yfrne.2012.01.001

Lassmann, H. (2005). Multiple sclerosis pathology: evolution of pathogenetic concepts. *Brain Pathology*, 217–222.

Micieli, G., Tosi, P., Marcheselli, S., et al. (2003). Autonomic dysfunction in Parkinson's disease. *Neurological Science, 24*(Supp), S32–S34.

MND Association of New Zealand. (2012). How common is MND? Retrieved June 18, 2012, from http://mnda.org.nz/common–mnd.asp?about

Motor Neurone Disease Association Australia. (2012). What is MND? Retrieved June 18, 2012, from http://www.mndaust.asn.au/

Mott, S., Dixon, M., Bird, G., et al. (2004). Pain as a sequela of Parkinson's disease. *Australian Family Physician, 33*(8), 663–664.

Mott, S., Kenrick, M., Dixon, M., et al. (2005). Sexual limitations in people living with Parkinson's disease. *Australasian Journal on Ageing, 24*(4), 196–201. doi: 10.1111/j.1741–6612.2005.00118.x

MS Research Australia. (2012). Living with MS. Retrieved March 20 2012, from http://www.msra.org.au/living-ms

Mythri, R. B., & Bharath, M. M. (2012). Curcumin: a potential neuroprotective agent in Parkinson's disease. *Current Pharmaceutical Design, 18*(1), 91–99.

Newland, P. K., Fearing, A., Riley, M., et al. (2012). Symptom clusters in women with relapsing-remitting multiple sclerosis. (Report). *Journal of Neuroscience Nursing, 44*(2), 66–71.

Oliver, D. (2007). Palliative care. In M. C. Kiernan (Ed.), *The motor neurone disease handbook* (pp. 186–195). Pyrmont: Australasian Medical Publishing Company.

Oliver, D., & Borasio, G. D. (2004). Palliative care for patients with MND/ALS. *European Journal of Palliative Care, 11*(5), 185–187.

Parkinsonism Society of New Zealand. (2012). Parkinson's New Zealand. Retrieved June 15, 2012, from http://www.parkinsons.org.nz/

Pender, M. P. (2004). The pathogenesis of primary progressive multiple sclerosis: antibody-mediated attack and no repair? *Journal of Clinical Neuroscience, 11*(7), 689–692. doi: 10.1016/j.jocn.2003.12.013

Polman, C. H., Reingold, S. C., Edan, G., et al. (2005). Diagnostic criteria for multiple sclerosis: 2005 revisions to the 'McDonald Criteria'. *Annals of Neurology, 58*(6), 840–846. doi: 10.1002/ana.20703

Porth, C. M. (2005). *Pathophysiology: concepts of altered health status*. Philadelphia: Lippincott, Williams & Wilkins.

Przedborski, S. (2007). Etiology and pathogenesis of Parkinson's disease. In J. Jankovic & E. Tolosa (Eds.), *Parkinson's disease and movement disorders* (pp. 77–92). Philadelphia: Lippincott, Williams & Wilkins.

Ravina, B., Camicoli, R., Come, P., et al. (2007). The impact of depressive symptoms in early Parkinson's disease. *Neurology, 69*(4), 342–347.

Ray, R. A., & Street, A. F. (2005). Who's there and who cares: age as an indicator of social support networks for caregivers among people living with motor neurone disease. *Health and Social Care in the Community, 13*(6), 542–552.

Ray, R. A., Brown, J. B., & Street, A. F. (first published online April 19, 2012). Dying with motor neurone disease, what can we learn from family caregivers? *Health Expectations*. doi: 10.1111/j.1369–7625.2012.00773.x

Reade, J. W., White, M. B., White, C. P., et al. (2012). What would you say? Expressing the difficulties of living with multiple sclerosis. *Journal of Neuroscience Nursing*, *44*(1), 54–63.

Renton, A., E., Majounie, E., Waite, A., et al. (2011). A hexanucleotide repeat expansion in C9ORF72 is the cause of chromosome 9p21–Linked ALS–FTD. *Neuron*, *72*(2), 257–268. doi: 10.1016/j.neuron.2011.09.010

Rodriguez-Proz, M. C., Matsubara, J. M., Clavero, P., et al. (2009). Deep brain stimulation and Parkinson's disease. In L. R. Squire (Ed.), *Encyclopedia of Neuroscience* (pp. 375–384). Sydney: Elsevier.

Sapir, S., Ramig, L., & Fox, C. (2008). Speech and swallowing disorders in Parkinson's disease. *Current Opinion in Otolaryngology & Head and Neck Surgery*, *16*, 205–210.

Savica, R., Grossardt, B. R., Bower, J. H., et al. (in press). Risk factors for Parkinson's disease may differ in men and women: An exploratory study. *Hormones and Behavior*. doi: 10.1016/j.yhbeh.2012.05.013

Talbot, K. (2007). Epidemiology of motor neurone disease. In M. C. Kiernan (Ed.), *The motor neurone disease handbook* (pp. 3–13). Pyrmont: Australasian Medical Publishing Company.

Talman, P., Forbes, A., & Mathers, S. (2009). Clinical phenotypes and natural progression for motor neuron disease: analysis from an Australian database. *Amyotrophic lateral sclerosis*, *10*, 79–84.

Tan, E. K., & Skipper, L. M. (2007). Pathogenic mutations in Parkinson Disease. *Human Mutation*, *28*(7), 641–653.

Taylor, B. V., Pearson, J. F., Clarke, G., et al. (2010). MS prevalence in New Zealand, an ethnically and latitudinally diverse country. *Multiple Sclerosis*, *16*(12), 1422–1431.

The EFNS Task Force on Diagnosis Management of Amyotrophic Lateral Sclerosis, Andersen, P. M., Abrahams, S., Borasio, G. D., et al. (2012). EFNS guidelines on the clinical management of amyotrophic lateral sclerosis (MALS) — revised report of an EFNS task force. *European Journal of Neurology*, *19*(3), 360–375. doi: 10.1111/j.1468–1331.2011.03501.x

Vucic, S., & Kiernan, M. C. (2007). Abnormalities in cortical and peripheral excitability in flail arm variant amyotrophic lateral sclerosis. *Journal of neurology, neurosurgery, and psychiatry*, *78*, 849–852.

Wallin, M. T., & Kurtzke, J. F. (2003). Trends in multiple sclerosis (MS) prevalence and incidence: geographic, racial, and ethnicity risk factors. *MS Q REP*, *22*(4), 1, 3–7.

Ward, C. (2005). Neuroleptic malignant syndrome in a patient with Parkinson's disease: a case study. *Journal of Neuroscience Nursing*, *37*(3), 160–162.

CHAPTER 18

Philip A. Stumbles
Prue Andrus
Christophe von Garnier

Chronic asthma

Learning objectives

When you have completed this chapter you will be able to:

- describe the pathogenesis of chronic atopic asthma and the clinical features observed during exacerbation of the disease
- explain the triggers for exacerbation of chronic atopic asthma and steps that can be taken to avoid them
- describe the approaches to long-term management of this condition
- explain the principles underpinning the approaches to nursing practice in the treatment of chronic atopic asthma
- understand the psychological issues that can affect the care of patients with this chronic disorder.

Key words

airway hyper responsiveness, asthma, exacerbation, bronchodilation, peak expiratory flow

INTRODUCTION

Asthma is a term that describes a collection of clinical disorders rather than a single disease that have in common reversible airflow limitation to the lungs in response to certain triggers. The complex nature of the disease is highlighted by the distinction between the clinical manifestations of the disease in adults compared with children. Although the prevalence of wheezing is considered to be high in children under the age of 6 years, approximately half will cease wheezing by adolescence (Holt, Macaubas, Stumbles, & Sly, 1999). The incidence of the disease then tends to decline towards adulthood, with the most current figures indicating that asthma is Australia's most widespread chronic health problem, with 8.2–13.9% of children (up to 15 years of age) and 8.6–12.4% of adults reporting doctor-diagnosed asthma with treatment in the previous 12 months between the 2003 to 2009 period (Australian Centre for Asthma Monitoring, 2011). Additional information from a 2007–2009 National Health Survey by the Australian Bureau of Statistics showed that up to 19%, or 3 888 952 Australians, have been diagnosed with asthma at some stage in their lives (Australian Centre for Asthma Monitoring, 2011).

The key underlying disease process occurring in asthma is inflammation of the airway walls and lung parenchyma, the triggering of which induces bronchial hyper responsiveness (BHR). The assessment of BHR by methacholine challenge testing is a mainstay of chronic or uncontrolled asthma diagnosis (Quaedvlieg, Sele, Henket, & Louis, 2009), and has a strong negative predictive power in excluding a diagnosis of asthma (American Thoracic Society, 2000). One of the most common triggers of BHR in adults is inhaled allergens, which is the underlying basis of atopic or eosinophilic asthma. According to the National Asthma Council of Australia, around 80% of people with asthma also have allergies (National Asthma Council of Australia, 2012), while data from the 2007–2008 National Health Survey indicate that sinusitis and rhinitis are the most common respiratory co-morbid condition amongst people with asthma (Australian Centre for Asthma Monitoring, 2011). Atopy is defined as the production of a particular type of antibody, termed IgE, to low levels of a variety of allergens; this is the underlying cause of allergic conditions such as rhinitis, atopic dermatitis (eczema) and allergic sensitisation to food allergens. Importantly in terms of chronic asthma, a diagnosis of atopy is strongly associated with the persistence of asthma into adolescence and adulthood. Individuals with allergic rhinitis or eczema or who are sensitised to house dust mites are considered to be at high risk for the development of asthma.

In addition to the atopic asthma 'phenotype', several other phenotypes representing asthma induced by non-atopic triggers represent a significant category of adult asthma sufferers; these include asthma exacerbations triggered by a variety of non-specific stimuli such as exercise, cold air, drugs (aspirin, NSAIDs), occupational exposures and active or passive cigarette smoke exposure (Wenzel, 2006). Respiratory infections such as respiratory syncytial virus, rhinovirus and influenza viral infections are also a common cause of asthma exacerbations in children, but cause a minority of exacerbations in adults (Johnston, 1998). Clinically, additional subtypes can be made based on the inflammatory phenotype, where 'eosinophilic' and 'non-eosinophilic' or 'neutrophilic' phenotypes can be diagnosed on the basis of the inflammatory cell types in induced sputum or bronchioalveolar lavage samples (Wenzel, 2006; Brooks, 2013). Although these inflammatory subtypes are not regularly identified in the day-to-day clinical management of the person with asthma, they may be useful in the design of new treatments for patients in which conventional anti-inflammatory therapies are not effective (Barnes, 2012). In Case Study 18.1, Charlene's asthma exacerbation developed subsequent to an influenza infection, which may have heightened her responsiveness to other environmental triggers including allergens.

The management of chronic asthma requires a comprehensive approach, the primary aim of which is to minimise the number and severity of asthma exacerbations. This will involve the identification of triggers, avoidance of triggers where possible, appropriate medications and education for patients, family and carers.

CASE STUDY 18.1

Charlene is a 23-year-old female with a history of atopic asthma. She was first diagnosed with asthma by her family general practitioner (GP) when she was an infant. During her childhood she has been hospitalised on several occasions for exacerbations of asthma. Charlene also experiences eczema and is allergic to nuts, however she has no other relevant clinical history.

Charlene experiences symptoms of asthma on most days and seeks medical treatment several times each year to treat exacerbations of asthma, usually related to respiratory viral infections. Her usual asthma management includes the use of a rapid acting beta-2-agonist inhaler and a low-dose inhaled glucocorticosteroid (see Figure 18.3, later in the chapter).

Charlene has recently moved away from her family for the first time. She has just commenced studies at university and now shares a house with three other students. She has noticed that since moving into shared accommodation that her asthma symptoms have worsened. The share house is in an older suburb, with poor heating and ventilation, and one of her house mates smokes cigarettes. She has recently had a respiratory bacterial infection following an influenza viral infection (treated with oral antibiotics and oral glucocorticosteroids) however her asthma symptoms are slow to improve. She has not attended university on many occasions as she has been tired, kept awake at night due to coughing. She is worried about her approaching exams and is feeling fatigued, stressed and having trouble controlling her asthma symptoms (wheezing, breathlessness, night time and early morning coughing).

At her mother's insistence Charlene attends her GP again for treatment of her worsening symptoms and subsequently is referred to the practice asthma nurse for a review of her action plan.

BEHAVIOURS THAT CONTRIBUTE TO THE DEVELOPMENT OF THE CONDITION

Pathophysiology

Over 90% of adults and 80% of children with asthma are diagnosed as atopic and therefore management of this condition requires knowledge of the factors that trigger an allergic response. In the patient with chronic or persistent asthma, the key physiological feature underlying this condition is BHR, which in the context of allergic asthma manifests as a heightened or exaggerated bronchoconstrictor response to aeroallergens. The underlying basis for this condition is a persistent inflammatory response into the airways that ultimately results in airway remodelling, narrowing of the airways and heightened responsiveness to allergic and non-allergic triggers. How this condition develops over the life of a patient is still poorly understood. However, it seems likely that genetically susceptible individuals are primed at birth (or even in utero) to develop an atopic response to one or more environmental allergens. An understanding of the nature of the inflammatory response is important in order to guide correct diagnosis of the disease and choice of treatment approaches (Holgate & Polosa, 2006).

It is interesting to note that the incidence of atopy and allergy in Australia, and other western and developing nations, is increasing. Again, the reason for this is not fully understood, but its basis is likely to be in the early year of life and may perhaps relate to the increasing 'cleanliness' of urban home environments in these regions: the so-called 'hygiene hypothesis'. For example, there is evidence to suggest that early exposure to the high bacterial loads in some farm environments can prevent the development of atopy and asthma (Holt, 2004). Other environmental factors may also be at play, including increased levels of pollution in metropolitan regions and the likelihood of an increasing effect of global warming: increased atmospheric CO_2 levels are known to stimulate pollinosis, which can increase the levels of allergens in the atmosphere, while changing climates will alter the geographic spread of allergens and the types of allergens to which people are exposed. It is therefore important to identify allergen triggers where possible, so that avoidance strategies for the patient can be put in place. However, it may also be important to establish whether the environmental conditions of the patient have also changed. In the case of Charlene in Case Study 18.1, moving into an environment with high levels of passive smoke exposure represented a high-risk environment. The environment into which the patient is moving should be taken into account when considering discharge from hospital of the stabilised patient, and all other potential trigger factors should be considered (see below).

However, it should also be noted that a lack of diagnosis for atopy does not preclude a diagnosis of asthma — this is particularly the case for children — and asthma can develop in response to a variety of non-allergenic triggers. These include cold air, exercise, stress, oesophageal reflux and responses to medications such as aspirin and non-steroidal anti-inflammatory drugs (NSAIDs). However, as Charlene has been diagnosed as atopic, it is likely that her exacerbation was triggered by an allergic response and we will therefore focus this discussion on the allergic triggers of asthma.

Allergen triggers

For patients with allergic asthma, it is well established that exposure to allergens can trigger an asthmatic response. In Australia and other developed countries, one of the most common indoor allergic triggers is allergens of the house dust mite (HDM) *Dermatophagoides pteronyssinus* and *Dermatophagoides farinae*. HDM allergens usually take the form of small protein molecules that are part of the mite or are excreted as waste products (Holt & Thomas, 2005). However, in addition to HDM, other common indoor allergens include animal dander from cats and dogs, cockroach allergens and occasionally moulds. Food allergens such as peanuts and seafood are also reported by some patients to induce asthma exacerbations, although this often occurs in conjunction with other more generalised food allergy reactions such as skin rashes and gut symptoms that occur as part of a systemic anaphylactic response (Department of Health and Ageing, 2004). Cat allergens are a particularly potent form of allergen: they are secreted by the sebaceous glands, salivary glands and uterus, stick to the hair and become airborne when hair is shed. About 50% of patients who are allergic to cats make IgE that binds to the cat allergen Fel d 1 — a uteroglobin (blastokinin) secreted by the uteruses of many mammals, the cat version of which is especially allergenic (Holt & Thomas, 2005). The most important outdoor allergens are the pollens of grasses, weeds (especially ragweed), olive, birch and conifers: patients may react to one or several of these allergens, but sensitisation will depend on geographical location.

Allergen avoidance

The case for allergen avoidance in the prevention of asthma is complex. However, in some cases, allergen avoidance or reduced allergen exposure can be effective in reducing asthma symptoms and requirement for medications. For example, patients with a proven allergy to HDM can take measures to kill mites or restrict their breeding and remove the allergens they produce. However, in some individuals there may not be a direct relationship between allergen exposure and development of asthma symptoms. This may be the case because the individual is sensitised to more than one allergen or that allergen exposure is exacerbated by exposure to other triggers, such as influenza virus infection, cigarette smoke or medications. This is likely to be the case for Charlene, as several factors may be involved in triggering her exacerbation and contribute to the severity of symptoms: moving into a different environment, exposure to passive cigarette smoke and a recent influenza infection. Care should be taken to reduce allergen exposure and triggers in the home environment when the patient is stabilised.

ALTERED MOBILITY AND FATIGUE — RELATIONSHIP TO ACTIVITIES OF DAILY LIVING

Below are some potential losses associated with chronic asthma (adapted from Miller, 2000, p. 527).

1 *General health status:* energy is compromised due to the difficulty on expiration (the energy required to breathe out) and poor oxygen absorption. Strength is compromised due to the lower levels of oxygen in the blood with no reserves to compensate when the muscles need more oxygen quickly. The ability to communicate (talk) can be compromised due to need of the body to inhale and exhale air, which is the most difficult part of breathing for the asthma sufferer. During the simple activity of walking, for example, the asthma sufferer may have difficulty in doing both activities. Even simple household activities and work activities can be difficult if the patient is having difficulty speaking and breathing at the same time.

2 *Diet/activity restrictions:* diet plays an important role in the long-term management of asthma. Food that contains allergens such as peanuts and the additives that are in different foods can trigger an acute episode in the patient. Activity restrictions are often a part of life — dietary restrictions may have impact on the amount of energy taken in by the patient, and also the type and place of activity are key players in the risk of an acute episode. Examples include working in an environment with a lot of dust or smoke and allergens or the ability to go on a picnic in spring, living in the city or the country. Participation in sport may be restricted, not just because of the exertion required, but also because of the timing — training in the evening in cold damp air may trigger an attack (National Asthma Council of Australia, 2006).

3 *Loss of certainty, predictability for day-to-day events:* because asthma is a lifelong disorder and one that can be set off at any time by many things, the asthma sufferer is often unable to plan ahead with any certainty. For example, buying very expensive tickets to a concert 3 months in advance may be risky — what if the asthma sufferer has an attack on the day of the concert? These sorts of issues face the asthma sufferer every day.

4 *Loss of independence and ability to care for self:* as with all sufferers of chronic illness, there is a desire to be independent but as the disease progresses more assistance is required, and maintaining some independence requires a great deal of self-motivation and support. Over a long time this situation can lead to some severe mental health problems and even clinical depression.

BODY IMAGE — IMPACT ON THE PERSON AND THEIR CARERS

Body image is very important in the management of chronic illness, both to the patient and to the family and carers. The thought that they are different from others has a very strong influence on the patient; all the secondary losses due to chronic asthma seem to gain in importance to the sufferer over time. While all or some of these losses can be real and cause interference in life they are able to be managed. The patient tends to see the whole picture as one rather than looking at the picture in small pieces. The nurse plays a vital role in helping the patient to look at their situation in a different way, although it must be remembered that the nurse can only lead and that the patient needs to take the responsibility in making the changes. Later in the chapter we will look at some ways of coping and how to work with these. The family and carers can become drawn into the negative thoughts and behaviours of the patient and then the situation can become pathologically unsound. If the family/carers become drawn in, the patient will often see that as agreement by the family/ carers that the situation is as bad and unsolvable as the patient thinks it is. Giving too much sympathy to the patient is also quite destructive at times, as this can be seen as a message that the situation is really bad. Nurses need to give empathy, rather than sympathy, as this is a more constructive way to communicate with the patient and the family/carers.

Some of the main areas of concern to the patient in regard to body image are loss of self-esteem and dignity, loss of sexual performance abilities, loss of relationships with others and loss of full potential of body function. All of these have a large impact on the individual and the nurse needs to be in tune with their patient to pick up on any hint of the above and then start to help the patient to address these and manage them in a positive way.

ISSUES OF QUALITY OF LIFE IN RELATION TO THEIR CONDITION

The first thing the nurse needs to understand is the meaning of stress and coping: stresses are demands placed on people in their everyday life; coping is a dynamic cognitive and behavioural strategy used to manage internal and external demands that are seen as difficult or as exceeding the patient's normal resources (Miller, 2000). The main approaches to treatment are to identify the coping methods and styles of the patient. Once these are known, the nurse can work with the patient in the adaptation of these for the current situation. Coping methods are behaviours that we all learn throughout our lives: we can learn coping in both positive and negative ways and we reuse the situations that are seen as similar to the one we are in now. The outcome is not always the way we want it to be and if maladaptive coping methods are used the outcome is also maladaptive. Coping occurs along a continuum and is dynamic, based on the stressor and other life events. The three most common coping styles people may use in life are:

1 *direct approach:* confronting the stressor by tackling (energetically fighting), vigilant focusing (obsessional alertness to details) or sensitisers (readily acknowledge emotions of hate, fear)
2 *avoidance:* minimising the threat or seriousness of a situation through minimisation, repression, denial or selective inattention
3 *non-specific defences:* combination of the above approaches.

These styles have their place in dealing with chronic illness, and it is the way they are chosen and used that determines the outcome. The positive and negative aspects of each

TABLE 18.1
Coping styles

COPING STYLE	POSITIVES	NEGATIVES
Direct approach	Take action Accurate emotional perception	Higher anxiety
Avoidance	Break from non-productive worrying Time to find reasons for hope	Problem solving and treatment are delayed True feeling unknown

approach are outlined in Table 18.1. As a general rule, flexibility is the best approach; denial (avoidance) may be helpful early in a traumatic process or when a threatening situation is uncontrollable. However, direct approach coping will be necessary as the process progresses so that the right treatment is sought and valued.

INTERVENTIONS TO ATTAIN COMPLIANCE

Interventions for chronic asthma focus on prevention of acute exacerbations through recognition and avoidance of the triggers, monitoring of symptoms and improving dosages and adherence to medication (Newman, Steed, & Mulligan, 2004). The major objective is to control asthma by achieving and maintaining airway function. A variety of therapeutic interventions can be employed to achieve this, and are best monitored by use of an asthma action plan.

Asthma action plans

An asthma action plan should be implemented in order to monitor the long-term use of medications and improve compliance. The plan should be reviewed regularly and adjusted according to progression of the disease. The individual plan must be fully explained to and understood by the patient. The patient may be included in the decisions on the action plan to take into consideration individual preferences; alternatively patients may prefer their action plan to be decided by their doctor.

An asthma action plan should include:

- guidance for identifying signs of worsening control
- clear instructions for how to respond to any given change in asthma control.

In adults, individualised asthma action plans have been shown to reduce absences from work, hospital admissions, emergency presentations to general practice, use of short-acting beta-2-agonists and to generally improve lung function.

An example of an asthma action plan as recommended by the Department of Health and Ageing can be seen in Figure 18.1. Other plans include those developed by the National Asthma Council of Australia to help both the patient and the carer recognise and respond appropriately to worsening asthma.

Asthma control

For asthma, control refers to control of the manifestations of disease rather than prevention or cure: asthma can be treated but not cured. This should include control of the clinical features of the disease, including lung function abnormalities, as well as reducing the inflammation that underlies the disease. Complete control of asthma for prolonged periods

My Asthma Action Plan

When my asthma is WELL CONTROLLED

- No regular wheeze, or cough or chest tightness at night time, on waking or during the day
- Able to take part in normal physical activity without wheeze, cough or chest tightness
- Need reliever medication less than three times a week (except if it is used before exercise)
- Peak Flow* above ☐

What should I do?

Continue my usual treatment as follows:

Preventer

Reliever

Combination Medication

Always carry my reliever puffer

When my asthma is GETTING WORSE

- At the first sign of worsening asthma symptoms associated with a cold
- Waking from sleep due to coughing, wheezing or chest tightness
- Using reliever puffer more than 3 times a week (not including before exercise)
- Peak Flow* between

☐ and ☐

What should I do?

Increase my treatment as follows:

See my doctor to talk about my asthma getting worse

When my asthma is SEVERE

- Need reliever puffer every 3 hours or more often
- Increasing wheezing, coughing, chest tightness
- Difficulty with normal activity
- Waking each night and most mornings with wheezing, coughing or chest tightness
- Feel that asthma is out of control
- Peak Flow* between

☐ and ☐

What should I do?

Start oral prednisolone (or other steroid) and increase my treatment as follows:

See my doctor for advice

How to recognise LIFE-THREATENING ASTHMA

Dial 000 for an ambulance and/or 112 from a mobile phone if you have any of the following danger signs:

- extreme difficulty breathing
- little or no improvement from reliever puffer
- lips turn blue

and follow the Asthma First Aid Plan below while waiting for ambulance to arrive.

A serious asthma attack is also indicated by:

- symptoms getting worse quickly
- severe shortness of breath or difficulty in speaking
- you are feeling frightened or panicked
- Peak Flow* below ☐

Should any of these occur, follow the Asthma First Aid Plan below.

Asthma First Aid Plan

1 Sit upright and stay calm.

2 Take 4 separate puffs of a reliever puffer (one puff at a time) via a spacer device. Just use the puffer on its own if you don't have a spacer. Take 4 breaths from the spacer after each puff.

3 Wait 4 minutes. If there is no improvement, take another 4 puffs.

4 If little or no improvement **CALL AN AMBULANCE IMMEDIATELY (DIAL 000** and/or **112** from mobile phone) and state that you are having an asthma attack. Keep taking 4 puffs every 4 minutes until the ambulance arrives.

See your doctor immediately after a serious asthma attack.

Dr name: .... Ph .... Signature ....

Parent/Carer .... Ph ....

Name: .... Date: .... Best Peak Flow*: .... Next Doctor's Appointment: ....

* Not recommended for children under 12 years

FIGURE 18.1 Asthma action plan. *Note*: From My Asthma Action Plan, used by permission of the Australian Government.

My Asthma Action Plan

This written Asthma Action Plan will help you to manage your asthma.
Your Asthma Action Plan should be displayed in a place where it can be seen by you and others who need to know.
You may want to photocopy it.

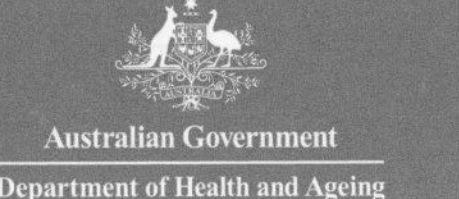

What happens in asthma?

Asthma inflames the airways. During an asthma attack, the air passages (airways) of the lungs become inflamed, swollen and narrowed. Thick mucus may be produced and breathing becomes difficult. This leads to coughing, wheezing and shortness of breath.

Asthma Triggers

Common asthma triggers are house dust mite, pollens, animal fur, moulds, tobacco smoke, and cold air. It is unusual but some foods may trigger asthma attacks.

Exercise is a common asthma trigger but can be well managed with pre-exercise medication and warm-up activities.

My known asthma triggers are:

....

....

....

....

Before exercise I need to warm up properly and take the following asthma medication:

....

....

....

....

Useful telephone numbers

- Asthma Foundation 1800 645 130 for information and advice about asthma management
- My pharmacy: ....

How your preventer medicine helps

Your preventer medicine reduces the redness and swelling in your airways and dries up the mucus. Preventers take time to work and need to be taken every day, even when you are well.

Preventer medications are: Qvar (beclomethasone), Flixotide (fluticasone), Intal Forte CFC-Free (sodium cromoglycate), Pulmicort (budesonide), Singulair (montelukast) and Tilade CFC-Free (nedocromil).

How your reliever medicine helps

Your reliever medicine relaxes the muscles around the airways, making the airways wider and breathing easier. It works quickly to relieve asthma symptoms, so it is essential for asthma first aid.

Reliever medications are: Airomir, Asmol, Epaq and Ventolin (all brands of salbutamol) and Bricanyl (terbutaline).

How your symptom controller helps

Symptom controllers can help people who still get symptoms even when they take regular preventer medicines. If you need a symptom controller, it should be taken with your preventer medication. It should not be taken instead of a preventer.

Like your reliever medicine, your symptom controller helps widen the airways. But while your reliever works for around 4–6 hours, symptom controllers work for up to 12 hours at a time. However, they are not good for quick relief of symptoms so they should not be used for asthma first aid.

Symptom controllers are: Foradile and Oxis (both brands of eformoterol), and Serevent (salmeterol).

There are **combination medications** that combine a symptom controller and a preventer in one puffer.

Combination medications are: Seretide (fluticasone and salmeterol) and Symbicort (budesonide and eformoterol).

Your GP can advise you on the availability under the Pharmaceutical Benefits Scheme of the drugs mentioned above.

My medications are

Preventer

....

Reliever

....

Symptom Controller

....

Combination Medication

....

Other Comments

....

....

....

....

....

....

....

....

....

....

reprinted November 2006

FIGURE 18.1 — cont'd

Characteristic	Controlled	Partly controlled (Any present in any week)	Uncontrolled
Daytime symptoms	None (2 or fewer/ week)	More than twice/week	3 or more features of partly controlled asthma present in any week
Limitations of activities	None	Any	
Nocturnal symptoms/ awakening	None	Any	
Need for rescue/ reliever treatment	None (2 or fewer/ week)	More than twice/week	
Lung function (PEF or FEV_1)	Normal	< 80% predicted or personal best (if known) on any day	

FIGURE 18.2 Levels of asthma control. *Source*: Global Initiative for Asthma. (2011). At-a-glance asthma management pocket reference. Retrieved from http://www.ginasthma.org/guidelines-pocket-guide-for-asthma-management.html

can be achieved with appropriate medications, allergen avoidance or reduction measures and lifestyle modifications. However, patients should also be aware of when their asthma is not optimally controlled. The Global Initiative for Asthma has developed a working scheme for determining how well an individual's asthma is controlled (Global Initiative for Asthma [GINA], 2011): this is based on identifying the levels of control as 'controlled, partly controlled and uncontrolled' (Figure 18.2). A change in the level of control should be identified as part of the action plan and should prompt immediate review of the maintenance treatment. An example of a medication management plan that can be initiated in order to regain control is shown in Figure 18.3. This involves a step-wise approach to medication based on the level of control of symptoms and typically involves a combination of approaches underpinned primarily by increasing doses of anti-inflammatory inhaled corticosteroids that are secondarily combined with long-acting beta-2-agonists bronchodilators. Other anti-inflammatory measures include the use of oral corticosteroids or leukotriene antagonists to control inflammation, as well as anti-IgE antibodies in more severe cases to block allergic inflammation mediated by this molecule.

Spirometry and peak expiratory flow measurements

Spirometry is a measurement of the time-dependent volume of air breathed into (inspiration) and out of (expiration) the lungs. The aim of spirometry is to detect the presence and variability of airflow obstruction, and to measure the degree of airflow limitation (referred to as obstruction) compared to either the predicted normal (reference value) or the individual's personal best value measured when their asthma is well controlled. Accurate measurement of respiratory function is necessary in the diagnosis of asthma and to effectively manage treatment. Spirometry generates flow-volume loops that indicate the amount of air a person can breathe in and out (volume) and the speed or flow rate at which this can be achieved (flow) with the forced expiratory volume in one second (FEV_1) being a key parameter to diagnose airflow limitation (obstruction). For the doctor, the

Reduce ←	Treatment Steps			→ Increase
Step 1	Step 2	Step 3	Step 4	Step 5
Asthma education Environmental control				
As needed rapid-acting β_2-agonist	As needed rapid-acting β_2-agonist			
Controller options	Select one	Select one	Add one or more	Add one or both
	Low-dose inhaled ICS*	Low-dose ICS plus long-acting β_2-agonist	Medium- or high-dose ICS plus long-acting β_2-agonist	Oral glucocorticosteroid (lowest dose)
	Leukotriene modifier †	Medium- or high-dose ICS	Leukotriene modifier	Anti-IgE treatment
		Low-dose ICS plus leukotriene modifier	Sustained release theophylline	
		Low-dose ICS plus sustained release theophylline		

* ICS = inhaled glucocorticosteroids
† = Receptor antagonist or synthesis inhibitors

FIGURE 18.3 Step-wise approach to treatment of uncontrolled asthma for adults, adolescents and children over 5 years. *Source*: Global Initiative for Asthma. (2011). At-a-glance asthma management pocket reference. Retrieved from http://www.ginasthma.org/guidelines-pocket-guide-for-asthma-management.html

shape of the flow volume loops indicates the nature and severity of the patient's asthma and whether the patient responds to bronchodilation following inhalation of a short-acting beta-2-agonist bronchodilator (Figure 18.4). A significant bronchodilator response occurs when either FEV_1 or FVC (forced vital capacity) increase by >200mL and >12%. In the right clinical context this allows the diagnosis of asthma.

Peak flow, or peak expiratory flow (PEF), is the measurement of the peak rate, or maximum rate, at which an individual can expel air from the lungs. Peak flow measurements provide an indication of airflow limitation (obstruction) and are usually scored as a percentage measurement of a person's 'best' result; that is, an average result recorded over a period of 1 or 2 weeks when their asthma is well controlled. The measurement can also be recorded as 'percentage predicted', the predicted value being a composite value of age, height, gender and ethnically matched non-asthmatic individuals. However, if a personal best value is known, this is generally a more reliable measure as it will take into account person–person variations. Peak flow measurements are an integral part of an asthma management plan and can be used for early detection of asthma worsening and assist to intensify medical treatment. As an example, when a PEF value falls below 80% of the predicted value, or personal best value if known (see Figure 18.2). PEF measurements can also be useful in monitoring responses to medications such as inhaled corticosteroids after a severe attack. In interpreting this type of monitoring, however, it is important that several readings are taken over a prolonged period of time, as a variability between readings can occur

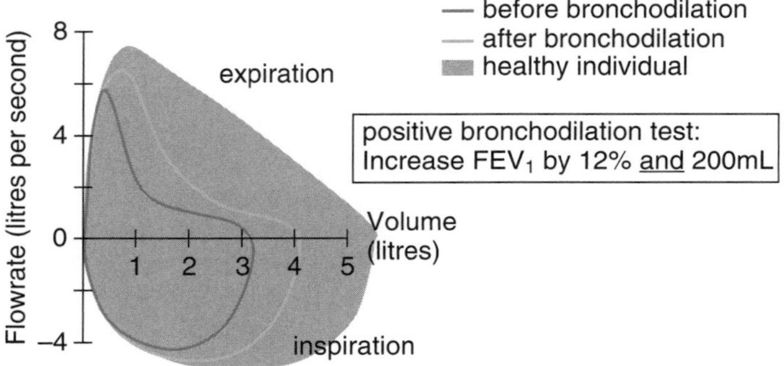

FIGURE 18.4 Spirometry for the diagnosis of airflow limitation (obstruction) and asthma with the bronchodilator response. FEV_1 = forced expiratory volume in one second; FVC = forced vital capacity.

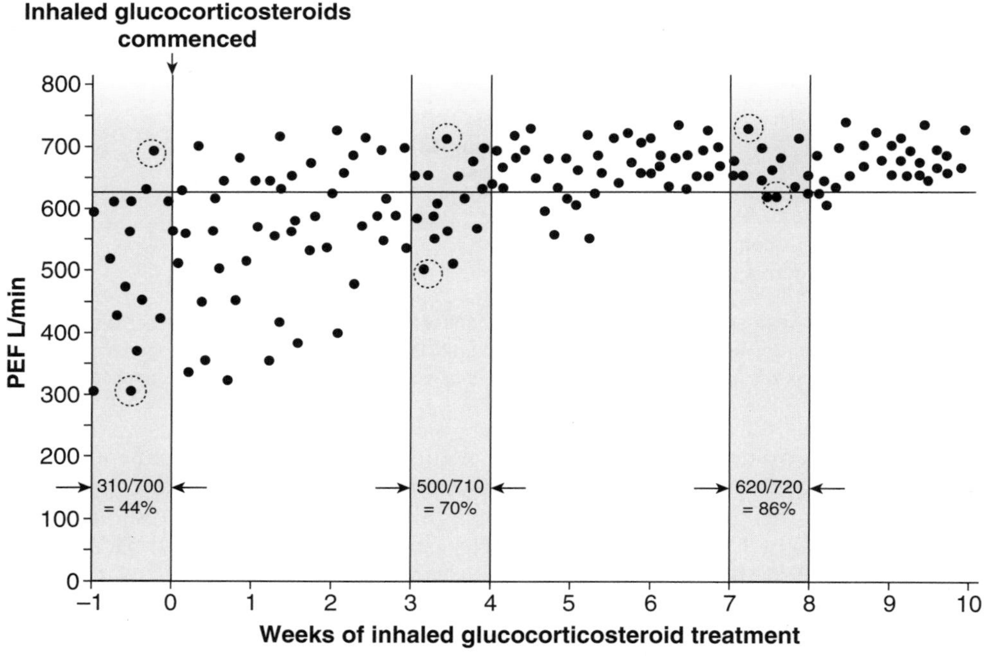

FIGURE 18.5 Measuring variability of peak expiratory flow. *Source*: Global Initiative for Asthma. (2011). At-a-glance asthma management pocket reference. Retrieved from http://www.ginasthma.org/guidelines-pocket-guide-for-asthma-management.html

(Figure 18.5). It is important to be aware that PEF values are not recommended for the diagnosis of asthma as other non-asthmatic respiratory conditions can cause a change in PEF values, and thus spirometry is the recommended diagnostic test. Patients should be advised to see a doctor if they are feeling unwell.

Successive spirometry measurements before and after bronchodilator use allow diagnosis of airway obstruction, enable measurement of the degree of airway obstruction, monitor the effects of treatments, demonstrate the presence and reversibility of airway obstruction to the patient, provide objective feedback to the patient about the presence and severity of asthma and accurately back-titrate preventive medication to determine the minimum effective dose (National Asthma Council of Australia, 2012).

FAMILY AND CARERS

Nursing management

In planning the nursing management of the person with asthma we have chosen to use nursing process as the framework for the nursing management. A detailed care plan is shown in Figure 18.6 (adapted from Gulanick & Myers, 2011).

EDUCATION FOR THE PERSON AND FAMILY

Education for the person with chronic asthma is critical. Education can empower the person to effectively self-manage and take responsibility for their chronic illness. The education process should begin with the initial diagnosis of asthma and continue throughout all subsequent interactions between the patient, family and healthcare professionals. The aim of education is to empower the patient to effectively manage their asthma in order to:

- achieve the optimum health (physical and psychological)
- reduce unplanned GP consultations, emergency room treatments and hospital admissions
- have the confidence to manage change in asthma conditions.

In adults the use of asthma self-management education programs will involve the following:

- written information about asthma
- monitoring of asthma control, based on PEF and/or symptoms
- a written asthma action plan (see Figure 18.1)
- regular review by a health professional (may include doctor, nurse or asthma educator). This will include review of medications, assessment of asthma control, discussion of triggers, consideration of lifestyle choices and discussion and provision of feedback to the patient about their overall control of asthma.

In addition, the person, family and friends should also be educated in what to do in case of an emergency asthma attack. The Asthma Foundations of Australia have developed an asthma first aid plan that provides a useful summary of what to do in case of emergency (Table 18.2).

Self-management interventions

Self-management interventions (SMI) in chronic asthma involve more than providing information to the patient. The key feature of these interventions is to increase patients' involvement and control in their treatment and its effect on their lives in order to improve rates of adherence to medications and to improve quality of life (Lawn & Schoo, 2010). It is a process developed over time in partnership between the patient and health professionals that enables the patient to actively participate in their asthma care with the doctor, nurse or asthma educator and will include:

- understanding the nature of asthma (chronic inflammatory disease)
- being actively involved in planning care and the review process

CHRONIC ASTHMA NURSING CARE PLAN	
Nursing diagnosis: Ineffective breathing pattern related to swelling and spasming of the bronchial tubes in response to allergies, drugs, stress, infection and inhaled irritants.	
Expected outcome: The patient to maintain optimal breathing patterns, as evidenced by regular respiratory rate or pattern.	
Ongoing assessment	
Interventions	**Rationale**
Assess respiratory rate and depth, monitor breathing pattern. Assess for use of accessory muscles, retractions and flaring of nostrils.	Respiratory rate and rhythm changes can be an early warning sign to impending respiratory difficulties.
Assess relationship of inspiration to expiration.	Reactive airways allow air to move into the lungs with greater ease than to move out of the lungs.
Monitor peak expiratory flow rates and forced expiratory volumes.	The severity of the exacerbation can be measured objectively by monitoring these values. The peak expiratory flow rate (PEFR) is the maximum flow rate that can be generated during a forced expiratory manoeuvre with fully inflated lungs. It measures in litres per second and requires maximal effort. When done with good effort it correlates well with forced expiratory volume in 1 second (FEV_1) measured by spirometry and provides a simple reproducible measure of airway obstruction.
Assess vital signs every hour as needed if patient in distress.	
Assess fatigue.	Fatigue may indicate increasing distress leading to respiratory failure.
Monitor oxygen saturation by pulse oximetry, maintaining the oxygen saturation above 90% or higher, with oxygen as ordered by the doctor.	
Monitor arterial blood gases (ABGs).	During a mild to moderate asthma attack, patients may develop a respiratory acidosis.
Assess breath sounds and note wheeze or other adventitious breath sounds.	Adventitious sounds may indicate a worsening condition or additional pathology such as pneumonia. Diminishing wheezing and inaudible breath sounds may indicate impending respiratory failure.
Assess level of anxiety.	Hypoxia and the sensation of not being able to breathe is very frightening and may cause worsening hypoxia.
Therapeutic interventions	
Interventions	**Rationale**
Encourage the patient to sit upright.	This position allows for adequate lung excursions and chest expansion.
Encourage slow deep breathing. Instruct patient to use pursed lip breathing for exhalation. Instruct to time breathing so that exhalation takes 2 to 3 times as long as inspiration.	Pursed lip exhalation facilitates expiratory airflow by helping to keep the bronchioles open. Prolonged expiration prevents air trapping.
Use beta-2-adrenergic agonist drugs by metered-dose inhaler (MDI) or nebuliser as prescribed.	Beta-2-adrenergic agonist drugs relax airway smooth muscle.
Administer medications as prescribed.	Corticosteroids are the most effective anti-inflammatory drugs for the reversible airflow obstruction. During severe attacks, anticholinergics may be effective when used in combination with beta-2-adrenergic agonists.

FIGURE 18.6 Chronic asthma nursing care plan (Gulanick & Myers, 2011).

Plan activity and rest to maximise patients energy.	Fatigue is common with the increase work of breathing from the ineffective breathing pattern.
Nursing diagnosis: Ineffective airway clearance related to bronchospasm, excessive mucous production and ineffective cough and fatigue.	
Expected outcome: Patients airway is maintained free of secretions as evidenced by normal/improved breath sounds and normal ABGs or oxygen saturation if 90% or greater on pulse oximeter.	
Ongoing assessment	
Interventions	**Rationale**
Auscultate lungs with each routine vital sign check.	This allows for early detection and correction of abnormalities.
Assess secretions noting colour, viscosity, odour and amount.	Thick tenacious secretions may indicate dehydration. Coloured or odours secretions may indicate bleeding or infection.
Assess cough for effectiveness and productivity.	Consider possible causes of an ineffective cough, respiratory muscle fatigue, severe bronchospasm, thick tenacious sputum.
Assess patient's physical capabilities and activities of daily living (ADLs).	Fatigue can limit ADLs.
Monitor pulse oxygen saturation and ABGs.	Hypoxia can result from increased pulmonary secretions.
Therapeutic Interventions	
Interventions	**Rationale**
Administer β-2-adrenergic agonists (e.g. albuterol) by MDI or nebuliser, as prescribed.	β-2-adrenergic agonist drugs relax airway smooth muscle.
Administer other medications as prescribed.	Corticoster oids are the most effective antiinflammatory drugs for the reversible airflow obstruction. During severe attacks, anticholinergics may be effective when used in combination with β-2-adrenergic agonists.
Encourage patient to cough and assist with effective coughing techniques: • sit patient upright • splint chest • patient to use abdominal muscles • use cough techniques as appropriate.	Promotes chest expansion. Promotes comfort. Ability for a more forceful cough.
Assist in mobilising secretions to facilitate airway clearance: • increase room.	Humidity will help liquefy
Nursing diagnosis: Anxiety related to respiratory distress, change in health status, changes in environment and routines, and coping with chronic illness.	
Expected outcome: Patients anxiety is reduced as evidenced by cooperative behaviour, demonstrates positive coping mechanisms and verbalised report of decreased anxiety.	
Ongoing assessment	
Interventions	**Rationale**
Assess anxiety level, including vital signs, respiratory status, irritability, apprehension and orientation	Anxiety can affect respiratory rate and rhythm.
Assess ability to relax.	
Assess oxygen saturation levels.	Anxiety increases with increasing hypoxia and may be an early warning sign of decreasing oxygen levels.
Assess theophylline level if patient is taking theophylline.	Theophylline increases anxiety.

FIGURE 18.6 — cont'd

(continued next page ...)

Therapeutic interventions	
Interventions	**Interventions**
Stay with patient and encourage slow, deep breathing.	
Explain importance of remaining calm.	Maintaining calmness decreases oxygen consumption and work of breathing.
Keep significant other informed of patient progress.	Information can help to relieve apprehension.
Avoid excessive reassurance.	Excessive reassurance may increase anxiety for many people.
Assist the patient with developing anxiety reducing skills (e.g. relaxation, deep breathing, progressive muscle relaxation, positive visualisation and reassuring self-statements).	Using anxiety-reduction strategies enhance the patient's sense of personal mastery and confidence.
Encourage patient to seek assistance from understanding significant other or healthcare provider if anxious feelings become difficult.	
Nursing diagnosis: Deficit knowledge related to ineffective past teaching or learning, and unfamiliarity with resources.	
Expected outcome: Patient verbalises understanding of disease process and treatment.	
Ongoing assessment	
Intervention	**Rationale**
Assess knowledge base of chronic asthma.	Asthma is a chronic disease and many new medications and treatments continue to be developed.
Assess educational, environmental, social and cultural factors that may influence teaching plan.	
Assess cognitive function and emotional readiness to learn.	
Therapeutic interventions	
Interventions	**Rationale**
Establish common goals with the patient.	
Actively include the patient in the decision process of the education and management.	
Instruct patient in anatomy and physiology of the respiratory system and provide information to appropriate level.	Information will assist the patient to understand the complexities of their airway problems.
Discuss the relation of the disease process of asthma related to signs and symptoms.	Information will assist the patient to understand the complexities of their airway problems.
Discuss the medications that the patient is taking including: • name of medication • action and role of each medication • dosage of medication • method of administration • care of the MDI • side-effects of medication • action on experiencing side effects • consequences of improper use • consideration of medications' influence with ADLs.	Return demonstration on MDI technique are necessary to ensure appropriate delivery of medications.
Discuss concept of energy conservation. Encourage resting as needed during activities, avoiding over exertion and fatigue, sitting as much as possible and alternating heavy and light tasks.	Learning self-management skills may reduce dyspnoea from fatigue.

FIGURE 18.6 — cont'd

Discuss Asthma Action Plan. Including signs and symptoms of infection and worsening asthma and when to contact healthcare provider.	
Discuss triggers and factors that lead to exacerbations of asthma and how to avoid them.	
Discuss effect of smoking and refer patient or significant others to cessation of smoking program or support group.	
Discuss importance of specific therapeutic measures as listed: • Breathing exercises *Exercise 1* 1. Lie supine, with one hand on chest and one on abdomen. 2. Inhale slowly through mouth, raising abdomen against hand. 3. Exhale slowly through pursed lips while contracting abdominal muscles and moving abdomen inwards.	This exercise strengthens muscles of respiration.
Exercise 2 1. Walk; stop to take a deep breath. 2. Exhale slowly while walking.	This exercise develops slowed, controlled breathing.
Exercise 3 1. For pursed-lip breathing, inhale slowly through nose. 2. Exhale twice as slowly as usual through pursed lips.	This exercise decreases air trapping and airway collapse.
• Cough: lean forward; take several deep breaths with pursed-lip method. Take last deep breath, cough through open mouth during expiration and simultaneously contract abdominal muscles.	Effective method that prevents waste of energy.
• Chest physiotherapy or pulmonary postural drainage. Demonstrate correct methods of postural drainage: positioning, percussions, vibration.	Facilitates expectoration of secretions and prevents waste of energy.
• Hydration: discuss importance of maintaining 1.5 to 2 L/day. • Humidity: discuss various forms of humidification.	Decreases viscosity of secretions. Prevents drying of secretions.
Discuss the need for regular consultation by healthcare team for review of management, prescriptions, ongoing education.	
Discuss available resources: • Asthma Foundation website. *(e.g. Carers Resources)* • National Asthma Council website *(e.g. Carers Resources).*	
Discuss the need for patient to obtain vaccines for pneumococcal pneumonia and yearly vaccine for influenza.	Vaccine decreases severity and occurrence of these diseases.
Discuss use of medical alert bracelet or other identification.	Alerts others to chronic asthma.
Include relevant others including family members in education to ensure patient has relevant knowledgeable help in time of crisis.	

FIGURE 18.6 — cont'd

TABLE 18.2

Asthma first aid plan. *Note:* Adapted from the Asthma Foundations of Australia (2005).

STEP 1	Sit the person upright and give them reassurance. Do not leave them alone.
STEP 2	Without delay, give 4 separate puffs of a blue inhaler (e.g. Ventolin). Give the medicine one puff at a time via a spacer device and ask the person to take 4 breaths from the spacer after each puff. If a spacer is not available, use the puffer on its own.
STEP 3	Wait 4 minutes. If there is no improvement, repeat steps 2 and 3.
STEP 4	If there is still little or no improvement call an ambulance.

Reflective questions

1 Consider how you would explain the benefits of an asthma action plan to a patient with chronic asthma who has not previously had an action plan. What are the key aspects of the plan that the patient, family and carers should understand?

2 What are some of the key triggers for asthma exacerbations and what measures could be taken to avoid these triggers? What education could be provided to the patient by the practice nurse to improve the home or work environment?

3 How would you explain the benefits of a preventative inhaler to a teenager, and what strategies could you take to educate and improve patient compliance with inhaler use?

- identifying activities that protect and promote health (including knowledge of medications and correct use of inhaler devices)
- monitoring the signs and symptoms of asthma
- managing the psychosocial impact of chronic illness upon lifestyle.

CONCLUSION

Asthma is a complex condition that requires careful diagnosis and management. The underlying pathology of this condition is inflammation of the airways driven by a variety of allergic and non-allergic stimuli. However, a high proportion of people with asthma suffer from an allergic condition called atopy; therefore, a key step in the care of the allergic asthmatic patient is the identification of allergic triggers of the disorder and taking steps to avoid or minimise exposure to these. The key principle of nursing management of chronic asthmatic patients is to restore airway function to the optimal level for the individual and to instigate a treatment regimen to maintain optimal lung function. A key component in the management of the chronic asthmatic patient is the development of an asthma management plan in conjunction with the patient and the doctor. This will aid in compliance with treatment in order to maintain optimal airway function, and help to identify signs and symptoms that will indicate when the condition is worsening and when treatment should be sought. Family and friends should also be educated as to the nature of this chronic condition, what to do in case of an acute exacerbation and ways that the patient's environment can be improved and maintained in order to minimise the risk of exacerbations occurring.

Recommended reading

Australian Centre for Asthma Monitoring. (2011). *Asthma in Australia 2011*. Canberra: Australian Institute of Health and Welfare. Available from http://www.aihw.gov.au/publication-detail/?id=10737420159

Corbridge, S. (2010). Asthma in adolescents and adults. *The American Journal of Nursing, 110*, 28–38.

Global Initiative for Asthma. (2011). At-a-glance asthma management pocket reference. Available from http://www.ginasthma.org/guidelines-pocket-guide-for-asthma-management.html

National Asthma Council of Australia. (2006). Asthma management handbook. Available from http://www.nationalasthma.org.au/handbook

National Asthma Council of Australia. (2012). What is asthma? Available from http://www.nationalasthma.org.au/understanding-asthma/what-is-asthma-

References

American Thoracic Society. (2000). Guidelines for Methacholine and Exercise Challenge Testing — 1999. *American Journal of Respiratory and Critical Care Medicine, 161*, 309–329.

Asthma Foundations of Australia. (2005). Asthma First Aid Plan. Retrieved January 30, 2013, from http://www.asthmaaustralia.org.au

Australian Centre for Asthma Monitoring. (2011). *Asthma in Australia 2011*. Canberra: Australian Institute of Health and Welfare. Retrieved January 30, 2013, from http://www.aihw.gov.au/publication-detail/?id=10737420159

Barnes, P. J. (2012). Severe asthma: advances in current management and future therapy. *The Journal of Allergy and Clinical Immunology, 129*, 48–59.

Brooks, C. R., van Dalen, C. J., Hermans, I. F., et al. (2013). Identifying leucocyte populations in fresh and cryopreserved sputum using flow cytometry. *Cytometry Part B-Clinical Cytometry, 84B*(2), 104–113.

Department of Health and Ageing. (2004). Asthma and allergy: A guide for health professionals. Retrieved January 30, 2013, from http://www.nationalasthma.org.au

Department of Health and Ageing. (2006). Asthma Action Plan. Retrieved January 30, 2013, from http://www.health.gov.au/internet/main/publishing.nsf/content/asthma-plan

Global Initiative for Asthma. (2011). At-a-glance asthma management pocket reference. Retrieved 30 January 2013 from http://www.ginasthma.org/guidelines-pocket-guide-for-asthma-management.html

Gulanick, M., Myers, J. L. (2011). *Nursing Care Plans: Nursing Diagnosis and Interventions*. (7th ed.). St Louis: Elsevier

Holgate, S. T., & Polosa, R. (2006). The mechanisms, diagnosis, and management of severe asthma in adults. *Lancet, 368*, 780–793.

Holt, P. G. (2004). The hygiene hypothesis: Modulation of the atopic phenotype by environmental microbial exposure. In E. Isolauri & W. A. Walker (Eds.), *Allergic diseases and the environment* (pp. 53–68). Switzerland: Nestec.

Holt, P. G., & Thomas, V. V. R. (2005). Sensitization to airborne environmental allergens: unresolved issues. *Nature Immunology, 6*, 957–960.

Holt, P. G., Macaubas, C., Stumbles, P. A, et al. (1999). The role of allergy in the development of asthma. *Nature, 402*(Supp.), B12–B17.

Johnston, S. L. (1998). Viruses and asthma. *Allergy, 53*, 922–923.

Lawn, S., & Schoo, A. (2010). Supporting self-management of chronic health conditions: Common approaches. *Patient Education and Counseling, 80*(2), 205–211.

Miller, J. F. (2000). *Coping with chronic illness: overcoming powerlessness.* Philadelphia: FA Davis

National Asthma Council of Australia. (2006). Asthma management handbook. Retrieved January 30, 2013, from http://www.nationalasthma.org.au/handbook

National Asthma Council of Australia. (2012). What is Asthma? Retrieved 30 January 2013 from http://www.nationalasthma.org.au/understanding-asthma/what-is-asthma-

Newman, S., Steed, L., & Mulligan, K. (2004). Self-management interventions for chronic illness. *Lancet, 364*(9444), 1523–1537.

Quaedvlieg, V., Sele, J., Henket, M., et al. (2009). Association between asthma control and bronchial hyperresponsiveness and airways inflammation: a cross-sectional study in daily practice. *Clinical and Experimental Allergy: Journal of The British Society for Allergy and Clinical Immunology, 39*, 1822–1829.

Wenzel, S. (2006). Asthma: defining of the persistent adult phenotypes. *Lancet, 368*, 804–813.

CHAPTER 19

Colleen Doyle
Rebecca Howard
Sandy Ward
Maree Daly

Chronic obstructive pulmonary disease

Learning objectives

When you have completed this chapter you will be able to:

- describe the main signs and symptoms of chronic obstructive pulmonary disease (COPD) and understand how common it is
- understand the mental health issues for the person with COPD
- describe the epidemiology of COPD
- understand the importance of self-management through attendance at pulmonary rehabilitation and patient education classes
- explain the main nursing principles relevant to the ongoing care of the person with COPD including palliation.

Key words

dyspnoea, exacerbation, hypoxaemia, pulmonary rehabilitation, mental health

INTRODUCTION

Chronic obstructive pulmonary disease (COPD) is one of the most common diseases in the world, yet public awareness of the disease is much lower than for other lung diseases such as asthma or emphysema. One reason for this relates to the language used to describe the disease. COPD is not one single disease but an umbrella term for chronic bronchitis and emphysema. In the past COPD has also been referred to as chronic obstructive airway disease (COAD), chronic obstructive lung disease (COLD), chronic airflow limitation (CAL) and chronic obstructive respiratory disease. This differing terminology can lead to confusion and may impact on public understanding. COPD is now the commonly accepted term for the disease.

In practice it may be difficult to differentiate between asthma, which is reversible airway obstruction, and COPD, which is irreversible airway obstruction. People with COPD experience breathlessness, coughing, wheeze, increased sputum production, sleep disturbance, fatigue and weight loss. Everyday tasks such as vacuuming, putting on shoes or even walking can become difficult due to breathlessness and the debilitating effects of the disease. Smoking is the main behavioural cause of COPD, but there is increasing evidence that some individuals have a genetic susceptibility to developing COPD. Occupational or environmental exposures to dust and fumes can also contribute to COPD. One of the most effective treatments for people with COPD is pulmonary rehabilitation, a program of exercise and education that can greatly improve quality of life. Influenza vaccinations are also very effective in protecting against exacerbations. There is increasing evidence for the effectiveness of cognitive behaviour therapy for managing depression and anxiety associated with the disease. Nurses should be aware that COPD is not a hopeless disease, and that much can be done to improve patients' quality of life.

WHAT IS COPD?

The World Health Organization (WHO) provides the following definition of COPD:

> Chronic obstructive pulmonary disease (COPD) is not one single disease but an umbrella term used to describe chronic lung diseases that cause limitations in lung airflow. The more familiar terms 'chronic bronchitis' and 'emphysema' are no longer used, but are now included within the COPD diagnosis.
>
> The most common symptoms of COPD are breathlessness, or a 'need for air', excessive sputum production, and a chronic cough. However, COPD is not just simply a 'smoker's cough', but an under-diagnosed, life threatening lung disease that may progressively lead to death. (WHO, 2012)

COPD is one of the most common diseases in the world. It is a term for a collection of lung diseases, all of which prevent the sufferer from breathing easily. In individuals with COPD, the lung is damaged and the airways are partly obstructed, making it hard to breathe. Emphysema and chronic bronchitis are two common types of COPD. The airflow limitation is usually progressive and is associated with an abnormal inflammatory response of the lungs to noxious particles or gases (Global Initiative for Chronic Obstructive Lung Disease [GOLD], 2010).

HOW IS COPD RELATED TO ASTHMA AND OTHER LUNG FUNCTION DISEASES?

Lung function diseases are all characterised by limitations to airflow, which is measured via spirometry, a respiratory function test (RFT, also known as a lung function test). The separation of asthma and COPD aligns with the current treatment of the two lung conditions as separate although overlapping diseases (see Figure 19.1). Currently accepted definitions emphasise the reversibility of asthma, which is highly responsive to treatment, while COPD is considered to be at the opposite end of the spectrum of airway disease, being poorly reversible and characterised by progressive airway narrowing (Jenkins, Thompson, Gibson, & Wood-Baker, 2005). Emphysema is a pathological diagnosis, and consists of alveolar dilation and destruction. Chronic bronchitis is defined as a daily cough with sputum production for at least 3 months for two or more consecutive years (McKenzie

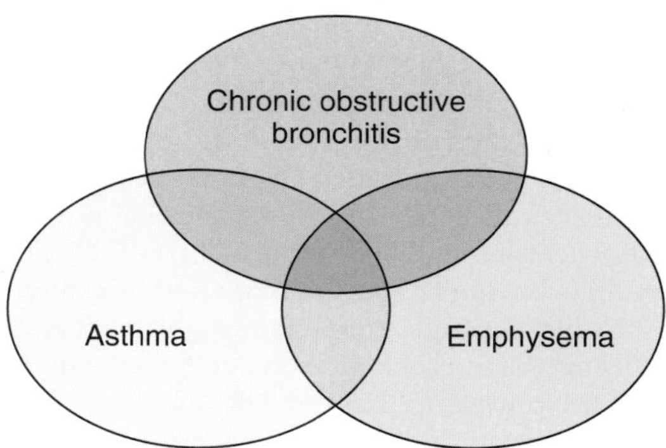

FIGURE 19.1 Overlapping lung diseases

et al., 2012). (Normal lungs produce about 30 millilitres of sputum daily, so sputum production on its own is not abnormal.) In practice, there may be considerable overlap between types of lung disease.

People with COPD commonly refer to their condition by lay terms such as 'asthma' or 'emphysema'; however, they usually have a combination of all three types of pathology in varying degrees. Chronic asthma stems from hyperactivity and thickening of airway walls over a prolonged period. The degree of reversibility on RFTs after bronchodilator administration distinguishes asthma (high degree of reversibility) from chronic asthma (low degree of reversibility). Emphysema involves the destruction of the peripheral airways including the alveoli, resulting in loss of lung elasticity, narrowing of the terminal airways and decreased surface area for gas exchange. During expiration, loss of elasticity may result in collapse of the terminal airways, which in turn increases work of breathing. In comparison, chronic bronchitis exhibits a persistent productive cough, due to hypertrophy and hyperplasia of the airway's mucus-producing cells. The upper airways are usually inflamed and swollen, resulting in debris and obstruction.

HOW COMMON IS COPD?

Worldwide, COPD is the fourth leading cause of death, responsible for almost 6% of all deaths. In high income countries, such as Australia and New Zealand, COPD accounts for 3.5% of deaths (WHO, 2012). In Australia in 2009, COPD was the fourth leading cause of death for men and sixth for women (Australian Institute of Health and Welfare [AIHW], 2012b). In New Zealand, COPD is the third leading cause of death for men and fourth for women and New Zealand has the fifth highest death rate from COPD in the world (Australian Lung Foundation [ALF], 2001). In a report published in 2003 (Town, Taylor, Garrett, & Patterson, 2003), COPD was identified as a significant New Zealand health issue affecting over 200 000 New Zealanders. Although there is an absence of reliable data on prevalence the report estimated that over $192 million was spent on COPD-related health costs and COPD affected approximately 15% of persons over the age of 45. The report highlighted the need for early detection, which is paramount, as in later stages the effects are irreversible.

According to the Australian Lung Foundation, in 2008, about 1.2 million Australians had symptomatic COPD. This is expected to increase to 2.6 million by 2050. Prevalence is increasing because of the ageing of the population, and public awareness remains low, resulting in under diagnosis (ALF, 2012). About 2.4% of Australians reported having bronchitis or emphysema in the 2007–2008 National Health Survey (Australian Bureau of Statistics [ABS], 2010), compared to 3.5% in 2001, 4.1% in 1995 and 3.0% in 1989. Although these estimates would contain some cases of bronchitis that were not chronic in nature, it is still likely to have underestimated the true prevalence of COPD in Australia. Other data puts the prevalence rate at 5.6% for the Australian population overall, and 8.2% for people over 30 (Access Economics, 2008; see also AIHW, 2011). The under-estimation in the self-reported data may be due to the fact that COPD is often not diagnosed until it begins to restrict a person's lifestyle and is moderately advanced and also some people with COPD are not aware of their diagnosis. Relatively few people at younger ages have bronchitis or emphysema, but the prevalence rises to 8% at the age of 75 years and over (ABS, 2010). COPD is very common among people who are admitted to hospital. COPD is involved in more hospital admissions than asthma.

COPD is also overwhelmingly more common than asthma as a cause of death. According to a recent AIHW report, in 2009 asthma accounted for 1.7 deaths per 100 000 people, compared to 23 deaths per 100 000 people attributed to COPD (AIHW, 2012a). Rates of hospitalisations in 2009 were similar, at 0.05% and 0.06% of all hospitalisations for asthma and COPD respectively (AIHW, 2006).

EPIDEMIOLOGY OF COPD

There is considerable stigma associated with having the disease COPD, due to the societal perception that COPD is caused by smoking and therefore the sufferers have 'brought it on themselves'. Surprisingly, only a minority of cigarette smokers develop COPD, although tobacco smoking is the single most important environmental determinant of COPD. Approximately 20% of smokers develop COPD (Sampsonas, Karkoulias, Kaparianos, & Spiropoulos, 2006). Among non-smokers, the prevalence of the disease is about 7%, indicating that there are genetic as well as environmental factors that play a role in the development of COPD. Therefore, while we can consider behaviours that contribute to the development of the condition, this would not give a complete picture of the determinants of COPD. Many determinants or risk factors are not 'behaviours' and as such are not easily avoided by the people with the disease. Risk factors may be associated with social status, cultural mores, occupational roles or other complex contributors.

The prevalence of COPD is generally higher in men than in women, attributable to the higher rates of smoking among men although the gender difference may be reducing (Viegi et al., 2006). However, there may also be gender differences in the susceptibility to deleterious effects of smoking, with men showing greater susceptibility, possibly due to additive effects of exposure to pollutants and occupational dusts or chemicals (Watson et al., 2006). With smoking rates among women increasing, COPD rates are also increasing among women. While COPD appears more prevalent in men, when smoking and occupational exposure are taken into account there is no gender difference.

Certain cultural groups smoke more than others. The prevalence of smoking in people from indigenous (Aboriginal and Torres Strait Islander, and Māori) backgrounds, some culturally and linguistically diverse backgrounds, people with mental disorders and substance use disorders and prisoners is greater than in the general population, increasing the susceptibility of such groups to COPD (Baker et al., 2006). Migrants constitute approximately 23% of the Australian population, and approximately 14% of the Australian population has emigrated from countries of non-English-speaking backgrounds (Baker et al., 2006; Page et al., 2007). Rates of smoking among those with mental health disorders are very high, with reported rates of 70–88% among those with psychotic disorders (Baker et al., 2006). The majority of individuals with alcohol and drug abuse problems also smoke, as do nearly all Australian prisoners with substance abuse problems (Baker et al., 2006).

Studies in the UK have shown a clear social class gradient for COPD with greater prevalence among people of lower socioeconomic status (SES). Low SES is associated with poorer health and higher mortality from most chronic conditions, and in Australia areas of low SES have higher rates of smoking, physical inactivity and obesity (AIHW, 2006). In New Zealand it is reported that COPD is considerably higher for the Māori population than for the non-Māori population and hospital admission occurs much earlier. Mortality from COPD tends to increase in Australia for both males and females with increasing geographic remoteness (AIHW, 2006).

As only up to 20% of smokers develop COPD, this subgroup may have a genetic susceptibility that interacts with exposure to tobacco smoke to impair lung function. The 'Dutch hypothesis' was formulated in the early 1960s when the alpha-antitrypsin gene was implicated in development of COPD. The Dutch hypothesis essentially pointed to endogenous factors (genes) playing a major role in the development of COPD, while alternative hypotheses have mainly considered exogenous factors and their contribution to the development of COPD. (The Dutch hypothesis holds that genetic susceptibility and allergens lead to both asthma and COPD. In contrast, the British hypothesis states that COPD is closely related to irritant exposure and to recurrent infections.) A recent review of the genetics of COPD indicated that while smoking contributes about 15% to the variability of lung function, genetic factors account for a further 40% (Wood & Stockley, 2006). Observations of differences in rate of decline in lung function, family aggregations of spirometric measures and higher rates of airflow obstructions among first-degree relatives of patients with COPD all point to genetic factors. Apart from the alpha-1-antitrypsin gene, recent research is beginning to uncover other genes implicated. Therefore it appears that both genetic susceptibility and environmental exposure may be important determinants of the development of COPD.

As is well known, cigarette smoking is a leading cause of preventable illness and death, accounting for 12% of the burden of disease in Australian men and 7% in Australian women (Mathers, Vos, & Stevenson 1999). Smoking contributes to COPD, heart disease and stroke, diabetes complications, asthma and various cancers, including lung disease. These diseases are all Australian national health priorities (Ministerial Council on Drug Strategy, 2004). At any time, many smokers want to quit. Less than 10% of Australian smokers consistently deny any interest in quitting (Borland, Balmford, & Hunt, 2004). As a result of physical dependence intention does not always translate into action and many quit attempts are unsuccessful. Cigarette smoking is a specific cause of COPD (American Thoracic Society, 2003). There is a dose–response relationship between the amount smoked and the observed accelerated decline in airway function (National Heart, Lung and Blood Institute [NHLBI] & WHO, 2001).

Although cigarette smoking is the strongest risk factor for developing COPD, there is increasing evidence that occupational exposure to airborne particles such as in coal mines, hard rock mines, tunnel work and concrete manufacture also increases the risk of developing COPD. There is substantial evidence that exposure to occupational dust and fumes is linked with airflow obstruction, and risk can be equated with dust-years of exposure (Blanc & Toren, 2007).

There is substantial evidence of an association between occupational exposure and the development of COPD. Most studies reported an annual decline in FEV_1 due to occupational exposures after adjustment for age and smoking of 7–8 mL per year (American Thoracic Society, 2003). Approximately 15% of chronic bronchitis or COPD is due to work-related factors (American Thoracic Society, 2003; Blanc & Toren, 2007). Dusty environments and smoking are both risk factors for developing COPD, but when combined, the risk of COPD increases greatly (Blanc & Toren, 2007). Matheson et al. (2005) indicated that 15–19% of COPD in smokers and up to 31% of COPD in never-smokers can be attributed to occupational exposure to dust. For workers who are heavily exposed to occupational dust and fumes, the magnitude of the effect can be greater than that of cigarette smoking alone (American Thoracic Society, 2003). Studies reviewed by Blanc and Toren indicated that exposures were to dust consisting of silica, coal, agricultural dusts, coke oven emissions and tunnelling dusts and fumes. Cement workers are at high risk of developing chronic respiratory symptoms and COPD (Mwaiselage, Bratveit, Moen, & Mashalla, 2005). Monso et al. (2004) found that there was a dose–response relationship between exposure to dust and endotoxins associated with animal farming and COPD in never-smoking animal farmers working inside confined buildings (Monso et al., 2004).

Air pollution, both outside and inside, is a risk factor for COPD. Outside, exposure to elevated air pollution levels is related to chronic bronchitis and lung dysfunction (Viegi et al., 2006). Viegi et al. (2006) reviewed the evidence for a link between air pollution and COPD. They found that suspended particulates and NO_x are associated with COPD mortality risk and COPD hospital admissions. Infections are the main risk factor for exacerbation of COPD (Garcia-Aymerich et al., 2000). No influenza vaccination is a known risk factor for exacerbation of COPD (Nichol, Baken, & Nelson, 1999), and a Cochrane review of the effect of influenza vaccine on high-risk patients showed that vaccination does protect against exacerbation (Poole, Chacko, Wood-Baker, & Cates, 2007).

Diet and nutrition can affect most chronic diseases, including COPD. Obesity is a risk factor for the development of a number of chronic diseases, including COPD (Thorn et al., 2006), and obesity is commonly found in association with COPD, particularly chronic bronchitis rather than emphysema. Individuals with COPD tend to lead a more sedentary lifestyle in attempts to control breathing difficulties, but the association between obesity and COPD is complicated. The concurrence of COPD and obesity increases the risk of cardiovascular disease two to three times, independent of hypertension and smoking (Poulain et al., 2006). On the other hand, weight loss and muscle wasting are common among patients with COPD, and should be managed as early as possible in order to prevent functional decline (Brug, Schols, & Mesters, 2004). One study showed that frequent consumption of cured meat is associated with increased risk for developing COPD (Jiang, Paik, Hankinson, & Barr, 2007). Cured meats such as bacon, sausage, luncheon meats and cured hams are high in nitrites, which are used as a meat preservative. Nitrites may cause nitrative and nitrosative damage to the lung, producing structural changes similar to emphysema (tobacco smoke is another major source of nitrite in the body). Several studies have suggested that dietary antioxidants and foods rich in antioxidants (i.e. fruits and vegetables) may protect the airways against oxidant-mediated damage that leads to COPD (Walda et al., 2002). Walda et al. found that in five population-based cohorts of men from Finland, Italy and the Netherlands, there was a protective effect of fruit and possibly vitamin E intake against COPD.

EFFECTS OF COPD ON PHYSICAL HEALTH

People with COPD experience a broad spectrum of symptoms, depending on their particular lung pathology, the severity of their illness and their adaptation to it. Early symptoms of COPD may include breathlessness (dyspnoea), cough, wheeze, increased production of phlegm (sputum), sleep disturbance and fatigue. Fatigue also features in the latter symptoms of COPD and is often associated with escalating dyspnoea, increasingly frequent exacerbations, muscle wasting, loss of appetite and/or weight and cor pulmonale (right-sided heart failure).

Significant airflow obstruction may be present before the individual is aware of any symptoms. As such, it is no surprise that people are often diagnosed with COPD quite late in the disease trajectory. COPD has a 'relapse remitting' course, which Lynn (2001) described as one of illness over many months or years with occasional dramatic exacerbations; each episode may cause death but the individual usually survives many such episodes before death. In the medium to latter stages of COPD, increasingly frequent hospital admissions are not uncommon, reflecting deteriorating lung function and increasing susceptibility to infection. Exacerbations tend to be more common in people with moderate to severe COPD and of greater consequence in those with advanced disease (Sherwood Burge, 2006).

Pathophysiology of breathlessness

COPD severity is classified by the degree of obstruction during expiration on RFTs. However, evidence suggests that there is little correlation between the degree of obstruction on RFTs and the physical impairment or degree of dyspnoea endured by the individual (Wolkove, Dajczman, Colacone, & Kreisman, 1989). Dyspnoea may vary from very mild breathlessness on exertion to rendering an individual housebound. A complex relationship of neural and biochemical factors controls our respiratory rate, which is further modulated by emotional facets such as tolerance of the individual to the sensation of dyspnoea, anxiety, previous experience and expectations. Intrapulmonary pathology (e.g. airway obstruction, impaired gas exchange, hyperinflation) together with extrapulmonary factors (e.g. deconditioning and muscle wasting) govern the biochemical factors that influence the central nervous system's control of respiration.

A fear of being dyspnoeic discourages people with COPD from participating in activities that result in breathlessness, which in turn causes further deconditioning and activity avoidance. This vicious cycle of deconditioning (see Figure 19.2) is a common phenomenon and may be further precipitated by musculoskeletal problems (e.g. arthritis), inconvenience (e.g. driving is quicker than walking) or lack of enjoyment of exercise (e.g. colder climates). The principal intervention for people with COPD who are deconditioned is a course of pulmonary rehabilitation, which is discussed later in this chapter.

Respiratory assessment should consider the many alternative causes of dyspnoea. There is a plethora of non-COPD causes of dyspnoea, including heart disease, anaemia, pulmonary embolism, pleural effusion and pneumothorax. Those that relate to COPD include, but are not limited to, airway obstruction from sputum or foreign objects, bronchospasm, fatigue and, in some cases, hypoxaemia. Worsening of dyspnoea may signify an exacerbation of COPD, which is often associated with increased sputum production and/or viscosity, wheeze, fever or pleuritic pain. Oxygen therapy is indicated in COPD during acute

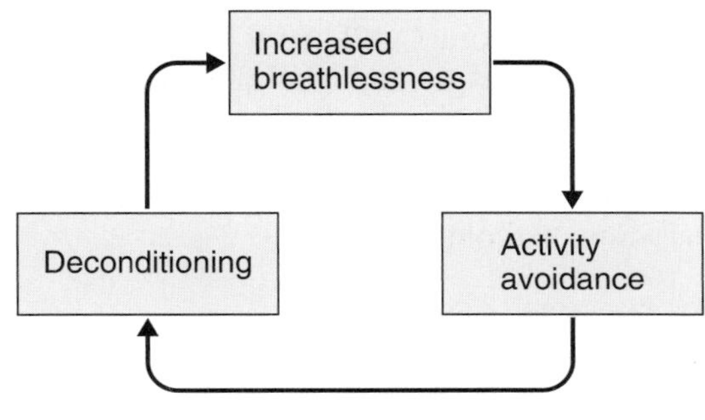

FIGURE 19.2 Cycle of deconditioning

exacerbations where oxygen saturations (SpO_2) are decreased (e.g. <92% on room air), or as a domiciliary therapy, where a person's partial pressure of oxygen (PaO_2) is <55 mmHg on arterial blood gases. Unless there is evidence of hypoxaemia, supplementary oxygen will not usually relieve dyspnoea, although this is a common lay misconception. In administering oxygen therapy for people with COPD, the nurse should always be mindful of the possibility of oxygen toxicity and carbon dioxide retention, and observe closely for signs of respiratory system depression. It should also be noted that when delivering oxygen therapy to patients with COPD who have had an episode of hypercapnic respiratory failure, high oxygen concentrations may worsen their condition due to suppression of hypoxic ventilatory drive (Smith, Roberts, Duggan-Brennan, Powrie, & Haffenden, 2009; Feller-Kopman & Schwartzstein, 2012). Although COPD patients with hypercapnic respiratory failure are not common (around 10%; Plant, Owen, & Elliott, 2000), it is recommended that *all patients* with low oxygen saturation do receive oxygen therapy, it is important to identify these patients as they particularly *need continuous assessment* while receiving oxygen therapy.

Altered mobility and fatigue

Regardless of the variation between individuals, dyspnoea is generally the most overt limitation on a person's activities of daily living (ADL). Around the time of diagnosis people often report earlier limitation in usual activities of exertion (e.g. climbing stairs, playing with grandchildren), while in latter stages household activities such as cleaning and cooking become increasingly difficult. Tasks that involve bending forwards, such as vacuuming, putting on shoes and making beds, are commonly reported as particularly challenging by people with COPD, perhaps due to the restriction of respiration in an already biomechanically-challenged thorax. Overhead chores such as pegging out washing or storing groceries in an overhead cupboard result in disproportionate dyspnoea, as does showering in a steamy, poorly ventilated bathroom. Tasks often need to be modified, or split into stages to avoid immediate limitation due to dyspnoea or fatigue.

Secondary impairment may result when a physical inability to walk, drive or catch public transport to shops leads to nutritional inadequacies. Weight loss associated with muscle wasting is common in the latter stages of COPD and further impedes exercise tolerance and respiratory function. Low body mass index (BMI) is a well-documented risk factor for poor prognosis in COPD (Schols, Slangen, Volovics, & Wouters, 1998) and, while the mechanisms for involuntary weight loss are not well understood (Ferreira, Brooks, Lacasse, & Goldstein, 2001), impaired swallowing function in advanced COPD is one likely contributor. Increasing dyspnoea makes the 3- to 5-second breath hold required for swallowing difficult, and may increase the risk of aspiration and chest infection. Inhaled respiratory medications often result in a dry mouth, which further hampers safe swallowing function. These factors may lead to avoidance of particular foods or of eating altogether, resulting in nutritional deprivation.

While the physical limitations from COPD vary between individuals, they also vary greatly within individuals as the relapse and remitting course of exacerbations lessen a person's usual physical capabilities. It should also be remembered that COPD is a disease of ageing, thus age-related changes such as reduced muscle strength and mass, fatigue, joint stiffness due to degenerative changes and bone loss are commonplace, and may not be related to the individual's lung pathology.

Measurement of physical health

Many best practice interventions for COPD, while improving dyspnoea and quality of life, do not alter physiological lung function. Hence assessment of the impact of interventions should focus on the initial goals of the intervention. That is, the use of tools that measure change in other outcomes such as BMI, dyspnoea, functional capacity, the number of exacerbations and quality of life may be more appropriate than repeating RFTs. The goal of many COPD interventions is to decrease dyspnoea; however, dyspnoea is subjective and difficult to quantify. Scales such as the Borg Scale of Dyspnoea (Mahler et al., 1987) and the Medical Research Council Scale of Dyspnoea (Bestall et al., 1999) have been validated for use in this population. The measurement of functional capacity is often achieved using the 6 Minute Walk Test (American Thoracic Society, 2002) or the Incremental Shuttle Walk Test (Singh, Morgan, Scott, Walters, & Hardman, 1992). These tests may also be used to assess for exertional desaturation or oxygen requirements, and are used by physiotherapists to prescribe exercise. It is worth remembering that physiological measurements of COPD (e.g. spirometry, 6 Minute Walk Test) do not necessarily correlate with the various symptoms of COPD. As such, quality-of-life tools and measures of dyspnoea may more accurately reflect a patient's perception of their disease severity or impairment, the impact of treatments and the fluctuations in symptoms (Yusen, 2001).

EFFECTS OF COPD ON MENTAL HEALTH AND QUALITY OF LIFE

Distinguishing between the physical symptoms of COPD, the behavioural, psychological and emotional reactions relating to adjustment and the psychological symptoms associated with the presence of a clinical disorder related to depression or anxiety can present a challenge to the health professional. The effect of COPD on an individual's quality of life (QOL) and mental and physical health are not independent from each other. Symptoms such as breathlessness, insomnia, fatigue, poor appetite, reduced activity levels, feelings of guilt and anger, irritability, reduced self-esteem, just to mention a few, may all affect QOL and be related to COPD, to adjusting to COPD or to anxiety and/or depression.

Also, physical deconditioning may lead to social isolation as friends and hobbies become inaccessible, resulting in loneliness and its associated symptom of depression (Kara & Mirici, 2004). Similarly, the anxiety that a person feels in anticipation of dyspnoea may prevent them being adequately motivated to attempt activity, resulting in further deconditioning and progressive dyspnoea. In addition, the presence of mental health conditions has been associated with longer hospitalisations, poorer survival rates, increased symptom burden and poorer physical and social functioning in COPD patients (Ng et al., 2007).

Quality of life

Having a chronic illness such as COPD will inevitably impact on QOL. WHO defines quality of life as an 'individual's perception of their position in life in the context of the culture and value systems in which they live and in relation to their goals, expectations, standards and concerns' (1997, p. 1). Thus defined, QOL is a broad concept that can be affected in a multitude of ways. In recognition of the breadth of this definition along with the considerable impact health status and illness can have on QOL, investigations often focus on health related quality of life (HRQOL) as a measure of QOL as it is affected specifically by health and healthcare (Kil, Oh, Koo, & Suk 2010).

While HRQOL is an important factor in and of itself, it also has a significant impact on a range of other variables. It is a prognostic factor in COPD, with poor HRQOL associated with higher mortality and greater risk of hospitalisation (Balcells et al., 2010). In a review, Tsiligianni and colleagues found the most significant factors associated with HRQOL to be dyspnoea, exercise tolerance and anxiety and depression (Tsiligianni, Kocks, Tzanakis, Siafakas, & van der Molen, 2011). A combination of depression and anxiety in a person with severe COPD has a more significant impact on HRQOL (Balcells et al., 2010). Other factors found to be related to reduced HRQOL included being female, being under or overweight, continuing to smoke, more severe COPD and the presence of co-morbidities (Tsiligianni et al., 2011).

Yusen (2001) describes health-related quality of life as a reflection of the health- and disease-related aspects, including the impact of disease, treatments and tests, of daily life and wellbeing. The goals of most interventions for COPD are, directly or indirectly, to improve quality of life.

In choosing a tool to measure QOL, the nurse should consider whether a respiratory disease-specific QOL tool, such as the Guyatt Chronic Respiratory Disease questionnaire (Guyatt et al., 1987) or the St George Respiratory Disease Questionnaire (Jones, Quirk, Baveystock, & Littlejohns, 1992), or a generic QOL tool is more appropriate. The domains included in the choice of tool should reflect the intervention and its goals. For example, an exercise and education program of pulmonary rehabilitation may use a disease-specific QOL tool that covers domains such as physical, emotional, knowledge, mastery and fatigue. The tool's domains encompass the degree of dyspnoea on activities, the impact of disease on ADL and the frustration and feelings of hope or despair in living with COPD. The choice of tool should depend on the purpose — to measure overall impact of COPD at one point in time, or to test and retest QOL in response to an intervention. Whichever instrument is chosen, it should be reliable and valid in the population that it is to be used for. For example, measuring QOL in a culturally and linguistically diverse population requires that the tool be either available in multiple languages, or validated when translated by an interpreter. Other considerations may include the literacy of the population, and whether the tool is designed to be administered by a healthcare professional or independently by the patients themselves.

Adjustment to illness

Symptoms of COPD can present years after smoking has ceased and can occur in the absence of known risk factors. For many people, recurrent chest infections or insidious dyspnoea leads to a diagnosis some time after initial symptoms arise. Being diagnosed with a chronic disease such as COPD can be understandably confronting and distressing. COPD is irreversible, incurable and progressive and the person diagnosed with COPD must make significant adjustments over multiple domains, including behavioural, emotional, psychological and social. The process of adjustment will be ongoing as the impact of the disease changes over time. In the behavioural domain, people with COPD may have to reduce their activity levels. The physical limitations from dyspnoea may require early retirement and a change of role in employment, social and family contexts. For people who have been active, independent and self-sufficient, the effect of COPD on their activities can be quite devastating (Falvo, 2005). People with COPD must also endure significant lifestyle changes, with the acquisition of new habits (e.g. medications, exercise, modified activities) and the suppression of old habits (e.g. smoking, poor self-care).

Being diagnosed with COPD may result in altered self-perception, including body image. Social roles and relationships may change. An individual's loss of independence and restrictions on recreational activities may result in irritability, a sense of hopelessness (Yusen, 2001), decreased confidence and lowered self-esteem. Frustration and powerlessness are also common in response to recurrent infections and the impossibility of predicting the timing or severity of exacerbations. There is evidence to demonstrate that acute exacerbations of COPD have a negative impact on health-related quality of life and exercise capacity (Carr, Goldstein, & Brooks, 2007) for the duration of the exacerbation and potentially for some time after if the recovery is prolonged. Perhaps the most difficult adjustment people with COPD must face is adaptation to the sensation of shortness of breath and the associated fear of breathlessness and, at the extreme end, the fear of dying.

Impact on the person and their family

The sequelae of COPD and its treatments often bring sufferers embarrassment and result in their avoidance of public situations. Breathlessness, a productive cough and the use of inhalers often lead to undue attention from the general public, so people with COPD avoid enclosed spaces such as public transport. Some of the common visible physical symptoms that the patient and family must adjust to include portable oxygen or walking aids, clubbed fingers, cushingoid features and bruising from steroid-based medications. Aside from dyspnoea, relinquishment of social activities with others may stem from more diverse causes such as:

- stress incontinence as a side-effect of pelvic floor pressure from frequent coughing
- travel restrictions, as persons with chronic hypoxaemia may not be able to fly due to atmospheric pressure changes at altitude
- a fear of 'holding up' the rest of the group due to low energy levels and fatigue.

Patients with COPD may also feel guilt, shame or anger about their illness and it is important to remember that COPD has a degree of stigma as a 'self-inflicted' illness (Sherwood Burge, 2006), which health workers should avoid reinforcing.

Inevitably these symptoms and their impact on ADL and life role require support and understanding from family and caregivers. Relationships can be compromised and strained due to effects of the illness on family members. Partners may have to take on the role of carer, thereby sacrificing some of their own needs. There may be anger towards the person with COPD if the illness is seen as being caused by their own behaviour, such as smoking. This may be accompanied by guilt about feeling angry. There may also be anger directed at others, such as employers, if the illness is seen to be a result of the occupational environment.

Family members may overestimate the impact of the disease and put their loved one in the sick role, reducing behavioural expectations, thereby reinforcing sickness behaviour and inadvertently contributing to deconditioning. Alternatively, some family members may not fully appreciate the impact of the disease on the activity levels of the person with COPD and hold unrealistic expectations of their capabilities (Falvo, 2005).

COPD may put considerable financial stress on a family if the person with the illness has ceased work and their partner has to alter their work arrangements in order to take on a caring role. There are also costs associated with medical treatment, hospitalisations and medication. A couples' intimate relationship may also be adversely affected. The person with COPD may feel anxiety about engaging in sexual activity due to the impact this has on their breathing (Falvo, 2005).

Depression and anxiety

Estimates of the prevalence of depression and anxiety in people with COPD vary widely, (depression: 8–80%; anxiety 6–74%) though the general consensus in the literature seems to be that the rates are high and that depression and anxiety are probably under-diagnosed and certainly under treated (Yohannes, Willgoss, Baldwin, & Connolly, 2010). Significant depressive symptoms have been reported in 16–74% of people with COPD (Ng et al., 2007). The variation in rates of depression and anxiety in people with COPD reported in the literature is in part related to the variety of measures used and whether they are diagnostic- or symptom-based. 'Clinically significant' levels of depression and anxiety have been reported at 40% and 36% respectively (Yohannes, Baldwin, & Connolly, 2000).

Depression may be 'reactive' to the situation and considered a consequence of physical disease, or be of more established biological cause (Gore, Brophy, & Greenstone, 2000). In a large cohort study, Hanania et al. (2011) found that rates of depression in COPD are higher than in the general population and also higher than in the population of smokers. This suggests that COPD is at least a contributing factor to the depression experienced in this population. Within COPD populations, these researchers found that depression is more prevalent in women, in people with more serious COPD, in people who are over 60 years of age and in those who continue to smoke.

Depression in COPD leads to reduced functional capability, magnifies morbidity and worsens functional and health status of patients (Hanania et al., 2011). Depression has been shown to have a negative impact on a range of health outcomes including mortality, continued smoking, length of hospital stay and physical and social functioning, even when confounders such as chronicity of COPD and socioeconomic variables are controlled for (Ng et al., 2007). An increased rate of exacerbations has also been associated with depression in COPD resulting in higher levels of healthcare use. Hanania et al. estimate that only one third of people with COPD and depression receive appropriate treatment and this is in spite of the observation that people with COPD and a depressive disorder are more likely to present with moderate to severe symptoms which can have a significant negative impact on functioning.

Anxiety is particularly common in COPD as a result of dyspnoea (Gore et al., 2000) and may be exacerbated by the vicious cycle of deconditioning (see Figure 19.2). A fear of becoming breathless leads to activity avoidance or fear of exercise, and results in further deconditioning. Anticipatory anxiety then results when the individual next attempts an activity that they perceive may result in breathlessness. Panic attacks and panic disorder are particularly prevalent in people with COPD, and rates are considerably higher than those found in the general population (Livermore, Sharpe, & McKenzie, 2010). Anxiety can be particularly difficult to identify in COPD patients due to the overlap of physiological symptoms in particular.

MANAGEMENT OF COPD

Management of psychological symptoms

Given the high prevalence of symptoms of anxiety and depression in people with COPD, it is unfortunate that current national and international treatment guidelines devote little, if any, content to the treatment of psychological symptoms (APA & ALF, 2011; GOLD, 2006; Qaseem et al., 2011). One reason that treatment guidelines focus overwhelmingly on the physical characteristics of the disease may be due to the lack of supporting evidence for effective treatments for the mental health component (Cafarella, Effing, Usmani & Frith, 2012). To date, there has not been sufficient investigation into treatments for anxiety and depression in people with COPD to warrant firm conclusions or evidence-based recommendations (Fritzsche, Clamor, & von Leupoldt, 2011). Over the coming years, this situation is likely to change as further research is undertaken and evidence begins to accumulate. In the meantime, it is possible to address the psychological aspects of COPD using what we already know.

First, given the prevalence rates and the impact of depression and anxiety on HRQOL, morbidity and mortality, the importance of monitoring patients with COPD for signs of depression or anxiety cannot be overstated. Deterioration in mood, increasing avoidance behaviour, high levels of fear and catastrophic or negative cognitions are all signs that suggest further assessment may be required. Screening instruments such as the Hospital Anxiety and Depression Scale (HADS) and the nine-item Patient Health Questionnaire (PHQ 9) are readily available and quick to administer. While these instruments are not intended to be diagnostic, they may indicate that a referral for more thorough assessment is warranted. There is an argument to be made that screening patients with COPD for depression and anxiety should be part of standard practice.

Pulmonary rehabilitation (PR) has been shown to improve HRQOL and depression levels in people with COPD (Bratas et al., 2010) and is routinely recommended for people whose COPD has become functionally disabling in order to reduce fatigue, improve exercise tolerance, reduce the progression of the disease and prolong life expectancy (Addy, 2007).

Unfortunately, depression and anxiety may impact a person's capacity to engage with PR, despite its effectiveness (Baraniak & Sheffield, 2011). For example, Addy (2007) has argued that for people with anxiety about breathlessness, their fear that increased activity levels will exacerbate the condition results in a reluctance to engage in PR. Such fear avoidance cycles can cause further disability through physical deconditioning. Addy recommends psychological treatment to address this problem using cognitive and behavioural interventions such as graded exposure.

Cognitive behaviour therapy (CBT) is an evidenced-based psychological intervention that includes a wide range of behavioural and cognitive strategies targeting particular symptoms and disorders. Graded exposure is an example of one such behavioural technique. While the evidence for the effectiveness of psychological interventions, including CBT, for the treatment of depression and anxiety in COPD patients is mixed (Baraniak & Sheffield, 2011), there is a strong evidence base for CBT in the treatment of anxiety and depression in the general population and CBT is also an effective treatment for anxiety and depression associated with chronic illness (Cafarella et al., 2012).

Although the research into treatment for depression and anxiety in people with COPD is sparse, there is an extensive body of research examining treatments for depression and anxiety in the general population, some of which have also been examined in people with co-morbid chronic diseases. Examples include pharmacological treatments, especially selective serotonin reuptake inhibiters (SSRIs), relaxation therapy, Interpersonal Psychotherapy (Cafarella et al., 2012) and mindfulness-based therapies such as mindfulness-based cognitive therapy (MBCT) (Addy, 2007). These all have the potential to ameliorate symptoms of depression and anxiety in people with COPD.

The treatment of depression and anxiety is the realm of the specialist, usually a psychologist, who will undertake a thorough psychological assessment and develop a targeted treatment plan with the patient. The role of the nurse may be to identify patients who may be at risk of developing anxiety or depression, to identify signs and symptoms that may warrant further investigation and to make appropriate onward referrals. The nurse may also provide a pivotal role in encouraging the patient to seek further treatment and to provide reassurance that treatment for anxiety and depression is available.

Education for the person with COPD and their family — pulmonary rehabilitation

Pulmonary rehabilitation (PR) is a structured program of education and exercise for people with chronic lung diseases that aims to improve self-efficacy in relation to their condition, increase exercise tolerance, decrease dyspnoea and improve QOL. The structure of programs varies, although evidence-based guidelines recommend at least twice-weekly outpatient attendance for 8 weeks (Australian Physiotherapy Association [APA] & Australian Lung Foundation [ALF], 2006).

PR is most commonly run by nurses and physiotherapists in a variety of healthcare settings, including acute care and community sites. While it is an ideal opportunity for multidisciplinary care of the individual, the role of the nurse may vary according to the diversity of other health professional disciplines that may be available and involved in the program. Historically, nurses with specialist skills have played primary roles in patient education within these programs (ALF, 2002). Guidelines suggest that the education component of programs should be multidisciplinary and include information on self-management and the prevention and treatment of exacerbations (Ries et al., 2007). According to Australian expert opinion (APA & ALF, 2006; ALF, 2002), education topics should include knowledge of the respiratory system and their condition, symptom recognition and management, the role of exercise, smoking cessation, correct use of medications, emotional management skills (including management of anxiety, depression and panic attacks), breathing control exercises, airway clearance strategies, energy conservation and nutrition. The exercise component of PR programs should include endurance and strength training exercises for both upper and lower limbs (Ries et al., 2007), as well as a home-based exercise program (APA & ALF, 2006).

Trials of PR have demonstrated clinically and statistically significant improvements in dyspnoea (Ries et al., 2007) and QOL domains, including fatigue, mastery, emotional function and dyspnoea (Lacasse et al., 2006; Ries et al., 2007). Improvements in functional exercise capacity and maximal exercise capacity have been widely demonstrated, although results are not always statistically significant (Lacasse et al., 2006). However, patients' perception of dyspnoea consistently improves (Lacasse et al., 2006), suggesting that PR results in improved perception and tolerance of dyspnoea regardless of objective change in exercise capacity. For patients with exercise-induced hypoxaemia, the use of supplementary oxygen during PR is recommended (Ries et al., 2007). There is evidence that functional improvements decline over 12–18 months if patients do not participate in a maintenance exercise program after completing a PR course (Ries et al., 2007; Ries et al., 2003). However, the optimal format (e.g. frequency, duration) for maintaining benefits has not yet been established.

Other issues to consider: palliative care for COPD

Historically, people with COPD have not routinely been referred to palliative care services for their end-of-life care. This may be because the timing of death in COPD is often uncertain until very late in the course of the disease (Lynn, 2001), unlike more typical palliative care diagnoses such as malignancy. However, recent literature has highlighted the relevance of palliative care in managing the end-of-life symptoms of COPD (Murray et al., 2005; Gore et al., 2000; Seamark, Seamark, & Halpin, 2007). Gore et al. (2000) describe COPD's course as a prolonged period of disabling dyspnoea, increasing hospital admissions and premature death. They further highlight that the experience of reduced QOL, psychological issues and unmet information requirements parallels that of lung cancer patients, who are more readily referred to palliative care services.

Features related to poor prognosis and possible consideration for palliative care include severe airflow obstruction ($FEV_1 < 30\%$ of predicted), severe dyspnoea at rest, hypoxaemia at rest on supplementary oxygen, hypercapnia ($PaCO_2 > 55$ mmHg), frequency of exacerbations, development of cor pulmonale, and unintentional and continuing weight loss or low BMI (Seamark et al., 2007; Budweiser et al., 2007; Lynn, 2001).

In COPD there is often no clearly identifiable point at which management changes from active to palliative in focus. Nursing care for end-of-life COPD should be specifically tailored to address symptoms, of which dyspnoea and anxiety are usually the most prominent. Unlike some other conditions, medications that would be considered part of active management, such as antibiotics, bronchodilators and steroids, may still play an important palliative role in the suppression of dyspnoea. Lynn (2001) describes the unique need for both disease-modifying and comfort-enhancing interventions simultaneously in end-stage COPD management. Constipation is also not unusual in the end-of-life phase (Seamark et al., 2007), particularly if opioids are being used for dyspnoea management. While there is evidence to support oral and parenteral opioids to treat advanced dyspnoea (Jennings et al., 2002), they should be used judiciously in COPD due to their depression of the respiratory system.

NURSING PRINCIPLES AND INTERVENTIONS

As the symptoms of COPD develop, the physical changes and their effects on a person's psychosocial wellbeing result in increased need for both physical and emotional support. The nurse's role in COPD management varies across healthcare settings and the acuity of disease spectrum. Regardless of the setting, nursing interventions should focus on minimising disease progression and maximising QOL. For example:

- Utilise interventions that encourage patient motivation. The relapse/remitting course of COPD means that, while symptoms are usually present in some form, the individual's care needs will fluctuate. The individual and/or their carers are responsible for their own care for a large proportion of the time and will benefit from enhanced self-efficacy skills to monitor and manage their condition. Patients should be encouraged to be involved in their care planning process to promote motivation, understanding and self-efficacy.
- Assess for insomnia and encourage appropriate sleep hygiene habits. Insomnia in COPD is multifactorial, and may be due to physiological COPD changes, age-related sleep pattern changes or medications, but is also a symptom of depression.
- Changes in mental health status and ability to cope should be monitored and reported. Kara and Mirici (2004) suggest monitoring for signs of loneliness and depression. Nurse interventions may include referrals to strengthen social networks and relieve stress of family burdens. Referral to a psychologist for therapy to treat anxiety or depression should also be considered.
- Encourage and educate regarding smoking cessation. Ironically, while smoking is often the causative factor of COPD, many patients with COPD who still smoke describe their continued habit as their last remaining pleasure in life, despite the knowledge that further harm will eventuate. Consider referral to smoking cessation specialist clinic where available.
- Provide support and education for family and caregivers as they too adjust to lifestyle and routine modifications.
- Encourage annual influenza vaccination and five-yearly pneumococcal vaccination (Sherwood Burge, 2006).
- Monitor functional capabilities. Encourage work simplification and activity modification where appropriate, and assess for increased care needs during exacerbations.

- During stable periods, encourage regular graduated exercise to maintain functional capabilities. Consider referral to a PR program if evidence of dyspnoea on exertion.
- Monitor BMI and nutritional status. Consider referral to a dietitian if overweight or underweight.
- Monitor airway clearance techniques. Consider referral to a respiratory physiotherapist if patient describes difficulty in clearing sputum.
- Encourage self-monitoring of symptoms and the discussion of an action plan with their treating medical practitioner, including signs to seek medical attention when symptoms worsen.
- Provide education on prevention of exacerbations, including the avoidance of risk factors such as cold weather, pollution exposure or contact with people with a bacterial or viral infection (Sherwood Burge, 2006).
- Assess use of inhaled medication devices and provide education to patient and carer to optimise drug administration. Misuse of inhaled devices may lead to inadequate drug dosing and suboptimal disease control (Rau, 2006). Reassess capability to use usual inhaled devices during exacerbations as diminished respiratory reserve may impede optimal device use.
- Titrate oxygen therapy as appropriate in the acute setting and monitor for side effects. Provide education regarding the use of domiciliary oxygen where prescribed, including safety considerations around the home.
- Monitor for signs of aspiration whether obvious (e.g. changes in quality of voice, or coughing/choking on eating or drinking), or more subtle (pocketing of food/fluid around mouth, recurrent chest infections, difficulty managing some food consistencies). If evidence or suspicion of aspiration, consider referral to speech pathologist.

Principles of nursing practice

The following principles of nursing practice apply to nursing patients with COPD:

- encourage medication compliance/optimise technique
- maximise functional ability/minimise further deconditioning
- recognise signs and symptoms of deterioration (and act promptly)
- educate patient/carer to recognise signs and symptoms
- support activity modification
- support symptom relief and comfort.

CONCLUSION

COPD is one of the most common diseases in the world. Emphysema and chronic bronchitis are two common types of COPD. The airflow limitation is usually progressive and is associated with abnormal inflammatory response of the lungs to noxious particles or gases. The nurse's role in COPD management as discussed in this chapter varies across the healthcare settings depending on the acuity of the disease. It is important that the nurse focus on minimising disease progression and at the same time working with the family and significant others to maximise the quality of life for the person.

CASE STUDY 19.1

Mr C, a 78-year-old man, was admitted to RN John's ward with an exacerbation of his COPD. His observations were initially stable and he was treated with intravenous antibiotics, oral corticosteroids and oxygen therapy via nasal prongs. He was breathless on minimal activity and required assistance with all his personal care and transfers.

During handover the following morning it was reported that Mr C's oxygen saturations had dropped overnight and his oxygen therapy was increased. When John assessed Mr C he found that he was drowsier than on the previous day, although his oxygen saturations had improved. John was concerned about possible carbon dioxide (CO_2) retention and reported his decreased conscious state to the treating doctor. Arterial blood gases (ABGs) confirmed a rising CO_2 and the doctor commenced Mr C on non-invasive ventilation (BiPAP) and decreased his fraction of inspired oxygen (FiO_2). His conscious state then required bed rest, full nursing care and frequent observations to monitor his respiratory and cardiovascular status while the BiPAP was in situ.

By the end of John's shift, Mr C's ABGs were improving and his BiPAP had reduced from continuous to intermittent. By the next day, Mr C's pH and CO_2 were within normal range and the BiPAP was ceased. The ward nurses continued to observe Mr C closely for the remainder of his admission, administering only low flow oxygen (<3 litres per minute) and accepting oxygen saturations of 88–92% to avoid further CO_2 retention.

CASE STUDY 19.2

Emma is a community health nurse working at a centre where an 8-week outpatient pulmonary rehabilitation program is run. Emma's role, together with a respiratory physiotherapist and an allied health assistant, includes pre- and post-program assessments in which comprehensive respiratory assessments are carried out and measures of exercise capacity are completed. During the assessments, Emma must not only assess the participants' respiratory system, but their overall health status, including their safety to exercise.

Emma encourages participants to set goals for themselves and monitors these each week. A team of allied health staff contribute to the program's education components including information on how to manage anxiety and depression symptoms. Emma provides information on respiratory medications, the use of respiratory devices, smoking cessation and action plans for symptom monitoring and the management of exacerbations. Throughout the 8 weeks Emma monitors each participant, taking regular observations and liaises closely with participants' general practitioners regarding symptoms and progress. At the conclusion, Emma assists participants to make a plan to maintain the physical benefits they have gained over the 8 weeks.

Reflective questions

1 Consider what information might be useful to a person with COPD who does not wish to undertake pulmonary rehabilitation.

2 People with COPD are commonly increasingly breathless during exacerbations. Consider how a person's care needs may change over the course of a 7-day hospital admission for an exacerbation of COPD.

3 A single mother who smokes is admitted with pneumonia and diagnosed with COPD.

(a) How may this new diagnosis affect this woman's emotional status?

(b) Discuss the nursing education interventions that should be addressed and the most appropriate times for these to take place.

4 Participants of pulmonary rehabilitation programs frequently have co-morbidities, often related to smoking. What other systems should be assessed to ensure that a person is able to participate in a group exercise situation?

Recommended reading

Cafarella, P. A., Effing, T. W., Usmani, Z., et al. (2012). Treatments for anxiety and depression in patients with chronic obstructive pulmonary disease: A literature review. *Respirology*, *17*, 627–638.

Cross, S. (2005). Managing exacerbations of chronic obstructive pulmonary disease. *British Journal of Nursing*, *14*(11), 607–609.

Gore, J. M., Brophy, C. J., & Greenstone, M. A. (2000). How well do we care for patients with end stage chronic obstructive pulmonary disease (COPD)? A comparison of palliative care and quality of life in COPD and lung cancer. *Thorax*, *55*, 1000–1006.

Kara, M. (2005). Preparing Nurses for the Global Pandemic of Chronic Obstructive Pulmonary Disease. *Journal of Nursing Scholarship*, *37*(2), 127–133.

The COPDX Plan. Available from http://www.mja.com.au/public/issues/178_06_170303/tho10508_all.html

References

Access Economics. (2008). *Economic impact of COPD and cost effective solutions*. Australian Lung Foundation.

Addy, K. B. E. (2007). The treatment of depression and anxiety within the context of chronic obstructive pulmonary disease. *Clinical Case Studies*, *6*(5), 383–393.

American Thoracic Society. (2002). ATS Statement: Guidelines for the six-minute walk test. *American Journal of Respiratory and Critical Care Medicine*, *166*, 111–117.

American Thoracic Society. (2003). American Thoracic Society statement: occupational contribution to the burden of airway disease. *American Journal of Respiratory and Critical Care Medicine*, *167*, 787–797.

Australian Bureau of Statistics. (2010). *National Health Survey, Summary of results, 2007–2008*. Commonwealth of Australia.

Australian Institute of Health and Welfare. (2006). *Chronic diseases and associated risk factors in Australia*. Canberra: Author, cat no PHE81.

Australian Institute of Health and Welfare. (2011). *Asthma in Australia with a focus chapter on chronic obstructive pulmonary disease*. AIHW Asthma Series no. 4. Cat. No. ACM 22. Canberra: AIHW.

Australian Institute of Health and Welfare. (2012a). *Australia's Health 2012: The thirteenth biennial health report of the Australian Institute of Health and Welfare*. Canberra.

Australian Institute of Health and Welfare. (2012b). Chronic respiratory conditions including asthma and COPD. Accessed 5 July 2012 from http://www.aihw.gov.au/chronic-respiratory-conditions/

Australian Lung Foundation. (2001). *Case Statement Chronic Obstructive Pulmonary Disease*. Australian Lung Foundation.

Australian Lung Foundation. (2002). *Evidence Base and Standards for Pulmonary Rehabilitation in Australia*. Adelaide: Australian Lung Foundation.

Australian Lung Foundation. (2012). Fact sheet: A report into the economic impact of chronic obstructive pulmonary disease (COPD) and cost effective solutions report. Accessed 5 July 2012 from http://www.lungfoundation.com.au/lung-information/publications/economic-impact-of-copd-2008.

Australian Physiotherapy Association and Australian Lung Foundation. (2006). Pulmonary Rehabilitation Toolkit. Accessed 1 July 2007 from http://www.pulmonaryrehab.com.au.

Baker, A., Ivers, R. G., Bowman, J., et al. (2006). Where there's smoke there's fire: high prevalence of smoking among some sub-populations and recommendations for intervention. *Drug and Alcohol Review*, *25*, 85–96.

Balcells, E., Gea, J., Ferrer, J., et al. & the PAC-COPD Study Group. (2010). Factors affecting the relationship between psychological status and quality of life in COPD patients. *Health and Quality of Life Outcomes*, *8*, 108.

Baraniak, A., & Sheffield, D. (2011). The efficacy of psychologically based interventions to improve anxiety, depression and quality of life in COPD: A systematic review and meta-analysis. *Patient Education and Counseling*, *83*, 29–36.

Bestall, J. C., Paul, E. A., Garrod, R., et al. (1999). Usefulness of the Medical Research Council dyspnoea scale as a measure of disability in patients with chronic obstructive pulmonary disease. *Thorax*, *54*, 581–586.

Blanc, P. D., & Toren, K. (2007). Occupation in chronic obstructive pulmonary disease and chronic bronchitis: an update. *The International Journal of Tuberculosis and Lung Disease*, *11*(3), 251–257.

Borland, R., Balmford, J., Hunt, D. (2004). The effectiveness of personally tailored computer-generated advice letters for smoking cessation. *Addiction*, *99*, 369–377.

Bratas, O., Espnes, G. A., Rannestad, T., et al. (2010). Pulmonary rehabilitation reduces depression and enhances heath-related quality of life in COPD patients especially in patients with mild or moderate disease. *Chronic Respiratory Disease*, *7*(4), 229–237.

Brug, J., Schols, A., & Mesters, I. (2004). Dietary change, nutrition education and chronic obstructive pulmonary disease. *Patient education and counselling*, *52*, 249–257.

Budweiser, S., Jorres, R. A., Riedl, T., et al. (2007). Predictors of survival in COPD patients with chronic hypercapnic respiratory failure receiving non-invasive home ventilation. *Chest*, *131*, 1650–1658.

Cafarella, P. A., Effing, T. W., Usmani, Z., et al. (2012). Treatments for anxiety and depression in patients with chronic obstructive pulmonary disease: A literature review. *Respirology*, *17*, 627–638.

Carr, S. J., Goldstein, R. S., & Brooks, D. (2007). Acute Exacerbations of Chronic Obstructive Pulmonary Disease in subjects completing pulmonary rehabilitation. *Chest* (Pre-published online) doi: 10.1378/chest.07-0269 Accessed 15 June 2007 at www.chestjournal.org

Falvo, D. (2005). *Psychosocial Aspects of Chronic Illness and Disability* (3rd ed.). Sudbury, MA: Jones and Bartlett.

Feller-Kopman, D., & Schwartzstein, R. (2012). Use of oxygen in patients with hypercapnia. Retrieved January 15, 2012, from http://www.uptodate.com/contents/use-of-oxygen-in-patients-with-hypercapnia

Ferreira, I. M., Brooks, D., Lacasse, Y., et al. (2001). Nutritional Intervention in COPD: A Systematic Overview. *Chest, 119*, 353–363.

Fritzsche, A., Clamor, A., & von Leupoldt, A. (2011). Effects of medical and psychological treatment of depression in patients with COPD – A review. *Respiratory Medicine, 105*, 1422–1433.

Garcia-Aymerich, J., Barreiro, E., Farrero, E., et al. (2000). Patients hospitalized for COPD have a high prevalence of modifiable risk factors for exacerbation (EFRAM study). *European Respiratory Journal, 16*(6), 1037–1042.

Global Initiative for Chronic Obstructive Lung Disease. (2010). Global strategy for the diagnosis, management and prevention of chronic obstructive pulmonary disease. Retrieved May 2, 2013, from http://www.goldcopd.org

Gore, J. M., Brophy, C. J., Greenstone, M. A. (2000). How well do we care for patients with end stage chronic obstructive pulmonary disease (COPD)? A comparison of palliative care and quality of life in COPD and lung cancer. *Thorax, 55*, 1000–1006.

Guyatt, G. H., Berman, L. B., Townsend, M., et al. (1987). A measure of quality of life for clinical trials in chronic lung disease. *Thorax, 42*(10), 773–778.

Hanania, N. A., Müllerova, H., Locantore, N. W., et al. (2011). Determinants of depression in the ECLIPSE chronic obstructive pulmonary disease cohort. *American Journal of Respiratory and Critical Care Medicine, 183*, 604–611.

Jenkins, C. R., Thompson, P. J., Gibson, P. G., et al. (2005). Distinguishing asthma and chronic obstructive pulmonary disease: why, why not and how? *Medical Journal of Australia, 183*(1), S35–S37.

Jennings, A. L., Davies, A. N., Higgins, J. P. T., et al. (2002). A systematic review of the use of opioids in the management of dyspnoea. *Thorax, 57*, 939–944.

Jiang, R., Paik, D. C., Hankinson, J. L., et al. (2007). Cured meat consumption, lung function, and chronic obstructive pulmonary disease among United States adults. *American Journal of Respiratory and Critical Care Medicine, 175*, 798–804.

Jones, P. W., Quirk, F. H., Baveystock, C. M., et al. (1992). A self complete measure of health status for chronic airflow limitation. The St George's Respiratory Questionnaire. *American Review of Respiratory Disease, 145*(6), 1321–1327.

Kara, M., & Mirici, A. (2004). Loneliness, Depression and Social Support of Turkish Patients with chronic obstructive pulmonary disease and their spouses. *Journal of Nursing Scholarship, 36*(4), 331–336.

Kil, S. Y., Oh, W. O., Koo, B. J., et al. (2010). Relationship between depression and health-related quality of life in older Korean patients with chronic obstructive pulmonary disease. *Journal of Clinical Nursing, 19*, 1307–1314.

Lacasse, Y., Goldstein, R., Lasserson, T. J., et al. (2006). Pulmonary rehabilitation for chronic obstructive pulmonary disease (review). *Cochrane Database of Systematic Reviews*, Issue 4. Art. No.:CD003793 doi: 10.1002/14651858.CD003793pub2

Livermore, N., Sharpe, L., & McKenzie, D. (2010). Panic attacks and panic disorder in chronic obstructive pulmonary disease: A cognitive behavioral perspective. *Respiratory Medicine, 104*, 1246–1253.

Lynn, J. (2001). Serving patients who may die soon and their families. The Role of Hospice and other services. *Journal of the American Medical Association, 285*(7), 925–932.

Mahler, D. A., Rosiello, R. A., Harver, A., et al. (1987). Comparison of clinical dyspnoea ratings and psychophysical measurement of respiratory sensation in obstructive airway disease. *American Review of Respiratory Diseases, 135*, 1229–1233.

Matheson, M. C., Benke, G., Raven, J., Sim, M. R., et al. (2005). Biological dust exposure in the workplace is a risk factor for chronic obstructive pulmonary disease. *Thorax, 60*, 645–651.

Mathers, C., Vos, T., Stevenson, C. (1999). *The burden of disease and injury in Australia.* Canberra: Australian Institute of Health and Welfare, cat no PHE17.

McKenzie, D., Abramson, M., Crockett, A. J., et al. on behalf of The Australian Lung Foundation. (2012). *The COPDX Plan: Australian and New Zealand Guidelines for the management of Chronic Obstructive Pulmonary Disease 2011.* The Australian Lung Foundation.

Ministerial Council on Drug Strategy. (2004). *Australian National Tobacco Strategy, 2004–2009: The Strategy.* Brisbane: Australian Government Department of Health and Ageing.

Monso, E., Riu, E., Radon, K., et al. (2004). Chronic obstructive pulmonary disease in never-smoking animal farmers working inside confinement buildings. *American Journal of Industrial Medicine, 46*, 357–362.

Murray, S. A., Kendall, M., Boyd, K., et al. (2005). Illness trajectories and palliative care. *British Medical Journal, 330*, 1007–1011.

Mwaiselage, J., Bratveit, M., Moen, B. E., et al. (2005). Respiratory symptoms and chronic obstructive pulmonary disease among cement factory workers. *Scandinavian Journal of Work, Environment and Health, 31*(4), 316–323.

National Heart, Lung and Blood Institute and World Health Organisation. (2001). *Global initiative for chronic obstructive lung disease: a collaborative project of the National Heart, Lung, and Blood Institute and World Health Organisation.* Bethesda, MD: National Institutes of Health.

Ng, T. P., Niti, M., Tan, W. C., et al. (2007). Depressive Symptoms and Chronic Obstructive Pulmonary disease. *Archives of Internal Medicine, 167*, 60–67.

Nichol, K. L., Baken, L., & Nelson, A. (1999). Relation between influenza vaccination and outpatient visits, hospitalisation and mortality in elderly persons with chonic lung disease. *Annual Internal Medicine, 130*, 397–403.

Page, A., Begg, S., Taylor, R., et al. (2007). Global comparative assessments of life expectancy: the impact of migration with reference to Australia. *Bulletin of the World Health Organization, 85*(6), 474–481.

Plant, P., Owen, J. L., Elliott, M. W. (2000). One-year period prevalence study of respiratory acidosis in acute exacerbations of COPD; implications for the provision of non-invasive ventilation and oxygen administration. *Thorax, 55*(7), 550–554.

Poole, P. J., Chacko, E., Wood-Baker, R. W. B., et al. (2007). Influenza vaccine for patients with chronic obstructive pulmonary disease. *Cochrane Data of Systematic Review*, 2006, Issue 1 Art. No:CD002733 doi: 10.1002/14651858.CD002733pub2

Poulain, M., Doucet, M., Major, G. C., et al. (2006). The effect of obesity on chronic respiratory diseases: pathophysiology and therapeutic strategies. *Canadian Medical Association Journal, 174*(9), 1293–1299.

Qaseem, A., Wilt, T. J., Weinberger, S. E., et al. (2011). Diagnosis and management of stable chronic obstructive pulmonary disease: A clinical practice guideline update from the American College of Physicians, American College of Chest Physicians, American Thoracic Society, and European Respiratory Society. *Annals of Internal Medicine, 155*, 179–191.

Rau, J. L. (2006). Practical Problems with Aerosol Therapy in COPD. *Respiratory Care, 51*(2), 158–172.

Ries, A., Bauldoff, G. S., Carlin, B. W., et al. (2007). Pulmonary Rehabilitation: Joint ACCP/AACVPR Evidence-Based Clinical Practice Guidelines. *Chest, 131*, 4–42.

Ries, A. L., Kaplan, R. M., Myers, R., et al. (2003). Maintenance after Pulmonary Rehabilitation in Chronic Lung Disease. *American Journal of Respiratory and Critical Care Medicine, 167*, 880–888.

Sampsonas, F., Karkoulias, K., Kaparianos, A., et al. (2006). Genetics of chronic obstructive pulmonary disease, beyond 1-antitrypsin deficiency. *Current Medicinal Chemistry, 13*, 2857–2873.

Schols, A. M. W. J., Slangen, J., Volovics, L., et al. (1998). Weight Loss is a Reversible Factor in the Prognosis of Chronic Obstructive Pulmonary Disease. *American Journal of Respiratory and Critical Care Medicine, 157*, 1791–1797.

Seamark, D. A., Seamark, C. J., Halpin, D. M. G. (2007). Palliative care in chronic obstructive pulmonary disease. *Journal of the Royal Society of Medicine, 100*, 225–233.

Sherwood Burge, P. (2006). Preventing exacerbations. How are we doing and can we do better? *Proceedings of the American Thoracic Society, 3*, 257–261.

Singh, S., Morgan, D., Scott, S., et al. (1992). Development of a shuttle walking test of disability in patients with chronic airways obstruction. *Thorax, 47*, 1019–1024.

Smith, S., Roberts, S. B., Duggan-Brennan, M., Powrie, K. E., & Haffenden, R. (2009). Emergency oxygen delivery 2: patients with asthma and COPD. *Nursing Times, 105*(11), 22–23.

Thorn, J., Bjorkelund, C., Bengtsson, C., et al. (2006). Low socio-economic status, smoking, mental stress and obesity predict obstructive symptoms in women, but only smoking also predicts subsequent experience of poor health. *International Journal of Medical Science, 4*(1), 7–12.

Town, I., Taylor, R., Garrett, G., et al. (2003). *The burden of COPD in New Zealand*. Wellington, NZ: Asthma and respiratory foundation of New Zealand Inc.

Tsiligianni, I., Kocks, J., Tzanakis, N., et al. (2011). Factors that influence disease-specific quality of life or health status of patients with COPD: A review and meta-analysis of Pearson correlations. *Primary Care Respiratory Journal, 20*, 257–268.

Viegi, G., Maio, S., Pistelli, F., et al. (2006). Epidemiology of chronic obstructive pulmonary disease: health effects of air pollution. *Respirology, 11*, 523–532.

Walda, I. C., Tabak, C., Smit, H. A., et al. (2002). Diet and 20-year chronic obstructive pulmonary disease mortality in middle-aged men from three European countries. *European Journal of Clinical Nutrition, 56*, 38–643.

Watson, L., Vonk, J. M., Lofdahl, C. G., et al. (2006). Predictors of lung function and its decline in mild to moderate COPD in association with gender: Results from the Euroscop study. *Respiratory Medicine, 100*, 746–753.

Wolkove, N., Dajczman, E., Colacone, A., et al. (1989). The relationship between pulmonary function and dyspnoea in obstructive lung disease. *Chest, 96*, 1247–1251.

Wood, A. M., & Stockley, R. A. (2006). The genetics of chronic obstructive pulmonary disease. *Respiratory Research, 7*(130). Retrieved May 2, 2013, from http://respiratory-research.com/content/7/1/130

World Health Organization. (1997). *WHOQOL; Measuring quality of life. Division of mental health and prevention of substance abuse*. Geneva: Author.

World Health Organization. (2012). Programmes and projects: chronic respiratory diseases. Retrieved January 15, 2012, from, http://www.who.int/respiratory/copd/en/

Yohannes, A. M., Willgoss, T. G., Baldwin, R. C., et al. (2010). Depression and anxiety in chronic heart failure and chronic obstructive pulmonary disease: prevalence, relevance, clinical implications and management principles. *International Journal of Geriatric Psychiatry, 25*, 1209–1221.

Yohannes, A. M., Baldwin, R. C., & Connolly, M. J. (2000). Depression and anxiety in elderly outpatients with chronic obstructive pulmonary disease: Prevalence, and validation of the BASDEC screening questionnaire. *International Journal of Geriatric Psychiatry, 15*, 1090–1096.

Yusen, R. (2001). What outcomes should be measured in patients with COPD? *Chest, 119*, 327–328.

CHAPTER 20

Angela M. Kucia
Elizabeth Birchmore

Coronary heart disease

Learning objectives

When you have completed this chapter you will be able to:

- describe modifiable biomedical and behavioural risk factors for coronary heart disease and secondary prevention strategies to address these risk factors
- demonstrate an awareness of issues that impact upon quality of life for people with coronary heart disease
- discuss the current evidence relating to the relationship of various psychological disorders and coronary heart disease
- identify management strategies that reduce symptoms in people with chronic coronary heart disease
- describe models of cardiac rehabilitation programs and community supports available to those with coronary heart disease.

Key words

cardiac rehabilitation, coronary heart disease, angina, risk factors, secondary prevention

INTRODUCTION

Coronary heart disease (CHD) is a disease characterised by reduced blood supply to the heart muscle, usually due to a narrowing of the coronary arteries as a result of atherosclerosis. In Australia and New Zealand, as in most Western nations, CHD is a major public health problem and accounts for a major proportion of health expenditure (Australian

Institute of Health and Welfare [AIHW], 2012; Hay, 2004). Although mortality from CHD has declined over the past two decades, we are now facing the challenge of managing chronic heart diseases in the long term, and thus there is a shift towards managing disability due to CHD and enhancing quality of life in addition to longevity (Access Economics [AE], 2005).

CHD may result in a condition known as angina pectoris, characterised by discomfort in the chest, which may radiate to the jaw, shoulder, back or arm. Typically, it is aggravated by exertion or emotional stress, and relieved by nitro-glycerine and rest. Although angina pectoris usually occurs in patients with coronary artery disease involving at least one large epicardial artery, it may also occur in persons with valvular heart disease, hypertrophic cardiomyopathy and uncontrolled hypertension. It can also be present in patients with normal coronary arteries and myocardial ischaemia related to coronary artery spasm or endothelial dysfunction (Gibbons et al., 2003).

Most patients with angina resulting from CHD can be managed with revascularisation procedures (coronary artery bypass surgery or percutaneous transluminal coronary angioplasty), medications and lifestyle modifications. For some patients with stable angina, or in whom revascularisation is not an option, medication management and lifestyle modifications are the only options for treatment of this chronic condition.

Caring for patients with CHD requires an in-depth knowledge of management options, including strategies for modification of biomedical and behavioural risk factors that contribute to this condition, and the contribution that the multidisciplinary team can make in terms of assisting patients to optimise their quality of life in the presence of this chronic disease.

Case Study 20.1 will be used as a framework to discuss the management of patients with coronary heart disease. Also refer to Box 20.1.

CASE STUDY 20.1

Peter Smedley is a 58-year-old man who has been admitted to the hospital after having a conscious collapse at work. He had complained of chest pain to his work colleagues. He thought it was indigestion following a 'business lunch' where he had eaten a large meal and consumed an undisclosed amount of alcohol. His colleagues noted that he appeared pale and sweaty and looked to be quite unwell. His boss insisted that an ambulance be called and shortly after the call was made, Peter had an unconscious collapse. Fortunately, his secretary had just undertaken a course in Basic Life Support and as Peter was unresponsive with no signs of life, she commenced cardiopulmonary resuscitation (CPR). The ambulance arrived within 8 minutes and found that Peter was in ventricular fibrillation. He was successfully defibrillated into sinus rhythm and it was evident from the recorded ECG trace that Peter had ST-segment elevation in the inferior leads indicating an inferior ST-elevation myocardial infarction (STEMI). Peter was taken directly to the coronary catheter laboratory where he underwent percutaneous coronary angioplasty and placement of a stent to his proximal right coronary artery (RCA). During the procedure, it was noted that the RCA had diffuse disease that was not ideal for angioplasty, particularly in the distal segment. It was decided that the residual coronary artery disease would be best managed with medical therapy.

CASE STUDY 20.1 — cont'd

Peter was transferred to the coronary care unit (CCU) where he was referred to the cardiac rehabilitation team and underwent routine screening for cardiovascular disease risk factors. Prior to this presentation, Peter had rarely consulted with his general practitioner (GP). He admits that a few years ago he was told he had high blood pressure and was prescribed some medication, but he didn't get around to having the prescription filled, and as he felt all right, he did not go back to the GP. He was uncertain whether there was any history of heart disease in his family as he was estranged from his parents, but his sister had told him that his father had died of a stroke or a heart attack — he wasn't sure which. He has smoked since he was 14 years of age and has contemplated giving up smoking as his work colleagues have been 'nagging' him to quit, but he finds it difficult to stop smoking because of the pressure he is under with his job. He doesn't undertake any regular exercise and is overweight. He doesn't know his cholesterol level and has never been tested for diabetes. It is noted his that his blood sugar on his arrival to hospital was 13 mmol/L.

Peter is divorced with no children and lives alone. He travels a lot with his job and as he was away from home so often, his wife found someone else. He doesn't have a strong social network, but keeps in touch with his sister and her family. He discloses that he drinks a bottle of wine every night which helps him to sleep and sometimes drinks during the day on occasions such as business lunches. He has difficulty controlling his stress levels and feels depressed and lonely sometimes, and bitter about his marriage break up. He says he is not an alcoholic but a couple of drinks keep him from thinking about things that upset him. Peter also admits that he has been having chest pains for a few weeks now, but thought it was indigestion. As he has residual coronary artery disease, it is possible that he may continue to have episodes of angina, particularly at times of higher myocardial oxygen demand, such as during exercise. Whilst stable angina is associated with a low risk of acute coronary events and increased mortality, the risk is still higher than their counterparts who do not have stable angina.

Peter needed to be educated about secondary prevention activities and actively involved in secondary prevention. The goals of management of established disease are to minimise the negative effects of the disease and to reduce the risk of further cardiovascular events. Introducing strategies to address modifiable risk factors that affect health status are core business for nurses involved in the management of patients with CHD. The best time to identify and raise awareness of the impact of the risk on cardiac disease is in the primary care setting. However, in reality, the opportunity to do this often presents following an acute event.

RISK FACTORS AND BEHAVIOURS THAT CONTRIBUTE TO THE DEVELOPMENT OF CHD

A number of clearly defined genetic, behavioural and biomedical risk factors are associated with CHD. Risk for CHD rises progressively according to the number of risk factors present in an individual. People with existing CHD are in the highest risk group for future cardiac events, so a more stringent approach to risk factor management through pharmacological and lifestyle interventions will be required.

BOX 20.1
Evidence in practice: the COURAGE study

For patients who present to hospital with an acute coronary syndrome due to abrupt occlusion of a coronary artery, there is no question that the culprit artery needs to be opened to allow blood flow to the muscle. The preferred management is percutaneous coronary angioplasty (PTCA), though fibrinolytic therapy is used if percutaneous intervention (PCI) is not readily available. However, in patients with stable coronary artery disease, the plan of care is not so clear-cut.

The COURAGE Study recruited 2287 patients with at least one severely stenosed coronary artery limiting blood flow to the heart muscle. Patients were randomised to (a) PTCA and stent or (b) medical therapy. PCI did not reduce the risk of death, myocardial infarction or other major cardiovascular events when added to optimal medical therapy (Boden et al., 2007). The lesson learnt from this study is that people with stable angina or a narrowed coronary artery have choices in the management of stable angina, and patient preference should be considered.

Cardiac risk factors are traditionally thought of as those that cannot be changed by lifestyle change or medical treatment, and those that are modifiable through interventions such as pharmacotherapy and/or lifestyle change. These modifiable risk factors may be further divided into biomedical or behavioural risk factors.

Non-modifiable biomedical risk factors include:

- age, with CHD predominantly affecting middle-aged and older Australians
- gender, with CHD being more common in men than women due to protective effects of oestrogen, until age 65, from which point women have equal risk to men
- family history of CHD, with the risk of CHD increasing if a first-degree relative is diagnosed with heart or blood vessel disease before the age of 60 (AE, 2005).

Although these risk factors cannot be modified, awareness of these risks may encourage patients to take positive steps in addressing other risk factors that are modifiable.

Modifiable biomedical risk factors include:

- dyslipidaemia, a metabolic derangement that can be hereditary or acquired, and contributes to many forms of disease, notably CHD
- hypertension, which is the greatest contributor to the burden of heart disease than any other modifiable risk factor (Begg et al., 2007)
- diabetes, which is also a major risk factor for stroke, peripheral arterial disease, nephropathy and retinopathy
- renal failure, which can be either a cause or a consequence of CHD. CHD is the major cause of death in people with end-stage renal failure (ESRD) and mortality from CHD is 30 times greater in people with ESRD than the general population (Sarnak et al., 2003).

Modifiable behavioural cardiovascular risk factors include:

- tobacco smoking, which increases blood pressure and clotting tendencies, with chemicals such as carbon monoxide and cyanide that are found in tobacco smoke leading to cardiovascular and lung damage

- poor nutrition or excessive food consumption, which can affect other risk factors such as being overweight and diabetes (AE, 2005)
- high consumption of alcohol and binge drinking, which are associated with hypertension, although low to moderate alcohol use may have health benefits (AE, 2005)
- physical inactivity, which is second only to tobacco smoking in terms of its impact on the burden of disease in Australia, and is the leading cause of disease in Australian women (AE, 2005)
- being overweight or obese, which is associated with an increased mortality that rises exponentially with the degree of increased body mass index (BMI), and contributes to co-morbid conditions due to obesity including hypertension, type II diabetes, sleep apnoea, osteoarthritis (which affects mobility), psychological disorders and social problems (Tonkin et al., 2005)
- depression, stress, social isolation, poor social support, which have been associated with the development of CHD (Bunker et al., 2003).

Depression is around three times more common in patients after an acute myocardial infarction than in the general community (Thombs et al., 2006), and depression is higher among people with heart disease living in the community when compared with those without heart disease (Lichtman et al., 2008).

Absolute risk assessment

Most cardiac patients tend to have multiple risk factors, thus multiplying the overall extent of the risk. Similarly, the presence of one disease, for example diabetes, can increase the risk of developing another. Measuring individual cardiovascular risk factors in isolation poorly estimates a person's likelihood of developing new or worsening current cardiovascular disease. Instead, absolute risk, the numerical probability of a cardiovascular event occurring within a 5-year period, is usually used. Visual tools such as the absolute risk factor assessment tool may also reinforce to patients the need for change, and provide encouragement to persist with lifestyle modification (National Vascular Disease Prevention Alliance [NVDPA], 2012). It should be noted that currently available absolute risk calculators may significantly underestimate cardiovascular risk in Aboriginal, Torres Strait Islander, Māori and Pacific Islander peoples (National Heart Foundation of Australia [NHFA], 2010).

CARDIAC REHABILITATION

Cardiac rehabilitation (CR) is described by the NHFA and the Australian Cardiac Rehabilitation Association (ACRA) (2004) as 'all measures used to help people with heart disease return to an active and satisfying life and to prevent recurrence of cardiac events'. It is an important component of CHD management. CR is usually first offered to in-hospital patients following an acute event, such as myocardial infarction or unstable angina, or following re-vascularisation procedures, but may also be made available to patients with stable angina, controlled heart failure and other vascular or heart disease or those awaiting cardiac investigation or intervention (NHFA & ACRA, 2004).

In the acute setting, CR begins as soon as is practical following admission, with the aim of moving the patient into the recovery phase as soon as possible after an acute event. This is often referred to as 'Phase 1' CR and involves initial contact and introduction to the service, basic information and reassurance, supportive counselling, guidelines for mobilisation and information on pharmacotherapy. Prior to discharge from hospital, patients should be fully informed of their risk factor status, and know what their specific biomedical target levels are. Discharge planning also begins soon after admission, including referral to outpatient CR (NHFA & ACRA, 2004) and general practitioner (GP) follow-up. CR aims to encourage patients and their families to embrace secondary prevention principles and goals, including compliance with pharmacotherapy, and facilitate the development of self-management skills to enhance long-term lifestyle change, particularly with regard to reducing risk of recurrent cardiac events. Patients are made aware of community resources and encouraged to utilise these resources in their long-term care. CR is generally continued as an outpatient and ongoing prevention approach (known as 'Phase 2' CR), but patients may access these services at different levels of the disease management continuum, depending upon factors such as the patient's readiness to take part in a CR program or availability of CR services (NHFA & ACRA, 2004).

Attendance to structured cardiac rehabilitation programs remains poor. Factors such as distance, early hospital discharge, early return to work, poor referral practices and patient preferences are often cited as the reasons for poor attendances. Furthermore, it seems that compliance with lifestyle modification falls by the wayside at about 6 months from the index event, when patients feel that they have been 'cured' of their disease (EUROASPIRE II, 2001). Developing partnerships between patients and clinicians and assisting patients to understand the long-term impact of risk factors on health may assist and enhance long-term secondary prevention strategies. Timing of the intervention is often a key factor on how an educational strategy may be received by the patient and family members. Thus consideration of variables that may affect the patient's ability to receive and process information must be taken into account when developing an educational program. The increasing use of internet resources, nurse led clinics and community care options are being developed to increase opportunities for other models of cardiac rehabilitation.

PATIENT EDUCATION: UNDERSTANDING THE DISEASE

Educational information about the cause of CHD and subsequent management options are usually available to the patient as print materials, supported by counselling and advice by health professionals, including medical and nursing staff, dietitians, pharmacists and social workers. Although it is recognised that patients need information to enable them to actively participate in their rehabilitation and management, in many instances patient education programs fail to influence patients' behaviour in relation to risk factor reduction. It is important for the nurse to ascertain which factors the patient considers are the major influences on their illness. Some patients demonstrate an internal locus of control; they feel responsible for becoming ill and believe that their lifestyle behaviour has caused their illness. Others exhibit an external locus of control in that they believe their illness is attributed to external factors over which they had no control. Those with an internal locus of control may be more amenable to behavioural change because they take some responsibility for the state of their health and physical recovery. It is important for nurses to recognise the health beliefs of individual patients and what they see as important information at each stage of their illness.

In Case Study 20.1, it is clear that Peter needs education about risk factors for CHD and to be actively involved in secondary prevention plans. As with most patients with CHD, Peter has multiple risk factors, thus multiplying the overall extent of the risk. Similarly, the presence of one disease, for example diabetes, can increase the risk of developing another. Risk factor information is interdependent; thus CR should present a holistic view rather than attempting to manage each risk as a stand-alone entity. When planning risk management strategies, the nurse involved in CR will include management of co-morbidities that impact on cardiovascular risk.

Peter has risk factors that can't be changed: he is a middle-aged male and has a family history of cardiovascular disease. Although Peter cannot change these risk factors, he needs to be aware that having them means that the presence of other risk factors exponentially elevates his risk of further cardiac events; thus it is in his best interests to address those risk factors that can be modified.

Smoking

In addition to long-term effects such as accelerated atherosclerosis, immediate cardiovascular effects of smoking include: temporary increases in blood pressure and heart rate; vasoconstriction; reduced oxygen delivered to tissues due to binding of carbon monoxide to haemoglobin in the bloodstream; increased clotting tendencies and potentiation of cardiac arrhythmias (NHFA, 2002).

A large number of people continue to smoke, despite stating that they wish they had never started smoking or could quit. Nicotine, found in cigarette smoke, is highly addictive but, clearly, psychological as well as physiological factors contribute to lack of success in quitting smoking.

The overall goals for addressing Peter's smoking are complete cessation of smoking and avoidance of second-hand smoke. Peter needs to understand the impact of smoking on his cardiovascular health, and to make a positive commitment to quitting. Evidence suggests that even brief episodes of counselling are effective in increasing cessation success (NHFA & Cardiac Society of Australia and New Zealand [CSANZ], 2012). Consideration should be given to referring Peter to Quitline or a smoking cessation program. These are often offered within CR services and are also available in the community. The Quit Program is a good resource for those planning to stop smoking.

Nicotine replacement therapy (NRT), available via a number of forms of delivery, should be considered for patients such as Peter who smoke more than 10 cigarettes per day. NRT can be used safely in smokers with stable CHD, but should be used with caution in people with recent myocardial infarction, unstable angina, severe arrhythmias or a recent cerebrovascular event.

NRT may be an option for Peter, although, given his CHD, the supervision of a medical practitioner, nurse practitioner or pharmacist is advisable. Bupropion (Zyban) is a non-nicotine oral therapy that can be used in combination with NRT for patients requiring additional assistance. Varenicline (Champix) is another oral therapy that activates dopamine receptors and blocks nicotine from attaching to these receptors (Zwar et al., 2011). In deciding whether or not to use pharmacotherapies to assist in smoking cessation, one must consider the high risk of continuing to smoke against the benefits and risks of pharmacotherapy. Pharmacotherapy alone will have less chance of success if not accompanied by behavioural and psychosocial support: Peter's psychosocial problems have to be addressed in planning his quit smoking process to maximise his chance of success.

Nutrition

Peter has recognised that his diet is poor. Nutritional goals for Peter include establishing and maintaining healthy eating, which include limiting saturated fatty acid (SFA) intake to <7% and trans fatty acid (tFA) intake to <1% of total energy. Although moderate amounts of lean meats, poultry, fish, reduced-fat dairy products and polyunsaturated or monounsaturated fats are permitted, Peter needs to consume mainly plant-based foods such as vegetables, fruits and legumes (dried peas, dried beans and lentils) and grain-based foods (preferably wholegrain) such as bread, pasta, noodles and rice. Phytosterols, more commonly known as plant sterols, are steroid compounds which occur in fruit, vegetables, nuts and seeds and are chemically similar to cholesterol. They act by inhibiting the absorption of cholesterol in the intestines, thus reducing the level of circulating cholesterols. The dietitian would recommend a diet high in these components as part of a healthy diet regimen for Peter, and given that Peter is overweight and has diabetes and hyperlipidaemia, it is advisable that he be referred to a dietitian.

Alcohol

The goal of management for Peter with regard to his alcohol use is low-risk alcohol consumption. It is extremely important to do a thorough alcohol assessment with Peter to ensure that he is not at risk of alcohol withdrawal during his hospitalisation and so that he can recognise how risky alcohol consumption can affect his CHD. Patients like Peter who have hypertension are advised to limit their alcohol intake to no more than two standard drinks per day for men, or one standard drink per day for women (NHFA & CSANZ, 2012). As with smoking, Peter's psychosocial situation is likely to have an impact upon his alcohol consumption; thus psychological and social management will play a big part in meeting the goal of low-risk alcohol consumption for Peter.

Physical activity

The NHFA and CSANZ (2012) advise that patients with CHD set a goal of progressing over time to at least 30 minutes of moderate-intensity physical activity on most, if not all, days of the week. Patients with unstable angina, uncontrolled or severe hypertension, severe aortic stenosis, uncontrolled diabetes, complicated acute myocardial infarction, uncontrolled heart failure, symptomatic hypotension (<90/60 mmHg), resting tachycardia or arrhythmias will need to have a clinical assessment of their exercise capabilities and may need to modify or defer physical activity until their condition has stabilised.

As is the case with many patients, Peter has had quite a sedentary lifestyle, and so building physical activity into his normal routine may seem quite daunting to him. The positive benefits of physical activity on recovery include improved confidence and morale and it usually enables patients to resume a normal lifestyle, which may include returning to work. Physical activity will also have a significant impact on reducing existing cardiac risk factors such as hypertension, hyperlipidaemia, obesity and insulin resistance. Physical activity will also have a positive impact on psychological health and wellbeing. A key step in motivating patients to engage in physical activity is to ensure that they are aware of the positive benefits on their heart health. A study by Jolliffe et al. (2001) demonstrated that physically active survivors of myocardial infarction are up to 25% less likely to die than their sedentary counterparts.

Peter will need an assessment prior to undertaking physical activity, and the nurse then needs to discuss his physical activity needs and capabilities with him. Peter has admitted to having a sedentary lifestyle and feels that his job is a barrier to opportunities for physical activity. The nurse needs to reassure Peter that physical activity does not have to be completed all at once: short bouts of 10 minutes' duration may be more suited to Peter's lifestyle. Peter is wondering how he will know when he is exercising appropriately. Moderate activity should cause a moderate noticeable increase in Peter's depth and rate of breathing, but he should still be able to talk comfortably.

Provision of some written guidelines for Peter regarding everyday physical activity tasks, such as a light-to-moderate walking program, water aerobics or cycling for pleasure, may encourage him to undertake physical activity regularly. Following discussion, Peter feels that he is more likely to undertake purposeful walking regularly than activities that need some organisation. During this time, the nurse may take the opportunity to explain to Peter how to recognise any early warning signs of ischaemia, such as breathlessness or chest discomfort, and together they can discuss strategies that may be used should symptoms reoccur. Peter should ensure that he carries a supply of sublingual or short-acting nitrate (anginine) during physical activity.

Relatives often become quite anxious when their loved one begins to return to activity as they are concerned that activity may cause another event. It is important that nurses caring for patients with CHD include family members in education consultations wherever possible to allay any fears or misconceptions that may restrict physical activity, including sexual activity, following discharge from hospital.

Early referral to an outpatient cardiac rehabilitation program is recommended for Peter, so his progress and response to a physical activity regimen can be monitored.

Healthy weight

Peter is overweight. The NHFA and CSANZ (2012) suggest that waist measurements of less than 94 cm for males and 80 cm for females and a BMI between 18.5 and 24.9 should be target goals for healthy weight to reduce cardiovascular risk. Peter is going to be referred to a dietitian and, in collaboration with the nurse and dietitian, Peter needs to set intermediate achievable goals. He wants to be able to make assessments of weight change, and so the nurse needs to teach Peter how to do waist measurement. The waist circumference is measured half way between the inferior margin of the last rib and the crest of the ilium in the mid-axillary plane at the end of expiration. Peter's weight and height are measured, and his healthy weight calculated according to BMI. Peter has already received information on nutrition and exercise, and he is reminded that for weight loss to occur, he must use up more energy (kilojoules) through regular physical activity and consume less energy from food and drinks (NHFA & CSANZ, 2012).

Lipids

Statins have been shown to be of benefit in patients with CHD regardless of their total or low-density lipid levels; thus early initiation of lipid-lowering therapy is recommended for all patients with CHD (except in exceptional circumstances), and is beneficial in high-risk groups such as those with diabetes. Target treatment goals for lipid therapy are low-density lipid-cholesterol (LDL-C) <1.8 mmol/L; high-density lipid-cholesterol (HDL-C) >1 mmol/L and triglyceride (TG) level <2.0 mmol/L (NHFA & CSANZ, 2012).

A dietitian has already been booked to see Peter, who has already received some healthy eating advice, but Peter is also in need of pharmacotherapy for this condition. Statins are the treatment of choice for lowering LDL-C cholesterol. Patients who are overweight and have type II diabetes, high TG level and/or low HDL-C may benefit from fibrate therapy, although caution should be exercised in using statins and fibrates together as there is a risk of myopathy. If this combination is used for Peter, he must be educated about reporting unusual muscular pain promptly. Ezetimibe is effective in reducing the concentration of LDL-C as monotherapy or as an adjunct to a statin. Peter has elevated TG levels and in addition to dietary changes needed in keeping his diabetes under control, he may benefit from marine omega-3 fortified food and drinks and/or marine omega-F3 capsules (NHFA & CSANZ, 2012).

Blood pressure

Around 30% of Australians have diagnosed hypertension (NHFA, 2010), and there is evidence to suggest that there is one person with untreated hypertension for every person treated with hypertension (Briganti et al., 2003). Moreover, of those on treatment, a high proportion still have elevated blood pressure levels (AE, 2005).

As Peter has hypertension, pharmacological and non-pharmacological strategies for reducing blood pressure need to be discussed with him. For patients with coronary heart disease, nurses often have an active role in ongoing blood pressure monitoring, and should be aware of these targets. As Peter has had some difficulty complying in the past, it is important that he understands that hypertension is a major risk in CHD: the higher the blood pressure, the greater the chance of Peter incurring an adverse event related to CHD, stroke, kidney disease, heart failure or death (NHFA & ACRA, 2004).

There are a number of pharmacological agents for the management of hypertension, but the first choice is normally angiotensin-converting enzyme inhibitors (ACEIs), or angiotensin II receptor antagonists (ARAs) if ACEIs are not tolerated. Other agents include calcium channel blockers (CCBs) and diuretics. Most patients will require a combination of medications to control hypertension, and the choice of therapy is often influenced by co-existing medical conditions and patient tolerance. Specialist nurses may be involved in the titration of pharmacotherapy and ongoing monitoring of hypertension.

Peter has admitted that his diet is not as good as it could be and that he eats a lot of fast foods. As sodium contributes to hypertension, Peter needs to be advised how to reduce his sodium intake by avoiding processed foods such as processed meats, commercial sauces, soups, packet seasoning, stock cubes, potato chips, salted nuts and takeaway foods that are high in salt, and increasing his intake of fresh fruit and vegetables. He also needs to be advised how to interpret the 'nutrition information' panel on food purchases and to choose foods labelled as 'no added salt', 'low salt' or 'salt reduced'.

Lifestyle modifications are an important component of hypertension management whether or not pharmacological agents are also used. Lifestyle modifications are going to be an integral part of Peter's hypertension management, with particular attention to the 'SNAP' (smoking, nutrition, alcohol, physical activity) risk factors (NHFA & CSANZ, 2012). Weight reduction is also an important factor.

Diabetes

Peter has been diagnosed with Type 2 diabetes, which commonly occurs in middle-aged adults and is often linked with obesity. The goal of Peter's diabetes management is to maintain an optimal blood sugar as indicated by an HbA_{1c} equal to or less than 7% (NHFA & CSANZ, 2012). Peter will need to start oral hypoglycaemics and he will receive education on diet and management of other risk factors that have an impact on his diabetes.

Compliance

The chronic nature of CHD will require the patient to take numerous medications, attend regular medical appointments and undertake numerous lifelong lifestyle changes. The degree to which the patient is able to commit to this regimen may determine their outcome in terms of ongoing symptoms and quality of life. Compliance requires patients to agree to and participate in a treatment program as advised by their treating doctor or health worker. Therefore in order to be compliant the patient must see that the advice or treatment prescribed will add value to their quality of life.

Non-compliance with cardiac medications following discharge from hospital is a huge problem. The benefit of statin therapy in patients with CHD has been clearly established and is now part of gold-standard therapy, but long-term patient compliance with these therapies is sub-optimal. Jackevicius, Mamdani and Tu (2002) reported that in a study of patients with CHD, only 40.1% were taking their medication 2 years after their cardiac event. The reasons for poor compliance rates are numerous and complex. Many of these are patient-related factors, but system difficulties may also have an impact.

A lack of awareness or understanding of the importance of taking a number of cardiac drugs is often the case, with many patients stopping their medications when they feel better. In a study by Kimble and Kunik (2002) of general aspects of angina self-management and quality of life in 95 patients with angina, 65% lacked knowledge about using sublingual nitrates to prevent symptoms and 32.6% took sublingual nitrates for symptoms other than chest pain. Medication regimens are often complicated, and cardiac patients are often required to take several different types of medications for long periods of time. Financially, the cost of purchasing medications, particularly for those on a fixed income, may be seen as prohibitive. Other factors are difficulties with language that affect the patient's ability to read the instructions on medication packaging, cognitive impairment and poor manual dexterity, particularly in the frail, aged patient, which makes them unable to open medication packaging or collect refilled prescriptions.

Patients are often labelled as poorly compliant with taking medications and adhering to recommended lifestyle change without much consideration being given to factors outside the patient's locus of control. These factors can be described as system factors. Poor communication between hospital and community care providers resulting from pressure on institutions to reduce length of stay may see patients being discharged without adequate dialogue between the different sectors of healthcare and the patient. Patients are often discharged with 2 or 3 days of medication and are often unable to access general practice due to difficult working hours, or lack of after-hours services.

The nurse can encourage Peter's compliance with medication by involving him in medication administration as soon as he is clinically stable. This will assist him to become familiar with the size, colour and shape of his medication prior to his having to be fully responsible for them. The nurse can then assess how Peter will be able to manage post-discharge and, if necessary, make recommendations for a delivery device to be monitored by a community pharmacist. Peter will be given a medication chart that explains what each of his medications is for, the time of the day that it is to be taken and any other special instructions that may be required. The nurse will discuss with Peter how he will manage his medication at home. If possible, Peter's family members will be included in education sessions. Peter may need to be referred to a community pharmacist for a Home Medication Management Review (HMMR) if issues related to poor compliance recur.

PSYCHOSOCIAL ASSESSMENT

Depression and anxiety

Depression is prevalent in populations with CHD. As well as being a predictor for the development of CHD, depression is predictive of adverse outcomes among patients with existing cardiac disease (Lett et al., 2004; Mallik et al., 2005). Furthermore, it may result in pathophysiological processes such as hypercortisolaemia, impaired platelet function, reduced heart rate variability, impaired vagal control and increased potential for arrhythmias (Rumsfeld & Ho, 2005; Lederbogen et al., 2001).

Anxiety may be responsible for an increased susceptibility to unhealthy lifestyles such as smoking, reduced physical activity due to feelings of exhaustion and weakness, restless behaviour and apprehension. Anxious states may result in elevated cholesterol, hypertension, diabetes, diaphoresis and reduced heart rate variability; instances of sudden cardiac death have been reported (Bunker et al., 2003).

Peter has given several clues in his history to suggest that he may be depressed. He needs a professional assessment for depression so that he can receive appropriate psychological and medical management. Nurses caring for patients with CHD should have skills that will assist them to identify patients who may be depressed, and refer them for specialised management as needed. There are a number of validated tools that can aid in this process (Beck et al., 1961; Hare & Davis, 1996, Zigmond & Snaith, 1983).

Peter has already received advice on regular physical activity, which may help to reduce his depression and anxiety, but he may need pharmacological therapy. Selective serotonin uptake inhibitors have been shown to be safe and efficacious in the management of CHD patients with depression. Tricyclic antidepressants should be avoided in CHD patients (NHFA & CSANZ, 2012).

Clearly, pharmacological management alone isn't going to solve Peter's problems. The nurse has a role in referring Peter to a social worker and counselling. It is likely that Peter will also have input from a psychiatrist or specialist mental health nurse. Cognitive behavioural therapy delivered by a mental health professional specifically trained in this form of therapy is also an effective management strategy (NHFA & CSANZ, 2012).

Social isolation and lack of social support

The absence of supportive family members and/or friends, participation in work, community or recreational activities and involvement in a social network are also risk factors for adopting an unhealthy lifestyle. There is strong and consistent evidence that social isolation and lack of social support are independent risk factors for CHD and worsen prognosis for patients with existing disease (Bunker et al., 2003).

When a crisis such as an acute cardiac event occurs, patients often find themselves surrounded by family members and friends who they wouldn't normally see in their regular day-to-day activities. The actual strength of that social support may not be evident until after discharge, when friends and family members fade into the background, as the crisis is no longer evident. Thus the nurse needs to carefully assess what support is likely to continue after discharge from hospital. If the patient lives alone, the nurse needs to assess how the patient will be able to function, and whether there are people who continuously support that person at home. Asking questions about practical things, such as whether they are able to go to the doctor unaided and who assists with shopping and other activities of daily living, may provide a better insight into their social context.

Aboriginal and Torres Strait Islander peoples are a particular at-risk group for the negative impact that social isolation and poor social support can have on the recovering cardiac patient. It is a time when they are often in an unfamiliar environment, away from their family members, and experiencing both language and cultural difficulties. Wherever possible, an Aboriginal Health Worker or Aboriginal Liaison Officer should be included as a member of the healthcare team.

Australians who have socioeconomic disadvantages are more likely to smoke, have diabetes and be obese, thus having a greater risk of death from cardiovascular disease. Aboriginal and Torres Strait Islander peoples have a high cardiovascular mortality and morbidity and are 2.6 times more likely to die from a vascular event than non-Indigenous Australians (AIHW & ABS, 2005). Similarly, Māori and Pacific people have poor cardiovascular health outcomes compared with non-indigenous New Zealanders (Bramley et al., 2004).

Peter has had a couple of his work mates visit during his hospital admission, but clearly they are not going to be able to offer him the type of support he is going to need. On the day prior to discharge, a chest pain action plan is discussed with Peter. All patients with

CHD should be discharged with a fast-acting nitrate and provided with a written action plan for chest pain that includes instructions to:

- rest and self administer short-acting nitrate
- tell someone nearby about the symptoms
- call an ambulance if symptoms are severe, get worse or last for more than 10 minutes (NHFA & CSANZ, 2012).

CONCLUSION

Peter attends the CR sessions and also seems to enjoy the CR exercise program. He joins a gym that specialises in exercise programs for people with IHD and heart failure. He has occasional angina, but thus far manages to control it with anginine and rest. He has been compliant with medication, has lost 10 kg, reduced his LDL and triglycerides and his diabetes is well controlled. His blood pressure has continued to be somewhat elevated and he is still undergoing some adjustments to his antihypertensive therapy.

He has cut back on his working hours and has a job in the office which does not involve frequent travel. The regular hours contribute to his being able to eat regular healthy meals (although he confesses that he occasionally has a meat pie or two). Now that he is home more often, he has bought a dog and goes for regular walks in the early evening with the dog, and his outlook on life seems much improved. He understands that he has chronic disease and that he is going to have to be compliant with medication and lifestyle changes for the rest of his life. He tells you that he suspects he won't have a long life, but he intends to live for as long as he can and be healthy and enjoy what he has. There will be a lot of challenges in Peter's future in maintaining this enthusiasm, but continued support from his health carers in managing this chronic disease will enhance Peter's chances of continuing with a positive outlook.

Working systematically through this case study, it can be seen that nurses and other members of the multidisciplinary health team can assist patients and their families to embrace secondary prevention principles and goals, including compliance with pharmacotherapy, and facilitate the development of self-management skills to embrace long-term lifestyle change, particularly with regard to reducing risk of recurrent cardiac events.

Reflective questions

1. The case study presented is set in a large tertiary institution with access to all the services required to support recovery and ongoing management. If this case study was set in a rural or remote centre, how do you think the options for management might differ?
2. Compliance with cardiovascular medication regimens is a problem that may lead to readmissions, recurrent events and poorer outcomes for patients with CHD. Do you think there may be particular groups of patients for who compliance is a problem, and if so, why?
3. Do you think that people with mental health issues may be at increased risk of CHD?
   (a) What aspects of mental illness and management might contribute to CHD?
   (b) What might be the barriers to reducing the risk of developing/worsening CHD in patients with mental health conditions?

Recommended reading

National Heart Foundation of Australia and the Cardiac Society of Australia and New Zealand. (2012). *Reducing risk in heart disease: an expert guide to clinical practice for secondary prevention of coronary heart disease*. Melbourne: National Heart Foundation of Australia. Retrieved August 22, 2012, from http://www.heartfoundation.org.au/SiteCollectionDocuments/Reducing-risk-in-heart-disease.pdf

National Vascular Disease Prevention Alliance. (2012). Guidelines for the management of absolute cardiovascular disease risk. Retrieved August 22, 2012, from http://www.heartfoundation.org.au/information-for-professionals/Clinical-Information/Pages/absolute-risk.aspx

New Zealand Guidelines Group and Heart Foundation New Zealand. (2002). Cardiac rehabilitation: Summary and Resource Kit. Wellington New Zealand. Retrieved August 24, 2012, from http://www.heartfoundation.org.nz/uploads/guidelines_resource_kit(1).pdf.

O' Flynn, N., Timmis, A., Henderson, H., et al., on behalf of the Guideline Development Group. (2011). Management of stable angina: summary of NICE guidance. *British Medical Journal, 343*, d4147.

Zwar, N., Richmond, R., Borland, R., et al. (2011). *Supporting smoking cessation: a guide for health professionals*. Melbourne: The Royal Australian College of General Practitioners. Retrieved August 24, 2012, from http://www.racgp.org.au/Content/NavigationMenu/ClinicalResources/RACGPGuidelines/smoking/Smoking-cessation.pdf

References

Access Economics. (2005). The shifting burden of cardiovascular disease. Retrieved August 24, 2012, from http://www.heartfoundation.org.au/SiteCollectionDocuments/HF-Shifting_burden-CVD-AccEcons-2005-May.pdf

Australian Institute of Health and Welfare. (2012). *Australia's Health 2012*. Australia's health series no.13. Cat. No. AUS156. Canberra: Australian Institute of Health and Welfare.

Australian Institute of Health and Welfare & Australian Bureau of Statistics. (2005). *The health and welfare of Australia's Aboriginal and Torres Strait Islander peoples 2005*. AIHW cat no IHW 14. ABS cat no 4704.0. Canberra: Australian Institute of Health and Welfare.

Beck, A. T., Ward, C. H., Mendelson, M., et al. (1961). An inventory for measuring depression. *Archives of General Psychiatry, 4*, 561–571.

Begg, S., Vos, T., Barker, B., et al. (2007). *The burden of disease and injury in Australia 2003*. Cat. no. PHE 82. Canberra: AIHW.

Boden, W. E., O'Rourke, R. A., Teo, K. K., et al. (2007). Optimal medical therapy with or without PCI for stable coronary disease. *The New England Journal of Medicine, 356*, 1503–1516.

Bramley, D., Riddell, T., Crengle, S., et al. (2004). A call to action on Maori cardiovascular health. *The New Zealand Medical Journal, 117*, 1197. Retrieved March 9, 2008, from http://www.nzma.org.nz/journal/117-1197/957/

Briganti, E. M., Shaw, J. E., Chadban, S. J., et al. (2003). Untreated hypertension among Australian adults: The 1999–2000 Australian diabetes, obesity and lifestyle study (AusDiab). *Medical Journal of Australia, 179*, 135–139.

Bunker, S. J., Colquhoun, D. M., Esler, M. D., et al. (2003). 'Stress' and coronary heart disease: psychosocial risk factors. *Medical Journal of Australia, 178*(6), 272–276. Retrieved March 7, 2008, from http://www.mja.com.au/public/issues/178_06_170303/bun10421_fm.html

EUROASPIRE II Euro Heart Survey Programme. (2001). Lifestyle and risk factor management and use of drug therapies in coronary patients from 15 countries. *European Heart Journal, 22*(7), 554–572.

Gibbons, R. J., Abrams, J., Chatterjee, K., et al., Task Force on Practice Guidelines (2003). ACC/AHA 2002 guideline update for the management of patients with chronic stable angina. *Circulation, 107*(1), 149–158.

Hare, D. L., & Davis, C. R. (1996). Cardiac depression scale: validation of a new depression scale for cardiac patients. *Journal of Psychosomatic Medicine*, *40*(4), 379–386.

Hay, D. R. (2004). Cardiovascular disease in New Zealand 2004. A summary of recent statistical information. Technical Report No. 82. The National Heart Foundation of New Zealand. Retrieved March 11, 2008, from http://www.nhf.org.nz/files/NHF6949%20TechReport.pdf

Jackevicius, C. N., Mamdani, M., & Tu, J. V. (2002). Adherence with statin therapy in elderly patients with and without acute coronary syndromes. *Journal of the American Medical Association*, *288*(4), 462–467.

Jolliffe, J. A., Rees, K., Taylor, R. S., et al. (2001). Exercise-based rehabilitation for coronary heart disease. Art No: CD001800. *Cochrane Database of Systematic Reviews*, Issue 1. doi: 10.1002/14651858.CD001800.

Kimble, L. P., & Kunik, C. L. (2002). Knowledge and use of sublingual nitroglycerin and cardiac-related quality of life in patients with chronic stable angina. *Journal of Pain and Symptom Management*, *19*(2), 109–117.

Lederbogen, F., Gilles, M., Maras, A., et al. (2001). Increased platelet aggregability in major depression? *Psychiatry Research*, *102*(3), 255–261.

Lett, H. S., Blumenthal, J. A., Babyak, M. A., et al. (2004). Depression as a risk factor for coronary artery disease: evidence, mechanisms, and treatment. *Psychosomatic Medicine*, *66*(3), 305–315.

Lichtman, J. H., Bigger, J. T., Jr., Blumenthal, J. A., et al. (2008). Depression and coronary heart disease: Recommendations for screening, referral, and treatment: A science advisory from the American Heart Association Prevention Committee of the Council on Cardiovascular Nursing, Council on Clinical Cardiology, Council on Epidemiology and Prevention, and Interdisciplinary Council on Quality of Care and Outcomes Research: Endorsed by the American Psychiatric Association. *Circulation*, *118*, 1768–1775.

Mallik, S., Krumholz, H. M., Lin, Z. Q., et al. (2005). Patients with depressive symptoms have lower health status benefits after coronary artery bypass surgery. *Circulation*, *111*(3), 271–277.

National Heart Foundation of Australia. (2002). Cigarette smoking. Retrieved March 8, 2008, from http://www.heartfoundation.org.au/document/NHF/Cigarette_Smoking_Aug_2002.pdf

National Heart Foundation of Australia and Australian Cardiac Rehabilitation Association. (2004). Recommended framework for cardiac rehabilitation 2004. Retrieved August 24, 2012, from http://www.heartfoundation.org.au/SiteCollectionDocuments/Recommended-framework.pdf

National Heart Foundation of Australia and the Cardiac Society of Australia and New Zealand. (2012). *Reducing risk in heart disease: an expert guide to clinical practice for secondary prevention of coronary heart disease*. Melbourne: National Heart Foundation of Australia. Retrieved August 22, 2012, from http://www.heartfoundation.org.au/SiteCollectionDocuments/Reducing-risk-in-heart-disease.pdf

National Heart Foundation of Australia (National Blood Pressure and Vascular Disease Advisory Committee). (2008). Guide to management of hypertension. Updated December 2010. Retrieved August 22, 2012, from http://www.heartfoundation.org.au/information-for-professionals/Clinical-Information/Pages/hypertension.aspx

National Vascular Disease Prevention Alliance. (2012). Guidelines for the management of absolute cardiovascular disease risk. Retrieved August 22, 2012, from http://www.heartfoundation.org.au/information-for-professionals/Clinical-Information/Pages/absolute-risk.aspx

Rumsfeld, J. S., & Ho, P. M. (2005). Depression and cardiovascular disease: A call for recognition. *Circulation*, *111*(3), 250–253.

Sarnak, M. J., Levey, A. S., Schoolwerth, A. C., et al. (2003). Kidney disease as a risk factor for development of cardiovascular disease: a statement from the American Heart Association Councils on Kidney in Cardiovascular Disease, High Blood Pressure Research, Clinical Cardiology, and Epidemiology and Prevention. *Circulation*, *108*, 2154–2169.

Thombs, B. D., Bass, E. B., Ford, D. E., et al. (2006). Prevalence of depression in survivors of acute myocardial infarction. *Journal of General Internal Medicine, 21*, 30–38.

Tonkin, A., Barter, P., Best, J., et al. (2005). National Heart Foundation of Australia and the Cardiac Society of Australia and New Zealand: Position statement on lipid management – 2005. *Heart, Lung and Circulation, 14*, 275–291.

Zigmond, A. S., & Snaith, R. P. (1983). The hospital anxiety and depression scale. *Acta Psychiatrica Scandinavica, 67*(6), 361.

Zwar, N., Richmond, R., Borland, R., et al. (2011). *Supporting smoking cessation: a guide for health professionals*. Melbourne: The Royal Australian College of General Practitioners. Retrieved August 22, 2012, from http://www.racgp.org.au/Content/NavigationMenu/ClinicalResources/RACGPGuidelines/smoking/Smoking-cessation.pdf

CHAPTER 21

Patricia M. Davidson
Phillip J. Newton
Peter Simon Macdonald

Chronic heart failure

Learning objectives

When you have completed this chapter you will be able to:

- describe the epidemiology and pathophysiology of chronic heart failure
- appreciate the burden of heart failure on the individual, their family and society
- discuss evidence-based strategies for the diagnosis and management of chronic heart failure
- reflect on the role of the nurse in the multidisciplinary care team
- identify the need for communication across the care continuum to improve outcomes for people with chronic heart failure.

Key words

chronic heart failure, nurse coordinated care models, nursing, self-care, symptom management

INTRODUCTION

Chronic heart failure (CHF) is a growing public health problem both in Australia and globally and is associated with significant morbidity, mortality and economic burden. This is particularly the case among those aged 65 years and older (Liao, Allen, & Whellan, 2008; Carlsen et al., 2012). Epidemiological data estimates the lifetime risk of developing CHF as 1 in 5 (Lloyd-Jones et al., 2002). The prevalence of CHF is predicted to increase in parallel with the ageing of the population and the continuing decrease in fatal coronary heart disease (CHD) (Lloyd-Jones, Camargo, Allen, Giugliano, & O'Donnell, 2003; National Heart Foundation of Australia, 2005; National Heart Foundation of Australia and the

Cardiac Society of Australia and New Zealand, 2011). Rising rates of inactivity, smoking, hypertension, diabetes, atrial fibrillation and obesity threaten to change the contemporary epidemiology of CHF and have significant implications for nursing management.

As you work through this chapter, it is important that you recognise that nurses and other health professionals play a critical role in preventing CHF, as well as treating and managing the condition. Several key principles underpin the structure of this chapter. Firstly, it is important to appreciate the pathophysiological and epidemiological basis of CHF to undertake informed clinical practice; secondly the role of the nurses in evidence-based practice strategies to prevent and manage CHF is emphasised; and thirdly the process of reflection in developing your clinical practice from prevention to palliation of CHF is emphasised.

There are no definitive data on the incidence and prevalence of CHF in Australia and available information is largely modelled from clinical trial and international data sets. In 2000, it was estimated that 325 000 Australians had symptomatic heart failure and another 214 000 Australians had asymptomatic left ventricular dysfunction (2.8% of the population) (Clark, McLennan, Dawson, Wilkinson, & Stewart, 2004). A survey of randomly selected residents in Canberra, aged between 60 and 86 years, was conducted between February 2002 and June 2003 (Abhayaratna et al., 2006). Participants enrolled in the study had a comprehensive clinical history, were examined by a cardiologist and received an echocardiogram. Consistent with other data sets, the incidence of CHF in the Canberra Heart Study increased with age (4.4 fold increase from the 60–64 years group to the 80–86 years group, $p < 0.0001$) (Abhayaratna et al., 2006). More recent data using linked, administrative datasets from Western Australia suggest that whilst the incidence (new onset) of CHF has decreased over the preceding two decades, the number of hospitalisations per year has increased during this same period (Teng, Finn, Hobbs, & Hung, 2010) and these findings are consistent with other contemporary studies.

Although you will encounter patients with CHF across the lifespan from paediatrics to gerontology, the majority of people you will deal with in your clinical practice will be older and suffering from multiple concurrent conditions, such as diabetes, depression, arthritis and chronic obstructive pulmonary disease. Preventing illness as well as assisting individuals to cope and adjust to living with a chronic illness is an important part of the nurses' role.

The prevalence and likely burden of CHF is important to consider giving the ageing of the Australian population, which is consistent with other western societies. In coming decades we will see a 3–4 fold increase in the number of Australians living over the age of 65 years (Australian Bureau of Statistics, 2005). This predicted increase will also be seen in those over the age of 85 years increasingly requiring the incorporation of a cardiogeriatric approach to care, recognising the physical, social and psychological aspects of ageing as well as biomedical issues. A cardiogeriatric approach is when best practices of cardiovascular and gerontological care are combined to tailor and target appropriate interventions to meet the needs of individuals and their families.

It is therefore important that you approach the person with CHF considering the range of physical, social, cultural, psychological and spiritual factors impacting on living with a chronic condition and not merely focus on the biomedical dimensions of CHF management. Considering issues such as cognitive impairment and physical frailty are just as important in developing nursing care plans for patients with CHF as a cardiovascular physical assessment. Over the past decade, there has been an increasing focus on managing CHF because of the high costs to the individual and the healthcare system, primarily stemming from frequent hospitalisations, many of which are avoidable through targeted disease management interventions (Stewart et al., 2012).

DEFINITION OF CHRONIC HEART FAILURE

In spite of the burden and prevalence of CHF, there is no international consensus on the definition of CHF. The National Heart Foundation/Cardiac Society of Australia and New Zealand defines CHF as a:

> … complex clinical syndrome with typical symptoms (e.g. dyspnoea, fatigue) that can occur at rest or on effort, and is characterised by objective evidence of an underlying structural abnormality or cardiac dysfunction that impairs the ability of the ventricle to fill with or eject blood (particularly during physical activity). A diagnosis of CHF may be further strengthened by improvement in symptoms in response to treatment.
>
> (Krum, Jelinek, Stewart, Sindone, & Atherton, 2011)

CAUSES OF CHRONIC HEART FAILURE

CHF is a complex clinical syndrome characterised by evidence of an underlying structural abnormality or cardiac dysfunction that impairs the ability of the ventricle to either fill or eject blood. The most common cause of CHF is CHD which is present in over 50% of newly diagnosed patients (Krum et al., 2011). Hypertension is present in approximately two-thirds of people with CHF. Less common is idiopathic dilated cardiomyopathy, representing 5–10% of the cases of CHF. Left ventricular hypertrophy contributes to the development of CHF, due to changes in the heart muscle caused by the stress of pressure and volume overload. Remodelling is characterised by a change in the dimensions of the left ventricle and the ventricular wall causing myocardial fibrosis, myocyte hypertrophy and hypertrophy of the coronary artery smooth muscle cells. The causes of CHF are broadly attributed to ventricular function and the capacity of the ventricles to contract and relax.

Systolic heart failure: impaired ventricular contraction

CHD, resulting in decreased perfusion of the myocardium, is the most common cause of systolic heart failure. Essential hypertension may also contribute to CHF through increasing afterload and accelerating the progression of CHD. People with non-ischaemic idiopathic dilated cardiomyopathy are often younger and there is often a familial association. Less common causes of systolic heart failure (where the heart does not pump effectively) include valvular heart disease, alcoholic dilated cardiomyopathy, peripartum cardiomyopathy, myocarditis and thyroid dysfunction.

Heart failure with preserved ejection fraction: impaired ventricular relaxation

Impaired ventricular relaxation results in the lack of ability of the ventricles to fill with blood, rather than a problem of pumping: that is why it is described as heart failure with preserved ejection fraction. The most common cause of heart failure with preserved ejection fraction is hypertension and is most common in elderly women. Diabetes is an important contributing factor for CHF and can also be associated with myocardial ischaemia (Lind et al., 2012). Heart failure with preserved ejection fraction can occur in conditions such as aortic stenosis (a condition where the opening of aortic valve is narrowed), hypertrophic (enlargement of constituent heart cells) and restrictive cardiomyopathy (where the heart chambers are unable to fill).

DELETERIOUS COMPENSATORY MECHANISMS IN CHRONIC HEART FAILURE

Systolic heart failure is associated with a decrease in cardiac output due to left ventricular dysfunction. The body in response to the reduced cardiac output activates several neurohormonal compensatory mechanisms. While the activation of these systems is effective in the short term, in the longer term they become ineffective and even deleterious leading to further progression of CHF. The activation of these systems stresses the failing ventricle resulting in further reduction in cardiac output and stroke volume. These systems also cause further changes in the structure of myocardium which is known as remodelling. Two of these mechanisms will now be considered.

Renin-angiotensin-aldosterone system

When the cardiac output falls, the kidneys respond by stimulating the renin-angiotensin-aldosterone system. This system leads to the retention of sodium and water. The mechanism of sodium and water is designed to compensate for a low volume state. In individuals with CHF alterations in tissue and organ perfusion are the consequence of lower circulation volume as a result of either reduced cardiac output caused by left ventricular dysfunction (systolic CHF) or abnormal filling (heart failure with preserved ejection fraction). Fluid retention is a common sign of CHF. If left untreated, retained fluid may manifest as oedema. The long term activation of the renin-angiotensin-aldosterone system may also contribute to the cardiac remodelling seen in CHF (Jackson, Gibbs, Davies, & Lip, 2000).

Sympathetic nervous system response

An early compensatory mechanism in CHF is the stimulation of the sympathetic nervous system. Cardiac output is initially maintained through vasoconstriction and increased heat rate. Again, while effective in the short term, the resulting increase in preload and afterload further reduces cardiac output which results in further ventricular dysfunction. The resulting tachycardia may increase the vulnerability of the CHF myocardium to arrhythmias.

The activation of the compensatory mechanisms in CHF, while effective in the short term, results in detrimental effects on heart function when prolonged.

To prevent this detrimental cyclical stimulation, these compensatory mechanisms have become the target of pharmacological management of CHF, particularly with the introduction of angiotensin converting enzyme (ACE) inhibitors, beta blockers and aldosterone antagonists, three of the common classes of drugs prescribed in CHF, particularly systolic CHF (National Heart Foundation of Australia and the Cardiac Society of Australia and New Zealand, 2011; Lindenfeld et al., 2010).

SIGNS AND SYMPTOMS OF CHRONIC HEART FAILURE

CHF is a condition which is associated with numerous signs and symptoms. Dyspnoea (shortness of breath) is the most common symptom associated with CHF. Initially dyspnoea occurs on exertion but as CHF worsens it may occur with minimal activity or at rest. Breathlessness that occurs at night waking the individual is known as orthopnoea. When pulmonary congestion is present patients may need to sleep on a number of pillows to decrease the sensation of dyspnoea. This may indicate fluid congestion in the lungs. Other signs and symptoms associated with CHF include fatigue and cachexia. Oedema can

TABLE 21.1
New York Heart Association Functional Class. *Note*: From Kossman (1964, p. 112).

Class I	No limitation: ordinary physical exercise does not cause undue fatigue, dyspnoea or palpitations.
Class II	Slight impairment of physical activity: comfortable at rest but ordinary activity results in fatigue, palpitations.
Class III	Marked limitation of physical activity: comfortable at rest but less than ordinary activity results in symptoms.
Class IV	Unable to carry out any physical activity without discomfort: symptoms of CHF are present even at rest with increased discomfort with any physical activity.

be present and reflected in a raised jugular venous pressure, ankle and sacral oedema, ascites and hepatomegaly indicating fluid retention. Other signs including tachycardia, displaced apex beat and a third heart sound are indicative of CHF. Heart murmurs can also be present indicating structural heart disease, such as mitral regurgitation. The New York Heart Association (NYHA) Scale, as described in Table 21.1, is a common way to classify the severity of CHF through the impact of symptoms on physical activity.

DIAGNOSIS OF CHRONIC HEART FAILURE

The diagnosis of CHF is based on clinical features, chest X-ray and assessment of ventricular function using methods such as echocardiography. As you can see above the signs and symptoms of CHF, such as fatigue and dyspnoea, can reasonably be associated with a range of other conditions, including physical deconditioning. As a consequence it is important that astute physical examination and appropriate diagnostic tests be instituted in order to:

- confirm the clinical diagnosis
- determine the structural or biochemical anomalies responsible for CHF
- identify exacerbating and precipitating factors and treat accordingly
- instigate appropriate therapeutic interventions
- determine the probable clinical course and prognosis.

Physical examination

The physical examination is important not only in diagnosing CHF but also in monitoring the condition. Key steps in the physical examination include:

- measuring blood pressure and heart rate both lying and standing
- assessment of heart rate and rhythm
- checking peripheral pulses and tissue perfusion
- examining the veins in the neck for elevated venous pressure
- listening to breath sounds and auscultation of the chest cavity
- listening to the heart for murmurs or extra heart sounds
- checking the abdomen for swelling caused by fluid build-up and for enlargement or tenderness over the liver
- assessing the legs and ankles for swelling caused by oedema
- measuring and recording body weight.

Whenever CHF is suspected the individual should undergo an electrocardiogram (ECG), chest X-ray and echocardiogram, even if the physical examination is normal. Biochemical and haematological tests such as full blood count, plasma urea, creatinine and electrolytes should be measured during the investigation period and subsequently if there are any changes in clinical status.

B-type natriuretic peptide (BNP) is secreted by the ventricles of the heart in response to excessive stretching of cardiac myocytes in the ventricles. Two forms of BNP (BNP and NT pro BNP) are currently able to be measured. The plasma concentrations of both forms of BNP are increased in patients with asymptomatic and symptomatic left ventricular dysfunction. Initially, BNP has been used in the emergency department to differentiate shortness of breath as being caused by CHF or by some other cause (Maisel et al., 2004). Recently, further research has demonstrated the feasibility and effectiveness of BNP levels as a biomarker, as well as an independent predictor of CHF (Biswas et al., 2012; Yamamoto et al., 2012). Higher BNP levels at admission have been associated with increased risk of acute myocardial infarction (AMI) and mortality (Kociol et al., 2012). Moreover, animal studies have suggested elevated levels of BNP contribute to the progression of CHF after AMI (Thireau et al., 2012). As further research is undertaken, further uses of BNP are being proposed including screening for CHF, treating CHF patients according to the BNP level and monitoring the effectiveness of the treatments. Box 21.1 summarises some of the key diagnostic approaches in CHF.

Electrocardiogram

The electrocardiogram depicts the electrical activity of the heart. It is unusual in CHF for the patient to have a normal ECG, although identification of abnormalities is not diagnostic. Common anomalies identified on the ECG include ST and T wave changes, atrial fibrillation and bundle branch blocks.

Chest x-ray

In CHF, the chest X-ray (CXR) can show an enlarged heart (cardiomegaly) and pulmonary venous congestion with upper lobe blood diversion. In severe cases interstitial oedema may

BOX 21.1
Diagnosis of heart failure

- An echocardiogram should be undertaken to confirm a clinical diagnosis, identify structural abnormalities and potentially reversible pathology such as valvular dysfunction or ischaemia.
- Coronary angiography should be considered in people with suspected myocardial ischaemia following the weighting of risks and benefits.
- Plasma B-type natriuretic peptide has been shown to improve diagnostic accuracy with a high negative predictive value.
- Endomyocardial biopsy may be indicated in patients where an inflammatory or infiltrative process is suspected.
- Diagnostic test to identify viable myocardium and reversible ischaemia such as radionuclide ventriculography, stress echocardiography or positive electron tomography.
- Assessment of thyroid function and assessment for concomitant conditions such as diabetes and hypertension.

be present and prominent vascular markings present in the perihilar region. The presence of pleural effusions in the basal areas may obscure the costophrenic angle. Kerley B lines (thin linear pulmonary opacities caused by fluid or cellular infiltration into the interstitium of the lungs) may be indicative of lymphatic oedema due to raised left atrial pressure. It is important to consider that a normal CXR does not exclude a diagnosis of CHF.

Echocardiogram

All patients with suspected CHF should have an echocardiogram. A standard echocardiogram is also known as a transthoracic echocardiogram (TTE) or a cardiac ultrasound. The echocardiogram gives information about the size, volume and thickness of the atria and ventricles as well as the presence or absence of regional wall motion abnormalities. An echocardiogram involves placing a transducer on the chest wall to capture of images of the heart. The echocardiogram allows imaging of valves and the degree of heart muscle contraction which can allow the determination of the indicator of the ejection fraction. The left ventricular ejection fraction is the amount of blood ejected in each heart beat and is an important predictor of outcome with a diagnosis of CHF. The echocardiogram can also allow detection of potentially correctable causes of CHF, such as valvular disease.

MANAGEMENT OF CHRONIC HEART FAILURE

Management of CHF involves prevention, early detection, slowing of disease progression, relief of symptoms, minimisation of exacerbations and prolongation of survival. Key therapeutic approaches or considerations include the implementation of both non-pharmacological and pharmacological strategies.

Pharmacological therapy

The pharmacological management of CHF aims to relieve symptoms and improve prognosis of CHF, primarily through modification of activation of the renin-angiotensin system that occurs in response to a decrease in cardiac output. The following pharmacological treatments are used:

- angiotensin-converting enzyme inhibitors (ACEIs) that prevent disease progression and prolong survival
- beta-blockers that prolong survival in symptomatic patients
- diuretics that provide symptom relief and restoration or maintenance of euvolaemia; often aided by daily self-recording of body weight and adjustments of diuretic dosage
- aldosterone receptor antagonists (aldosterone antagonists)
- angiotensin II receptor antagonists and digoxin in patients who remain symptomatic.

Device therapy

Technological advances have assisted in improving the quality of life of people with CHF. The cost and complexity associated with implantation limit the access of these therapies to large numbers of people with CHF.

- Biventricular pacing has been shown in patients with New York Heart Association Class II or IV and wide QRS complexes to improve activity tolerance and quality of life, as well as reducing mortality (Cleland et al., 2005; Tang et al., 2010).

- Implantable cardioverter defibrillators, which have been shown to reduce the risk of sudden cardiac death in patients with CHF and low left ventricular ejection fractions (Moss et al., 2002).
- Ventricular assist devices (VADs) are designed to assist either the right (RVAD) or left (LVAD) ventricle, or both at once (BiVAD). These are mechanical pumps that are implanted to help the heart's weakened ventricle pump blood throughout the body. In Australia, VADs are used as a bridge to transplantation, while in countries such as the United States they are used as destination therapy.

Surgical therapy

Surgical approaches in CHF include myocardial revascularisation and cardiac transplantation. Although cardiac transplantation is an effective option, access to this therapy is limited through donor shortage and issues in patient selection (Berry et al., 2011).

Team management approach to chronic heart failure management

An important focus on CHF care is supporting individuals in the community. As a consequence CHF is often managed away from acute hospitals by community-based teams and general practitioners. Current CHF guidelines recommend the use of a team management approach to CHF. Whilst the composition of this team will vary between institutions due to a number of reasons including resources and models of care, a typical CHF team will generally include CHF specialist nurses, cardiologists and the general practitioner. Other allied health workers who may be involved includes pharmacists, social workers, occupational therapists, physiotherapists and dietitians.

Based on evidence from systematic reviews and meta-analyses it is possible to identify broad elements that are common to the most effective programs. These include:

- involvement of health professionals and other providers from a range of disciplines using a team approach across healthcare sectors
- implementation of evidence-based management guidelines, including systems for optimisation of pharmacological and non-pharmacological therapy
- monitoring of signs and symptoms to enable early identification of decompensation and/or deterioration, and effective protocols for symptom management
- inclusion of patients and their families in negotiating the aims and goals of care
- development and implementation of individualised management plans
- promotion of and support for self-care (e.g. taking medicines, following lifestyle management advice about smoking cessation, physical activity and exercise programs, nutrition and limiting alcohol use and monitoring and interpreting symptoms), the use of behavioural strategies to support patients in modifying risk factors and adhering to their management plans
- continuity of care across healthcare services, including acute care, primary care and community care
- monitoring of program outcomes and systems to ensure continuous quality improvement.

A range of challenges are faced by health professionals in educating CHF patients including cognitive impairment and co-morbidities. These challenges highlight the need to move away from traditional education strategies and move to a model with multiple sessions and reinforcing of information. In fact, a failure to adhere to the recommended treatment regimen is a major cause for decompensation and hospitalisation. A range of supplementary tools, including written, audio and visual strategies, are available to provide and reinforce information. When undertaking this process it is important to consider factors such as impaired vision and hearing or health literacy issues which may impact upon the ability of the patient to interact with this information. The nurse should engage with the patient to be sure that they are able to:

- identify key health providers, particularly their general practitioner, and have current methods of contacting these people
- engage family members as much as possible in their care plan
- demonstrate knowledge of the name, dose and purpose of each medication or at least have a comprehensive list of medications and a reliable system of dosing and monitoring adherence, such as a dosette box
- understand the rationale of daily weights and have a system of recording these
- have a mechanism for monitoring signs and symptoms of worsening CHF
- have an action plan to contact providers or undertake self-management strategies in response to specific symptoms, such as dyspnoea and orthopnoea, or weight changes.

MANAGING ACUTE DECOMPENSATED HEART FAILURE

The aim of supportive and disease management strategies in CHF is to prevent decompensation, particularly to the extent requiring hospitalisation. Effective symptom management and recognition are key factors in decreasing the risk of decompensation. The management of acute decompensated heart failure is complex and involves recognition of precipitants, such as pneumonia. Symptomatic management involves the use of oxygen, diuretics, vasodilators such as morphine and nitrates and, where indicated, inotrope therapy. Adjunctive therapies include non-invasive mechanical therapies such as continuous positive airway pressure (CPAP) via mask, or bilevel non-invasive positive-pressure (BiPAP) ventilation to decrease pulmonary congestion. When the exacerbation is associated with haemodynamic decompensation patients may require inotropic support, intubation and ventilation, intra-aortic balloon counter pulsation. In severe cases of decompensated heart failure, VADs may be indicated as a bridge to transplantation or as destination therapy.

STRATEGIES TO MANAGE CHRONIC HEART FAILURE ON A DAILY BASIS ACROSS THE DISEASE CONTINUUM

Optimally, the approach to CHF management should reflect a team management approach. This should occur from the primary care setting, where the practice nurse collaborates with the general practitioner through to the specialist setting where nurses coordinate a range of health professionals in providing evidence-based management. A range of nurse-coordinated programs, including home-based and clinic-based strategies, as well as telephone support and internet-based strategies have been shown to improve the outcomes of people with heart failure (Stewart et al., 2012; Inglis et al., 2010).

Box 21.2 summarises key considerations in CHF management. The important role of nurses in coordinating and managing care of the person with CHF cannot be

BOX 21.2
Key characteristics of coordinated chronic heart failure programs

- Comprehensive assessment of the needs of patients and their family focussing on physical, social, cultural, psychological and existential issues.
- Negotiation of goals of treatment and the developing of a treatment plan.
- Promotion of adherence to evidence-based therapies and strategies to promote access.
- Coordination and communication between patients, their families and care providers.
- Provision of information and counselling strategies, tailored to individual needs.
- Promotion of self-care, including titration of diuretic therapy in appropriate patients (or with family member/caregiver assistance).
- Adoption of behavioural strategies to increase adherence such as diaries and medication management strategies.
- Monitoring and follow-up after hospital discharge or after periods of instability.
- Instigation of action plans and processes for monitoring signs and symptoms, particularly fluid overload as monitored by daily weights.
- Implementation of social support and consideration of financial considerations.

overemphasised. Key skills required by the nurse working with CHF include expert cardiovascular knowledge, proficient clinical assessment skills and the capacity to communicate effectively with patients, their families and a range of providers.

EVIDENCE-BASED TREATMENT GAP

Despite the evidence for the improvement of morbidity and mortality for both pharmacological and non-pharmacological management strategies for CHF, utilisation of these therapies is often sub-optimal (Zannad et al., 1999). Possible explanations for this are the complexity of CHF management and the increasing evidence that there needs to be an established infrastructure to support the implementation of evidence-based practice into usual clinical care (Caldwell & Dracup, 2001; Fuat, Hungin, & Murphy, 2003; Phillips, Marton & Tofler, 2004; Clark et al., 2007).

Many contemporary healthcare systems are configured for acute, reactive care rather than planned, proactive, systematic management of chronic conditions (Phillips et al., 2004). Further, the perceived disparity between clinical trial and community populations potentially preclude doctors from prescribing therapies, particularly within elderly populations (Fuat et al., 2003; Phillips et al., 2004; Clark et al., 2007; McMurray, 2000; Lloyd-Williams et al., 2003).

PALLIATIVE AND SUPPORTIVE STRATEGIES IN CHRONIC HEART FAILURE

People with severe CHF and of advanced age are treatable and are fortunate to have access to a range of therapies. The poor prognosis associated with heart failure mandates that clinicians engage with patients and their families in advance care planning and providing adequate symptom management (Davidson et al., 2010). Living with a life limiting illness means that people may experience a range of physical, psychological and existential symptoms impacting on functional status and diminished quality of life (Bekelman et al., 2007). In addition families and significant others also experience a significant treatment burden. Therefore, people should only be considered palliative when all therapeutic options have been explored within the context of the clinical condition and the patient's needs and value systems (Pantilat & Steimle, 2004). The treatment gap in CHF means that many people fail to receive evidence-based treatments and as a consequence many people suffer and die unnecessarily. Therefore whenever assessing patients with CHF for a palliative approach it is important that clinicians consider whether the patient has been assessed for reversible conditions, particularly ischaemia and anaemia, has had a trial of evidence-based therapies appropriate to their condition and importantly undergone specialist CHF assessment from both the medical and the nursing perspectives. Increasingly it is evident that communication strategies, such as advance care planning, are integral in ensuring that the patient and their families are aware of their condition and prognosis, yet are supported to manage their condition within a context of hope. Supporting patients and their families to negotiate transitions in the CHF illness trajectory are critical roles of nurses and should be prominent goals of therapy.

BOX 21.3
Summary points

- CHF is a common condition primarily affecting older people and is associated with poor prognosis, significant symptom burden and high healthcare costs.
- The commonest cause of CHF is CHD which can largely be prevented through addressing modifiable risk factors, such as smoking, inactivity and obesity.
- Diagnosis of CHF should be undertaken using objective measures such as echocardiography.
- Promoting self-management is an important part of CHF care planning.
- Symptom monitoring and treatment is important in avoiding decompensation.
- Heart failure has a substantial evidence base to guide management and nurses play a critical role in care.
- People with CHF often have a poor prognosis so that palliative care is an important component of management.

CONCLUSION

CHF is a common and burdensome condition, particularly in the elderly. The high risk of mortality and co-morbidity burden underscores the importance of providing accurate information about prognosis and advance care planning to avoid unnecessary and futile treatments. As health professionals negotiate the plan of care with patients and their families it is important to consider the aetiological and pathophysiological factors that impact on disease progression as well as psychological and social factors that impact on the capacity to adhere to recommended treatment strategies. We are fortunate to have evidence-based practice guidelines to guide the management of CHF, yet a treatment gap challenges optimal outcomes for people with CHF. As hospitalisation for decompensated CHF is a frequent event, discharge planning and follow-up in the outpatient and community setting using an interdisciplinary approach is critical. Integrating optimal medical therapy with strategies to promote self-care and communication across the care continuum is necessary to optimise patient outcomes. Monitoring and enhancing adherence with the treatment plan and promoting symptom monitoring and action plans are important strategies in improving patient outcomes, including improving quality of life, increasing functional status, reducing hospitalisation and health service utilisation and cost as well as prolonging survival.

CASE STUDY 21.1

Mavis Brown, a 74-year-old female patient, was admitted from home with progressive increase in breathlessness, orthopnoea and ankle oedema over the previous 3 weeks. She has a history of diabetes, osteoarthritis and glaucoma. Her ECG confirmed sinus tachycardia and evidence of a previous acute myocardial infarction. Her chest X-ray confirmed cardiomegaly and interstitial oedema. Chest auscultation revealed bibasal crepitations and her jugular venous pressure was elevated. Her current medications included aspirin, a lipid lowering agent and ACE-inhibitor therapy.

Case study questions

1. What do you consider is the most likely cause of Mavis' breathlessness?
2. Do you think it is probable that Mavis has CHF? If so, how will this be definitively diagnosed?
3. What would be the treatment strategies to relieve her symptoms?
4. What are the key self-management strategies that prevent fluid overload in people with CHF?

CASE STUDY 21.2

Bruce Fletcher is an 81-year-old retired plumber who presents to his GP complaining of chronic fatigue, and with a 4-week history of breathlessness when walking his dog. He has recently started using three pillows in his bed due to night-time wheeze and coughing. On examination his blood pressure (BP) is 135/85 mmHg, his heart rate is 80 beats per minute at rest and regular and a third heart sound can be heard. His weight is 80 kg, increased by 4 kg since it was last measured 6 months ago. Echocardiography documents global systolic dysfunction and his left ventricular ejection fraction is 28%. He is referred to the nurse-led heart failure clinic for education and support.

Case study questions

1. What are the important self-management strategies to discuss with Bruce?
2. What is the likely structural abnormality in the heart contributing to Bruce's symptoms?
3. What would be the medication regimen you would anticipate that Bruce would be prescribed?
4. What are considerations for medication adherence in CHF?

Reflective questions

1 What are the factors contributing to the burden of CHF in contemporary society?
2 What is the role of self-management in CHF?
3 What are the signs and symptoms signalling decompensation in CHF?
4 What is the role of advance care planning and shared decision making in CHF?

Recommended reading

Krum, H., Jelinek, M. V., Stewart, S., et al. (2011). 2011 Update to National Heart Foundation of Australia and Cardiac Society of Australia and New Zealand Guidelines for the prevention, detection and management of chronic heart failure in Australia, 2006. *The Medical Journal of Australia, 194*(8), 405–409.

Riegel, B., Lee, C. S., & Dickson, V. V. (2011). Self care in patients with chronic heart failure. *Nature Reviews Cardiology, 8*(11), 644–654.

Allen, L. A., Stevenson, L. W., Grady, K. L., et al. (2012). Decision Making in Advanced Heart Failure A Scientific Statement From the American Heart Association. *Circulation, 125*(15), 1928–1952.

Lainscak, M., Blue, L., Clark, A. L., et al. (2011). Self-care management of heart failure: practical recommendations from the Patient Care Committee of the Heart Failure Association of the European Society of Cardiology. *European Journal of Heart Failure, 13*(2), 115–126.

National Heart Foundation of Australia. (2010). Multidisciplinary care for people with chronic heart failure. Principles and recommendations for best practice. Available at http://www.heartfoundation.org.au/SiteCollectionDocuments/Multidisciplinary-care-for-people-with-CHF.pdf

References

Abhayaratna, W. P., Smith, W. T., & Becker, N. G., et al. (2006). Prevalence of heart failure and systolic ventricular dysfunction in older Australians: the Canberra Heart Study. *Medical Journal of Australia, 184*(4), 151–154.

Australian Bureau of Statistics. Population projections, Australia 2004 to 2101. Canberra 2005. Retrieved August 8, 2013, from http://www.abs.gov.au/Ausstats/abs@.nsf/mf/3222.0

Bekelman, D. B., Havranek, E. P., Becker, D. M., et al. (2007). Symptoms, depression, and quality of life in patients with heart failure. *Journal of Cardiac Failure, 13*(8), 643–648.

Berry, G. J., Angelini, A., Burke, M. M., et al. (2011). The ISHLT working formulation for pathologic diagnosis of antibody-mediated rejection in heart transplantation: evolution and current status (2005–2011). *The Journal of heart and lung transplantation: the official publication of the International Society for Heart Transplantation, 30*(6), 601.

Biswas, S. K., Sarai, M., Toyama, H., et al. (2012). Role of 123I-BMIPP and serum B-type natriuretic peptide for the evaluation of patients with heart failure. *Singapore Medical Journal, 53*(6), 398–402.

Caldwell, M. A., & Dracup, K. (2001). Team management of heart failure: The emerging role of exercise, and implications for cardiac rehabilitation centers. *Journal of Cardiopulmonary Rehabilitation, 21*(5), 273–279.

Carlsen, C. M., Bay, M., Kirk, V., et al. (2012). Prevalence and prognosis of heart failure with preserved ejection fraction and elevated N-terminal pro brain natriuretic peptide: a 10-year analysis from the Copenhagen Hospital Heart Failure Study. *European Journal of Heart Failure, 14*(3), 240–247.

Clark, R. A., Driscoll, A., Nottage, J., et al. (2007). Inequitable provision of optimal services for patients with chronic heart failure: a national geo-mapping study. *Medical Journal of Australia, 186*(4), 169.

Clark, R. A., McLennan, S., Dawson, A., et al. (2004). Uncovering a hidden epidemic: A study of the current burden of heart failure in Australia. *Heart Lung and Circulation, 13*, 266–273.

Cleland, J. G. F., Daubert, J.-C., Erdmann, E., et al. (2005). The effect of cardiac resynchronization on morbidity and mortality in heart failure. *New England Journal of Medicine, 352*(15), 1539–1549.

Davidson, P. M., Macdonald, P. S., Newton, P. J., et al. (2010). End stage heart failure patients — palliative care in general practice. *Australian Family Physician, 39*(12), 916.

Fuat, A., Hungin, A. P. S., & Murphy, J. J. (2003). Barriers to accurate diagnosis and effective management of heart failure in primary care: Qualitative study. *British Medical Journal, 326*, 196–200.

Inglis, S., Clark, R., McAlister, F., et al. (2010). Structured telephone support or telemonitoring programmes for patients with chronic heart failure. *Cochrane Database of Systematic Reviews* Issue 8. Art. No.: CD007228.

Jackson, G., Gibbs, C., Davies, M., et al. (2000). ABC of heart failure. *Pathophysiology BMJ, 320*(7228), 167–170.

Kociol, R. D., Greiner, M. A., Hammill, B. G., et al. (2012). B-type natriuretic peptide level and postdischarge thrombotic events in older patients hospitalized with heart failure: insights from the Acute Decompensated Heart Failure National Registry. *American Heart Journal, 163*(6), 994–1001.

Kossman, C. (Ed.). (1964). *Diseases of the heart and blood vessels; nomenclature and criteria for diagnosis*. Boston: Little Brown.

Krum, H., Jelinek, M. V., Stewart, S., et al. (2011). Update to National Heart Foundation of Australia and Cardiac Society of Australia and New Zealand Guidelines for the prevention, detection and management of chronic heart failure in Australia, 2006. *The Medical Journal of Australia, 194*(8), 405.

Liao, L., Allen, L. A., & Whellan, D. J. (2008). Economic burden of heart failure in the elderly. *Pharmacoeconomics, 26*(6), 447–462.

Lind, M., Olsson, M., Rosengren, A., et al. (2012). The relationship between glycaemic control and heart failure in 83,021 patients with type 2 diabetes. *Diabetologia, 55*(11), 2946–2953.

Lindenfeld, J., Albert, N., Boehmer, J., et al. (2010). HFSA 2010 comprehensive heart failure practice guideline. *Journal of Cardiac Failure, 16*(6), e1–e194.

Lloyd-Jones, D. M., Camargo, C. A., Allen, L. A., et al. (2003). Predictors of long-term mortality after hospitalization for primary unstable angina pectoris and non-ST-elevation myocardial infarction. *American Journal of Cardiology, 92*(10), 1155–1159.

Lloyd-Jones, D. M., Larson, M. G., Leip, E. P., et al. (2002). Lifetime risk for developing congestive heart failure: the Framingham Heart Study. *Circulation, 106*(24), 3068–3072.

Lloyd-Williams, F., Mair, F., Shiels, C., et al. (2003). Why are patients in clinical trials for heart failure not like those we see in everyday practice. *Journal of Clinical Epidemiology, 56*(12), 1157–1162.

Maisel, A., Hollander, J. E., Guss, D., et al. (2004). Primary results of the Rapid Emergency Department Heart Failure Outpatient Trial (REDHOT). A multicenter study of B-type natriuretic peptide levels, emergency department decision making, and outcomes in patients presenting with shortness of breath. *Journal of the American College of Cardiology, 44*(6), 1328–1333.

McMurray, J. (2000). Heart failure: we need more trials in typical patients. *European Heart Journal, 21*, 699–700.

Moss, A. J., Zareba, W., Hall, W. J., et al. (2002). Prophylactic Implantation of a Defibrillator in Patients with Myocardial Infarction and Reduced Ejection Fraction. *New England Journal of Medicine, 346*(12), 877–883.

National Heart Foundation of Australia and the Cardiac Society of Australia and New Zealand. (2011). *Guidelines for the prevention, detection and management of chronic heart failure in Australia (Chronic Heart Failure Guidelines Expert Writing Panel)*. Melbourne: Author.

National Heart Foundation of Australia. (2005). *The shifting burden of cardiovascular disease in Australia*. Melbourne: Author.

Pantilat, S. Z., & Steimle, A. E. (2004). Palliative care for patients with heart failure. *JAMA: The Journal of the American Medical Association, 291*(20), 2476–2482.

Phillips, S. M., Marton, R. L., & Tofler, G. (2004). Barriers to diagnosing and managing heart failure in primary care. *Medical Journal of Australia, 181*(2), 78–81.

Stewart, S., Carrington, M. J., Marwick, T., et al. (2012). Impact of home versus clinic-based management of chronic heart failure: the WHICH? (Which Heart failure Intervention is most Cost-effective & consumer friendly in reducing Hospital care) multicenter, randomized trial. *Journal of the American College of Cardiology, 60*, 1239–1248.

Tang, A. S. L., Wells, G. A., Talajic, M., et al. (2010). Cardiac-resynchronization therapy for mild-to-moderate heart failure. *New England Journal of Medicine, 363*(25), 2385–2395.

Teng, T.-H. K., Finn, J., Hobbs, M., et al. (2010). Heart Failure: Incidence, case-fatality and hospitalization rates in Western Australia between 1990 and 2005. *Circulation: Heart Failure, 3*, 236–243.

Thireau, J., Karam, S., Fauconnier, J., et al. (2012). Functional evidence for an active role of B-type natriuretic peptide in cardiac remodelling and pro-arrhythmogenicity. *Cardiovascular Research [Research Support, Non-U.S. Gov't], 95*(1), 59–68.

Yamamoto, E., Sato, Y., Sawa, T., et al. (2012). Correlation between serum concentrations of B-type natriuretic peptide and albumin in patients with chronic congestive heart failure. *International Heart Journal, 53*(4), 234–237.

Zannad, F., Briancon, S., Juilliere, Y., et al. (1999). Incidence, clinical and etiologic features and outcomes of advanced chronic heart failure: The EPICAL study. *Journal of the American College of Cardiology, 33*(3), 734–742.

CHAPTER

22

Ann Bonner
Bettina Douglas

Chronic kidney disease

Learning objectives

When you have completed this chapter you will be able to:

- recognise the stages associated with chronic kidney disease
- understand the physical, psychological and social impact of chronic kidney disease
- describe the effects of chronic kidney disease on quality of life
- understand the importance of patient self-management in achieving optimal health
- consider the nursing role in patient education for people with renal health breakdown.

Key words

chronic kidney disease (CKD), kidney replacement therapy (KRT), patient education, quality of life, self-management

INTRODUCTION

Chronic kidney disease (CKD) is a serious global health problem and, in its later stages, requires people to invest considerable time to manage their health, including modifying their diet, managing numerous medications, undergoing kidney replacement therapy (KRT) (if required) and attending medical and hospital appointments. CKD, its treatment and concomitant complications have a significant impact on a person's lifestyle, family responsibilities, ability to work and financial status (Australian Institute of Health and Welfare [AIHW], 2011a). CKD endures for the rest of a person's life, often for many decades, so the burden on an individual and their family is immense and frequently under-recognised by health professionals.

This chapter includes a review of CKD and an exploration of its effects on mobility, fatigue, body image and quality of life. CKD is also associated with numerous co-morbid chronic conditions, particularly cardiovascular disease and diabetes. The importance of adherence, patient education and the impact on families and carers will be discussed. Nurses have a crucial role in providing healthcare and may lead the multidisciplinary CKD team. The goal of the multidisciplinary team is to support people to engage in effective self-management of CKD and its associated complex treatment regimens. As CKD is a major concern for indigenous people in Australia and New Zealand, Case Study 22.1 will be used to examine the development, impact and consequences of living with reduced kidney function.

UNDERSTANDING CHRONIC KIDNEY DISEASE

The kidneys have remarkable functional reserve. Up to 80% of the glomerular filtration rate (reflected in creatinine clearance measurements) may be lost with few obvious changes in the functioning of the body. A person is born with about 2 million nephrons and can survive without dialysis until almost 90% of the nephrons are lost. In the majority of cases the individual passes through the early stages of CKD without recognising the disease state because the remaining nephrons hypertrophy to compensate. CKD is defined as either kidney damage or a glomerular filtration rate (GFR) ≤60 mL/min/1.73 m^2 for more than 3 months. Globally since 2005, the agreed definition of kidney damage is the presence of pathological abnormalities or markers of damage, including abnormalities in blood or urine tests or imaging studies (Levey et al., 2005; Kidney Health Australia, 2012).

CKD is characterised by a progressive loss of kidney function over time, and the development and progression of cardiovascular disease (Thomas, 2011). It results from a number of conditions that cause permanent loss of nephron function and a decrease in GFR. A five-stage classification system for describing the severity of CKD has been developed. This uses GFR to describe the phases of CKD and guides clinical interventions (Table 22.1).

In the early stages of CKD, polyuria results from the decreased ability of the kidneys to concentrate urine. This is most noticeable at night, and the patient must arise several times to urinate (nocturia). During stage 3, when about 50% of nephron function has been destroyed, hypertension, elevated urea and creatinine levels and anaemia develop (Castner, 2010). These effects are summarised in Figure 22.1.

The prognosis and course of CKD are highly variable depending on the aetiology, patient's condition and age and adequacy of healthcare follow-up. Some individuals live normal, active lives with stable CKD, whereas others may progress to end-stage kidney disease (ESKD). Haemodialysis, peritoneal dialysis or kidney transplantation, collectively known as kidney replacement therapy (KRT), are required when the clinical manifestations become life-threatening; this is during stage 5.

In Australia and New Zealand, the exact number of people with CKD is not known but Kidney Health Australia estimates that one in nine people over the age of 25 years have at least one clinical sign of CKD. The major causes of ESKD, however, are well known, and these are diabetes mellitus (35% Australia, 51% NZ), glomerulonephritis (22% Australia, 22% NZ) and hypertension (14% Australia, 12% NZ) (Grace, Hurst, & McDonald, 2011). Other significant causes include polycystic kidney disease, reflux nephropathy and analgesic nephropathy.

Between 1989 and 2009, Australia's population increased by 30%. During the same period the number of men starting treatment for ESKD increased by 202% and the number of females starting treatment for ESKD increased by 128% (AIHW, 2011b). Aboriginal and

CASE STUDY 22.1 Part 1

Lillian is a 53-year-old Aboriginal and Torres Strait islander (ATSI) woman. She has attended this general practice for some time and recently had an annual health check. At that visit a number of issues were identified. Lillian has known stage 3b CKD with microalbuminuria secondary to reflux nephropathy. Her kidney function is fairly stable, but she has high blood pressure, has gained some weight and has raised cholesterol. Lillian is married to a man of British origin. They live in their own home and have two adult children who live in the same city. They both receive Centrelink payments: he gets the age pension and she receives a carer's payment since he had a stroke 2 years ago. Lillian says she does not know of any family members with diabetes.

On reading her medical notes, Lillian is taking perindopril and lercanidipine for high blood pressure, atorvastatin (a lipid lowering drug) and vitamin D. She does not know the names of her tablets and is vague about why they were prescribed. She wonders if she really needs to keep taking them and she is not sure if they are doing her any good.

Lillian was referred to the nurse practitioner-led kidney clinic at the local hospital. This was because her urine albumin/creatinine ratio (ACR) has remained high despite treatment with perindopril (an angiotensin-converting enzyme inhibitor). Albuminuria is a recognised marker of risk for kidney disease progression (Johnson et al., 2012b). The referral to specialist healthcare is consistent with the best practice guidelines for the management of chronic kidney disease in primary healthcare (Kidney Health Australia, 2012).

	AT LAST VISIT	NOTES/COMMENTS
Weight	74 kg	Has gained about 10 kg weight in past 5 years
Height	157 cm	
Body mass index (BMI)	30 kg/m^2	Obese*
Blood pressure	153/93	Target BP < 130/80
Urinalysis	Protein positive, otherwise no abnormalities	
Urine albumin/creatinine ratio (ACR) (RR < 1.0)	121 mg/mmol	This is defined as macroalbuminuria
Smoking status	Former smoker	
Haemoglobin (RR 115–160)	125 g/L	
Serum creatinine (RR 40–100)	118 micromol/L	
eGFR (RR > 60)	44 mL/min/1.73 m^2	

*The current World Health Organization (WHO, 2006) definition maintains the cut-off points for BMI classification should be maintained across different population groups. There is evidence that health risk does increase at lower BMI in Asian populations. The implications of this for other population groups are unclear. This is a topic that is still being researched.

TABLE 22.1

Staging of CKD. Combines kidney function stage (stages 1–5) with description of kidney damage (albuminuria) and clinical diagnosis to specify CKD fully (e.g. stage 2 CKD with microalbuminuria, secondary to diabetic kidney disease). Colour coding refers to Clinical Action Plan applicable (refer to source). *Note*: From: *Chronic Kidney Disease (CKD) Management in General Practice* (2nd edition). Kidney Health Australia, Melbourne, 2012.

		ALBUMINURIA STAGE		
Kidney function stage	GFR (mL/min/1.73 m^2)	Normal (urine ACR mg/mmol) Male: <2.5 Female: <3.5	Microalbuminuria (urine ACR mg/mmol) Male: 2.5–25 Female: 3.5–35	Macroalbuminuria (urine ACR mg/mmol) Male: >25 Female: >35
1	≥90	Not CKD unless haematuria, structural or pathological abnormalities present		
2	60–89			
3a	45–59			
3b	30–44			
4	15–29			
5	<15 or on dialysis			

Torres Strait Islander (ATSI) peoples in Australia and New Zealand Māoris are disproportionately affected by ESKD — up to 30 times the national average. While the high prevalence of diabetes in ATSI peoples is a factor in the high rate of CKD (AIHW, 2011c) low birth weight, cigarette smoking as well as social and economic disadvantage are significant contributors to adverse health outcomes (AIHW, 2011a; Thomas, 2011). CKD also affects children and adolescents, with 364 young people between 0 and 19 receiving KRT at the end of 2010. The cause of CKD in young people varies with age but glomerular nephritis is the most common (32%) (Kennedy et al., 2011).

CKD AND ACCELERATED CARDIOVASCULAR DISEASE

While people are understandably concerned about the risk of progression of CKD to ESKD, even in the early stages of CKD the risk of cardiovascular disease is even more significant. In fact for people with CKD, the risk of dying from a cardiovascular event is much greater than requiring dialysis or a transplant (Chronic Kidney Disease Prognosis Consortium, 2010; Kidney Health Australia, 2012).

Therefore key goals of management of CKD are to:

1 identify the cause of CKD to exclude any treatable kidney disease
2 reduce progression of kidney disease by treating high blood pressure and albuminuria
3 reduce cardiovascular risk
4 avoid nephrotoxic medications or volume depletion.

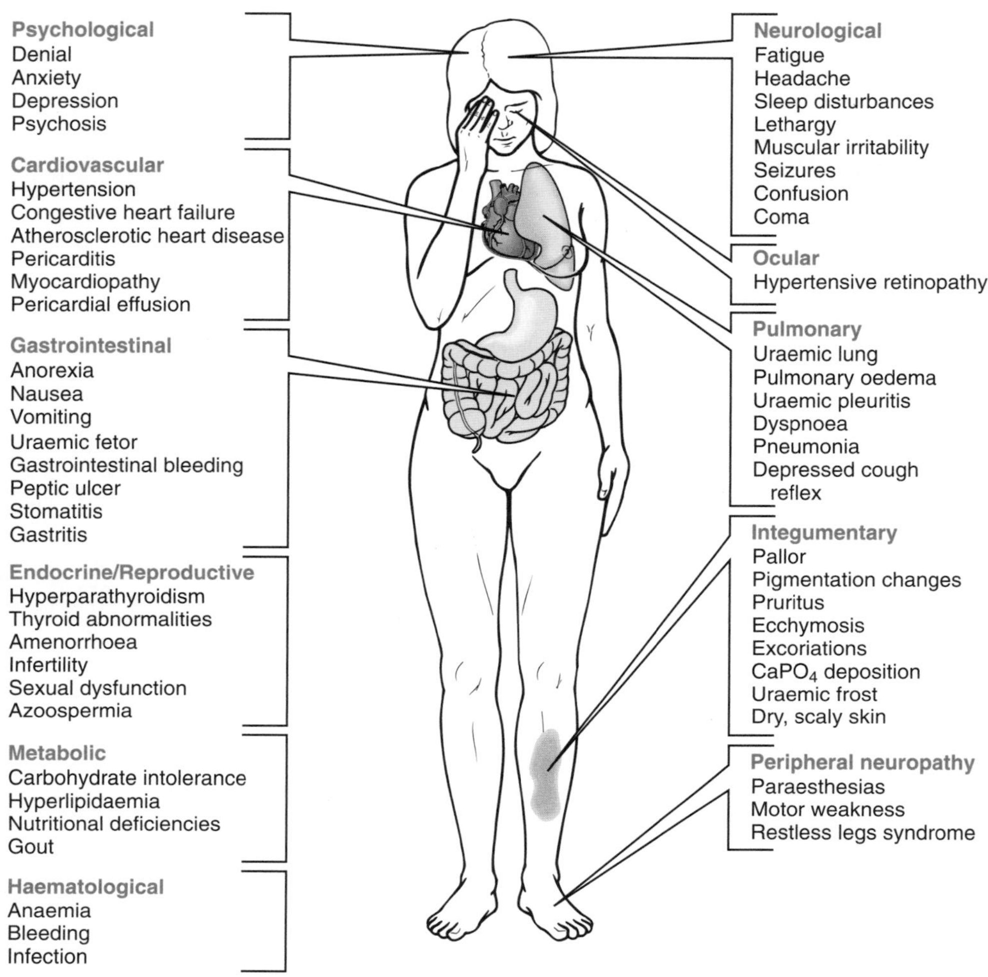

FIGURE 22.1 Clinical manifestations of uraemia. *Note*: From Brown & Edwards (2012, Fig 46.5, p. 1302).

SCREENING FOR CHRONIC KIDNEY DISEASE

An annual kidney health check is recommended for those at risk of CKD (see Table 22.2). In its simplest form a kidney health check will have three components:

1 urine albumin creatinine ratio (ACR)
2 serum creatinine measurement, leading to an estimated GFR (eGFR)
3 blood pressure (BP) measurement.

CKD can only be diagnosed if the urine ACR or eGFR tests are abnormal on at least two out of three separate occasions. Since 2005, all pathology services in Australia and New Zealand automatically report eGFR for adults having serum creatinine measurements. This calculates an eGFR using the patient's age and sex as well as the creatinine (Johnson et al., 2012a). Like all clinical measurements there are many variables that influence eGFR. An

TABLE 22.2

Early detection of CKD using Kidney Health Check *Note*: From: *Chronic Kidney Disease (CKD) Management in General Practice* (2nd edition). Kidney Health Australia, Melbourne, 2012.

<table>
<tr><th>INDICATION FOR TESTING*</th><th>RECOMMENDED TESTS</th><th>FREQUENCY OF TESTING</th></tr>
<tr><td>Smoker</td><td rowspan="7">Urine ACR§
eGFR blood pressure</td><td rowspan="7">Every 1–2 years**</td></tr>
<tr><td>Diabetes</td></tr>
<tr><td>Hypertension</td></tr>
<tr><td>Obesity</td></tr>
<tr><td>Established cardiovascular disease†</td></tr>
<tr><td>Family history of CKD</td></tr>
<tr><td>Aboriginal or Torres Strait Islander origin aged ≥30 years‡</td></tr>
</table>

*Whilst being aged 60 years of age or over is considered to be a risk factor for CKD, in the absence of other risk factors it is not necessary to routinely test these individuals for kidney disease.

**1 year for individuals with hypertension or diabetes.

†Established cardiovascular disease is defined as a previous diagnosis of coronary heart disease, cerebrovascular disease or peripheral vascular disease.

‡See source text for more detail re: indications for testing in ATSI peoples.

§If urine ACR positive arrange two further tests over 3 months (preferably first morning void). If eGFR < 60 mL/min/1.73 m^2 repeat within 14 days.

unexpected finding calls for a careful assessment before assuming the presence of CKD (Thomas, 2011).

DELAYING PROGRESSION

The single most important intervention to delay progression of CKD is to achieve good blood pressure control. The target BP for people with diabetes and/or albuminuria is consistently <130/80. Otherwise BP should be consistently <140/90 (Kidney Health Australia, 2012; National Vascular Disease Prevention Alliance, 2012).

Although medication may be introduced early, therapeutic lifestyle change is an important element of delaying progression and preventing complications (Thomas, 2011). Lifestyle changes include cessation of smoking, increased physical activity, weight loss and reduced dietary sodium intake. The nurse should encourage the patient to set realistic goals, plan strategies and give positive reinforcement for achievements. Smoking cessation is an important goal for anyone with CKD. Large population studies have shown that smoking is a significant risk factor for future ESKD and smoking cessation reduced this risk (Hallan & Orth, 2011).

Patients with CKD and albuminuria (see Case Study 22.1) may be prescribed an angiotensin-converting enzyme inhibitor (ACEI) or an angiotensin receptor blocker (ARB) even if their blood pressure is normal. These classes of drugs have been shown to protect the kidneys by reducing albumin loss as well as through the blood pressure-lowering effect (Turner, Bauer, Abramowitz, Melamed, & Hostetter, 2012).

There is limited evidence that intensive treatment of other co-morbidities such as diabetes actually slows progression of CKD once it has developed. However, achieving good glycaemic control is an important goal for patients with CKD because it helps prevent other complications of diabetes such as retinopathy (Turner et al., 2012).

Not all people with CKD require a referral to a renal unit. Indications for referral to a nephrologist are:

- eGFR < 30 mL/min/1.73 m^2
- persistent significant albuminuria (urine ACR ≥ 30 mg/mmol)
- a consistent decline in eGFR from a baseline of <60 mL/min/m^2 (a decline of >5 mL/min/m^2 over a 6-month period which is confirmed on at least three separate readings)
- glomerular haematuria with macro-albuminuria
- CKD and hypertension that is hard to get to target despite at least three antihypertensive agents.

These indications for referral should also take into consideration the individual patient's circumstances and preferences.

The book, *Chronic Kidney Disease Management in General Practice,* provides contemporary explanations useful for nurses working in either primary healthcare or acute hospitals across Australia and New Zealand regarding care for people with CKD (Kidney Health Australia, 2012). Anyone presenting with signs of acute nephritis (oliguria, haematuria, hypertension and oedema) should be treated as a medical emergency and referred without delay.

PREVENTING COMPLICATIONS

People with CKD are susceptible to deterioration in remaining kidney function due to dehydration and nephrotoxic substances. It is important for nurses to be aware that the kidneys are less able to regulate urinary concentration and are more sensitive to dehydration. Intravenous fluids may be needed for diagnostic and/or therapeutic interventions that require fasting. In addition, radio-opaque contrast used in coronary angiography (and similar procedures) is nephrotoxic, and decisions to use contrast will be weighed up in view of the risks and benefits to the individual patient. Many medications (e.g. gentamicin, vancomycin) will require dose adjustment and monitoring to ensure patient safety. Others such as metformin must be used with caution in earlier stages of CKD and discontinued in patients with a creatinine clearance of less than 30 mL/min (Thomas, 2011).

TREATING COMPLICATIONS

As CKD progresses, the complications of CKD manifest, usually around late stage 3 and stage 4. These complications are as a result of anaemia and abnormal bone and mineral metabolism. Management involves medication (iron supplements and erythropoietin-stimulating agents for anaemia; calcitriol and phosphate binders for bone and mineral metabolism) (Turner et al., 2012). Some patients will need sodium bicarbonate to correct acidosis or Resonium A for hyperkalaemia.

The patient may require dietary advice to maintain a healthy nutrition status. The broad guidelines for patients with CKD are in line with the recommendations for the general population. They need to be particularly conscious of limiting sodium (salt) and avoiding saturated fats. Referral to a dietitian is required if the patient needs specific advice about managing protein or potassium intake or if there are several conditions that have an impact on nutrition. Patients in stages 4 and 5 CKD should be referred to a dietitian to prevent malnutrition and manage the symptoms of uraemia (Ash et al., 2006). It is important to note that protein restriction (<0.8 g/kg/day) is not recommended practice in Australia.

THE PATIENT WITH END-STAGE KIDNEY DISEASE

When renal function deteriorates to the point of ESKD (stage 5) people make a decision about the type of treatment they would like. There are essentially two options: conservative care or KRT. Conservative care is typically chosen by people aged over 65 years who have several co-morbid chronic health conditions and who are likely to have shorter life expectancies (Morton, Turner, Howard, Snelling, & Webster, 2012). Conservative care involves providing symptom support, often in collaboration with a palliative team (Harrison & Watson, 2011). From a patient and family perspective, symptom management and quality of life are deemed important when considering this option (Johnston & Noble, 2012).

KRT includes haemodialysis, peritoneal dialysis and renal transplantation. The choice of dialysis modality is influenced by a number of factors, including the preference of a fully informed patient, absence of medical and surgical contraindications and resource availability. If the patient is willing and suitable it is suggested that peritoneal dialysis is preferable to haemodialysis to better preserve residual kidney function and allow graded introduction of dialysis (Stanley, 2010). Peritoneal dialysis (PD) is performed by introducing 2–3 litres of a sterile dextrose-containing solution (dialysate) into the peritoneal cavity. There are several different techniques for PD; the most common is automated peritoneal dialysis (APD) where the patient connects to a small machine every night.

Haemodialysis (HD) involves access to the vascular system (usually an arteriovenous fistula is formed and cannulated), an extracorporeal circuit, dialyser and technological equipment. Typically, a patient will receive a minimum of 4 hours of treatment on three occasions each week. HD can be undertaken in three different clinical settings: 'in-centre', in satellite haemodialysis units or at home. 'In-centre' refers to therapy provided to people who are medically unstable and require significant care with on-site nephrology support; the *centre* is located *in* a hospital within a recognised renal unit. Satellite haemodialysis encompasses lower acuity care located in hospitals with no formal nephrology unit or community-based units where self-care is encouraged (Agar, MacGregor, & Blagg, 2007). If a person is suitable to undertake haemodialysis at home, then the number of hours is flexible and they are encouraged to dialyse for five or six times a week, often overnight.

The last type of KRT is renal transplantation, and is an option for most patients with ESKD, either before or after the initiation of dialysis. The donor kidney is placed in the iliac fossa and native kidneys are not removed. Immunosuppression (e.g. prednisone, mycophenolate and cyclosporin) is required to prevent rejection.

ALTERED MOBILITY AND FATIGUE

No matter what the stage of CKD, people experience a range of burdensome symptoms (often worse that those experienced by cancer sufferers) that affect all body systems (Murtagh, Addington-Hall, & Higginson, 2007), and they are required to invest considerable time in managing their health, including modifying their diet, managing numerous medications, undergoing KRT (if required) and attending medical and hospital appointments. CKD, its treatment and concomitant complications also impact significantly on a person's lifestyle, family responsibilities, their ability to work and financial status. The impact of CKD and its treatment on physical, emotional, social and overall health related quality of life is, therefore, profound.

At least 45% of people with CKD, particularly those who are in stages 4 and 5, develop anaemia (Gandra et al., 2010). Anaemia causes decreased energy, tiredness, shortness of breath and weakness. In addition, anaemia in CKD contributes to significant co-morbid complications such as left ventricular hypertrophy, congestive heart failure and ischaemic heart disease (Schmid & Schiffl, 2010). As a consequence, people have increased hospitalisations and a shorter life expectancy (Palmer et al., 2010). There is a reduced capacity of people with CKD to engage in activities of daily living (White et al., 2010) which is likely to be due to a number of factors including anaemia, fatigue, lengthy treatment commitments and debilitating co-morbid conditions. The capacity to perform routine living chores and to participate in and enjoy everyday life is reduced as a result of having CKD (Bonner, Wellard, & Caltabiano, 2009). Not surprisingly a person's ability to engage in exercise is reduced (Bennett et al., 2010).

Fatigue is a complex, subjective experience and is reported by 70–97% of people with CKD (Murtagh, Spagnolo, Panocchia, & Gambaro, 2009; Bossola, Vulpio, & Tazza, 2011). Despite advances in renal healthcare, fatigue remains ranked as one of the most troublesome symptoms for people with CKD (Danquah, Zimmerman, & Diamond, 2010). Factors associated with the fatigue experienced in CKD include prescribed medications and their side effects; nutritional deficiencies; physiological alterations, such as obstructive sleep apnoea (Kidney Health Australia, 2012); abnormal urea and haemoglobin levels; and psychological factors such as depression, sleep dysfunction and those associated with haemodialysis treatment (O'Sullivan & McCarthy, 2009).

BODY IMAGE

CKD can result in both physical and psychological changes in body image. There is limited research, however, exploring the patient's perception of body image in CKD. Physical changes are common and are not restricted to those directly affecting the renal system, as other body systems are also involved (see also Figure 22.1). Alterations in body image are often due to external changes in skin, body weight, mobility, side effects of medications and the presence of KRT devices. In children, growth retardation occurs due to the effects of uraemia on growth hormone production (Fine, 2010). Internal or psychological alterations such as fatigue, depression and altered feelings of wellbeing also occur. Both external and internal alterations in body image may contribute to a decreased quality of life and adherence with treatment.

When CKD progresses to stage 5 and KRT is commenced, other physical alterations to a person's body image occur due to the presence of dialysis access devices and a number of surgical procedures. These access devices could be one or more of (or in some situations both) a peritoneal dialysis (PD) catheter, an arteriovenous fistula (AVF) or an external vascular catheter. A PD catheter and extension set protrudes from the body by approximately 15–30 cm and often requires adjustments to the type of clothing worn to accommodate its presence (e.g. underpants, location of belts or waist bands). An AVF is an internal surgical anastomosis of an artery and a vein (commonly radial artery and cephalic vein) and results in arterial blood flowing straight into the vein. The AVF causes the vein to dilate, and when repeatedly cannulated for haemodialysis, can result in tortuous and/or aneurysmal dilations and changes in body image (Richard & Engebretson, 2010). Vascular catheters can be temporary or permanent and are often visible. Lastly, scars as a result of previous, and often numerous occasions of, surgery for access devices and/or kidney transplantation can also affect an individual's body image.

Nurses need to understand, assess and recognise the impact of CKD on an individual's actual or perceived alterations in body image. Assisting individuals to verbalise their feelings and to provide supportive strategies is an important facet of providing renal nursing care.

QUALITY OF LIFE

The experience of living with CKD (a chronic, life-altering illness) involves many challenges for patients and their families in achieving a satisfactory quality of life (QOL) (Untas et al., 2011) and is related to the ramifications of CKD and its treatment on the physical, cognitive, psychological and social aspects of their lives (Soni, Weisbord, & Unruh, 2010). Regardless of the stage of CKD it is crucial for healthcare professionals to strive to keep the QOL of patients at the highest possible level (Finkelstein, Wuerth, & Finkelstein, 2009).

It is difficult to adequately assess QOL, as it is a subjective and individual experience. For example, a person who is blind with bilateral leg amputations, diabetes, renal failure and requiring haemodialysis may well rate their QOL as quite good. Nevertheless, QOL is important to assess. In CKD common tools used in both clinical practice and research to assess QOL are Medical Outcomes Survey Short Form, Kidney Disease Quality of Life and Choices Health Experience Questionnaire (Unruh, Weisbord, & Kimmel, 2005). Overall, it is well documented that people with CKD have much lower QOL scores compared with people of normal health, due to physical, psychological and social changes to daily life (Untas et al., 2011).

The many physical symptoms and complications of CKD can adversely affect QOL. These include anaemia, challenges of fluid and dietary restrictions, fatigue, adequate sleep, numerous symptoms associated with renal failure (see Figure 22.1), other health problems (e.g. diabetes, congestive heart failure, infection etc.) and chronic pain. All contribute to the stress associated with living and coping with CKD and its treatment. Treatment of ESKD with transplantation is linked to improvements of QOL (Rambod, Shabani, Shokrpour, Rafii, & Mohammadalliha, 2011).

Alterations in body image together with the physical and psychosocial complications of CKD have an impact on an individual's sexuality. Diabetes (a leading cause of CKD) as well as a number of medications (e.g. antihypertensive agents) interfere with sexual function. Other factors, such as endocrine, vascular and hormonal changes, are also involved in sexual dysfunction. Patients describe decreased interest in and frequency of intercourse and difficulties with erection. Difficulties with sexual arousal are among the most bothersome of symptoms reported by people with CKD, particularly for those on dialysis (Yong et al., 2009). Using a non-judgmental approach will assist nurses in early identification of sexual dysfunction and timely referral for support.

The impact of CKD on the psychological wellbeing of people is significant. For instance, it has been reported that people with CKD experience high levels of stress and anxiety, feeling scared or fearful and experience feelings of guilt, frustration, worry and powerlessness (Shin, 2011). Depression is the most common psychological problem seen effecting 1 in 5 people with CKD and 1 in 3 people on dialysis (Hedayati, Yalamanchili, & Finkelstein, 2012). There is strong evidence linking depression and CKD with a reduced QOL (Abdel-Kader, Unruh, & Weisbord, 2009). There are many causes of depression in CKD patients, such as stresses associated with the disease, medications used to treat CKD, increased need to see health professionals and hospitalisation or simply as a result of feeling unwell (Kring & Crane, 2009). Depression can be a response to loss, and CKD patients have sustained multiple losses, including role within the family and workplace, renal function and mobility, physical skills, cognitive abilities and sexual function (Finkelstein et al., 2009). At present there is a reliance on pharmacotherapy to treat depression in CKD as there is very limited evidence to support the effectiveness of psychosocial interventions in the treatment of depression in patients with CKD (Hedayati et al., 2012). Selective serotonin reuptake inhibitors are commonly prescribed as these drugs are extensively metabolised in the liver, making them safe for patients with CKD.

TABLE 22.3
Common psychological and sociological problems

PSYCHOLOGICAL	SOCIOLOGICAL
• Depression • Anger • Denial • Helplessness • Anxiety • Loss of control • Burden • Fear of death • Feelings of guilt	• Role change in family • Employment status • Ability to continue education • Financial status • Reduced social network and activities • Change in residential location • Holiday and recreation

The social impact of CKD is immense. At a personal level, there is an increase in social isolation and relationship difficulty, lack of independence (Shin, 2011) and financial problems often due to unemployment (Apostolou et al., 2007). Unemployment and reliance on government social welfare benefits are high. For children and adolescents, these complications affect their ability to attend and actively participate at school. Temporary or permanent relocation to larger regional or urban healthcare facilities is also experienced by patients living in rural and remote locations and this also affects QOL. Being able to take vacations when and where an individual desires is also affected by CKD and its treatment. At the family level, there is an impact on the quality of life of caregivers as well as financial impact on the family (Wiedebusch et al., 2010). Having adequate social support networks (home, work and renal unit) has been consistently linked to improved health outcomes (Untas et al., 2011). At a societal level, CKD health expenditure is a considerable socioeconomic burden on a country. Table 22.3 summarises the common psychological and sociological problems experienced by people with CKD and ESKD.

The effect of adding KRT into the demands of daily life with ESKD is considerable for most people and is considered to be one of the most stressful of all other illnesses and treatment regimens (Chanouzas, Ng, Fallouh, & Baharani, 2012). While haemodialysis treatment itself typically lasts for 4 hours, three times per week, every week of the year, there are also other demands, such as travelling to and from the dialysis unit, waiting for staff/machine availability, completing pre-dialysis assessment, cannulation of fistula, etc. This often means 8 to 10 hours need to be allowed for each treatment session, and this allocation of time needs to fit around usual activities of daily life such as work, family and school commitments. Peritoneal dialysis makes similar demands on time (approximately 4 hours per day) but PD treatment is typically undertaken on a daily basis (i.e. 365 days of the year). Consequently the demands of KRT is considerable and results in a highly abnormal everyday life (Cohen, Holder-Perkins, & Kimmel, 2007).

Rehabilitation is about the return of lost function and is an aspect of nursing care provided to people with CKD/ESKD. Given the repeated and frequent contact nephrology nurses have with people over long periods of time, they are in an ideal position to provide rehabilitation. Common rehabilitative interventions include the teaching, coaching and supporting strategies to assist people in increasing their movement along a continuum towards self-management (Bonner, 2012). The rehabilitative continuum typically begins with teaching people about CKD and its management through to complete independence by undertaking dialysis self-care at home. The point on this continuum is individualised for each person depending on their health, personal and home situations.

Promoting QOL is a key aspect of nursing care for people with CKD. Adequate and timely assessment and working collaboratively with patients is necessary to optimise QOL. No single strategy or plan will work for everyone but support, encouragement, education, rehabilitation and promoting self-care are fundamental elements of renal nursing care. Of importance for nurses is to assist patients to acquire and maintain a sense of control as they adjust to living with CKD. Learning to manage the illness, finding a balance between illness and normalcy and reaching an acceptance of the illness is crucial to achieving an optimal QOL. It is crucial that nurses ask people for their own assessments of how they are doing, what their relationships are like in their families and what life is like for them. For some patients, allocating selective attention to various aspects of living with CKD has enabled them to exert control over their health (Birmelé et al., 2012). Selective attention may also influence the decisions patients make about self-care and compliance with recommended treatments; this strategy may well enable some cognitive and behavioural control that allows individuals to adjust to living with kidney failure. The challenge for all health professionals involved in caring for people with CKD is to devise interventions that meaningfully increase QOL.

SUPPORTING EFFECTIVE SELF-MANAGEMENT IN CHRONIC KIDNEY DISEASE

CKD, regardless of stage, requires people to adhere to complex treatment regimens. Initially they are asked to modify their lifestyle (stop smoking, reduce weight, limit alcohol intake and increase exercise), take numerous medications (e.g. antihypertensive agents, statins, glycaemic agents, etc.) and possibly perform self-monitoring activities at home (e.g. blood pressure, weight, blood glucose levels, etc.). As their CKD progresses, they will be asked to make further adjustments, have regular pathology investigations performed and attend clinic appointments more frequently (see Table 22.4). Once they start KRT, their schedule is dominated by the activities required to stay alive (see above).

With the increasing number of patients with CKD has come the need to develop new roles for nurses to help manage this group of patients. Nurses are actively involved in patient care at all stages of CKD: as practice nurses in primary healthcare settings, nurses working in renal outpatient clinics and dialysis units. Increasingly CKD clinics are being led by nurse practitioners (Barrett et al., 2011; Smith & Thorp, 2011; Wong, Chow, & Chan, 2010). In Australia, the CKD nursing role has coincided with the development of the advanced and extended role of nurse practitioner, with the first CKD nurse practitioner that commenced in 2007.

The principles and strategies developed in other chronic disease areas such as asthma, diabetes and heart failure are similar to those required to develop and support effective CKD self-management (Lawn, McMillan, & Pulvirenti, 2011). For the nurse working with patients with CKD, this means that assessment must include consideration of the social environment and supports available (Pagels, Weng, & Wengstrom, 2008). Often multiple therapeutic lifestyle changes are indicated but it is unrealistic to expect that all can or will be adopted. The nurse will assess the patient's readiness to self-manage and work collaboratively with them to set goals. Compromise is often necessary to make sure goals are achievable.

Information giving must be at a level and pace appropriate for the individual (Morton, Howard, Webster, & Snelling, 2011). (See 'Education for the person and family' below.) Because there is so much to take in, a written management plan for the patient to take away and refer to can help them remember what has been discussed (Ormandy, 2008).

For some patients with poorly controlled BP, self-monitoring and recording their BP readings can be helpful. When they bring their record to an appointment it can be used to

TABLE 22.4

Outline of expected self-management behaviours for CKD/ESKD

	CKD	HOME DIALYSIS (HAEMODIALYSIS AND PERITONEAL DIALYSIS)	HOSPITAL HAEMODIALYSIS	TRANSPLANT
Therapeutic lifestyle change	• Stop smoking* • Healthy diet, no added salt • Safe alcohol • More exercise • +/– fluid restriction	• Stop smoking • Healthy diet plus adjustments as indicated by blood results • Safe alcohol • More exercise • +/– fluid restriction, depending on urine output	• Stop smoking • Healthy diet plus adjustments as indicated by blood results — likely to need potassium restriction • Safe alcohol • More exercise • Most likely to need fluid restriction	• Continue to be a non-smoker • Healthy diet, no added salt • Safe alcohol • More exercise • Unlikely to need fluid restriction — have to avoid dehydration • Sun protection
Home observations	BP Weight (if fluid management an issue)	Temperature, pulse, BP Weight		Temperature, pulse, BP Weight Urinalysis
Medications	Antihypertensives, diuretics Lipid-lowering agents Phosphate binders Vitamin D analogue Sodium bicarbonate	Antihypertensives, diuretics — can often be decreased Lipid-lowering agents Phosphate binders	Antihypertensives, diuretics — can often be decreased Lipid-lowering agents Phosphate binders	Immunosuppressive drugs (usually a combination of three) plus a number of other drugs to minimise the side effects. These are weaned as the transplant is established, but some medication continues for the duration of the transplant Other medications as required by the individual
	Iron Folic acid Erythropoietin-stimulating agent Other medications as required by the individual	Vitamin D analogue Iron Folic acid Erythropoietin-stimulating agent Other medications as required by the individual	Vitamin D analogue Iron Folic acid Erythropoietin-stimulating agent Other medications as required by the individual	
Dialysis access	Once dialysis is imminent	Care of AVF/Tenckhoff catheter. Self-cannulation for home haemodialysis	Care of AVF. Some patients self-cannulate	Once transplant is working, Tenckhoff catheter will be removed. AVF remains in situ
Dialysis procedure		Have to do procedure, maintain equipment, problem solving to the ability of the individual	In many centres patients are encouraged to participate in self-care as able	

*In most transplant centres, current smokers will not be accepted for the active transplant waiting list.

assess the accuracy of clinic BP measurements (so called White Coat hypertension) or to work out optimum medication timing and if there are any other factors (e.g. obstructive sleep apnoea or stress management) to be addressed. Ambulatory 24-hour blood pressure monitoring is increasingly recommended for assessment of hypertension and to monitor a person's response to therapy (National Vascular Disease Prevention Alliance, 2012).

On return visits the patient should be given positive reinforcement for their achievements and encouragement to persevere. It is important to build confidence and self-efficacy, as each gain is an opportunity to set new goals (Birmelé et al., 2012). Active and sustained follow-up by the nurse helps maintain momentum and give support. This may be through telephone calls, reminder notices and invitations to patient education seminars. Depending on local arrangements, home dialysis patients are followed up with home visits and may be able to get access to telephone assistance out of hours.

Not everyone can self-manage effectively. The approach described makes assumptions about and demands on literacy, cognitive and social skills, motivation and self-efficacy. For patients who are unable or unwilling to engage in self-management, the healthcare team must develop strategies that will provide the best possible outcome for the individual.

Blaming and labelling patients who do not follow their healthcare providers' advice should be avoided. In CKD and ESKD patient care, the label of 'non-compliance' can have far-reaching repercussions. For example, it may be viewed unfavourably when being assessed for transplantation as it is assumed that someone who is non-compliant with CKD and dialysis treatments will not follow post-kidney transplant instructions.

Family and carers

People with CKD often require the support of family and friends to manage their illness and treatment (particularly KRT) at home and be the principal caregiver. Existing family and marital relationships are altered by the complex and burdensome treatments associated with CKD and its treatment (Kelly, 2010; Nygårdh, Wikby, Malm, & Ahlstrom, 2011). The moment CKD and its treatment regimen enter the lives of family members and friends, significant adjustments to the roles they have in the relationship are required. There is the uncertainty about whether the person's health will become worse, how long treatment will be needed for, whether dialysis will effectively manage the condition or cause more problems, whether the person will die from CKD and when or if the person will get a kidney transplant. In addition, family members may experience guilt if the CKD is as a result of an inherited condition (e.g. polycystic kidney disease, Alport's syndrome).

Although home dialysis, whether peritoneal or haemodialysis, can be performed independently, evidence suggests that adult caregivers often assume some, if not total, responsibility for the dialysis regimen (Horsburgh, Laing, Beanlands, Meng, & Harwood, 2008). Caregivers not only provide physical and technical support but they also provide emotional support. For these caregivers, particularly spouses, KRT contributes to additional stress, fatigue, home responsibilities and a negative reaction to their partner's situation (Gayomali, Sutherland, & Finkelstein, 2008). Family members are constantly watching the person under care, juggling activities to meet all responsibilities, advocating or intervening on behalf of their loved one, modifying home routines to fit in with the KRT and encouraging their loved one to perform self-care and to adhere to the treatment regimen (Horsburgh et al., 2008).

One unique aspect for family members and friends associated with CKD is organ donation. With the shortage of deceased donors, living related and living unrelated kidney organ donation rates have increased in both Australia and New Zealand (Clayton, Campbell, Hurst, McDonald, & Chadban, 2011). Living relatives (i.e. parents, child, sibling, etc.) are still the most common source of living donors but living unrelated donors (e.g. spouse, significant other, close friend, etc.) have also increased the pool of available kidneys. While the donor's autonomy must be respected by healthcare professionals, the explicit or implicit pressure on family members, spouses or close friends to donate is an additional and largely not well understood and acknowledged burden associated with the experience of living with someone with CKD.

It is not surprising that the burden of CKD on caregivers has been the focus of research but there are rewards for being a caregiver; for many families, interpersonal relationships can be sustained and developed further. Nurses require an understanding of the impact of CKD on family members and others. Ongoing assessment, assisting family members and exploring the degree to which an individual family caregiver is involved in the care of their loved one are important components of providing holistic care. The type and amount of care provided by family members may alter over time due to the changing burden of CKD (i.e. different stages of CKD). Strategies such as providing professional support and early intervention to reduce the burden, strain and fatigue, increased social support services in the home and referral to other health professionals are important components of renal nursing care (Kelly, 2010).

Education for the person and family

The patient with CKD has a continuum of education needs. From the diagnosis of CKD to dialysis and transplantation there is much to learn in relation to their disease and how to manage it. Pre-dialysis education is particularly important (Morton, Howard, Webster, & Snelling, 2011) but when patients were asked to rate their level of knowledge, about one-third reported limited or no understanding of their CKD (Finklestein et al., 2008). Recently Wright and colleagues (Wright, Wallston, Elasy, Ikizler, & Cavanaugh, 2011) found that many topic areas important to supporting patients to perform self-care were in fact not well understood by patients with CKD. Older patients remember less and patients misconstrued 48% of what they thought they remembered. Importantly, the more information that was given, the less was correctly recalled.

There are more potential sources of information. Even if the patient doesn't access the internet, it is almost certain that friends and/or family do. Some of the information on the internet is excellent, but much is confusing, misleading or even dangerous. It is useful to ask patients what they know and create opportunities to clarify incorrect or misunderstood information. Some people will have friends or family members who have had CKD/ESKD and they may need explanation of current treatments and clinical practices.

According to Lloyd (2010, p. 11) in order:

> to understand how knowledge is constructed [of kidney disease and its treatment] it is important to understand how an individual interacts with one of the basic building blocks — information and the process of gathering information.

Bonner and Lloyd (2012, in press) found that people are likely to be information practitioners who receive or engage with knowledge and experiences at various times in their renal disease journey. 'Receivers' were people with CKD who do not interact with information but merely acquire it passively; being passive is their way of coping with kidney disease. In contrast, 'engagers' actively sought out and interacted with information and they used information to better understand and cope with kidney disease and its treatment.

When teaching patients about CKD or KRT, information is provided at a level and pace appropriate for the individual. This is easier to do when in a one-on-one situation. If conducting group education, attention must be given to meeting a variety of individual needs. Education seminars involving the renal multidisciplinary team are also provided. The seminars have been shown to help patients choose the most suitable KRT for them (Morton et al., 2011).

One of the challenges of nursing patients with ESKD is to provide effective patient education to people who are uraemic, often elderly and almost always very anxious. If a patient begins dialysis in a hospital haemodialysis unit, the dialysis nurses will explain what is happening to them. The patient will learn about how their self-care practices will have to adapt and change as they make the transition to their new treatment modality. They will be shown the dialysis area and where the patients are weighed and introduced to the pre-dialysis assessment (weight, temperature, pulse, blood pressure).

The patient will be told not to take any antihypertensive medications before the first dialysis, but to bring all medications so the nursing staff can obtain a complete list. Some 'antihypertensives' may be taken for heart failure and the patient will need to have a personalised medication plan. There will be further teaching as medications are adjusted (e.g. sodium bicarbonate may be stopped, water-soluble medications should be taken after dialysis) and new ones are started.

Initial concerns are likely to relate to the AVF which is being cannulated for the first time and may be soft and inclined to 'blow'. Patients should be shown how to apply pressure to the needle sites and given extra sterile gauze to take home in case of bleeding.

Once their dialysis routine is established, their diet and fluid intake will be reviewed by a dietitian. Depending on residual kidney function, the patient will be given diet advice that will maintain safe blood levels of potassium between treatments without compromising their nutritional status and that takes into account individual and cultural preferences.

PD home training is usually done as an outpatient (Jose et al., 2011). The patient has the Tenckhoff catheter inserted about a month before the anticipated need to start dialysis. The PD nurses are involved in teaching about pre-operative preparation and post-operative care of the catheter site. It is especially important to prevent and treat constipation as this interferes with the functioning of the catheter.

Learning to perform the PD exchange, connect to the APD machine and associated procedures is done at the patient's own pace. Most patients are ready to self-manage at home within 2 weeks. However, if there are barriers to learning (e.g. language, anxiety, etc.), it may take longer. The degree to which problem solving is taught is determined by the nurses' assessment of the patient's ability to take this on. For some patients the main focus is to make sure they recognise when problems occur, such as an infected catheter exit site or peritonitis, and what action to take, for example contact the GP or ring the PD unit.

Patients starting PD will also have changes to their medications and diet and fluids. Because APD provides dialysis constantly, the diet tends to be more relaxed in relation to potassium, but they must be careful to have adequate protein intake to replace the protein lost in the dialysate. Also, because of the dextrose in the dialysate there is a tendency to gain body weight.

Home HD training is a more complex series of learning activities and commonly takes about three months to complete. In addition to everything that the hospital haemodialysis patient learns about their self-management, the home HD patient must master a range of technical activities as well. This includes water treatment and machine maintenance as well as the dialysis procedure itself. The patient and their support person will be competent in emergency procedures, such as what to do in case of adverse reactions (such as hypotension), power or water failure.

Following transplantation, the kidney transplant recipient stays in hospital until surgically recovered. The patient will have a period of daily outpatient appointments, which then taper off to alternate daily, to weekly and so on until the kidney function is well established and stable. Before discharge, the patient will be educated about their new immunosuppressive medications, including what each one is for, how to recognise them, when they should be taken and which side effects to be aware of. In addition, a patient

CASE STUDY 22.1 Part 2

Because of the presence of macroalbuminuria, Lillian's BP target was established as <130/80. On discussion with the NP Lillian said she was not taking her tablets every day because she didn't know if they were really necessary. The NP explained the importance of achieving good blood pressure control and the need for indefinite treatment with tablets. They also discussed the ways to ensure a routine so she would remember to take them each day.

Lillian has gained a lot of weight and they talked about the importance of avoiding further weight gain and, if possible, losing weight. This was more challenging as Lillian said that her husband was a very fussy eater and preferred traditional British food. She said that her neighbour often suggested they should go for an early morning walk together, so she resolved to start doing that once or twice each week.

The NP arranged to see Lillian again in a month to check her BP, review blood tests including a lipid profile and provide further education and support for lifestyle change.

Reflective questions

1 What are the different stages of CKD and what are the priorities of healthcare for each stage?
2 How does CKD impact on the individual, family and wider community?
3 Why is it important for people with CKD to engage in effective self-management?

will learn to monitor the wellbeing of the kidney by doing a daily weight, urinalysis and BP.

CONCLUSION

This chapter has explained the key aspects of CKD, ESKD and KRT and its effect on aspects of daily life such as mobility, fatigue and quality of life. This was followed by a discussion of body image, adherence and the impact of CKD and KRT on family and carers. Nurses should develop strategies that better support people to self-manage this chronic and complex health condition, and that effective patient education is of prime importance when providing nursing care to people with CKD.

Recommended reading

Australian Institute of Health and Welfare (AIHW) National Centre for Monitoring Chronic Kidney Disease publications on CKD and related topics; see www.aihw.gov.au.

Castner, D. (2010). Understanding the stages of chronic kidney disease. *Nursing, 40*(5), 24–32.

Johnston, S., & Noble, H. (2012). Factors influencing patients with stage 5 chronic kidney disease to opt for conservative management: a practitioner research study. *Journal of Clinical Nursing, 21*(9/10), 1215–1222.

Lewis, A., Stabler, K., & Welch, J. (2010). Perceived informational needs, problems, or concerns among patients with stage 4 chronic kidney disease. *Nephrology Nursing Journal, 37*(2), 143–149.

Strand, H., & Parker, D. (2012). Effects of multidisciplinary models of care for adult pre-dialysis patients with chronic kidney disease: a systematic review. *International Journal of Evidence–Based Healthcare, 10*, 53–59.

References

Abdel-Kader, K., Unruh, M., & Weisbord, S. (2009). Symptom burden, depression, and quality of life in chronic and end-stage kidney disease. *Clinical Journal of American Society of Nephrology, 4*(6), 1057–1064.

Agar, J., MacGregor, M., & Blagg, C. (2007). Chronic maintenance hemodialysis: making sense of terminology. *Hemodialysis International, 11*, 252–262.

Apostolou, T., Hutchison, A., Chak, W., et al. (2007). Quality of life in CAPD, transplant and chronic renal failure, patients with diabetes. *Renal Failure, 29*(2), 189–197.

Ash, S., Campbell, K., MacLaughlin, H., et al. (2006). Evidence based practice guidelines for the nutritional management of chronic kidney disease. *Nutrition & Dietetics, 63*, S33–S45.

Australian Institute of Health and Welfare. (2011a). *End Stage Kidney Disease in Australia. Total Incidence 2003 – 2007.* Cat no PHE 143. Canberra: Australian Institute of Health and Welfare.

Australian Institute of Health and Welfare. (2011b). *Projections of the Incidence of Treated End Stage Kidney Disease in Australia 2010 – 2020.* Cat no PHE 150. Canberra: Australian Institute of Health and Welfare.

Australian Institute of Health and Welfare. (2011c). *Chronic Kidney Disease in Aboriginal and Torres Strait Islander People.* Cat no. PHE 151. Canberra: Australian Institute of Health and Welfare.

Barrett, B., Garg, A., Goeree, R., et al., (2011). A nurse-coordinated model of care *versus* usual care for stage 3/4 chronic kidney disease in the community: A randomized controlled trial. *Clinical Journal of the American Society of Nephrology, 6*, 1241–1247.

Bennett, P., Breugelmans, L., Barnard, R., et al., (2010). Sustaining a hemodialysis exercise program: a review. *Seminars in Dialysis, 23*(1), 62–73.

Birmelé, B., Le Gall, A., Sautenet, B., et al., (2012). Clinical, sociodemographic, and psychological correlates of health-related quality of life in chronic hemodialysis patients. *Psychosomatics, 53*(1), 30–37.

Bonner, A. (2012). Other chronic illness. In K. Mauk (Ed.), *Rehabilitation Nursing: A Contemporary Approach to Practice* (pp. 359–372). Sudbury: Jones and Bartlett.

Bonner, A., & Lloyd, A. (2012, In press). Exploring the information practices of people with end stage kidney disease. *Journal of Renal Care.*

Bonner, A., Wellard, S., & Caltabiano, M. (2009). Determining patient activity levels in chronic and end stage kidney disease. *Journal of Nursing & Healthcare of Chronic Illness, 1*, 39–48.

Bossola, M., Vulpio, C., & Tazza, L. (2011). Fatigue in chronic dialysis patients. *Seminars in Dialysis, 24*(5), 550–555.

Brown, J., & Edwards, H. (2012). *Lewis's Medical-Surgical Nursing* (3rd ed.). Elsevier: Sydney.

Castner, D. (2010). Understanding the stages of chronic kidney disease. *Nursing, 40*(5), 24–32.

Chanouzas, D., Ng, K., Fallouh, B., & Baharini, J. (2012). What influences patient choice of treatment modality at the pre-dialysis stage? *Nephrology Dialysis Transplantation, 27*(4), 1542–1547.

Chronic Kidney Disease Prognosis Consortium. (2010). Association of estimated glomerular filtration rate and albuminuria with all-cause and cardiovascular mortality in general population cohorts: a collaborative meta-analysis. *The Lancet, 75*(9731), 2073–2081.

Chronic Kidney Disease (CKD) Management in General Practice (2nd edition). Kidney Health Australia, Melbourne, (2012).

Clayton, P., Campbell, S., Hurst, K., et al., (2011). Transplantation. Chapter 8. In S. McDonald & K. Hurst (Eds.), *The 34th ANZDATA Registry 2011 Report*. Adelaide: Australia and New Zealand Dialysis and Transplant Registry.

Cohen, S., Holder-Perkins, V., & Kimmel, P. (2007). Psychosocial issues in end-stage renal disease patients. In J. T. Daugirdas, P. G. Blake, & T. S. Ing (Eds.), *Handbook of dialysis* (4th ed.). (pp. 455–461). Philadelphia: Lippincott, Williams & Wilkins.

Danquah, F., Zimmerman, L., & Diamond, P. (2010). Frequency, severity, and distress of dialysis-related symptoms reported by patients on hemodialysis. *Nephrology Nursing Journal, 37*, 627–638.

Fine, R. (2010). Etiology and treatment of growth retardation in children with chronic kidney disease and end-stage renal disease: a historical perspective. *Pediatric Nephrology, 25*(4), 725–732.

Finkelstein, F., Wuerth, D., Finkelstein, S. (2009). Health related quality of life and the CKD patient: Challenges for the nephrology community. *International Society of Nephrology, 76*(9), 946–952.

Gandra, S., Finkelstein, F., & Bennett, A., et al., (2010). Impact of erythropoiesis stimulating agents on energy and physical function in nondialysis CKD patients with anemia: A systematic review. *American Journal of Kidney Disease, 55*, 519–534.

Gayomali, C., Sutherland, S., & Finkelstein, F. (2008). The challenge for the caregiver of the patient with chronic kidney disease. *Nephrology Dialysis Transplant, 23*(12), 3749–3751.

Grace, B., Hurst, K., & McDonald, S. (2011). New patients commencing treatment in 2010. Chapter 2. In S. McDonald & K. Hurst (Eds.), *The 34th ANZDATA Registry 2011 Report*. Adelaide: Australia and New Zealand Dialysis and Transplant Registry.

Hallan, S., & Orth, S. (2011). Smoking is a risk factor in the progression to kidney failure. *Kidney International, 80*, 516–523.

Harrison, K., & Watson, S. (2011). Palliative care in advanced kidney disease: a nurse-led joint renal and specialist palliative care clinic. *International Journal of Palliative Nursing, 17*(1), 42–46.

Hedayati, S., Yalamanchili, V., & Finkelstein, F. (2012). A practical approach to the treatment of depression in patients with chronic kidney disease and end-stage renal disease. *Kidney International, 81*(3), 47–55.

Horsburgh, M., Laing, G., Beanlands, H., et al. (2008). A new measure of 'lay' care-giver activities. *Kidney International, 74*(2), 230–236.

Johnson, D. W., Jones, G., Mathew, T., et al. (2012a). Chronic kidney disease and automatic reporting of estimated glomerular filtration rate: new developments and revised recommendations. *Medical Journal of Australia, 197*(4), 222–223.

Johnson, D. W., Jones, G., Mathew, T., et al. (2012b). Chronic kidney disease and measurement of albuminuria or proteinuria: a position statement. *Medical Journal of Australia, 197*(4), 224–225.

Johnston, S., & Noble, H. (2012). Factors influencing patients with stage 5 chronic kidney disease to opt for conservative management: a practitioner research study. *Journal of Clinical Nursing, 21*(9/10), 1215–1222.

Jose, M., Johnson, D., Mudge, D., et al. (2011). Peritoneal dialysis practice in Australia and New Zealand: A call to action. *Nephrology, 16*(1), 19–29.

Kelly, M. (2010). Who cares … for the carers? *Journal of Renal Care, 36*(1), 16–20.

Kennedy, S., McTaggert, S., McDonald, S., et al. (2011). Paediatric report. Chapter 11. In S. McDonald & K. Hurst (Eds.), *The 34th ANZDATA Registry 2011 Report*. Adelaide: Australia and New Zealand Dialysis and Transplant Registry.

Kring, D., & Crane, P. (2009). Factors affecting quality of life in persons on hemodialysis. *Nephrology Nursing Journal, 36*(1), 15–24.

Lawn, S., McMillan, J., & Pulvirenti, M. (2011). Chronic condition self-management: Expectations of responsibility. *Patient Education & Counseling, 84*(2), e5–e8.

Levey, A. S., Eckardt, K.-U., Tsukamoto, Y., et al. (2005). Definition and classification of chronic kidney disease: A position statement from Kidney Disease: Improving Global Outcomes (KDIGO). *Kidney International, 67*, 2089–2100.

Lloyd, A. (2010). *Information literacy landscapes: Information literacy in education, workplace and everyday contexts*. Cambridge: Woodhead Publishing.

Morton, R., Howard, K., Webster, A., et al. (2011). Patient information about options for treatment (PINOT): A prospective national study of information given to incident CKD stage 5 patients. *Nephrology Dialysis Transplant, 26*(11), 1266–1274.

Morton, R., Turner, R., Howard, K., et al. (2012). Patients who plan for conservative care rather than dialysis: A national observational study in Australia. *American Journal of Kidney Diseases, 59*(3), 419–422.

Murtagh, F., Addington-Hall, J., & Higginson, I. (2007). The prevalence of symptoms in end-stage renal disease: A systematic review. *Advances in Chronic Kidney Disease, 14*, 82–99.

Murtagh, F., Spagnolo, A., Panocchia, N., et al. (2009). Conservative (non dialytic) management of end-stage renal disease and withdrawal of dialysis. *Progress in Palliative Care, 17*(4), 179–185.

National Vascular Disease Prevention Alliance (2012). Guidelines for the management of absolute cardiovascular disease risk. National Stroke Foundation. Retrieved July 12, 2012, from http://www.kidney.org.au/LinkClick.aspx?fileticket=A%2bRjUoFXdMg%3d&tabid=635&mid=1584

Nygårdh, A., Wikby, K., Malm, D., et al. (2011). Empowerment in outpatient care for patients with chronic kidney disease — from the family member's perspective. *BMC Nursing, 10*, 21.

Ormandy, P. (2008). Information topics important to chronic kidney disease patients: a systematic review. *Journal of Renal Care, 34*(1), 19–27.

O'Sullivan, D., & McCarthy, G. (2009). Exploring the symptom of fatigue in patients with end stage renal disease. *Nephrology Nursing Journal, 36*(1), 37–47.

Pagels, A., Weng, M., & Wengstrom, Y. (2008). The impact of a nurse-led clinic on self-care ability, disease-specific knowledge, and home dialysis modality. *Nephrology Nursing Journal, 35*(3), 242–248.

Palmer, S., Navaneethan, S., Craig, J., et al. (2010). Meta-analysis: Erythropoiesis-stimulating agents in patients with chronic kidney disease. *Annals of Internal Medicine, 153*, 23–33.

Rambod, M., Shabani, M., Shokrpour, N., et al. (2011). Quality of life of hemodialysis and renal transplantation patients. *Health Care Manager, 30*(1), 23–28.

Richard, C. J., & Engebretson, J. (2010). Negotiating living with an arteriovenous fistula for hemodialysis. *Nephrology Nursing Journal, 37*(4), 363–374.

Schmid, H., & Schiffl, H. (2010). Erythropoiesis stimulating agents and anaemia of end-stage renaldisease. *Cardiovascular & Hematological Agents in Medicinal Chemistry, 8*, 164–172.

Shin, L. (2011). The impact of dialysis on rurally based Maori and their whanau/families. *Nursing Praxis in New Zealand, 27*(2), 4–9.

Smith, D., & Thorp, M. (2011). Nurse-coordinated care in CKD: Time for translation into practice? *Clinical Journal of American Society of Nephrology, 6*, 1229–1231.

Soni, R., Weisbord, S., & Unruh, M. (2010). Health-related quality of life outcomes in chronic kidney disease. *Current Opinion in Nephrology and Hypertension, 19*, 153–159.

Stanley, M. (2010). Peritoneal dialysis *versus* haemodialysis (adult). *Nephrology, 15*, S24–S31.

Thomas, M. (2011). Chronic kidney disease: the six red flags. *Medicine Today, 12*, 14–26.

Turner, J., Bauer, C., Abramowitz, M., et al. (2012). Treatment of chronic kidney disease. *Kidney International, 81*, 351–362.

Unruh, M. L., Weisbord, S., & Kimmel, P. (2005). Health-related quality of life in nephrology research and clinical practice. *Seminars in Dialysis, 18*, 82–90.

Untas, A., Thumma, J., Rascle, N., et al. (2011). The associations of social support and other psychosocial factors with mortality and quality of life in the dialysis outcomes and practice patterns study. *Clinical Journal of American Society of Nephrology*, *6*, 142–152.

White, S., Dunstan, D., Polkinghorne, K. R., et al. (2010). Physical inactivity and chronic kidney disease in Australian adults: The AusDiab study. *Nutrition, Metabolism & Cardiovascular Disease*, *21*, 104–111.

Wiedebusch, S., Konrad, M., Foppe, H., et al. (2010). Health-related quality of life, psychosocial strains, and coping in parents of children with chronic renal failure. *Pediatric Nephrology*, *25*(8), 1477–1485.

Wong, F., Chow, S., & Chan, T. (2010). Evaluation of a nurse-led disease management programme for chronic kidney disease: a randomized controlled trial. *International Journal of Nursing Studies*, *47*(3), 268–278.

World Health Organization. (2006). Global database on body mass index. Retrieved May 9, 2012, from http://apps.who.int/bmi/index.jsp?introPage=intro_3.html

Wright, J., Wallston, K., Elasy, T., et al. (2011). Development and results of a kidney disease knowledge survey given to patients with CKD. *American Journal of Kidney Disease*, *57*(3), 387–395.

Yong, D., Kwok, A., Wong, D., et al. (2009). Symptom burden and quality of life in end-stage renal disease: A study of 179 patients on dialysis and palliative care. *Palliative Medicine*, *23*(2), 111–119.

CHAPTER

23

Michelle Woods

Chronic diseases of the bowel

Learning objectives

When you have completed this chapter you will be able to:

- explain the pathophysiology of irritable bowel syndrome and inflammatory bowel disease, including Crohn's disease and ulcerative colitis
- outline the nursing role when caring for a patient diagnosed with irritable bowel syndrome or inflammatory bowel disease
- describe the clinical manifestations of inflammatory bowel disease
- describe the effects that altered body image may have on a patient diagnosed with inflammatory bowel disease
- highlight the patient-centred interventions that may be considered when working with patients diagnosed with irritable bowel syndrome.

Key words

biopsychosocial condition, Crohn's disease, inflammatory bowel disease, ulcerative colitis, supportive care

INTRODUCTION

This chapter discusses chronic diseases of the bowel, including Crohn's disease or regional enteritis, ulcerative colitis and irritable bowel syndrome. More specifically, the principles and practices of supportive care for patients who have been diagnosed with inflammatory bowel disease (IBD) or with irritable bowel syndrome (IBS) will be presented.

IBD is a collective group of disorders that are chronic and incurable and characterised by inflammation in the intestinal tract. Crohn's disease (CD) and ulcerative colitis (UC) are two prominent and distinctive inflammatory bowel disorders. The disorders share the challenging characteristics of being largely unpredictable in the cycle of relapses (acute exacerbations) remission and in the severity in symptoms. Both are associated with high morbidity and decreased quality of life (QOL) (Longobardi, Jacobs, & Bernstein, 2003).

Epidemiological studies across developed countries highlight a rise in prevalence of these two disorders (Cummings, Keshav, & Travis, 2008). IBD is said to affect one in 400 people in the United Kingdom (Edge, 2006; Johnson, 2007) and smaller population studies in New Zealand and Australia (Wilson et al., 2010) indicate a rising annual incidence rate of IBD. Interestingly, the increased prevalence in Asia (Loftus, 2004), with a previously low incidence rate, supports the impact of environmental factors associated with the aetiology of IBD.

IBS is a chronic functional bowel disorder and is identified as having a similar rise in prevalence to IBD. It is estimated that IBS prevalence is 10–15% in the United Kingdom and 20–25% in the United States (American Gastroenterological Association, 2002; Wilson, Roberts, Roalfe, Bridge, & Singh, 2004). In Australia, a population-based study found that approximately 9% of participants meet the Rome II criteria for IBS (Boyce, Talley, Burke, & Koloski, 2006; see Box 23.1 later in this chatper).

While there is no cure for IBD or IBS, the rising prevalence has a substantial impact on the global economic burden (Access Economics, 2009). The nature of chronic bowel diseases and the age of onset tend to hinder the normal evolution of independent adulthood (Fuller-Thompson & Sulman 2006). This impingement affects psychological wellbeing and challenges for health professionals, patients and families in the provision of best practice of care for sustaining an optimal QOL. The issues arising from psychological, nutritional and other life issues that arise in association with chronic illness and IBD have been noted as the most challenging for clinicians (Gibson, 2009). Nurses play an integral role in facilitating patients' treatment goals. These goals involve non-pharmacological and pharmacological interventions and aim for intervals long in remission and short in acute exacerbations.

The role of the nurse in caring for people at risk and living with IBD and IBS is directly involved with primary, supportive and restorative care. For instance, a patient may confide in a primary care nurse, completing a chronic conditions care plan, that she is having multiple bowel motions per day, is periodically bloated and these symptoms are interfering with her capacity to work effectively in her current employment. Through further subjective assessment questions, the nurse identifies that the patient meets the Rome III criteria (see Box 23.1) for IBS and discusses these concerns with the patient and a medical practitioner for further review.

BOX 23.1
Rome III diagnostic criteria for irritable bowel syndrome

At least 3 months, with onset at least 6 months previously, of recurrent abdominal pain or discomforts* associated with two or more of the following:

- improvement with defecation; and/or
- onset associated with a change in frequency of stool; and/or
- onset associated with a change in form (appearance) of stool.

*Discomfort means an uncomfortable sensation not described as pain.

An acute care nurse may look after a patient experiencing an acute exacerbation of UC that results in a total colectomy with an ileal pouch–anal anastomosis who requires intravenous medications and supportive parenteral feeding. A specialist IBD nurse and/or nurse practitioner may monitor and provide support for a CD patient post-ileostomy. Additional interventions over time may include supporting the patient and their family in a collaborative plan that foresees strategies to decrease their risk for future exacerbation of CD.

Specific interventions vary on the nurse's practice arena, level of specialisation and advancement in practice. Intervention range may include, but is not limited to: initial assessment of IBD and IBS; preparations and ordering of diagnostic investigations; education and identification of factors contributing to the patient's capacity to adhere to medication; and providing and referring patients to support services. Central to all nurses is their role in facilitating the patient and their family/carer's understanding and efficacy that is necessary in living with a functionally challenging disease.

As with all chronic conditions, patients may become complex in their care needs and need a multidisciplinary care team to provide optimal care. An IBD patient may interact with the following healthcare providers: general practitioner; medical specialist; gastroenterologist; rheumatologist; practice nurse; nurse practitioner; stoma and/or IBD specialist nurse; dietitian; and psychologist. Further discussion and guidance regarding multidisciplinary teams can be found in Chapter 2.

INFLAMMATORY BOWEL DISEASE: TWO DISTINCTIVE DISORDERS

A nurse's capacity to provide quality nursing care for patients living with IBD is enhanced by a sound understanding of the aetiology, pathophysiology, disease trajectory and treatment options. CD and UC come under the heading of IBD as two distinct diseases with similar characteristics and symptoms. The main difference between Crohn's disease and ulcerative colitis is the *location* and *nature* of the inflammatory changes (Nightingale, 2007).

CD is a chronic inflammatory condition non-specific to a single area of the gastrointestinal (GI) system, affecting the whole bowel wall resulting in transmural lesions (Metcalf, 2002). The most common sites affected are the terminal ileum, jejunum and colon (Bliss & Sawchuk, 2005). The inflammation process is frequently discontinuous with normal bowel separating portions of diseased bowel.

In the earliest stages of the disease inflammation promotes lesion formation in the intestinal sub-mucosa, which over time traverses the intestinal wall to eventually involve the mucosa and serosa (Huether, 2006). These lesion formations lead to thickening of the intestinal wall and on inspection can be likened to a cobblestone (Huether, 2006). This leads to intestinal wall lumen narrowing and associated stricture development. The affected areas are in many cases regional, as they may affect one particular area of the bowel, skip a section and then represent as another affected area. These discontinuous areas are classified as 'skip lesion' (Bliss & Sawchuk, 2005).

The diagnosis of CD is confirmed by symptom history and clinical evaluation. Patient symptoms will vary due to the severity of inflammation and the area of bowel affected (Normile, 2004). Symptoms include increased frequency of bowel motions, abdominal pain, rectal bleeding (although rare), weight loss, reduced appetite and faecal incontinence (Huether, 2006; Younge & Norton, 2007).

The urgency of diarrhoea (bloody in colonic Crohn's) is often associated with mucus. Stricturing or narrowing of the intestine in CD can lead to obstructive symptoms

TABLE 23.1
Distinguishing features of Crohn's disease and ulcerative colitis

KEY FEATURES	CROHN'S DISEASE	ULCERATIVE COLITIS
Symptoms	Diarrhoea, fever, sores around the anus, abdominal pains and cramps, pain and swelling in the joints, anaemia, fatigue, loss of appetite, weight loss	Bloody diarrhoea, mild fever, inflamed rectum, abdominal pains and cramps, fatigue, loss of appetite, weight loss, pain and swelling in joints
Affected area	Mouth to anus	Colon only
Rectum involvement	Rectum sparing	Always
Inflammation of GI layers	Transmural	Mucosal layers only
Lesions	Granulomas	Granulomas are rare
Frank and occult bleeding per rectum	Up to 1/3 no evidence of bleeding	Most often frank blood
Cure	Incurable Maintenance therapy is used to reduce the chance of relapse	Through colectomy only Maintenance therapy is used to reduce the chance of relapse

associated with abdominal pain, constipation and vomiting. In more severe exacerbations anorexia, weight loss and anaemia lead to fatigue.

To exclude anaemia and infections both acute and chronic, pathology investigations include full blood count, inflammatory markers such as C-reactive protein and erythrocyte sedimentation rate (ESR). Stool cultures provide evidence to exclude infections such as *Clostridium difficile* toxin (Mowat et al., 2011). Confirmation of a diagnosis is through the utilisation of ileocolonoscopy and biopsy of the colonic and terminal ileal disease (Morrison, Headon, & Gibson, 2009).

UC is a chronic disease of the bowel that affects the mucosa and sub-mucosa of the colon and rectum. In most cases, the inflammatory process is confined to the rectum and sigmoid colon. However, it may progress to involving the entire colon, stopping at the ileocaecal junction (LeMone & Burke, 2008). The inflamed mucosa becomes oedematous, abscesses form and eventually the bowel mucosa becomes ulcerated. The ulcerations destroy the bowel mucosa and subsequently the patient may experience the primary symptom of bloody diarrhoea with the passage of mucus. Associated symptoms are lower abdominal cramping associated with urgency, called tenesmus (Johnson, 2007). Similar to CD, other manifestations include fatigue, weakness, nausea and anorexia. Typically the symptoms may last for days or weeks, followed by a period of remission. UC can be mild, moderate or severe. Classification is based on the number of bowel motions per day, associated abdominal pain, bleeding from the rectum, elevated temperature, elevated ESR and a drop in haemoglobin (King, 2007).

See Table 23.1 summarising the distinguishing features of CD and UC.

MANIFESTATIONS

The underlying autoimmune process of IBD does not confine to the bowel and extra intestinal manifestations occur in other body systems and organs. These may involve the dermatological system, ocular system, joints or the hepatobiliary system. Complications of IBD can be the result of severity in inflammation such as small bowel obstruction, toxic megacolon, fistulas and fissures, perforation and gastrointestinal blood loss (Thoreson & Cullen, 2007).

Both UC and CD are associated with an equivalent increased risk of colonic carcinoma (LeMone & Burke, 2008) Patients with UC have 7–30 times more prevalence of carcinoma of the colon than the general population. Factors attributing to increased risk of carcinoma of the colon are the duration of the colitis and the extent of colitis involvement (Thoreson & Cullen, 2007).

Demographics and aetiology

The exact cause of IBD is not known but rather the model in understanding the aetiology is multifactorial where an autoimmune response is strongly correlated with a genetic predisposition and triggered by modifiable and environmental risk factors.

Non-modifiable risk factors

The non-modifiable risk factors (Thoreson & Cullen 2007; Loftus, 2004) are detailed below.

- Gender: females tend to have a predominance of CD, whereas males tend to have a higher incidence of UC.
- Age: both CD and UC are most commonly diagnosed in late adolescence and early adulthood; however, the diagnosis may occur at any age.
- Race/ethnicity: studies comparing the prevalence of IBD among different ethnic groups suggests genetic predispositions. There is also strong evidence to suggest that CD does have some genetic predisposition, with between 12 and 18% of patients having some family history of the disease (Metcalf, 2002).
  - IBD has been recorded to be 2–4 times greater in Jewish populations as compared to other ethnic groups. Caucasians have a higher incidence of IBD. Ethnic and racial differences may be more related to lifestyle and environmental influences than genetic differences.

Modifiable risk factors

Modifiable risk factors (behaviours that contribute to disease probability) are detailed below.

- Cigarette smoking: implications for increased risk for CD (Thoreson & Cullen, 2007).
- Dietary: considerable speculation but inconsistent findings regarding the role food antigens may have as a trigger for the inflammatory reaction in IBD. A number of studies have implicated cow's milk, refined sugar, decreased vegetable intake and high fat intake as dietary risk factors for the development IBD (Punyanganie de Silva, Lund, Chan & Hart, 2011).
- Non-steroidal anti-inflammatories: studies linked to risk for the development of IBD and may exacerbate underlying IBD (Ananthakrishnan et al., 2012).
- Psychosocial factors: stress as an independent factor does not appear to directly contribute to a diagnosis of IBD. However stress may have a role in the exacerbation of symptoms possibly via activation of the enteric nervous system and the elaboration of pro-inflammatory cytokines (Johnson, 2007).

Treatment

Non-pharmacological

Nutritional therapy becomes a central focus in treatments of IBD (Mowat et al., 2011). It is essential for patients to have referral and access to a specialised dietitian with appropriate supplementation instituted as indicated (Nightingale, 2007). Patients are at risk for malnutrition secondary to the disease by avoiding foods perceived by the patient as triggering symptoms and pain and disease sequelae of malabsorption. In addition, long-term administration of steroids adversely results in poor bone mineralisation resulting in osteoporosis and predisposing children and adolescents to retarded growth (Mowat et al., 2011). Osteoporosis is due to: the relationship between inflammatory responses and an increase in bone breakdown; the use of corticosteroids as a treatment option; and diminished vitamin D and calcium levels due to malabsorption (Razack & Seinder, 2007).

Patients are particularly at risk for malnutrition in times of acute exacerbations — pain, nausea and diarrhoea. Malnutrition is the result of anorexia, malabsorption, fluid and electrolyte disturbance and side effects from medications (Razack & Seinder, 2007). Patients with CD are susceptible to large amounts of fluid loss due to malabsorption and consequently a reduction of essential electrolytes, especially potassium and magnesium (Normile, 2004; Ruthruff, 2007). Fluid and electrolyte balances are of paramount concern and, if possible, patients should be encouraged to drink between one and two litres of fluid per day to counteract these large losses (Ruthruff, 2007). Due to the involvement of all layers of the gastrointestinal wall and subsequent damage to intestinal mucosa, diets high in fat or milk and milk products are poorly absorbed (Bliss & Sawchuk, 2005) and are therefore often avoided.

Subsequently, malnutrition leads to fatigue and an inability to carry out some activities of daily living. Assessment for risk for malnutrition can be validated through such tools as Malnutrition Universal Screening Tool (MUST) available at http://www.bapen.org.uk/pdfs/must/must_full.pdf (last retrieved July 2012). Of particular importance is the distal bowel's involvement and receptor sites in the absorption of solely bile salts, vitamin B12 and magnesium. With both CD and UC impaired absorption results in nutritional deficiencies.

The most common nutritional deficiencies are:

- calories, protein and fat
- calcium
- vitamin D
- iron
- folic acid
- vitamin B12
- electrolytes and fluid.

In general there is no specific diet that has been found to be efficacious and patients should be encouraged to eat a balanced and nutritionally dense diet as tolerated (Eiden, 2003). Specific requirements are based on individual assessments and recommendations made based on symptoms and patient preferences. Specific dietary considerations include lactose intolerance, presence of bowel stricture/luminal narrowing and ostomies.

In specific circumstances protein and caloric support is indicated such as in perioperative care of patients with significant weight loss. In severe cases of CD intestinal failure is an indication for parenteral nutrition due to the extremely poor absorption rates of fluids and electrolytes (Bliss & Sawchuk, 2005). Element liquid feeding is an alternative to steroids and may be a consideration for children and adolescents to ensure optimal growth before fusion of epiphyses prohibits growth. This treatment option appears to have an anti-inflammatory effect and does require considerable motivation and dietetic support (O'Sullivan and O'Morain, 2001).

Pharmacological treatment

The goals of IBD treatment are to induce and maintain remission of both clinical symptoms and mucosal inflammation, and to re-establish the intestinal barrier, so as to reduce relapse and complication and to improve QOL. The treatment goal for long remission and symptom-free intervals is often enhanced by the anti-inflammatory and immunosuppressant agents. Treatment is initiated and monitored through a stepwise approach and more recently a top-down approach (Morrison, Headon, & Gibson, 2009).

5-Amino salicylic acid (5-ASA) drugs, such as sulfasalazine and mesalazine, are anti-inflammatory drugs indicated for mild-to-moderate symptoms of UC. The maintenance of remission and their intestinal inflammation in CD is controversial and tends to be limited to reduction of post-surgical reoccurrence limited to the small bowel if used in high doses (Gearry, Ajlouni, Nandurkar, Iser, & Gibson, 2007).

The use of antibiotic therapy, including metronidazole and ciprofloxacin, have an important role in treating secondary complications in IBD, such as abscess and bacterial overgrowth (Ruthruff, 2007). Long-term administration of antibiotics has been used in CD patients who have fistulas or recurrent abscesses near their anus. Patients whose active disease is successfully treated with antibiotics may be kept on these as maintenance therapy as long as the medications remain effective.

Corticosteroids are generally administered for severe exacerbations or 'flare-up' periods of the disease, and are usually continued for up to 3 weeks before being slowly tapered prior to discontinuation (Ruthruff, 2007). The route and dose of corticosteroids is determined by the severity of the symptoms and the therapeutic response to other drug therapies (Bliss & Sawchuk, 2005). The anti-inflammatory properties of corticosteroids suppress the symptoms of the disease and allow for affected areas to repair; however, patients require close monitoring due to the serious side effects of these drugs.

The anti-inflammatory properties of corticosteroids suppress the symptoms of the disease and allow for affected areas to repair; however, patients require close monitoring due to the adverse reactions of these drugs. Notable steroid adverse reactions include changes to body appearance such as acne, weight gain and distribution of fat deposits to the face, neck and abdomen. Daily disturbance in function include poor quality of sleep and metabolic changes can lead to impaired glucose tolerance and steroid induced diabetes.

Immunomodulators, such as azathioprine and mercaptopurine, are the long-term maintenance medication therapy for patients with more than mild CD and for chronically active or frequently relapsing UC where 5-ASA drugs sustained maintenance (Mowat et al., 2011). The goal of using this class of medication is to control active inflammation, allow for the withdrawal of steroids and ultimately to maintain long-term remission of CD and UC. Because immunomodulators weaken or modulate the activity of the immune system, decreasing the inflammatory response, patients are at risk for serious and opportunistic infections (Morrison, et al., 2009).

The chronic nature of CD and UC results in many patients exploring and engaging alternative treatment options and remedies to relieve their symptoms. While acupuncture, reflexology and aromatherapy are considered appropriate stress reduction techniques, some therapies may interact with prescribed medications, and therefore the patient should be instructed to discuss these therapies with their medical provider, nurse or pharmacist in the first instance (Bliss & Sawchuk, 2005). Notably, patients are at risk for overnight remedies promising 'quick relief' from IBD. Many products marked as 'bowel cleansing' can put patients at risk for electrolyte imbalances and disruption to bowel flora.

Surgery

Surgical intervention is often required for patients experiencing severe symptoms and episodes of the disease, and those who are unresponsive to conservative management strategies. Surgical therapy is a consideration for patients living with CD and up to 80% of patients with a 20-year trajectory of CD will have at least one bowel surgery (Thoreson & Cullen, 2007).

Surgery is usually required to stop bleeding, close fistulas, bypass obstructions or remove the affected areas of the intestine (Carter, Lobo, & Travis, 2004).

Indications are considered in relation to the length of time a patient has had the disease and the site within the gastrointestinal tract. Surgery may be considered as an option for UC patients who do not respond to other forms of treatment. Some patients with UC require a total colectomy with an ileal pouch–anal anastomosis (LeMone & Burke, 2008).

IRRITABLE BOWEL SYNDROME

> It's terrible. The symptoms are sometimes constant. There's diarrhoea and abdominal pain or constipation and bloating. I can't commit to anything too far in advance or anything that is regularly occurring. Wherever I go I need to find out where the toilets are; I often feel embarrassed.
>
> (patient quote)

IBS is a chronic functional bowel disorder characterised by the relapse and remission of abdominal pain or discomfort, bowel dysfunction and abdominal bloating (Agrawal & Whorwell, 2006; American Gastroenterological Association, 2002; Gastroenterology Society of Australia, 2003). Bowel dysfunction associated with IBS may occur in four different forms: constipation predominant (sluggish); diarrhoea predominant (hyperactive); alternating between constipation and diarrhoea (alternating); and non-extreme (Alison, 2002). A diagnosis of IBS is made by the exclusion of an organic disease and is based on diagnostic criteria. The Rome III IBS symptom-based diagnostic criteria are used to diagnose IBS (see Box 23.1) (Drossman, 2006).

In developed countries the majority of patients diagnosed with IBS are women, and typically first presentation with clinical symptoms is between 30 and 50 years of age (Boyce et al., 2006). IBS is one of the most common GI diseases and accounts for approximately 50% of referrals to gastroenterology outpatient clinics (Smith, 2006). The aetiology of IBS is understood as a biopsychosocial disorder and multifactorial in nature (Agrawal & Whorwell, 2006; Camileri & Choi, 1997). The altered bowel function, motility and sensation in the small bowel and colon are modulated from the central nervous system, referred to as the brain–gut axis (Smith, 2006). Multiple factors predisposing a person to IBS have been identified and categorised as: genetics; dietary factors, such as lactose intolerance; inflammation, such as yeast infection; and neurotransmitter, such as serotonin imbalances (Lembo, 2006).

The perception of stress initiates and/or exacerbates intensity of gastrointestinal motility that leads to a heightened perception of sensation. Unaddressed chronic and severe psychosocial factors result in poor resolution of IBS symptoms (Bennett et al., 1998), which exemplifies the biopsychosocial relationship of chronic conditions (Frankel, Quill, & McDaniel, 2003).

It is unlikely that psychological factors cause IBS, but the evidence suggests that depression and anxiety exert a strong influence on patients living with IBS compared to non-IBS suffers. Associations have been made between psychiatric disturbances and IBS pathogenesis. Seeking consultation for IBS symptoms is clearly dependent on the number of symptoms reported (especially abdominal pain) and has also been shown to correlate with high depression and anxiety scores (Graff, Walker, & Bernstein, 2009). Sexual and physical abuse may play a role in IBS as well. Reports from specialty clinics to which patients with severe cases of IBS are referred indicate that a significant percentage of women with IBS have a history of abuse (Thompson, 2002). Difficulty arises in interpreting the implications of co-morbidity between IBS and psychiatric disorders as primary or secondary (reactionary) (Smith, 2006).

Treatment

Non-pharmacological

Foods can be related to symptoms where GI stimulants or irritants such as spicy and fatty foods, caffeine and unrefined carbohydrates cause contraction of the intestine and cramping (Alison, 2002; Gunn, Cavin, & Mansfield, 2003). The GI deficiency of lactulose reduces intolerance to dairy foods and patients with lactose intolerance find that symptoms decrease when they have a limited amount of dairy products (Gastroenterology Society of Australia, 2003).

Gibson and Shepherd (2010) provide evidence of clinical trials restricting rapidly fermenting short-chain carbohydrates (FODMAP) in the control of functional gut symptoms. It is now widely accepted that this approach in restricting for patient with nil persistent symptoms has a durable effect in controlling symptoms (Gibson, 2009). Referral to a dietitian is warranted if patients need advice on the application of an elimination diet to assess trigger foods.

Similarly with IBD: non-pharmacological strategies such as relaxation therapy, hypnotherapy, short-term psychodynamic psychotherapy and cognitive behavioural therapy have been shown to decrease symptom distress (Taylor & Taylor, 2011).

Pharmacological

Medications provide partial relief of symptoms depending on the patient's symptom presentation. Therapy focuses on symptomatic relief of pain, diarrhoea and constipation (Agrawal & Whorwell, 2006; American Gastroenterological Association, 2002; Gastroenterology Society of Australia, 2003). However, many IBS patients have no long-lasting relief of symptoms after drug treatment. Over-the-counter medications such as paracetamol and ibuprofen can provide some relief for pain, but ibuprofen can cause gastritis.

CHRONIC DISEASES OF THE BOWEL: NURSING IMPLICATIONS

Nursing is a discipline in the understanding of human responses to the human conditions of illness, disease and injury. As a prime caregiver and advocate for patient self-management, the nurse needs to be able to demonstrate patient-centred care that is responsive to complex and challenging disorders. The nurse works in partnership with patients towards the patient outcome of self-management, which is:

> engaging in activities that protect and promote health, monitoring and managing of symptoms and signs of illness, managing the impacts of illness on functioning, emotions and interpersonal relationships and adhering to treatment regimens (Grunman & Von Korff, 1996, p. 1).

The effects of IBD and IBS on QOL include: overall health; vitality; sexual function; sleep; social functioning; and bodily pain. Nursing assessment identifies how these factors are related to behaviours that contribute to the development of the condition, alter mobility and body image and behaviours that sustain remission.

Behaviours that contribute to the development of the condition or sustain remission

Assessment of a patient's knowledge and understanding of their disease, its process, triggers, support systems and a patient's attributes of resilience and capacity to sustain treatment protocols in remission is key to establishing a collaborative care plan (Box 23.2). Furthermore, the role in chronic condition management may be one of identifying lifestyle behaviours that put the patient at risk for optimal health, such as cigarette smoking. A chronic condition management plan is only as good as the level of patient engagement in problem solving and negotiating achievable actions that are patient-centred. The role of the nurse, therefore, is in facilitation, whereby through a process of negotiation and

BOX 23.2
Steps for developing a collaborative management plan

1. Determine specific goals according to the problems and ability of the patient to self-manage. Such goals may include:
   - increase knowledge concerning their illness, lifestyle factors and treatment options
   - reduce illness symptoms
   - use symptom action plan and diaries
   - increase concordance with management strategies
   - improve function
   - reduce impact on social, emotional and personal life.
2. Prioritise goals in collaboration with the patient. Patient preferences are central but are influenced by the capacity for self-management and the available resources.
3. Determine outcomes for each of the goals using the SMART principles; that is, patient outcomes that are:
   - specific
   - measurable
   - achievable
   - reliable
   - timely.
4. Decide on the timeframe and responsibility for achievement of goals and/or monitoring. Where multiple health professionals are involved it is necessary to clearly identify the roles and responsibilities of each person. The control of this process must rest with the patient where possible. Progress monitoring, including frequency of review, must also be documented.
5. Select appropriate interventions to achieve goals using the decision-making principles.

(Royal Australian College of General Practitioners, 2006)

information sharing, treatment options and choices are discussed (Rogers-Clark, McCarthy, & Martin-McDonald, 2005).

Document the plan in the patient's notes and give the patient a copy. This may be in the form of a formal care plan into which other healthcare providers have input, a diagnosis-specific diary or monitor, or a centre-specific record (Royal Australian College of General Practitioners, 2006).

Small achievable steps are as follows (but limited to):

- ensuring sufficient rest and sleep and avoiding exhaustion
- chewing food very slowly, and avoiding overeating
- ingesting food only when emotionally calm and real hunger is present
- avoiding foods that are known triggers, such as coffee, tea, soft drinks, alcohol and so forth
- maintaining relationships with friends and family
- engaging in work and activities that are rewarding.

The chronic nature of IBD and at times increased disease activity are indicators of stress, depression and poor psychological health for patients (Fuller-Thompson & Sulman, 2006). Anxiety may not only relate to the diagnosis and symptom control, but also be associated with issues such as loss of income and an increase in family expenditure due to the cost of medical appointments, hospitalisation and medications (Normile, 2004). Nurses are in a prime position to assess patients and provide an environment where the patient and caregiver can freely discuss concerns, worries and fears. In periods of time when the patient is not managing with sustaining a plan or is exhibiting signs and symptoms of depression and anxiety a referral to a psychologist may aid the patient and their family in developing coping skills.

For patients living with IBS, the nature of the problems can be identified by the patient writing a diary of their food intake and symptoms, including the number and type of stools and the presence, severity and duration of pain. Patient awareness of these factors and symptom pattern recognition will greatly enhance self-assessment and provide the impetus to change behaviours and treatment options that can ultimately affect their condition. For example, in menstruating women, symptoms typically increase in severity immediately before or at onset of menses (Heitkemper et al., 2003). Through the course of managing IBS, patients also need to know signs and symptoms that would indicate further investigation. These have been identified as rectal bleeding, significant weight loss, fat substance in stool, diarrhoea at night and fever. Faecal occult blood testing is not an appropriate test for people with IBS symptoms (Gastroenterology Society of Australia, 2003).

Altered mobility, body image and fatigue

The stigma attached to bowel disease, as for any disease that is not visible, often means that the patient may decline to discuss symptoms, fears and concerns (Johnson, 2007; Rogers-Clark, McCarthy & Martin-McDonald, 2005). Altered body image (which may lead to low self-esteem) due to either the disease itself (pallor, skin lesions) or the side effects of treatment (weight gain from drug therapy) has a huge impact on wellbeing.

During an acute exacerbation, patients may feel lethargic or dirty, and changes in their physical appearance, secondary to weight gain due to corticosteroid treatment or weight loss due to chronic diarrhoea and malnutrition, may affect their willingness to engage in social activities. Diarrhoea and the subsequent odour are often a concern. Deodorisers and wipes should be kept close by to ensure that the dignity of the patient is maintained. Another factor to consider is perianal skin care, because often this area becomes excoriated and uncomfortable due to frequent diarrhoea (Bliss & Sawchuk, 2005). Skin integrity should also be a strong focus for the nurse. Redness and tenderness near the anus and surrounding perineum are aggravated by diarrhoea (Ruthruff, 2007).

Faecal incontinence and urgency for bowel movements can inhibit patients' confidence in employment, travel and social interactions. Consumer support web-based organisations such as Crohn's & Colitis Australia offer patients support with problem-solving ideas. For example, the *Can't Wait Card* aids people living with Crohn's or colitis (IBD) to gain access to a toilet in times of urgency (see http://www.cantwait.net.au/, retrieved July 2012). The National Institute of Clinical Excellence (2007) recommends that the patient continuing to have faecal incontinence should be referred to a specialist. Practical advice for patients with faecal incontinence includes, but is not limited to:

- eat small, frequent meals
- reduce intake of fibre, spicy and fried food
- avoid caffeine and other stimulants (artificial sweeteners)
- use simple pelvic floor exercises
- try neutralising sprays
- take an emergency kit when you go out
- wear clothes that conceal accidents
- when travelling know your journey and plan your route.

Fatigue is multifactorial and can be attributable to a number of reasons requiring a comprehensive assessment and investigative pathology. Fatigue can be attributable to poor sleep throughout a night due to nocturnal diarrhoea and abdominal pain. Other factors include malnutrition and iron deficit anaemia. In times of an acute exacerbation restricted activity and bed rest are to be encouraged (Bliss & Sawchuk, 2005) during symptomatic episodes. Surgical interventions, such as a resection of the affected area or formation of a stoma, can lead to impaired body image and is a challenging impairment to bodily function (Metcalf, 2002). Nurses can aid in stoma management and/or refer the patient to specialist nurses.

The impact of IBD and IBS on sexuality and sexual function is significant (Access Economics, 2009). Principles in assessing and addressing QOL and altered body image pertaining to sexuality and sexual function are addressed in Chapter 7. See Box 23.3 regarding how to measure the QOL.

Interventions to attain compliance

A key component of the treatment regimen for IBD is medication management, because medication therapy may induce remission (Normile, 2004) and reduce the incidence of relapse. In addition, the adherence of oral vitamins such as vitamin D and calcium is recommended in promoting bone health (Punyanganie de Silva et al., 2011). Clear review of the patient and family knowledge and verification of medications is necessary to enhance their understanding of the indication and rationale. Equally important is assessing the patient's beliefs in medication administration and side effects experienced. In addition, assessment of complementary alternative therapies is necessary to identify the drug interactions (Bliss & Sawchuk, 2005).

Notably the efficacy of medications in sustaining patients in remission is enhanced through the consistency of administration. Improving patient understanding of the disease may assist in identification of the precursory signs and symptoms, which may in turn reduce relapse rates (Younge & Norton, 2007). For instance, studies have shown 5-ASA

BOX 23.3
Measuring quality of life

VALIDATED QUESTIONNAIRES USEFUL TO ASSESS QUALITY OF LIFE AND GUT HEALTH

IBS-Quality of life (IBS-QOL)	Validated for assessment of QOL specific to IBS: 34 questions
Inflammatory Bowel Disease Questionnaire (IBDQ)	Validated for assessment of health-related quality of life (HRQOL) in adult patients with IBD
Bowel Disease Questionnaire (BDQ)	Validated to distinguish patients with functional and organic GI disease
Health Status Questionnaire (HSQ-12)	Validated for assessment of HRQoL in the general population
Short Form Health Survey SF-12 (SF-12)	Validated for assessment of HRQoL in the general population

(Bischoff, 2011)

drug regimens have a relatively low compliance rate (Morrison, et al., 2009). Problem solving with a UC patient not adhering to daily administration may involve changing the delivery from twice a day administration to once a day and/or highlighting the association of decreased risk of colorectal cancer with the consistent administration of 5-ASA drugs (Mowat et al., 2011).

Core interventions that may promote compliance include: access to support groups; rapid access and triage to health services; and patient and family educational strategies (Metcalf, 2002; Ruthruff, 2007). Support groups provide an avenue for patients to share their experiences and have the ability to develop coping skills and strategies (Metcalf, 2002). Support groups can attempt to overcome the isolation and fear associated with IBD and offer additional support to that provided from family and friends (Younge & Norton, 2007).

Education and family and carer support

While medical treatment aims at controlling inflammation, education centres on patient self-management, where the patient ultimately becomes the expert in managing their condition with the assistance of support networks. As with any chronic disease, patients with IBD must manage their treatment regimens as well as any symptoms which may arise. This requires focus and commitment while they still try to maintain a 'normal' life (Rogers-Clark et al., 2005).

Anticipatory guidance related to outcomes and disease process as well as disease trajectory and management may also be provided. However, it is important to discuss this information once the patient has demonstrated a readiness to learn more (Lubkin & Larsen, 2006). Ongoing support and education pertaining to medication management, diet nutrition and lifestyle changes are the prime focus of the nurse. Keeping patients informed about recommended dietary intakes, pain management, fluid intake and associated stress management techniques, including low-impact exercises and relaxation strategies, will provide significant emotional support (Ruthruff, 2007) (Box 23.4).

The role of the nurse specialist in the field of IBD is now recognised in many countries (Johnson, 2007), with nurses working alongside patients and their families to provide support, assistance and education (Edge, 2006). However, if access to a clinical nurse specialist is not available it is important for the patient and their family to have regular contact

BOX 23.4
Education for the person and family

A patient-centred approach to care for patients with IBS that explores the patient's illness experience and knowledge of their condition is aimed at facilitating self-management of their condition.

There are six interactive components of patient-centred care.

1. Exploring both the disease and the illness experience (FIFE) including:
   - their Feelings, such as fear about being ill
   - their Ideas about what is wrong with them
   - the Functional impact of their problems
   - their Expectations about what should be done.
2. *Understanding the whole person.* Over time the healthcare provider will come to know the patient and the patient's context-of-life setting and stage of personal development.
3. *Finding common ground.* To develop an effective management plan, the patient, healthcare provider and other appropriate health professionals must come to an agreement about:
   - the nature of the problems and priorities
   - the goals of treatment
   - the role of the patient and other healthcare providers.
4. *Incorporating prevention and health promotion.* It is important to find common ground for opportunities for disease prevention and health promotion.
5. *Enhancing the patient–healthcare provider relationship.* The development of the patient–healthcare provider relationship is essential.
6. *Being realistic.* Skills of priority setting, resource allocation and teamwork can be used to effect efficient time management. It is also important to make goals and timeframes for their achievement realistic.

(Royal Australian College of General Practitioners, 2006)

with their general practitioner, and visit a dietitian. The patient and family may also choose to join a community support group related to IBD.

Family support and education in conjunction with patient education is an essential area of focus. For example, families of patients with Crohn's disease must not only deal with the debilitating effects of this condition, but also the possible long-term effects, which include ongoing hospital admissions and, at times, surgical interventions and stoma formation (Normile, 2004).

Quality of life

Younge and Norton (2007) suggest that 88.5% of individuals with Crohn's disease experience a significantly diminished QOL due to the chronic nature of the condition. It is therefore a disease that is difficult for the patient to deal with because, as mentioned previously, most patients are diagnosed during the prime of their life. QOL may become affected due to the isolating nature of the disease, as some individuals claim they have lost control over their body.

Although IBS is not a life-threatening condition it can have a disabling impact upon the patient's health and lifestyle (Robinson et al., 2006). Patients with IBS commonly report that symptoms interfere with work, social activities and personal relationships (Smith, 2006). The patients who experience constipation-dominant IBS describe the straining of stool as leaving them with the feeling of incomplete evacuation. Patients in the diarrhoea-predominant group experience an increase in gut motility and secretions often leading to urgency and often faecal incontinence (Boyd-Carson, 2004). Non-gut symptoms reported include lethargy, heartburn, backache, nausea, urinary problems, weakness, palpitations and loss of appetite (Gastroenterology Society of Australia, 2003). It is the summation and chronicity of these symptoms and presence of pain that reduces patients' QOL on multiple levels, including diminished physical, social and emotional wellbeing (Lacy et al., 2007).

Finally the evaluation of QOL in living with a chronic condition can be further validated, measured through the utilisation of QOL surveys and assessment tools (Box 23.3) that include disease specific questions. These can be utilised to support a program targeted at the patient living with IBD and IBS or as individual markers in living with a chronic and challenging condition.

CONCLUSION

Living with a chronic bowel disease can be a debilitating and frustrating experience, as the patient and their family members come to terms with symptom control and management. While there is no one single treatment modality, supportive care of patients and their family members focuses on careful explanation, reassurance and education relating to diet, lifestyle factors and pharmacological interventions. Continuity of care is of utmost importance for these patients, and nurses are in a prime position where they can provide this care, based on individualised managed care plans.

Reflective questions

1 You are a practice nurse working in a rural general practice and have observed that the patients coming into the practice with Crohn's disease and UC have high rates of depression. To the best of your knowledge there are no resources for support, including no dietitian, in the town. Explore how you would, firstly, validate the need to address your observation and, secondly, what actions you could take to address your observation.

2 As a practice nurse in this rural clinic you observe that the compliance of long-term medications is low. Develop a list of the classes of medications indicated for IBD; design a table for patients so that they can view the rationale, the benefits, the potential side effects, what needs to be monitored and when and solutions to aid in daily compliance to a medication regimen.

3 Today in the rural practice you are working in the 'drop-in clinic'. A recently retired 45-year-old female tourist enters your facility and asks for information relating to IBS. She has been recently diagnosed with this condition, and she is concerned about her dietary regimen while travelling. Her husband is concerned about her abdominal bloating and flatulence. What information would you give her?

CASE STUDY 23.1

You are a school nurse at a high school and Amy, a 15-year-old female student, comes into your clinic because she cannot complete her exams. She states that she has terrible diarrhoea — foul smelling and bloody. She is fearful of faecal incontinence, as this would be humiliating and embarrassing. She states that this happened a year ago and she was diagnosed with UC. Amy states, 'I went on medications and then it went away and I thought I would not have to worry about it again'. She states that she has hidden the symptoms of abdominal pain and weight loss for the past month, but she cannot continue to hide them. She did recall that her parents and boyfriend had pestered her to take the medications but she did not see the point.

Amy says she is feeling isolated and none of her friends know that she has this 'disease'. She asks for your help. She currently does have a GP but has not kept up with appointments.

In assessment, you confirm that Amy has a fair understanding of UC but does not understand the chronic nature of UC. She has not taken her Sulfasalazine for 6 months.

Case study questions

1. What are the knowledge deficits and behaviours contributing to Amy's reason for seeking care?
2. Discuss how you would establish a collaborative management plan with Amy.
3. Discuss the specifics of the following nursing interventions you utilise when working with Amy: clinical; educational; advocacy; referral; case management.

CASE STUDY 23.2

You are a community nurse taking care of Allan who is 4 days post-operative for a bowel resection. He had resection of the terminal ileum and a hemicolectomy, removing the caecum and appendix surgery, and did not necessitate an ostomy.

Allan is a 33-year-old male with a 10-year history of Crohn's disease. He has his own business and has managed his Crohn's via conservative therapy with medications and diet. Intermittent flare-ups have increased substantially over the past 2 years and he attributes this to increased stress with his business. He has controlled episodes of relapses with steroids. Over the past year he has lost 15 kg and is malnourished.

Post-surgery Allan is now taking immunosuppressants, immunomodulators (6 mercatpopurine and azathioprine) and antibody therapy (infliximab) for prevention of recurrence after surgery.

As you change his dressing Allan states that he is overwhelmed and does not know how he is going to manage. Allan confides in you: 'It has just hit me — I am worried that my children will get this ...'. In addition he was told by the gastroenterologist that his bone density test is showing signs of osteoporosis.

CASE STUDY 23.2 — cont'd

Case study questions

1 Describe what you would assess to aid Allan in his adjustment post-operatively and setback with Crohn's disease.
2 Explain the rationale for his new medication regimen.
3 What focus and resources would you utilise to problem solve with Allan and his family?
4 Alan shares that he is fearful of losing his relationship with his wife secondary to sexual dysfunction. How would you explore this further with Allan?

Recommended reading

Brown, A. C., Rampertab, S. D., & Mullin, G. E. (2011). Existing dietary guideline for Crohn's disease and ulcerative colitis. *Expert Review of Gastroenterology and Hepatology*, *5*(3), 411–425.

Cronin, E. (2011). Advances in the management of Crohn's disease. *Nurse Prescribing*, *9*(10), 499–506.

Duncan, J. (2011). Nursing assessment in inflammatory bowel disease. *Gastrointestinal Nursing*, *9*(1), 14–20.

Gethins, S., Duckett, T., Shatford, C., et al. (2011). Self-management programme for patients with long-term inflammatory bowel disease. *Gastrointestinal Nursing*, *9*(3), 33–37.

Taylor, N. S., & Taylor, K. M. (2011). Complementary and alternative medicine in inflammatory bowel disease. *Gastrointestinal Nursing*, *9*(6), 32–39.

Related websites

Associations

American College of Gastroenterology: http://www.acg.gi.org/

American Gastroenterological Association: http://www.gastro.org/

Crohn's & Colitis Australia: http://www.crohnsandcolitis.com.au/

Gastroenterological Society of Australia (GESA): http://www.gesa.org.au/about.asp?id=5

International Foundation for Functional Gastrointestinal disorders: http://www.iffgd.org

Irritable Bowel Syndrome Association: http://www.aboutibs.org; http://www.ibsassociation.org/

Self-help and support groups

IBD Support Australia: http://www.ibdsupport.org.au/about-ibd

Irritable Bowel Syndrome Self-help and Support Group: http://www.IBSgroup.org

Clinical trials

Center Watch Clinical Trials Listing Service: http://www.centerwatch.com/patient/studies/CAT90.html

Commercial sites

IBS village (Novartis): http://www.ibsvillage.com

References

Access Economics. (2009). Working with IBD, June 2009. Retrieved July 2012, from http://www.crohnsandcolitis.com.au/content/Final_IBD_report_9_June.pdf

Agrawal, P., & Whorwell, P. (2006). Irritable Bowel Syndrome: Diagnosis and Management. *British Medical Journal, 332*, 280–283.

Alison, F. (2002). Irritable Bowel Syndrome (IBS). *Journal of Community Nursing, 16*(6), 32–36.

American Gastroenterological Association. (2002). American Gastroenterological Association Medical Position Statement: Irritable Bowel Syndrome. *Gastroenterology, 123*, 2105–2107.

Ananthakrishnan, A., Higuchi, L., Huang, E., et al. (2012). Aspirin, nonsteroidal anti-inflammatory drug use, and risk for Crohn disease and ulcerative colitis: a cohort study. *Annals of Internal Medicine, 156*, 350.

Bennett, E., Tennant, C., Piesse, C., et al. (1998). Level of chronic life stress predicts clinical outcome in irritable bowel syndrome. *GUT, 43*, 256–261.

Bischoff, S. (2011). 'Gut Health' – a new objective medicine? *BioMed Central, 9*, 24. Retrieved July 2012, from http://www.biomedcentral.com/1741-7015/9/24

Bliss, D., & Sawchuk, L. (2005). Nursing management: Lower Gastrointestinal Problems. In D. Brown & H. Edwards (Eds.), *Lewis's Medical Surgical Nursing; Assessment and Management of Clinical Problems* (pp. 1056–1106). Sydney: Elsevier.

Boyce, P., Talley, N., Burke, C., et al. (2006). Epidemiology of the functional gastrointestinal disorders according to Rome II criteria: an Australian population-based study. *International Medicine Journal, 36*, 28–36.

Boyd-Carson, W. (2004). Irritable bowel syndrome: assessment and management. *Nursing Standard, 18*(52), 47.

Camileri, M., & Choi, M. (1997). Review article: irritable bowel syndrome. *Ailment Pharmacology and Therapeutics, 11*, 3–15.

Carter, M., Lobo, A., & Travis, S. (2004). IBD Section, British Society of Gastroenterology: Guidelines for the management of inflammatory bowel disease in adults. *Gut, Suppl. 5*, V1–V16.

Cummings, F., Keshav, S., & Travis, S. (2008). Medical management of Crohn's disease. *BMJ (Clinical Research Ed.), 336*, 1062–1066.

Drossman, D. (2006). *Rome III: New Criteria for the Functional GI Disorders*. Paper presented at the AGA Symposium, California.

Edge, V. (2006). A Lifelong Journey. *Nursing Standard, 20*(35), 20–21.

Eiden, K. (2003). Nutritional Considerations in Inflammatory Bowel Disease. *Practical Gastroenterology, 5*, 33–54.

Frankel, R., Quill, T., & McDaniel, S. (Eds.) (2003). *The Biopsychosocial Approach: Past, Present, Future*. Rochester: University of Rochester Press.

Fuller-Thomson, E., & Sulman, J. (2006). Depression and inflammatory bowel disease: findings from two nationally representative Canadian surveys. *Inflammatory Bowel Disease, 12*(8), 697–707.

Gastroenterology Society of Australia. (2003). *Irritable Bowel Syndrome*. Sydney: Digestive Health Foundation.

Gearry, R., Ajlouni, Y., Nandurkar, S., et al. (2007). 5-Aminosalicylic acid (mesalazine) use in Crohn's disease: a survey of the opinions and practice of Australian gastroenterologists. *Inflammatory Bowel Diseases, 13*(8), 1009–1015.

Gibson, P. (2009). Overview of inflammatory bowel disease in Australia in the last 50 years. *Journal of Gastroenterology and Hepatology, 24*(Suppl. 3), S63–S68.

Gibson, P., & Shepherd, S. (2010). Evidence-based dietary management of functional gastrointestinal symptoms: The FODMAP approach. *Journal of Gastroenterology and Hepatology, 25*, 252–258.

Graff, L. A., Walker, J. R., & Bernstein, C. N. (2009). Depression and anxiety in inflammatory bowel disease: a review of comorbidity and management. *Inflammatory Bowel Disease, 15*, 1105–1118.

Grunman, J., & Von Korff, M. (1996). *Indexed Bibliography on Self Management for People with Chronic Disease*. Washington DC: Centre for Advancement in Health.

Gunn, M., Cavin, A., & Mansfield, J. (2003). Management of irritable bowel syndrome. *Postgraduate Medical Journal, 79*(929), 154–158.

Heitkemper, M., Cain, M., Jarret, M., et al. (2003). Symptoms across the menstrual cycle in women with irritable bowel syndrome. *American Journal of Gastroenterology, 98*, 420–430.

Huether, S. (2006). Alterations of Digestive Function. In K. McCance & S. Heuther (Eds.), *Pathophysiology: the Biologic basis for Disease in Adults and Children* (pp. 1385–1445). St Louis: Elsevier.

Hurlestone, D., & Brown, S. (2007). Techniques for Targeting Screening in Ulcerative Colitis. *Postgraduate Medical Journal, 83*, 451–460.

Johnson, H. (2007). Inflammatory Bowel Disease. *Practice Nurse, 33*(7), 35–39.

King, J. (2007). Does my Patient have Ulcerative Colitis or Crohn's Disease? *Nursing 2007, 37*(3), 30.

Lacy, B., Weiser, K., Noddin, L., et al. (2007). Irritable bowel syndrome: patients' attitudes, concern and level of knowledge. *Ailment Pharmacology and Therapeutics, 25*, 1329–1341.

LeMone, P., & Burke, K. (Eds.), (2008). *Nursing care of patients with bowel disorders.* In P. LeMone & K. Burke, *Medical-Surgical Nursing, Patient Thinking in Patient Care* (4th ed., pp. 753–823) New Jersey: Pearson Education.

Lembo, A. (2006). A 54-year-old woman with constipation – Predominant Irritable Bowel Syndrome. *The Journal of American Medical Association, 295*(8), 925–933.

Longobardi, T., Jacobs, P., & Bernstein, C. (2003). Work losses related to inflammatory bowel disease in the United States: results from the National Health Interview Survey. *The American Journal of Gastroenterology, 98*, 1064–1072.

Loftus, E. (2004). Clinical epidemiology of inflammatory bowel disease: incidence, prevalence, and environmental influences. *Gastroenterology, 126*(6), 1504–1517.

Lubkin, I., & Larsen, P. (Eds.), (2006). *Chronic Illness, Impact and Interventions* (6th ed.). Sudbury, MA: Jones & Bartlett Publishers.

Malnutrition Universal Screening Tool (MUST). Retrieved July 2012 from http://www.bapen.org.uk/pdfs/must/must_full.pdf.

Metcalf, C. (2002). Crohn's Disease: An Overview. *Nursing Standard, 16*(22), 45–54.

Morrison, G., Headon, B., & Gibson, P. (2009). Update in inflammatory bowel disease. *Australian Family Physician, 38*(12), 956–961.

Mowat, C., Cole, A., Windsor, A., et al. (2011). Guidelines for the management of inflammatory bowel disease in adults. *Gut, 60*(5), 571–607.

Nightingale, A. (2007). Diagnosis and management of inflammatory bowel disease (IBD). *Nurse Prescribing, 5*(7), 289–296.

Normile, L. (2004). Disorders of the Intestines and Rectum. In J. Neal & S. Guillet (Eds.), *Care of Adults with a Chronic Illness or Disability: A Team Approach*. St Louis: Elsevier.

Nunn, P. (2003). What nurses think of IBS patients: then and now. *Gastrointestinal Nursing, 1*(1), 17–18.

Punyanganie de Silva, S., Lund, E., Chan, S., et al. (2011). Is Diet Involved in the Etiology of Ulcerative Colitis and Crohn's Disease? A Review of the Experimental and Epidemiological Literature. *Inflammatory Bowel Disease Monitor, 12*(1), 14–22.

O'Sullivan, M., & O'Morain, C. (2001). Liquid diets for Crohn's disease. *Gut, 48*, 757.

Rayhorn, N., & Rayhorn, D. (2002). An In-depth Look at Inflammatory Bowel Disease. *Nursing 2002, 32*(7), 37–43.

Razack, R., & Seinder, D. (2007). Nutrition in Inflammatory Bowel Disease. *Current Opinion in Gastroenterology, 23*, 400–405.

Robinson, A., Lee, V., Kennedy, A., et al. (2006). A randomised control trial of self-help interventions in patients with a primary care diagnosis of irritable bowel syndrome. *Gut, 55*, 643–648.

Rogers-Clark, C., McCarthy, A., & Martin-McDonald, K. (Eds.) (2005). *Living with Illness, Psychosocial Challenges for Nurses.* Sydney: Elsevier.

Royal Australian College of General Practitioners. (2006). Chronic Conditions Self Management Guidelines. Retrieved August 29, 2012, from http://www.racgp.org.au/Content/NavigationMenu/ClinicalResources/RACGPGuidelines/SharingHealthCare/20020703ahp.pdf

Ruthruff, B. (2007). Clinical Review of Crohn's Disease. *Journal of the American Academy of Nurse Practitioners, 19,* 392–397.

Smith, G. (2006). Irritable bowel syndrome: quality of life and nursing interventions. *British Journal of Nursing, 13*(21), 1152–1156.

Taylor, N. S., & Taylor, K. M. (2011). Complementary and alternative medicine in inflammatory bowel disease. *Gastrointestinal Nursing, 9*(6), 32–39.

The National Institute of Clinical Excellence. (2007). Faecal incontinence: the management of faecal incontinence in adults. Retrieved July 2012, from http://www.nice.org.uk/nicemedia/pdf/CG49NICEGuidance.pdf

Thompson, W. (2002). IBS in men: A different disease? *Practical Gastroenterology, 26*(13), 13–21.

Thoreson, R., Cullen, J. J. (2007). Pathophysiology of Inflammatory Bowel-Disease: An Overview. *Surgery Clinics of North America, 87,* 575–585.

Wilson, S., Roberts, L., Roalfe, A., et al. (2004). Prevalence of irritable bowel syndrome: a community survey. *British Journal of General Practice, 54,* 495–502.

Wilson, J., Hair, C., Knight, R., et al. (2010). High incidence of inflammatory bowel disease in Australia: a prospective population-based Australian incidence study. *Inflammatory Bowel Diseases, 16*(9), 1550–1556.

Younge, L., & Norton, C. (2007). Contribution of Specialist Nurses in Managing Patients with Irritable Bowel Syndrome. *British Journal of Nursing, 16*(4), 208–212.

CHAPTER

24

Isabelle Ellis
Keryln Carville

Non-melanocytic skin cancers and melanoma

Learning objectives

When you have completed this chapter you will be able to:

- summarise the epidemiology of skin cancer
- outline the diagnostic procedures for skin cancer
- identify the potential problems and measures used to manage these for patients with skin cancer
- describe the principles of wound management for non-melanocytic skin cancer and melanoma
- outline health education strategies for the prevention of skin cancer.

Key words

squamous cell carcinoma, basal cell carcinoma, melanoma, Marjolin's ulcer, skin cancer

INTRODUCTION

Skin cancer is the most common form of cancer, especially in Australia and New Zealand. Skin cancer can be broadly classified as either melanoma or non-melanocytic skin cancer. The Australian Institute of Health and Welfare (AIHW) estimated that in 2012 there would be 12 510 new cases of melanoma, which makes it one of the three most common forms of registrable cancer. Comparisons can be made with other malignant conditions: for men the most common cancer estimate in 2012 was prostate cancer with 18 560 new cases expected; bowel cancer was next with 8760 new cases, followed by melanoma of the skin with 7440 new cases. Women most commonly were estimated to be diagnosed with breast cancer, 14 560 new cases, followed by bowel cancer, 7080 new cases and, again, third was melanoma of the skin with 5070 new cases (AIHW, 2012). Incidence data on non-melanocytic skin cancer is not routinely collected by the Australian state and territory cancer registries. However, in 2007 over 434 000 people were treated for one or more non-melanocytic skin cancer, either squamous cell carcinoma (SCC) or basal cell carcinoma (BCC) and 448 people died of the disease (Australian Institute of Health and Welfare & Australasian Association of Cancer Registries, 2008). This makes the incidence of skin cancer in Australia more than ten times that of the other three major forms of cancer combined. In Australia about 80% of all new cases of cancer are skin cancers (The Cancer Council Australia, 2012).

BEHAVIOURS THAT CONTRIBUTE TO THE DEVELOPMENT OF SKIN CANCER

Skin cancer is generally thought to be preventable, as exposure to sunlight is now widely accepted as the highest environmental risk factor for all types of skin cancer. Although the causative relationship between sunlight exposure and skin cancer is not fully understood, there is evidence to indicate a correlation between sunburn and skin cancer (Helfand, 2003). A person's susceptibility to sunburn is related to the amount of sun exposure and their skin tone. Fair-skinned and auburn-haired people experience sunburn more readily than people with darker complexions given the same exposure (Carter, Marks, & Hill, 1999). It is believed that episodes of sunburn in childhood and the cumulative effect of sun exposure pose the greatest risk (Helfand, 2003).

Although information about the risk of sun exposure is believed to be readily available, research has shown that 70% of children and adults are not protected adequately from exposure to sunlight in the high risk areas of north west Australia where the UV index reaches 11 on most days during the dry season between May and October (Woloczyn et al., 2010). An American cross-sectional survey of 10 000 teenagers found that 83% of respondents experienced at least one episode of sunburn during the previous summer (Helfand, 2003). The Cancer Council of Australia (2007) recommends that protective measures should be employed throughout life and there are calls to regulate the solarium industry to ensure that fair skinned people and minors are prohibited from using them (Gordon, Hirst, Gies, & Green, 2008).

BASAL CELL CARCINOMA AND SQUAMOUS CELL CARCINOMA

Basal cell carcinoma (BCC) is the commonest form of skin cancer and accounts for two-thirds of all non-melanocytic skin cancers. It is most commonly found in males and those aged over 40, and is usually found on the face (AIHW, 2001). A BCC usually presents as a persistent non-healing lesion, scaly spot or pinkish-red growth. It usually begins as a small waxy nodule with rolled translucent pearly borders and telangiectatic vessels may be visible. The BCC arises from the single layer of basal cells that line the basement membrane which separates the dermis from the epidermis. It is categorised as a nodular, pigmented, superficial, morpheaform or sclerotic lesion and fortunately it rarely metastasises; instead it invades and erodes adjoining tissues (Vargo, 2006). Left unchecked a BCC can cause destruction to the tissues and result in significant loss of tissue and disfigurement.

Squamous cell carcinoma (SCC) is also a common form of skin cancer. It tends to be of greater concern than BCC as it is an invasive cancer and may metastasise via the lymph and bloodstreams. Virtually all reported cases are among people over 40 years of age, with a higher incidence among persons 70 years and above (AIHW, 2001). An SCC usually presents as a rough, thickened, scaly lesion. The lesion may be asymptomatic or may tend to bleed. Although an SCC usually appears on sun-damaged skin it may arise from a pre-existing skin lesion such as scarred or ulcerated lesions or actinic keratoses (lesions of sun exposed skin) or leukoplakia (premalignant lesions of the mucous membranes). Alternatively, it may first appear on areas of skin with no evident sun damage. An SCC is a tumour of the keratinising cells of the epidermis. It can appear anywhere on the skin or mucous membranes and it is characterised as non-invasive (superficial) or invasive (Vargo, 2006).

PRESENTATION AND DIAGNOSIS OF NON-MELANOCYTIC SKIN CANCERS

General practitioners (GPs) are the gatekeepers to the health system in Australia and elsewhere; most people will access diagnostic services for skin lesions through their GP. The patient may present to their GP with a sinister looking lesion or a non-healing ulcer. According to Winterbottom and Harcourt (2004), there are a number of factors that lead people to seek medical advice, but none of the participants with skin cancer interviewed for their study sought medical help until others had persuaded them to do so, despite significant symptoms. These authors revealed that most of the participants in their study self-diagnosed their lesions and considered them to be relatively minor problems.

Two participants' comments illustrate this point well (Winterbottom & Harcourt, 2004, p. 229):

> It started like a pimple … and I thought I had been bitten, I was putting antiseptic on it, trying to get rid of it (participant with BCC).
>
> Certain members of my family used to have various bits and pieces like that so I wondered if it was hereditary (participant with SCC).

A diagnosis of BCC and SCC requires a biopsy of the lesion (punch, shave or excision) and histopathological examination of the tissue. Regional lymph nodes should be examined for suspected SCC metastases.

MEDICAL TREATMENT

The definitive goal of medical interventions for non-melanocytic skin cancers is to remove the tumour completely. This can be achieved by: surgical excision — by Moh's micrographic surgery, in which the tumour is removed layer by layer until the tissue margins are tumour free; or electrosurgery, in which the tumour is destroyed or removed by electrical energy; or cryosurgery, in which liquid nitrogen is used to freeze the tumour; or by radiation therapy.

Surgery for most non-melanocytic skin cancer is conducted as a minor outpatient procedure or admission to a day surgery unit. However, the visible nature of the disease and the types of treatment available mean that patients are often left with visible scars or disfigurement. Although not as life-threatening as a diagnosis of melanoma, non-melanocytic skin cancers, and in particular SCC, have the potential to be fatal if they go untreated. Chemotherapy and radiation therapy may be employed in the treatment of advanced BCC or SCC metastases. It has been identified that patients who received their surgery soon after diagnosis experience reduced stress when compared to those who have to wait for treatment (Winterbottom & Harcourt, 2004).

MALIGNANT MELANOMA

Malignant melanoma is a serious form of skin cancer. Along with breast cancer melanoma is the most common cancer in those aged 15–44 years and affects males more commonly than females (Australian Institute of Health and Welfare & Australasian Association for Cancer Registries, 2010). Melanoma presents as a skin lesion commonly on the back in men and on the extremities in women. It can also present as dark areas under the nails or on the membranes that line the mouth, anus or vagina (The Cancer Council Australia, 2012). The ABCDE classification (**a**symmetry, **b**order irregularity, **c**olour variation, **d**iameter greater than 6 mm and **e**levation of the lesion) is a useful prompt for identification of skin changes related to melanomas and aids clinical diagnosis (Vargo, 2006). Melanoma prognosis is highly dependent on the clinical stage or extent of the tumour burden at diagnosis (Markovic, Erickson, Rao, Weenig, & Pockaj, 2007). The depth of invasion is the most important histological prognostic factor, along with the presence of ulceration. Once a melanoma breaks through the basement membrane of the epidermis it has the potential to grow horizontally along the junction between the epidermis and the dermis. It can disseminate to any organ but this occurs most commonly in skin and subcutaneous tissue, lymph nodes, brain, bone, liver and the gastrointestinal tract (Vargo, 2006).

Melanoma classification has changed over time. Currently the 2002 American Joint Committee on Cancer Melanoma TNM (*Primary Tumor, Regional Lymph Nodes, Distant Metastasis*) Staging Classification is frequently used. This classification assesses the primary tumour depth, lymph node involvement and the location of metastases.

Presentation and diagnosis of melanoma

As with non-melanoma skin cancer, patients access melanoma diagnosis through their GP. Patients self refer or can be referred by a skin clinic. Delay in seeking treatment is considered to be one of the factors that influences prognostic outcomes. Research by Tsao, Bevona, Goggins and Quinn (2003) which used a population based approach to calculate the risk of moles turning into melanomas estimated that there was a very low likelihood of moles becoming melanomas in the Caucasian or white population for people under the age of 20; however, with increasing age, the risk rose sharply. Men over the age of 60 years were most likely to develop melanoma. They calculated the risk per mole as approximately 1 : 33 000 in this age group. Moles are common and even in high risk groups there is a low likelihood that any one mole will become a melanoma.

There is little research on what factors lead people to access their GP for skin cancer diagnosis. In a small qualitative study by Winterbottom and Harcourt (2004) it was found, as was the case for BCC and SCC, that patients needed to be urged by others to seek medical help. Many of their study participants failed to recognise the significance of their presenting lesions. A larger grounded theory study by Walter, Humphreys, Tso, Johnson and Cohn (2010) identified that seeking help was often prompted by another person or noticing rapid changes in a mole.

There was a sense of denial illustrated well by this patient's comment (Winterbottom & Harcourt, 2004, p. 230):

> I had such a long period of just picking it, thinking it would go away. I continued and therefore my hankies were covered in blood and everything else. Just ridiculous (participant with MM).

A diagnosis of melanoma is confirmed by biopsy and histopathological examination of the primary lesion and sentinel lymph node biopsy (SLB) or regional lymph nodes if deemed warranted. The number of lymph nodes affected and the tumour burden within the lymph nodes are important diagnostic features. Detailed inspection of the skin is also performed to identify satellite or in-transit metastases. Satellites are discontinuous foci of the tumour located within 5 cm of the primary tumour and in-transit metastases are discontinuous foci found more than 5 cm from the primary tumour. The presence of either of these markers indicates a poor prognosis (Markovic et al., 2007).

Medical treatment

The principal medical intervention for melanoma depends on the stage of the disease at diagnosis. The surgical intervention for a Stage 1 tumour, or small lesion of less than 1 mm thickness with no ulceration, involves excision of the tumour. Research has shown that a margin of 1 cm is sufficient for patients with a small lesion with no lymph involvement; in these patients there is a low risk of metastases (Markovic et al., 2007).

Patients with a Stage II primary tumour of intermediate thickness, between 1 and 4 mm, require a 2 cm excision margin (Markovic et al., 2007). The local recurrence rate has been found to be influenced by the presence or absence of ulceration and the site of the primary tumour. The highest rate of recurrence has been found to be where the primary tumour was on the head and neck, or the distal extremity (Markovic et al., 2007). An SLB is indicated if lymph node involvement is suspected on clinical examination, and then lymph node dissection is indicated. Further investigations such as a computerised axial tomography scan, magnetic resonance imaging, a positron emission tomography scan and a chest X-ray will be ordered.

Stage III tumours may be treated with local excision and systemic chemotherapy or radiation therapy, although neither of these adjuvant therapies has been successful to date in curing melanoma. A systematic review of medical treatments in melanoma in 2011 concluded that despite 'decades of clinical research' patients are still experiencing poor outcomes with advanced melanoma. It is recommended that these patients be enrolled in clinical trials as there is promise in the recent combination of treatment options such as chemotherapy, immunotherapy and targeted gene therapy (Garbe, Eigentler, Kielholz, Hauschild & Kirkwood, 2011).

The interdisciplinary team will assess patients for Stage IV tumours and, if identified, a decision will be made on the likelihood of surgical excision rendering the patient disease-free. In this case a complete surgical resection will be considered. If surgery is unlikely to be successful, the patient will be considered for palliative care.

Surgical excision of local recurrences and in-transit metastases is the most effective therapy (Markovic et al., 2007). The number and location of metastases are the best indicators for long-term survival. However, long-term survival for those with metastases of the lung, brain and liver has been, on average, 2 years or less.

MARJOLIN'S ULCER

A Marjolin's ulcer is the relatively rare but aggressive transformation of a chronic wound into a degenerative malignant skin lesion (Cohen, Dieglemann, & Lindblad, 1992). The resultant epidermoid cancer is more frequently an SCC, although BCCs and melanomas have also been reported (Dupree, Boyer & Cobb, 1998). Jean Nicolas Marjolin gave his name to this malignant transformation in 1828 when he noted the malignant degeneration of a burn scar (Trent & Kirsner, 2003). Since then the term has been used to describe malignant alterations in all types of chronic wounds and includes burns, osteomyelitis, leg ulcers, pressure ulcer and fistulae. It has been estimated that 1.7% of chronic wounds

CASE STUDY 24.1

Janine Jones is a 51-year-old office worker. She lives with her husband in Tasmania now that both of her sons have moved into their own flat. Janine has had an irregular-shaped mole on the anterio-tibial region of her right leg for a long time. She can't remember exactly when her husband joked about it looking like a pig with a curly tail; possibly as long as a year ago. But she has always had moles on her arms and legs. Mostly they are fairly regular in shape. About 5 years ago she went to a clinic and had a mole scan at her mother's insistence and they said she should 'keep an eye on them' but there didn't seem to be any that were 'sinister'. Not knowing what 'keep an eye on them' meant Janine had forgotten about her moles. More recently the one on her leg had bled; she thought she must have nicked it shaving but now it doesn't seem to be healing. She decided she should make an appointment to see her GP for some specialist advice on wound healing.

After inspecting Janine's skin the GP took a punch biopsy of the mole and sent it through for histology. That afternoon the call came and Janine was advised that she needed to come into hospital to have the mole removed; it was a melanoma.

Janine was admitted for excision of primary ulcerated tumour with satellite metastases.

CASE STUDY 24.2

Max Smart is a 70-year-old man who has had poorly controlled diabetes type II for more than 15 years. Max retired about 5 years ago and lives on his own in a small cottage. Max has two cats and a dog who he is very fond of and a lovely garden that occupies most of his time.

Max has a history of peripheral vascular disease and peripheral neuropathy and is prone to lower limb ulcers, which can be difficult to heal. In the last 6 months Max has had an ulcer on his left lower leg that has been particularly difficult to heal despite visits to the GP twice a week for dressings. The wound margins of the ulcer are poorly demarcated and there appears to be a nodular lump next to the distal edge. The nurse in the clinic has been measuring the wound area using a clear acetate sheet and the wound appears to be getting larger. The clinic nurse has been taking a digital image of the wound once a fortnight.

The GP thinks it is time to admit Max to hospital to try to get his diabetes under control and to facilitate education by the diabetes educator and review by the podiatrist and the nutritionist. Prior to admission a wound swab and a wound biopsy are taken.

Max's wound biopsy results come back positive for squamous cell carcinoma. He will require cryosurgery to treat the lesion.

will transform into a Marjolin's ulcer (Trent & Kirsner, 2003), and 30% to 40% of these will metastasise (Habif, 2004). The aetiology of Marjolin's ulcers is considered to be the prolonged cellular mitotic activity that occurs during attempts to re-epithelialise the chronic wound (Menendez & Warriner, 2006). The diagnosis and treatment of a Marjolin's ulcer is aligned with that of SCC, BCC and melanoma.

NURSING MANAGEMENT

The nursing management of patients who are to undergo treatment for potentially life-threatening skin cancer should be directed towards enhancing patients' coping skills. Strategies that can be used include hopeful and goal-oriented thinking. The provision of comprehensible information about the disease has also been shown to alleviate anxiety (Dolan et al., 1997; Winterbottom & Harcourt, 2004). In Janine's case the information on the stage of the tumour and the existence of satellite metastases will be needed. Janine may be shocked that her mole is actually a potentially life-threatening skin cancer. The nurse would manage information giving in the following ways:

- develop a trusting therapeutic relationship with Janine and her husband to alleviate anxiety and increase information uptake
- provide answers to the questions relating to the medical diagnosis and the treatment options that have been outlined to Janine
- maintain and communicate a positive outlook to assist Janine and her family to remain hopeful.

Max also has a potentially life-threatening skin cancer. Although his prognosis is better than Janine's he will require the nurse to manage information giving sensitively as well. Janine has family responsibilities and Max has three pets who he cares for. It is important for the nurse to recognise that they may be more concerned about the impact of their conditions on their loved ones than on themselves in the early stages of their care journey.

Optimal wound management is also a prime requisite.

Wound management

The presence of a malignant wound is visible evidence of the existence and progression of the malignancy. Anxiety and depression are frequently associated with the presence of these wounds and can impact significantly on the individual's coping mechanisms and quality of life. The care of a person with a malignant wound can present considerable challenges to the patient, their carers and health professionals as the disease exacerbates. Malignant wounds can present as either fungating or ulcerating lesions and at times protruding nodular growths and cavity formation may co-exist. Comprehensive and ongoing assessment of the person, their wound and their healing environment is a fundamental requirement for planning and implementing optimal wound management. In Max's case the healing environment is compromised by his poorly controlled diabetes. The nurse would promote wound healing in the following ways:

- encourage Max to maintain his blood sugar within normal limits
- encourage Max to consume a diet high in essential vitamins and minerals
- apply the appropriate pressure bandages to reduce lower limb oedema
- assist with ambulation to maintain the calf pump.

A holistic and multidisciplinary approach to symptom control of presenting problems is a principal activity. Potential problems associated with malignant wounds include:

- alterations in body image
- discomfort or wound pain
- bleeding
- infection
- increased exudate
- malodour.

Alterations in body image

Preservation of body image and self-esteem are overriding principles in the care of persons with malignant wounds. Quality of life can be severely reduced by ineffectual wound management protocols. Bulky dressings or those that require frequent changes because they fail to contain exudate or malodour significantly impair a person's psychological and physical wellbeing, while the use of conformable, skin-toned dressings may help to camouflage visible lesions on exposed sites. Head and neck tumours are particularly confronting, and wound management protocols should be directed towards optimising osmesis. Skilled orthotists employed within many specialised maxillo-facial units may assist in producing custom-made cosmetic orthotics, which can assist with the camouflage of significant facial defects. In cases of facial lesions significant removal of tissue and extensive reconstructive surgery may be required. Surgical reduction or 'debulking' of extensive fungating tumours may be a possibility and can improve bodily function and appearance, although this may prove to be a temporary solution.

In Janine's case the nurse would instigate care to manage the situation in the following ways:

- recognise that Janine may be distressed by the large scar on her leg
- encourage family members to continue to visit
- schedule dressing changes prior to visiting times to maximise Janine's comfort and reduce her distress
- assist with fitting and maintenance of any orthotic devices that have been fashioned.

Discomfort or wound pain

Comprehensive assessment will indicate whether discomfort or pain is related to the disease process or wound management protocols, and both aetiologies require appropriate and adequate pain relief. Pain related to wound management regimens or dressing changes must be eradicated or minimised. Analgesia should be offered prior to dressing changes. Irradiated skin can also be very sensitive or itchy and should be assessed for signs of inflammation, desquamation and ulceration (Carville, 2005). Patients with irradiated skin require gentle skin care protocols and the frequent application of moisturisers in the form of lotions or emollients to exposed skin. It they are undergoing active radiation therapy they should avoid all metallic agents, including silver- and zinc-impregnated dressings. All patients with irradiated skin damage should be advised to avoid skin trauma, sun exposure and irritant chemicals. An increasing range of non-adherent and silicon-backed dressings and tapes can lessen deafferentation pain associated with removal of adhesive agents. The use of roller or tubular bandages and secure garments for dressing retention may be a more acceptable option.

In both Janine's and Max's case the nurse would assess any discomfort or pain relating to their surgical procedure and prior to any dressing changes.

Bleeding

Disseminated disease can result in erosion of capillaries or major blood vessels, with resulting haemorrhage. Potential or actual bleeding in malignant wounds can be extremely distressing for patients, carers and staff. Protection of fragile tissues and avoidance of local trauma or unnecessary debridement of tissues in close approximation to major blood vessels is warranted. Dry eschar can protect underlying vascular structures, while debridement can increase the risk of haemorrhage. However, increased bacterial proliferation and autolysis of moist necrotic tissue may increase malodour and the risk of infection. Therefore, conservative debridement of moist necrotic tissue may be required. Autolytic debridement offers a more conservative approach and the use of topical antimicrobial agents such as cadexomer iodine or honey dressings affords additional antimicrobial protection. However, hydrogels and wound honey do add to the fluid burden of some wounds and this may be undesirable. Hypertonic saline agents should be avoided when there is potential bleeding. Topical agents that promote haemostasis in malignant wounds include the firmer calcium alginate dressings, cautery with silver nitrate sticks or solution and ostomy hydrocolloid powders that contain gelatine or pectin (Stomahesive and Hollihesive powders). Surgical haemostatic agents such as Surgicel are also useful but expensive and not readily available in many care settings. Topical adrenaline 1:1000 solution is occasionally prescribed. However, its vasoconstriction properties can lead to tissue necrosis if not used with due care (Grocott, 2000). The prescribed use of oral or topical fibrinolytic inhibitors have also proved to be useful in controlling bleeding (Dean & Tuffin, 1997). Application of dressings such as foams and absorbent pads as well as the wearing of loose-fitting garments may offer the wound some added protection against friction forces.

Infection

The presence of necrotic tissue and hypoxia in a malignant wound increases the risk of wound infection. Anaerobic and aerobic bacteria can proliferate in moist necrotic tissues and can exacerbate malodour and lead to an increase in exudate (Grocott, 2000). The classic local signs of pain, erythema, oedema, heat, increased exudate or purulence indicate infection. However, other local signs may indicate a level of increased colonisation, commonly referred to as 'critical colonisation'. These changes include changes in the nature (friable and hypergranulated) and colour (bright red or grey) of granulation tissue; increased pain, pain or exudate; static healing; rolled edges of the wound; and possible bridging of the tissues (Gardner, Frantz, & Doebbeling, 2001; Sibbald et al., 2003). Systemic antibiotics may be required but the efficacy is reduced when infection presents in poorly vascularised tumours. The use of topical antimicrobials in the form of 'tissue-friendly' solutions and dressings is prudent in suspected wound infection. Cadexomer iodine (Lodosorb), silver impregnated dressings, 'wound' honey, hypertonic saline impregnated dressings and povidone-iodine or chlorhexidine-impregnated tulle gras are some of the antimicrobial dressings available.

Increased exudate

Uncontrolled exudate and the need for frequent dressing changes reduce the person's quality of life, increase fatigue and increase the resources needed to care appropriately. There is also an increased risk of infection, maceration of tissues and malodour. Extra-absorbent dry dressings such as Zetuvit, Mesorb or Exu-Dry are useful, as are a large range of incontinent or sanitary pads. Wound or ostomy appliances for containment of fistulae output or large amounts of exudate that may be associated with fungating tumours provide a cost-effective and less fatiguing alternative to frequent dressing changes.

Malodour

Malodour is a particularly distressing complication of malignant wounds for all involved in the care or support of patients. Malodour can result from infection, faecal fistulae drainage, autolysis of necrotic tissue or poor wound hygiene. Malodour impacts significantly upon body image and quality of life, and wound management should be directed towards eliminating or controlling malodour (Young, 2005). Identification and management of the causative problem is crucial. Malodour is managed environmentally, systemically (when the aetiology is infection) and topically. Environmental control of malodour is best achieved by providing good ventilation, disposal of waste products and prudent use of air deodorisers. Topical management options include: the use of topical antiseptic dressings (as previously discussed) and activated charcoal dressings such as Actisorb Plus, Lyofoam C and CarboFlex. Topical antimicrobial dressings reduce the bacterial load in the wound and the activated charcoal dressings adsorb or attract volatile odours, gases and microorganisms (Lee, Anand, Rajendran, & Walker, 2006). A wide variety of ostomy or wound appliances is useful for containment of offensive exudate. Dry black tea bags used as a secondary or tertiary dressing have been reported to provide an additional benefit in the control of malodour when more orthodox dressings prove ineffectual or are not available (Ng & Lee, 2002).

Education for the person, family and community

There is a large body of evidence that reducing sun exposure reduces the risk of skin cancer of all types. Carter, Marks and Hill (1999) propose that a 20% reduction in lifetime UVR exposure will have more than a 30% reduction in non-melanocytic and a 30% reduction in melanoma skin cancers, with a decreased number of deaths (59 per annum in the non-melanocytic group and 249 per annum in the melanoma group) in Australia. Most of the mass media campaigns promote the use of sunscreen and the wearing of protective clothing and hats as personal protective measures. The Cancer Council's 'slip slop slap' campaign (slip on a shirt, slop on sunscreen and slap on a hat) is an example of this. These campaigns have been effective at raising awareness of the key messages (Smith et al., 2002): a telephone survey of a random sample of 800 parents of children under 12 in New South Wales reported a 95% awareness of the key messages. However, the most effective measure to reduce sun exposure is sun avoidance, particularly between the hours of 10 a.m. and 3 p.m. Studies have shown that intermittent sun exposure rather than chronic exposure increases the risk of melanoma. Childhood sun exposure has been shown to be a significant risk factor in melanoma sufferers, particularly in women who burned then tanned (Helfand, 2003). Like all health promotion campaigns targeting behaviour modification, the key is to translate awareness of the benefits into personal action. Nurses have a role in this in a number of ways:

- providing accurate information to parents and prospective parents in the antenatal and early childhood settings
- providing targeted brief interventions to reinforce messages in primary care settings and during clinical contact
- conducting local health promotion campaigns to reinforce mass media messages in community settings.

Reflective questions

1 A woman with varicose veins has a non-healing leg ulcer. You have taken a swab and it comes back with normal commensals. What other investigations are warranted?

2 What strategies could be used to encourage teenagers to adopt 'SunSmart' behaviours?

3 What features of a melanoma may lead you to suspect that the patient may have a poor prognosis?

Anti skin cancer messages need to include the following information:

- the use of sunscreen should not be an alternative to seeking shade between 10 a.m. and 3 p.m.
- apply adequate broad-spectrum sunscreen 20 minutes before going outdoors to give protective elements time to bond to the skin
- apply broad-spectrum sunscreen to all exposed skin surfaces daily for children before any outdoor play
- adequate sunscreen is 2 mg of sunscreen for each square centimetre of exposed skin: approximately one teaspoon per limb
- wear a wide-brimmed hat and clothing to cover exposed skin
- wear close-fitting glasses to protect eyes against sun damage.

CONCLUSION

Skin cancer is a major cause of morbidity and mortality. GPs have more than 1 000 000 consultations a year for skin cancer (The Cancer Council Australia, 2012). In 2009, 85 000 hospitalisations for non-melanocytic skin cancer were reported, more than 1:10 of the total hospitalisations for all types of cancer (Australian Institute of Health and Welfare & Australasian Association of Cancer Registries 2010). The estimated cost of treating melanoma and non-melanocytic skin cancers has been calculated to be more than $300 million per year (AIHW, 2005). Reducing the incidence of skin cancer requires individuals to take lifelong personal protective action for themselves and their children. Early detection is the key to a good outcome for non-melanocytic and melanoma skin cancers. This can be achieved by regular skin inspection and needs to be accompanied by personal action supported by encouragement to seek treatment when suspect lesions are found.

Recommended reading

Carville, K. (2005). *Wound care manual* (pp. 117–126). Perth: Silver Chain Foundation.

Garbe, C., Eigentler, T., Kielholz, U., et al. (2011). Systematic review of medical treatment in melanoma: current status and future prospects. *The Oncologist, 16*, 5–24.

Markovic, S., Erickson, L., Rao, R., et al. (2007). Malignant melanoma in the 21st Century, part 2: staging, prognosis and treatment. *Mayo Clinic Proceedings, 82*(4), 490–513.

Trent, J., & Kirsner, R. (2003). Wounds and malignancy. *Advances in Skin and Wound Care, 16*(1), 31–34.

Young, C. (2005). The effects of malodorous fungating malignant wounds on body image and quality of life. *Journal of Wound Care, 14*(8), 359–361.

References

Australian Institute of Health and Welfare. (2001). *Cancer in Australia 2001. AIHW cat no CAN23.* Canberra: Author.

Australian Institute of Health and Welfare. (2005). *Health system expenditures on cancer and other neoplasms in Australia 2000–2001. Health and Welfare Expenditure series no 22 cat no HWE 29.* Canberra: Author.

Australian Institute of Health and Welfare. (2012). *Cancer in Australia: an overview. AIHW Cancer Series no 74 cat no CAN70.* Canberra: Author.

Australian Institute of Health and Welfare and Australasian Association of Cancer Registries. (2008). *Cancer in Australia: an overview. Cancer Series no 46 cat no CAN 42.* Canberra: Australian Institute of Health and Welfare.

Australian Institute of Health and Welfare and Australasian Association of Cancer Registries. (2010). *Cancer in Australia: an overview. Cancer Series no 60 cat no CAN 56.* Canberra: Australian Institute of Health and Welfare.

Carter, R., Marks, R., & Hill, D. (1999). Could a national skin cancer primary prevention campaign in Australia be worthwhile? An economic perspective. *Health Promotion International, 14*(1), 73–82.

Carville, K. (2005). *Wound care manual.* Perth: Silver Chain Foundation.

Cohen, K., Dieglemann, R., & Lindblad, W. (1992). *Wound healing: Biochemical and clinical aspects.* Philadelphia: Saunders.

Dean, A., & Tuffin, P. (1997). Fibrinolytic inhibitors for cancer-associated bleeding problems. *Journal of Pain and Symptom Management, 13*(1), 20–24.

Dolan, N., Ng, J., Martin, G., et al. (1997). Effectiveness of skin cancer control educational intervention for internal medicine housestaff and attending physicians. *Journal of Internal Medicine, 12,* 531–536.

Dupree, M., Boyer, J., & Cobb, M. (1998). Marjolin's ulcer arising from a burns scar. *Cutis, 62*(1), 49–51.

Gardner, S., Frantz, R., & Doebbeling, B. (2001). The validity of the clinical signs and symptoms used to identify localised chronic wound infection. *Wound Repair and Regeneration, 9,* 178–186.

Garbe, C., Eigentler, T., Kielholz, U., et al. (2011). Systematic review of medical treatment in melanoma: current status and future prospects. *The Oncologist, 16,* 5–24.

Gordon, L., Hirst, N., Gies, P., et al. (2008). What impact would effective solarium regulation have in Australia? *Medical Journal of Australia, 189*(7), 375–378.

Grocott, P. (2000). The palliative management of fungating malignant wounds. *Journal of Wound Care, 9*(1), 4–9.

Habif, T. (2004). *Clincal dermatology: A colour guide to diagnosis and therapy* (4th ed.). St Louis: Elsevier.

Helfand, M. (2003). *Counseling to prevent skin cancer: a summary of the evidence (No. 03-521B).* Washington: Agency for Healthcare Research and Quality.

Lee, G., Anand, S., Rajendran, S., et al. (2006). Overview of current practices and future trends in the evaluation of dressings for malodorous wounds. *Journal of Wound Care, 15*(8), 344–346.

Markovic, S., Erickson, L., Rao, R., et al. (2007). Malignant melanoma in the 21st Century, part 2: staging, prognosis and treatment. *Mayo Clinic Proceedings, 82*(4), 490–513.

Menendez, M., & Warriner, R. (2006). Marjolin's ulcer: Report of two cases. *Wounds, 18*(3), 65–70.

Ng, P. L., & Lee, G. Y. (2002). A case report of an innovative strategy using tea leaves in the management of malodorous wounds. *Singapore Nurses Journal, 29*(3), 16–18.

Sibbald, R. G., Orsted, H., Schultz, G, et al. (2003). Preparing the wound bed: Focus on infection and inflammation. *Ostomy/Wound Management, 49*(11), 24–51.

Smith, B., Ferguson, C., McKenzie, J., et al. (2002). Impacts from repeated mass media campaigns to promote sun protection in Australia. *Health Promotion International, 17*(1), 51–60.

The Cancer Council of Australia. (2007). All about skin cancer. Retrieved July 29, 2007, from http://www.cancer.org.au/content.cfm?randid=960742.

The Cancer Council Australia. (2012). Skin Cancer. Retrieved February 6, 2013, from http://www.cancer.org.au/preventing-cancer/sun-protection/about-skin-cancer.html

Trent, J., & Kirsner R. (2003). Wounds and malignancy. *Advances in Skin and Wound Care, 16*(1), 31–34.

Tsao, H., Bevona, C., Goggins, W., et al. (2003). The transformation rate of moles (melanocytic nevi) into cutaneous melanoma: a population based estimate. *Archives of Dermatology, 139*(3), 282–288.

Vargo, N. (2006). Cutaneous malignancies: BCC, SCC, and MM. *Dermatology Nursing, 18*(2), 183–200.

Walter, F., Humphreys, E., Tso, S., et al. (2010). Patient understanding of moles and skin cancer and factors influencing presentation in primary care: a qualitative study. *BMC Family Practice, 11*, 62.

Winterbottom, A., & Harcourt, D. (2004). Patients' experience of the diagnosis and treatment of skin cancer. *Journal of Advanced Nursing, 48*(3), 226–233.

Woloczyn, M., Trzesinski, A., Takahashi, M., et al. (2010). Sun protective behaviours of beach goers in the North West. *Health Promotion Journal of Australia, 21*(2), 146–148.

Young, C. (2005). The effects of malodorous fungating malignant wounds on body image and quality of life. *Journal of Wound Care, 14*(8), 359–361.

CHAPTER 25

Tiffany Northall

Ageing and disability (osteoarthritis and osteoporosis)

Learning objectives

When you have completed this chapter you will be able to:

- outline the major risk factors for the development of osteoarthritis and osteoporosis in the ageing population
- describe the impact that osteoarthritis and osteoporosis have on the function and wellbeing of ageing persons within the community
- outline current approaches to reducing the impact of these conditions on members of the older population
- suggest nursing practices that will promote health and mobility in older persons experiencing the effects of osteoarthritis and osteoporosis
- develop strategies to support the families of clients experiencing the effects of osteoarthritis and osteoporosis.

Key words

activities of daily living, ageing, education, nursing practice, wellbeing

INTRODUCTION

The majority of the population in Australia and New Zealand anticipate a lifetime of independence and good health that allows them to maintain a self-directed lifestyle. However, living a healthy and productive life does not necessarily protect the individual from varying levels of disability later in life due to the natural changes of ageing, life's physical stressors and individual genetic make-up. Osteoarthritis, rheumatoid arthritis and

CASE STUDY 25.1

John is a 70-year-old retired plumber. John's father was a plumber and when John was 16 he began his plumbing apprenticeship with his father. He continued to work as a plumber until his retirement 10 years ago. John worked hard throughout his life and his plumbing business was successful. As a result he and his wife Cathy have an income from his superannuation that, while modest, allows them to live comfortably. He and his wife own a single storey home with a large garden which John enjoys maintaining.

John has always been physically active; he realised early in his plumbing career that he needed to exercise regularly and pay attention to body mechanics in order to be able to carry out his work effectively. Despite this, the physical nature of his job resulted in John having several injuries over his working life and he has now developed osteoarthritis in his spine and knees. The pain and mobility impairments from his osteoarthritis limit his ability to perform the activities of daily living. He finds sleeping, driving, walking, gardening, vacuuming and doing the laundry particularly difficult.

Five years ago John was diagnosed with bowel cancer. He received successful treatment for this and has an annual colonoscopy for monitoring. He does not smoke or drink alcohol and has a family history of type 2 diabetes and arthritis.

osteoporosis affect more than 6 million Australians, mostly among people aged 65 years and over (Dixon & Penm, 2006; Rahman, Bhatia, & Penm, 2005). As Australia's population ages, more people are likely to experience disability as a result of these conditions. Even if the disability does not interfere with daily function and mobility, in combination with other changes of ageing and age-related diseases, the effects of these conditions and their management can prove to be challenging for the person, their family and health providers, and result in increased levels of disability.

In this chapter there will be a focus on the effects of osteoarthritis and osteoporosis on two older people and their families through the use of case studies. The case studies will assist you to understand how nursing practices can promote health and wellbeing for persons experiencing disability and challenge as a result of the effects of these conditions.

OSTEOARTHRITIS

Behaviours that contribute to the development of osteoarthritis

Osteoarthritis is a disease that becomes more common over the age of 45. It affects 1.6 million Australians and is more common in women, with 4 out of 10 women over the age of 75 reported to have the disease (Australian Institute of Health and Welfare [AIHW], 2010). It is characterised by the deterioration of the articular cartilage that covers and protects the ends of the bones in joints. Where a healthy person has a balance between cartilage breakdown and production, the person with osteoarthritis loses this balance and degeneration exceeds regeneration. This results in painful bone-on-bone contact in the joints and the development of bony spurs and cysts on the bone surface, leading to joint deformity (Rooney, 2004). Lifestyle behaviours that are known to contribute to the development of osteoarthritis are obesity, misalignment of bones and joints, joint trauma and injury, repetitive occupational joint use and physical inactivity (Rahman et al., 2005, p. 26; Rooney, 2004; Swift, 2012a). John's situation illustrates a number of controllable and non-controllable factors that have placed him at greater risk of developing osteoarthritis. The uncontrollable factors include his age and his genetic disposition or family history. Being male does reduce his risk but this does not prevent osteoarthritis developing (AIHW, 2010; Rahman et al., 2005; Rooney, 2004). His efforts to control his weight over a lifetime have possibly reduced the onset of disability in the light of other biomechanical factors. John has had a physically strenuous working life as a plumber and has experienced multiple but relatively minor spinal injuries. However, both his occupation and the frequency of back injuries have made him aware of the benefits of body mechanics, weight control, exercise and activity to maintain mobility and independence. Until he retired he was physically active but his recent surgeries and therapy have reduced his exercise capacity and thus increased his risk of disability. While his treatment for cancer has been successful to date, it has constrained his lifestyle and reduced his energy levels.

Altered mobility and fatigue

Each person with osteoarthritis experiences their own challenges in maintaining mobility and managing the activities of daily living. The most problematic issue in the development of osteoarthritis is pain and it is the pain that limits mobility and function and contributes to fatigue affecting activity levels (Swift, 2012b). Physiological changes to joints also contribute to altered physical function, depending on the joint affected (Mann, 2012). Nursing assessment of people with osteoarthritis should include function, mood, mobility and pain assessments (National Institute for Health and Clinical Excellence [NICE], 2008).

A third of Australians with arthritis report that the disease limits their ability to perform the activities of daily living (AIHW, 2010). At this time John is not experiencing severe limitations in his bathing, grooming or dressing although he has made some changes to his clothing to compensate for reduced spinal mobility and he is no longer able to get into or out of a bathtub. Showering is not a problem for John as there is no need to step into a raised shower and the alcove is large enough to move around in freely.

While older women report greater levels of immobility and discomfort as a result of osteoarthritis than men, more women live alone and thus have less access to assistance from others with activities of daily living (Murtagh & Hubert, 2004). John is experiencing some mobility deficits as a result of his pain and joint restrictions. Living with Cathy offers the potential for support with activities of daily living yet it is John that provides physical support to his wife. This increases the physical demands on John that have the potential to increase his fatigue on particularly 'bad' days, when his pain becomes disabling. John's responses to the pain and reduced mobility are reported as typical of men affected by osteoarthritis, where mobility within the home and their community are of primary concern, whereas women have reported greater concerns with fine motor skill performance (Burks, 2002). John's outward responses to his pain include periods of solitude and silence and irritation that he is unable to perform some of the activities he planned around the house.

One of Western society's benchmarks of outward independence is the ability to drive, but driving necessitates getting into and out of a car, which requires spinal, hip and knee mobility (Burks, 2002). In addition, driving requires manipulation and coordination of the joints, especially the hips, knees and to some extent the ankles. It also requires the driver to sit in a restricted space. Although back pain is associated with activity limitation and work absence, there is very little evidence of the impact of back pain on older adults yet the prevalence of osteoarthritis increases with age. A systematic review of the literature by

Dionne, Dunn and Croft (2006) suggests that older adults complain less of back pain yet experience increasing frequency and severity of back pain with advancing age. This anomaly they attribute to an increase in tolerance for pain and/or increasing co-morbidities that also contribute to pain and disability. Therefore many older adults accommodate back pain into their collective discomforts from other problems or disorders rather than focusing on a single pain source (Dionne, Dunn, & Croft, 2006).

The pain of osteoarthritis is not limited to the hours a person is awake and mobile. The ageing adult will experience changes in sleep patterns, including earlier retiring and earlier waking and a reduced number of hours sleep to about 6.5 hours. Frequent awakenings are also common but tend to increase with concurrent medical conditions (Wolkove, Elkholy, Baltzan, & Palayew, 2007). John finds that he must get out of bed more frequently due to age-related nocturia and this reduces the duration of his restorative sleep. The pain and stiffness he experiences in his spine from sleeping in a single position for a prolonged time further interferes with the duration and quality of his sleep. To reduce the impact of broken sleep on Cathy, John sleeps in the spare bedroom. However, fewer hours of sleep, more frequent awakenings and physical discomfort have a cumulative effect on his vitality the following day. He experiences greater levels of fatigue with daytime pain and thus has less energy to mobilise, which is necessary to reduce joint stiffness and pain and prevent further disability.

Key points

- A third of Australians with arthritis report that the disease limits their ability to perform the activities of daily living (AIHW, 2010).
- Pain and joint stiffness affect mobility, independence, sleep and lifestyle.
- Holistic nursing assessment should be practiced.

Body image

John has maintained weight control throughout his life and his attention to body mechanics and exercise to support his vulnerable spine has resulted in an upright posture. Exercise not only has helped with his overall fitness but can also help to alleviate pain, promote confidence and improve quality of life (Swift, 2012a). However, John is concerned about his increasing physical vulnerability and for future wellbeing and mobility. He has seen his contemporaries develop deformities of the knee joint (genu valgum and genu varum), necessitating the use of canes or walking aids, and a number have needed joint replacement of the knees or hips.

The outward changes apparent to Cathy and his children include John's hesitancy and deliberate movements with position change, his need to ensure that there is a suitable chair to support his back at family outings but mostly his slow walking pace when he rises from the chair because of the discomfort that improves within a short distance. This change in pace frequently evokes negative comments from his children suggesting that he is 'just acting too old' or that he is 'getting slow'. While their comments can be thoughtless, they are also indicative of their anxiety resulting from the physical changes in their once active and energetic father, whom they saw as invincible during their growing years. The negative comments also reinforce John's concerns for his future mobility and independence and erode his hope of improvement.

While John lives independently in the community, he requires monitoring following the treatment for bowel cancer. This involves periodic day admissions for colonoscopy. Although admission and preparation for surgery have a focus on the immediate problem (cancer monitoring) the nursing assessment also needs to consider the impact of John's osteoarthritis during the procedure and his care in the postoperative period. He presents as a self-caring retiree who is fully mobile and in no apparent pain. However, the nursing assessment should consider the impact of the surgery and the intraoperative positioning of the patient as well as the anaesthetic recovery time, when John will be lying in a single position until he is conscious. Both of these factors can increase his potential for back pain during the recovery period that can be confused with the pain of surgical trauma. Periods of inactivity such as during an anaesthetic can result in increased stiffness and pain for people with osteoarthritis (Walker, 2011).Therefore, as a day-surgery client John will not mobilise as readily or as quickly following the anaesthetic-induced rest. As a result greater mobility support is indicated than his admission appearance may suggest.

Quality of life

Quality of life has been studied among many populations and is an individual or personal measure. Little is known of the effect of osteoarthritis on the quality of life of older persons. However, some suggest that the associated pain reduces a person's quality of life significantly and is linked to the existence of various psychological problems such as anxiety, depression and feelings of helplessness (Jakobsson & Hallberg, 2006; Swift, 2012b). In a survey of adults 75 years and older with osteoarthritis ($n = 168$) and those without osteoarthritis ($n = 246$), Jakobsson and Hallberg (2006) found that pain and reduced ability to perform the activities of daily living significantly reduced the older person's quality of life. The stiffness, pain and fatigue caused by osteoarthritis can have an effect on a person's ability to perform the activities of daily living (Swift, 2012b). However, there was no difference in reports of mood depression between those who did and did not have osteoarthritis. It is suggested that as a person ages they develop alternative views on life that assist in accommodating health and physical change. People who see their doctor for osteoarthritis report experiencing pain for more than 3 months before they sought medical advice (Birrell et al., 2000, as cited in Swift, 2012b). The reasons for this as suggested by Schofield (2008) is that older adults view pain as a part of ageing and as a result often do not report the symptoms of osteoarthritis until quality of life and function is significantly impacted.

Some evidence suggests that older persons with osteoarthritis who have strong social support experience improved quality of life (Jakobsson & Hallberg, 2002). Yet a study with 81 community-dwelling and socially interactive seniors found only a small influence of social support on reported quality of life (Kee, 2003). The factors that improved quality of life among these independent seniors were perceptions of control through routine and regularity of activities and daily living. The lower influence of social support was suggested to be a result of the participants' immersion in social activities that had become a natural part of their lives (Kee, 2003). John and Cathy have a close relationship with their two adult children but there is no extended family support as neither has married and there are no grandchildren. John's siblings live interstate and Cathy's brothers are deceased. As they both worked throughout their adult lives in a business that required 24-hour attention, there was little time or opportunity to develop social relationships outside the industry. Retirement has meant selling the property and moving away from lifetime neighbours and occupational contacts. Both John and Cathy face increasing social isolation that can have a negative impact on their quality of life, especially as they are not actively involved in social activities outside their immediate family and small circle of lifetime friends.

Where pain and reduced ability to perform the activities of daily living interfere with independence, there will be a negative impact on the quality of life. Participating in leisure activities can provide a diversion from the symptoms of arthritis; however it may be necessary to modify some activities. Janke, Jones, Payne, and Son (2011) found that people with arthritis were willing to find new standards of participating in leisure activities if pain or symptoms became a limiting factor. As prolonged periods of immobility can increase pain, people with arthritis reported a need to take more regular stops when travelling and driving so that they could exercise (Janke et al., 2011). These are issues that also affect John's life as he must limit his driving episodes to no more than 2 hours at a time. Prolonged sitting, even on occasional air flights to see his interstate family, increases his pain and fatigue at his destination, limiting his independence and quality of life.

Key points

- Stiffness, fatigue and pain from osteoarthritis can affect the ability to carry out the activities of daily living.
- Symptoms of osteoarthritis can cause anxiety, depression and feelings of helplessness which affect quality of life.

Interventions to attain self-management

Increasing interest in health self-management in our community is also associated with increasing availability of health information, especially through the internet. More seniors are looking for non-invasive approaches to manage their chronic health conditions, especially osteoarthritis. There are a number of non-pharmacological and pharmacological interventions that persons like John can use to manage the pain and retain optimum mobility. Non-pharmacological interventions include exercise, physical therapy, joint protection, heat and cold therapy, hydrotherapy, acupuncture, nutrition and weight reduction (Swift, 2012b).

Exercise has been found to have both psychological and physiological benefits for older adults. In the presence of osteoarthritis, exercise strengthens the supporting skeletal muscles that stabilise the joints which can help reduce pain and improve mobility and quality of life (Swift, 2012b). Exercise also increases cardiac efficiency and improves endurance and stamina. Exercise may be low impact, such as stretching to maintain the flexibility of the joints and swimming, but for more able older adults, it can include power walking or aerobic exercise. While exercise is suggested to reduce pain and improve physical function of knee joints, every older adult has their own motivators for and barriers to exercising that may include other co-morbidities, home care commitments and a lack of research evidence that guides the prescription of intensity and duration of the exercise (Fransen et al., 2007). There are a number of programs and opportunities for older community members to participate in aqua-aerobics or aquatic exercise (also known as hydrotherapy). However, participation does require the resources to access the programs. For John it would mean a 60-minute round trip due to the lack of public transport and the cost of the fuel for daily or regular participation would become prohibitive. However, for seniors living within walking or commuting distance, aquatic exercise has been found beneficial, although it does not provide long-term pain relief for knee or hip osteoarthritis (Bartels et al., 2007; Wang et al., 2006).

Rest is needed to reduce pain and to allow recovery after exercise (Walker, 2011). It is also suggested that joints can be protected through attention to body mechanics and posture and avoiding prolonged use of individual joints such as digging in the garden for long periods. More intensive or heavier activities should be broken into shorter periods, alternating with rest and lighter activities (Walker, 2011). The use of assistive devices such as garden trolleys and washing trolleys will protect joints from heavier workloads. Footwear that has a wide heel and uppers that cover the foot provide more structural protection to the foot bones and ankle joints and can reduce the pain of walking and exercise. Thermal therapy, such as the application of heat packs, can reduce muscle spasm and improve circulation but care must be taken with their use for older clients due to the risks of thermal burns associated with reduced peripheral sensation.

John has made some home modifications to accommodate his reduced mobility. Rather than bathing, he showers and rather than using lace-up shoes, he finds that ankle boots and loafers are easier to put on. The use of a long-handled shoehorn assists him to get his socks on without bending over to his toes. At this stage he does not need home aids such as rails in the shower and toilet but he purchases chairs with care to ensure that they provide him with the spine support he needs. He has found that sitting on a gel pillow reduces pressure on his coccyx when driving and flying and these have reduced his spinal discomfort. His last car purchase was influenced by the height of the car seat from the ground and the width of the door to get in and out.

Over-the-counter medications are frequently used to self-treat the milder symptoms associated with osteoarthritis. While some non-steroidal anti-inflammatory medications (NSAIDs) require a prescription, many people self-medicate with readily available analgesics and herbal supplements. Paracetamol is a commonly used pharmacological treatment for osteoarthritis pain (Swift, 2012b). However, there is some evidence that non-prescription NSAIDs (such as ibuprofen) are more effective on moderate pain but there is greater risk of gastric distress with their use (Schofield, 2008; Towheed et al., 2007a).

John has been influenced by media advertising to try glucosamine with chondroitin as a self-treatment for the pain of osteoarthritis. While as a combination supplement this over-the-counter preparation is more expensive than glucosamine alone, he was willing to try it. He has found, like a number of participants in clinical trials, that this medication reduced his knee pain significantly (Martin, Sell, & Damter, 2012). However, others report minimal or no improvement in the pain, suggesting that the effects of this supplement are individual (Towheed et al., 2007b; Distler & Anguelouch, 2006).

There is increasing access to alternative therapies for people with osteoarthritis but individuals should be advised to seek the services of qualified practitioners of these therapies to ensure that there will be no interactions with other prescribed medications or adverse effects on other physical disorders. Acupuncture has been incorporated by doctors in a number of general practices and can be used with some effect to control the pain of peripheral osteoarthritis (Kwon, Pittler, & Ernst, 2006; Swift, 2012b). While John is able to access many non-pharmacological treatments and adopt those that are suited to his resources and lifestyle these are also discussed collaboratively with his general practitioner (GP).

Key points

- Promote self-management by providing information.
- Comprehensive treatment regimens should be developed in consultation with the person's GP.
- Non-pharmacological interventions include exercise, physical therapy, alternative therapies, joint protection, heat and cold therapy, hydrotherapy, acupuncture, nutrition and weight reduction.
- Pharmacological interventions include over-the-counter and prescription medications.

Family and carers

John remains an independent retiree with mobility and physical limitations. His disability has little direct impact on his family except for his inability to undertake larger household repairs for his children (such as mowing and exterior painting). While he remains physically capable he is able to control his lifestyle to a high degree. However, the increasing frailty of Cathy and his own vulnerability related to his episode with cancer places John at risk of becoming physically less able to manage if he becomes incapacitated as a result of illness or injury, or by becoming a full-time carer to Cathy if she has an accident or fall.

While his children do not have families or children of their own, they do both work to support themselves and maintain their own homes. Their ability to provide supportive or full-time care for their parents in the near future appears limited at this time. John and Cathy would do well to plan for such a contingency or look to alternative living arrangements (a smaller residence or access to home care/support), should one of them become disabled.

As John is monitored closely following his cancer and prostate surgeries, he has regular health assessments with his GP and has his annual influenza immunisations with the practice nurse. This has been an ideal opportunity to discuss non-pharmacological options and evaluate his self-management strategies with both health practitioners.

Education for the person and family

John, like many of his contemporaries, has access to information about osteoarthritis through the internet. However, the large amount of information can prove to be confusing and conflicting at times. Individuals such as John and his family would be best advised to use the resources of established support groups such as Arthritis Australia (http://www.arthritisaustralia.com.au/) which provide up-to-date information sheets on varying self-management strategies as well as the latest medical and scientific evidence presented in accessible language. Education should include an understanding of the processes of osteoarthritis, pain and mobility management, strategies to maintain mobility (such as activity and exercise) and short- and long-term therapies (pharmacological and surgical). Community health centres and practice nurses can provide information about free community education on self-management of osteoarthritis within the individual's own community for those who feel unable to use internet resources.

OSTEOPOROSIS

Osteoporosis is when the bone loses minerals faster than the body can replace them, thereby reducing bone density. The reduction in bone density makes the bone brittle and more prone to fractures. It is the associated fractures that lead to the morbidity of osteoporosis (World Health Organization [WHO], 2004). Common fractures associated with osteoporosis are forearm, humerus, hip and spine with hip fractures having the highest associated morbidity and mortality (WHO, 2004).

Behaviours that contribute to the development of osteoporosis

All people are at risk of developing osteoporosis, especially in their later years. In 2007–08 it was reported that 692 000 Australians had been diagnosed with the disease (Australian Institute of Health and Welfare, 2011). Internationally one in every three women and one in every five men over the age of 50 will be affected by an osteoporotic fracture (McCloskey, 2009). In the normal ageing process the bones lose calcium, making them less dense. The outer layers of bone also become thinner, yet they do not lose size. However, the decrease in bone mass leads to a decrease in the strength of the bones. Until the age of about 20, there is either an increase in mineral deposition (calcium and phosphorus) or balance between deposition and absorption (bone formation and resorption) but this balance begins to fail from the age of 35 years (Swann, 2012). There are some factors that place individuals at higher risk of developing osteoporosis and a number of strategies that can

CASE STUDY 25.2

Leila is a 73-year-old widow who lives with her extended family in an urban area. Following the death of her husband Thomas 10 years ago Leila moved in with her daughter and son-in-law, assisting with the care of Leila's three grandchildren, who have now completed their education and left home. Through her early childhood and young adulthood Leila experienced periodic economic and nutritional deprivations because of the transient work habits of her family. She felt fortunate to have met and married Thomas who had a trade and provided for her and her young family. Leila cared for her family and worked locally in a market garden. She developed strong relationships with the other women who worked in the garden.

Leila has been generally well during her life, plagued only by seasonal influenza complicated by her ongoing cigarette smoking. She was smoking up to two packets per week from the age of 14 until her first hospitalisation. At age 55 she underwent a hysterectomy and bilateral oophorectomy because of fibroid growth with associated uterine bleeding.

Leila has had several falls at home, two that resulted in fractures and the need for hospitalisation. Three years ago Leila sustained a Colles fracture of the right wrist that required closed reduction. At the time she was assessed for osteoporosis, which was confirmed. Six months ago Leila fell while getting out of the car and sustained a fractured head of femur that was repaired with a hemiarthoplasty. Her recovery from surgery was problematic and she has returned to her daughter's home frail and highly anxious when mobilising.

prevent onset. A number of unmodifiable risk factors linked to the development of osteoporosis include ageing, being post-menopausal, family history of the disease, poor vitamin D intake and low body weight (Swann, 2012). The behaviours that can increase the potential for developing osteoporosis include low calcium intake, physical inactivity, tobacco consumption and excessive consumption of alcohol. Osteoporosis can also develop as a result of the use of corticosteroids (for the treatment of lung diseases and asthma), early menopause through surgery (total hystero-oophorectomy), rheumatoid arthritis, thyroid disease malabsorption syndromes (liver disease and inflammatory bowel disease) and physical disability (Swann, 2012).

Key points

- Risk factors linked to the development of osteoporosis include ageing, being post-menopausal, family history of the disease, poor vitamin D intake and low body weight.
- Behaviours that can increase the potential for developing osteoporosis include low calcium intake, physical inactivity, tobacco consumption and excessive consumption of alcohol.

When considering Leila's health and social history it can be seen that she has a history of nutritional deficits during her childhood but these have not continued into adulthood. Maintaining a diet that is high in calcium and vitamin D is particularly important for women over the age of 45 to help maintain bone health (Nazarko, 2011). A full nursing history of her intake with a focus on her intake of calcium-rich foods (milk, cheese, yoghurt, nuts and bread) will highlight any current deficiency. Vitamin D is found in oily fish and dairy foods; however most of the vitamin D we need is produced by exposing the skin to sunlight (Nazarko, 2011). Leila's history of working outdoors had stood her in good stead but the nursing assessment should focus on current outdoors activity to maintain vitamin D production. Most significantly Leila underwent a hysterectomy and bilateral oophorectomy almost 20 years ago. This is also the expected age for menopause, which results in decreased production of oestrogen, a hormone that is central to maintaining bone mass (Simon, Ravnikar, Hess, & Murphy, 2007). Questioning Leila revealed that she had not received or asked for post-menopausal hormone replacement therapy which would have lowered her risk of developing osteoporosis (Nazarko, 2011). Her decision to stop smoking almost 20 years ago and her minimal intake of alcohol at periodic family celebrations have eliminated these as risks to the development of osteoporosis. Perhaps the most telling factor in Leila's history is the two fractures she has sustained as a result of minimal trauma and the subsequent diagnosis of osteoporosis.

Altered mobility and fatigue

Leila and her family face a number of challenges in relation to her mobility. Where immobility increases the impact and severity of osteoporosis, increasing activity and mobility increase the risk of Leila falling and sustaining more fractures and pain. The previous hip and Colles fractures that Leila has experienced are indicators of osteoporosis as they are often caused by a fall from standing height or less (Australian Institute of Health and Welfare, 2011). The pain, mobility impairment and disability that can result from these fractures impeded recovery and increase the risk of developing further complications (Australian Institute of Health and Welfare, 2011).

Leila has returned from hospital where she received assistance and instruction on using a walking frame from the physiotherapist and nurses. However, her right wrist has residual weakness from the previous Colles fracture and this adds to her insecurity with walking. Leila requires someone to walk beside her because she fears her right hand will not grip the walker securely and her loss of independent mobility has become a source of personal stress, as she is acutely aware of the demands she is making on her family. This acts as a disincentive to walking distances because of her slow pace and she has declined suggestions that she go outdoors and sit in the gardens because she is afraid that her daughter will not hear her if she falls. The self-imposed limitations on her walking have reduced Leila's exercise tolerance and increased her levels of fatigue during activities such as bathing and walking to the kitchen for meals.

Leila's hip fracture is not the only source of her daily activity problems. The loss of strength from the fracture of her wrist has reduced her ability to turn on taps in the shower and bathroom, to be able to button or tie clothing and to grip the hairbrush to brush her own hair into the style she prefers. Where Leila once enjoyed preparing and cooking meals, she is no longer able to manipulate kitchen utensils or carry heavy pots or containers of food.

Body image

Leila accepts most of the changes of ageing that she is experiencing but her family take pains to ensure that her clothing is suitable for her ability. Her family pretend not to notice her occasional dishevelled appearance, as they know she has difficulty dressing herself and she cannot brush her hair well with her left hand. However, they take pains not to restrict her attempts to complete her own care.

Quality of life

Leila's increasing frailty and reliance upon others for her safety and care have reduced her perception of her quality of life. She had imagined that she would share her later years in the company of Thomas sharing memories and their achievements raising their family. Her loss of her husband and her loss of independence related to her osteoporosis contribute to an alteration in her perceived quality of life. These responses are similar to those reported by Adachi et al. (2010), where pain, fatigue and mobility impairments were linked to lower reported quality of life among women with osteoporosis.

Interventions to attain self-management

Because of her increasing age and decreased mobility Leila and her family have accepted that she will need support to maintain and strengthen her current level of self-management. An assessment by the Aged Care Assessment Team (ACAT) of the home and family resources (structural, physical and emotional) has identified that there are no structural changes to be made as Leila's son-in-law has made some changes to facilitate Leila's comfort over the years. There are gentle ramps where there were access steps, the shower and toilet have handrails, and tiled flooring throughout the home is non-slip although a hard surface to fall on. These all facilitate Leila's mobility and participation in family and outdoor activity.

While Leila had been managing her medications independently, since her last fall her daughter is monitoring the medications by dispensing daily doses in labelled containers kept on the kitchen table with reach.

Education for the person and family

Following the ACAT assessment Leila and her family participated in a conference with her doctor, nurse, occupational therapist and physiotherapist, at which they learned about a number of strategies they could implement to support Leila's recovery and reduce further disability. The family were helped to understand how the osteoporosis developed and its link to pain, disability and fractures. One of their primary goals as a family became the prevention of further falls and fractures. Leila's risk of falling was assessed against factors identified by Flores (2012). The factors include previous history of falling, diseases and disorders that affect balance and strength, sensory deficits, environmental factors and medication use (Flores, 2012). Leila has a previous history of falls and while she does not have orthostatic hypotension or arthritis she has some gait impairment and muscle weakness as a result of her previous fractures. Leila does not take any medication that may increase her risk of falls and her home environment has been adjusted to reduce environmental falls. While this was of some comfort to Leila, it was only one factor. To improve posture, muscle strength and coordination to prevent future falls Leila and her daughter began day rehabilitation at a local health centre where the physiotherapist taught Leila how to use and exercise her muscles effectively. The occupational therapist taught Leila how to exercise and use her right hand more effectively to dress and groom herself. Leila's daughter learned effective ways of getting her mother in and out of the shower and chairs at home and the types of utensils that would allow her mother to participate in food preparation again.

Leila and her family also learned that to prevent fractures and to prevent further bone loss, Leila needed to maintain an exercise program that actually challenged her bones. As she had already sustained two fractures, she was not a suitable candidate to undertake high-impact or resistance exercises (Osteoporosis Australia [OA], n.d.). They learned that weight-bearing exercises were most effective (Bonaiuti et al., 2007; OA, n.d.). Although

Reflective questions

1 What are the nursing considerations when looking after a client who has osteoarthritis in both hips and knees?

2 Consider strategies that a person with osteoarthritis may adopt at home to promote independence.

3 What are the risk factors for developing osteoporosis?

Leila found the exercise regimen tiring at first, over time her exercise endurance increased and she gained greater confidence in walking and self-care.

A review of the prescribed medications by the nurse identified the need for some further education on their effective use. Medications specifically related to the osteoporosis included a bisphosphonate preparation and paracetamol. The bisphosphonate preparation is used to reduce bone loss but it can cause pain when swallowing (McBane, 2011). Bisphosphonate has been associated with gastro-intestinal complications and administration recommendations include taking with a full glass of water and remaining upright for 30 minutes after administration (Lewiecki, 2011). The nurse encouraged Leila to talk to her doctor about developing a comprehensive medication regimen including an individual pain management plan to help her self-manage her disease.

Information and contact details for OA in their state were provided so that Leila and her family could access further information and advice on the disease and strategies to manage it in the future. Leila's daughter was also provided with information as having family history of maternal osteoporosis is a risk factor for developing the disease (Swann, 2012).

CONCLUSION

In this chapter you have seen how two older people have experienced disability as a result of lifestyle diseases that affect and will continue to affect millions of Australians directly or indirectly in the future. Many residents in aged care facilities have one or both of these diseases, limiting their mobility and participation in wider society. Too often these limits are considered a 'natural' part of ageing and thus not amenable to change and improvement. As this chapter has illustrated, there are a number of strategies that individuals and families can implement to prevent the onset of these diseases or reduce the severity of them. Nurses have a critical role in promoting independence and mobility through education and considered physical support.

Acknowledgment: the author would like to thank Leonie Williams and Belinda Harpin for their contribution to this chapter.

Recommended reading

Australian Institute of Health and welfare. (2010). *A snapshot of arthritis in Australia 2010.* Canberra, ACT: Author.

Chiodo, B. (2007). Preventing osteoporosis – healthy bones for life. *Journal of Community Nursing, 21*(5), 22–26.

Swann, J. I. (2012). Osteoporosis: the fragile bone disease. *British Journal of Healthcare Assistants, 6*(2), 59–62.

Swift, A. (2012a). Osteoarthritis 1: physiology, risk factors and causes of pain. *Nursing Times, 108*(7), 12–15.

Swift, A. (2012b). Osteoarthritis 2: pain management and treatment strategies. *Nursing Times, 108*(8), 25–27.

References

Adachi, J. D., Adami, S., Gehlbach, S., et al. (2010). Impact on prevalent fractures on quality of life: baseline results from the global longitudinal study of osteoporosis in women. *Mayo Clinic Proceedings, 85*(9), 806–813.

Australian Institute of Health and Welfare. (2010). *A snapshot of arthritis in Australia 2010*. Canberra, ACT: Author.

Australian Institute of Health and Welfare. (2011). *A snapshot of osteoporosis in Australia 2011*. Canberra, ACT: Author.

Bartels, E. M., Lund, H., Hagen, K. B., et al. (2007). Aquatic exercise for treatment of knee and hip osteoarthritis (Review). The Cochrane Collaboration. The Cochrane Library, Issue 2. Retrieved October 15, 2012, from http://www.thecochranelibrary.com

Birrell, F., Croft, P., Cooper, C., et al. (2000). Health impact of pain in the hip region with and without radiographic evidence of osteoarthritis: a study of new attenders to primary care. The PCR Hip Study Group. *Annals of the Rheumatic Diseases, 59*(11), 857–863.

Bonaiuti, D., Shea, B., Iovine, R., et al. (2007). Exercise for preventing and treating osteoporosis in postmenopausal women (Review). The Cochrane Collaboration. The Cochrane Library, Issue 2. Retrieved October 15, 2012, from http://www.thecochranelibrary.com

Burks, K. (2002). Health concerns of men with osteoarthritis of the knee. *Orthopedic Nursing, 21*(4), 28–34.

Dionne, C. E., Dunn, K. M., & Croft, P. R. (2006). Does back pain prevalence really decrease with increasing age? A systematic review. *Age and Ageing, 35*, 229–234.

Distler, J., & Anguelouch, A. (2006). Evidence-based practice: Review of clinical evidence on the efficacy of glucosamine and chondroitin in the treatment of osteoarthritis. *Journal of the American Academy of Nurse Practitioners, 18*, 487–493.

Dixon, T., & Penm, E. (2006). *Health expenditure for arthritis and musculoskeletal conditions in Australia 2000–2001*. Canberra: Australian Institute of Health & Welfare.

Flores, E. K. (2012). Falls risk assessment and modification. *Home Health Care Management & Practice, 24*(4), 198–204.

Fransen, M., McConnell, S., & Bell, M. (2007). Exercise for ostearthritis of the hip or knee (Review). The Cochrane Collaboration. The Cochrane Library, Issue 2. Retrieved October 17, 2012, from http://www.thecochranelibrary.com

Jakobsson, U., & Hallberg, I.R. (2002). Pain and quality of life among older people with rheumatoid arthritis and/or osteoarthritis: a literature review. *Journal of Clinical Nursing, 11*(4), 430–443.

Jakobsson, U., & Hallberg, I. R. (2006). Quality of life among older adults with osteoarthritis. *Journal of Gerontological Nursing*, (August), 51–60.

Janke, M. C., Jones, J. J., Payne, L. L., et al. (2011). Living with arthritis: using self management of valued activities to promote health. *Qualitative Health Research, 22*(3), 360–372.

Kee, C. (2003). Older adults with osteoarthritis. Physiological status and physical function. *Journal of Gerontological Nursing, 29*(12), 26–34.

Kwon, T. D., Pittler, M. H., & Ernst, E. (2006). Acupuncture for peripheral joint osteoarthritis. A systematic review and meta-analysis. *Rheumatology, 45*, 1331–1337.

Lewiecki, M. (2011). Safety of the long term bisphosphonate therapy for the management of osteoporosis. *Drugs, 71*(6), 791–814.

McBane, S. (2011). Oseoporosis: a review of current recommendations and emerging treatment options. *Formulary, 46*, 432–439.

McCloskey, E. (2009). *FRAX identifying people at high risk of fracture*. Switzerland: International Osteoporosis Foundation.

Mann, C. (2012). Recognising and meeting the needs of people with osteoporosis. *Primary Health Care, 22*(7), 32–39. Retrieved Octpber 18, 2012, from http://web.ebscohost.com/ehost/pdfviewer/pdfviewer?vid=4&sid=9f76e5fb-62a5–4020–8288–9ad423caea25%40sessionmgr10&hid=28

Martin, M. S., Sell, S. V., & Damter, J. (2012). Glucosamine and chondroitin and appropriate adjunct treatment of symptomatic osteoarthritis of the knee. *Orthopaedic Nursing, 31*(3), 160–166.

Murtagh, K. N., & Hubert, H. B. (2004). Gender differences and physical disability among an elderly cohort. *American Journal of Public Health, 94*(8), 1406–1411.

National Institute for Health and Clinical Excellence (NICE). (2008). *Osteoarthritis: National clinical guideline for care and management in adults*. London: Royal College of Physicians. Retrieved June 2013 from http://www.nice.org.uk/nicemedia/pdf/CG059FullGuideline.pdf

Nazarko, L. (2011). Silent epidemic: helping people live with osteoporosis. *British Journal of Healthcare Assistants, 5*(3), 111–116.

Osteoporosis Australia. (n.d.). Stop the next fracture. Consumer guide – managing osteoporosis. Osteoporosis Australia. Retrieved October 18, 2012, www.osteoporosis.org.au

Rahman, N., Bhatia, K., & Penm, E. (2005). *Arthritis and musculoskeletal conditions in Australia: with a focus on osteoarthritis, rheumatoid arthritis and osteoporosis. Arthritis series no. 1*. Canberra: Australian Institute of Health & Welfare.

Rooney, J. (2004). Oh, those aching joints. What you need to know about arthritis. *Nursing, 34*, 58–63.

Schofield, P. (2008). Pain management in osteoarthritis. *Practice Nurse, 35*(6), 20–25.

Simon, J. A., Murphy, D., Ravnikar, V. A., et al. (2007). Hysterectomy and surgical menopause. A management plan based on expert opinion. *Contemporary OB/GYN, 52*(9), 1–8.

Swann, J. I. (2012). Osteoporosis: the fragile bone disease. *British Journal of Healthcare Assistants, 6*(2), 59–62.

Swift, A. (2012a). Osteoarthritis 1: physiology, risk factors and causes of pain. *Nursing Times, 108*(7), 12–15.

Swift, A. (2012b). Osteoarthritis 2: pain management and treatment strategies. *Nursing Times, 108*(8), 25–27.

Towheed, T. E., Maxwell, L., Judd, M. G., et al. (2007a). Acetaminophen for osteoarthritis (Review). The Cochrane Collaboration. The Cochrane Library, Issue 2. Retrieved October 17, 2012, from http://www.thecochranelibrary.com

Towheed, T. E., Maxwell, L., Anastassiades, T. P., et al. (2007b). Glucosamine therapy for treating osteoarthritis (Review). The Cochrane Collaboration. The Cochrane Library, Issue 2. Retrieved October 17, 2012, from http://www.thecochranelibrary.com

Wang, T., Belza, B., Thompson, F. E., et al. (2006). Effects of aquatic exercise on flexibility, strength and aerobic fitness in adults with osteoarthritis of the hip or knee. *Journal of Advanced Nursing, 57*(2), 141–152.

Walker, J. (2011). Management of osteoarthritis. *Nursing Older People, 23*(9), 14–19.

World Health Organization. (2004). WHO Scientific Group on the Assessment of Osteoporosis at Primary Health Care Level. Summary Meeting Report, Brussels, Belgium, 5–7 May 2004. Retrieved January 15, 2013, from http://www.who.int/chp/topics/Osteoporosis.pdf

Wolkove, N., Elkholy, O., Baltzan, M., et al. (2007). Sleep and ageing: 1 Sleep disorders commonly found in older people. *Journal of the Canadian Medical Association, 176*(9), 1299–1304.

CHAPTER 26

Rhonda Griffiths

Principles of practice for supportive care: diabetes

Learning objectives

When you have completed this chapter you will be able to:

- differentiate between type 1, type 2 and gestational diabetes mellitus
- state the principles of management for each classification
- state the acute and chronic complications of diabetes mellitus
- state precautions to be adopted prior to, during and following exercise
- list the topics to be included in education for people with diabetes mellitus.

Key words

diabetes mellitus, management, diabetic complications, patient education, dietary modification and exercise

Glossary

AGEs: Advanced glycosylation end-products.
BGL: Blood glucose level.
CSII: Continuous subcutaneous insulin infusion.
DKA: Diabetic ketoacidosis.
DM: Diabetes mellitus.
GDM: Gestational diabetes mellitus.
HbA_{1c}: Glycoslated haemoglobin.
HBGM: Home blood glucose monitor.
IGT: Impaired glucose tolerance.
OGTT: Oral glucose tolerance test.
SBGM: Self-blood glucose monitoring.

INTRODUCTION

Diabetes mellitus (DM) is a metabolic disorder that affects an estimated 250 million people worldwide. Australian data indicates that 900 000 people (4.9% of the population) have been diagnosed with diabetes (Australian Institute of Health and Welfare [AIHW], 2011); however, only half the people with type 2 DM are diagnosed (Dunstan et al., 2002). In addition, 6% of Australians have impaired glucose tolerance (IGT) which is a precursor to type 2 DM (Dunstan et al., 2002). The incidence of DM is increasing, and there is currently no cure.

There are two primary forms of DM. About 10–15% of people have type 1 and 85–90% have type 2 DM (AIHW, 2011). There is a third form that is increasing in incidence. Gestational diabetes mellitus (GDM) is first diagnosed during pregnancy and is increasingly common in developed countries. GDM is also considered to be a precursor to type 2 DM, and up to half the women diagnosed with GDM develop type 2 DM over the 20 years following pregnancy (Lee, Hiscock, Wein, Walker, & Permezel, 2007). Regardless of the type, DM is characterised by chronic hyperglycaemia with disturbance of carbohydrate, fat and protein metabolism resulting from defects in insulin secretion and insulin action independently or in combination. This chapter focuses on the management of type 1 and type 2 DM. Guidelines for the management of GDM can be found in midwifery textbooks and journal articles.

Type 1 and type 2 DM are different disease processes. An individual can have type 1 or type 2, but never both. People with type 1 DM require exogenous insulin to sustain life because their pancreas does not produce any insulin; this group is insulin *dependent*. Type 2 DM occurs when the pancreas produces insufficient insulin and/or the body cannot use insulin effectively (insulin resistance). People with type 2 and GDM do not require exogenous insulin to sustain life, but many do inject insulin to improve their glycaemic control which improves quality of life; this group is insulin *requiring*.

The incidence of type 2 DM is not distributed equally across the community, with some ethnic groups being over-represented. Australians from Aboriginal and Torres Strait Islander communities are particularly at risk with up to 50% of people in some communities having DM (AIHW, 2011; Dunstan et al., 2002). The incidence of GDM is also increasing, and is estimated to be around 5% of pregnancies in Australia, although incidence rates as high as 20% are found among Aboriginal and Torres Strait Islander women and women from high-risk populations such as from the Indian sub-continent, Asia and Pacific islands (AIHW, 2002).

DM presents as a combination of symptoms and signs that include thirst, polyuria, polydipsia, blurred vision and, in type 1 diabetes, weight loss. In severe cases diabetic ketoacidosis (DKA) (for type 1) or the non-ketotic hyperosmolar state (type 2) may be present which, if not treated as an emergency, can result in death.

The goal of treatment is to assist the person with DM to achieve and maintain a blood glucose level (BGL) that is as close to physiological levels as possible, delaying onset and reducing the severity of diabetes related complications and decreasing the associated morbidity and mortality. A combination therapy of diet, medication and exercise, supported by education designed to meet the needs of each person, is the most effective way to achieve this goal. Two large landmark studies have demonstrated an association between poor control of blood glucose and the onset and progression of complications for type 1 DM (The Diabetes Control and Complications Trial Research Group, 1993) and type 2 DM (Stratton et al., 2000), also identifying the optimal BGLs for both types of DM. These studies remain the benchmark because the cost and scale of these studies will probably preclude them being replicated.

DIAGNOSIS OF DIABETES

Type 1 diabetes

Type 1 DM is the result of destruction of beta-cells in the pancreas. This destruction can occur for some time before clinical symptoms are obvious, although the progression of symptoms is rapid once the remaining beta-cells are unable to meet the body's demand for insulin (American Diabetes Association, 2007; Craig et al., 2011; De Fronzo, Ferrannini, Keen, & Zimmet, 2004). Type 1 is the most common form of DM among children and young adults, although onset can occur at any age (Craig et al., 2011). The incidence of the disorder varies around the world. The highest incidence is reported in Scandinavian countries and the lowest in Oriental groups and populations living in the tropics. The disorder is also extremely rare among American Indian tribes (Karvonen, Viik-Kajander, Libman, LaPorte, & Tuomilehto, 2000).

Type 1 DM has been associated with genetic determinants, environmental factors and acquired factors including autoimmune reactions. Autoimmune reactions appear to play a significant role as up to 70% of newly diagnosed people will have islet cell antibodies (De Fronzo et al., 2004). Some researchers have identified a peak in diagnosis in the winter months, although that is not consistent across all countries. Nevertheless, the seasonal incidence of the disorder suggests that viral infection is one cause (De Fronzo et al., 2004). The term *idiopathic diabetes* describes forms of type 1 diabetes with no known aetiology (American Diabetes Association, 2007). Discovering a cure for type 1 DM is a priority for researchers investigating the disorder; however at this stage there is no cure and no preventive measures can be taken. It is important for nurses to be aware that, unlike type 2 DM, obesity and lack of exercise do not contribute to the development of type 1 diabetes.

Type 2 diabetes

Type 2 is the most common form of DM and in some groups, including the America Indian tribes and population in the South Pacific, it is the only form of diabetes (De Fronzo et al., 2004). People with type 2 DM do not usually require insulin to survive, although many do use insulin to improve glycaemic control and quality of life (American Diabetes Association, 2007).

Although the aetiology of type 2 DM is not clear, there is a strong familial tendency to develop the disorder, particularly when combined with life style factors such as obesity. Women who have previously developed GDM have a increased risk of developing type 2 DM (Lee et al., 2007). Unlike type 1 DM, the beta-cells are not destroyed by autoimmune processes and DKA rarely occurs spontaneously, although it may occur in conjunction with stress or other illness, such as infection (American Diabetes Association, 2007). Individuals who are overweight or obese, who do not exercise and eat a diet high in fat are particularly at risk of developing type 2 DM. People who have an increased percentage of abdominal body fat, but who may not be obese by traditional measures, are also at risk because abdominal obesity is strongly associated with insulin resistance. Abdominal fat is also associated with increased cardiovascular disease (Aguilar-Salinas et al., 2006; Riddle & Karl, 2012). Increasing age is also a factor, therefore some lean elderly people will develop type 2 DM in old age. Insulin resistance is a distinguishing feature of the disorder and some people may have normal or elevated insulin levels (Bonadonna, Cucinotta, Fedele, Riccardi, & The Metascreen Writing Committee, 2006).

The metabolic syndrome, which is strongly associated with insulin resistance, describes a cluster of symptoms and signs associated with type 2 DM and cardiovascular disease, namely abdominal obesity, dyslipidaemia, insulin resistance, hyperglycaemia, impaired fibrinolysis and hypertension (Katzmarzyk, Church, Janssen, Ross, & Blair, 2005; Riddle & Karl, 2012, p. 2101; Rewers et al., 2004). The risk of developing diabetes or a cardiovascular event increases as the levels for these indicators increase above the normal range (Aguilar-Salinas et al., 2006; Bonadonna et al., 2006). DM is associated with increased morbidity and mortality, and people with DM and insulin resistance are at higher risk of mortality from cardiovascular disease (Bonadonna et al., 2006; Riddle & Karl, 2012).

There are two myths about type 2 DM which unfortunately continue to be perpetuated by some health professionals, despite the evidence that DM is a common cause of death in Australia (Australian Bureau of Statistics, May 2012). The first is that levels of blood glucose that are in the low range of elevated are not significant. You may hear individuals say that they have '... a touch of sugar, but nothing to worry about'. In fact, any elevation of blood glucose above the normal range places the person at risk of developing all of the chronic complications (discussed later in this chapter) associated with DM. The second myth is that type 2 DM can be cured. With effective management, including weight loss, increased exercise, dietary changes and medications, the blood glucose level may return to the normal range. However, the pathological processes associated with type 2 DM will manifest at any time if the individual does not continue to follow the recommended lifestyle practices.

DIAGNOSTIC CRITERIA

DM must be considered as the cause when the fasting BGL is above 7. 0 mmol/L, or random levels of 11.1 mmol/L or above (Colagiuri, Girgis, Eigenmann, Gomez, & Griffiths, 2009). If there is doubt about the diagnosis, an oral glucose tolerance test (OGTT) is usually performed. Following an overnight fast, an intravenous blood sample is collected and a 50 or 75 gram glucose drink is consumed. Blood samples are collected at 1 hour and 2 hours following the glucose drink. The BGL will remain elevated in the person with diabetes (World Health Organization, 1999).

Type 1 diabetes

The signs and symptoms of type 1 DM develop rapidly (over days to weeks) and include: hyperglycaemia; excessive thirst; frequent urination; excessive hunger; nausea and vomiting; weight loss; and blurred vision (Craig et al., 2011). People with type 1 DM may be acutely ill when diagnosed, frequently presenting as a medical emergency with hyperglycaemia over 15 mmol/L, ketone bodies in the urine and signs of acidosis and severe dehydration. A detailed description of the signs, symptoms and management of severe hyperglycaemia will not be provided here, therefore you are advised to consult one of your texts if you need to revise that information. An OGTT infrequently is not necessary to confirm the diagnosis as the random BGL will be above 11 mmol/L.

Type 2 diabetes

The onset of type 2 DM is usually insidious and may occur over years. The symptoms are similar to type 1 (hyperglycaemia; excessive thirst; frequent urination; excessive hunger; nausea and vomiting and blurred vision) although weight loss is rarely present: in fact the majority of people with type 2 DM are overweight or obese. As previously stated, DKA is also rarely seen in people with type 2 DM. The diagnosis is confirmed by a fasting BGL, a non-fasting BGL or the OGTT.

The incidence of type 2 DM in children and adolescents is increasing in developed countries. Young people who develop mature onset diabetes of the young (MODY) commonly have a family history of type 2 DM and occasionally they present with DKA, although these young people do not have insulin cell antibodies as is the case with type 1 diabetes (Alberti et al., 2004; Fajans & Bell, 2011).

INTERVENTIONS

The management of DM involves medications (insulin and/or oral medications), dietary modification, exercise and self-management education. While the principles of dietary modification and exercise are common to all types of DM, the medication regimen is varied according to the type of DM and the person's level of control. People with type 1 DM are not treated with oral medications (Craig et al., 2011). They have an individualised insulin regimen designed to maintain their BGL as close as possible to physiological levels and that also reflect their lifestyle. People with type 2 DM may be prescribed oral medications and/or insulin, depending on their BGL (Colagiuri et al., 2009).

This section provides an overview of management. DM is a complex disorder that is associated with other disease processes, for example cardiac disease and stroke, and leads to complications in almost all body systems. Therefore you are advised to consult specialised resources to assist you to develop appropriate care plans for people with DM.

Medication management

Type 1 diabetes

In the person without DM, insulin release is stimulated by the ingestion of food containing carbohydrates. Therefore, the objective of treatment is to have small amounts of insulin circulating at all times supplemented with larger doses after meals. A regimen of insulin injections is prescribed to mimic the physiological insulin secretion pattern of people who do not have DM.

The most common regimens for people with type 1 DM are either:

1 a combination of meal-time (rapid-acting) and background (long-acting) insulin therapies, or
2 a continuous subcutaneous infusion of insulin (CSII).

Insulin is administered by subcutaneous injection using a needle and syringe, an insulin pen device or, more recently, continuous subcutaneous insulin infusion by an infusion pump worn by the person (National Institute for Health and Clinical Excellence [NICE], 2011). Current forms of insulin must be injected as they are rendered inert by digestion. However, new forms of oral (The Diabetes Prevention Trial — Type 1 Study Group, 2005) and inhaled (McElduff & Yue, 2007; Rosenstock, Cappelleri, Bolinder, & Gerber, 2004; Rosenstock et al., 2010; Skyler et al., 2004) insulin are being tested.

Insulin was originally extracted from the pancreas of cattle or pigs. Current forms of insulin are produced in a laboratory which overcomes some of the side effects associated with insulin from animal sources. The name and time of onset, peak and duration of action of insulin available in Australia is presented in Table 26.1 (MIMS Australia Pty Ltd, 2012).

Insulin doses are individualised depending on the person's response. It is important to note that insulin requirements in all patients are dynamic and therefore require frequent monitoring and dose adjustment to achieve the best possible glycaemic control. Early in

TABLE 26.1
Types of insulin

	ONSET	PEAK	DURATION
Mixed insulin preparations			
Insulin Neutral 30% + Isophane 70% inject subcutaneous Brand name: Mixtard 30/70	30 mins	2–12 hrs	24 hrs
Insulin Neutral 30% + Isophane NPH 70% 100 units/mL inject subcutaneous Brand name: Humulin 30/70	More rapid than NPH alone	2–12 hrs	16–18 hrs
Insulin Neutral 50% + Isophane 50% 100 units/mL inject subcutaneous Brand name: Mixtard 50/50	30 mins	4–8 hrs	24 hrs
Analogue insulin preparations			
Rapid-acting insulin			
Insulin Aspart 100 units/mL Brand name: NovoRapid	0–20 mins	1–2 hrs	4–5 hrs
Insulin Lispro 100 units/mL Brand name: Humalog	0–20 mins	1–2 hrs	4–5 hrs
Insulin Glulisine 100 units/mL Brand name: Apidra	0–20 mins	1–2 hrs	4–5 hrs
Long-acting insulin			
Insulin Detemir 100 units/mL Brand name: Levemir	0.5–1 hr	3–8 hrs	Up to 24 hrs
Insulin Glargine 100 units/mL Brand name: Lantus	1–2 hrs	None	24 hrs
Mixed insulin preparations			
Insulin Aspart 30% + Protamine 70% 100 units/mL Brand name: NovoMix 30	0–20 mins	1–4 hrs	24 hrs
Insulin Lispro 25% + Lispro Protamine 75% 100 units/mL Brand name: Humalog Mix 25	0–20 mins	1–4 hrs	24 hrs
Insulin Lispro 50% + Lispro Protamine 50% 100 units/mL Brand name: Humalog Mix 50	0–15 mins	2 hrs	16–18 hrs
Human insulin preparations			
Short-acting insulin			
Insulin Neutral HM 100 units/mL inject subcutaneous Brand name: Humulin R	30 mins	2–4 hrs	6–8 hr
Insulin Neutral HM 100 units/mL inject subcutaneous Brand name: Actrapid	30 mins	2.5–5 hrs	8 hrs
Intermediate-acting insulin			
Insulin Isophane 100 units/mL inject subcutaneous Brand name: Protaphane	1.5 hrs	4–12 hrs	24 hrs
Insulin Isophane NPH 100 units/mL inject subcutaneous Brand name: Humulin NPH	1 hr	4–10 hrs	16–18 hrs

the diagnosis of type 1 DM there is often a phase when there is some residue insulin secretion and insulin replacement therapy may not be required for a brief period of time. This phenomenon is commonly referred to as the 'honeymoon' period (Harmel & Mathur, 2004) and is a result of the beta cells in the pancreas rallying to produce the last of the person's insulin prior to their complete destruction. This phenomenon can prove challenging for patients and their families as the diabetes goes into remission. Support and education is the key to successfully negotiating this period in the disease process.

Background or long-acting insulin

Long-acting insulin is used specifically to control the release of stored glucose from the liver, and therefore control the fasting BGL. Recent developments have enabled the design of new insulin analogues which have long-acting profiles that are more useful in the management of DM, particularly for people with type 1. Insulin Glargine (Lantus®) (Ratner et al., 2000; Wang, Carabino, & Vergara, 2003) and Insulin Detemir (Levemir®) (Hermansen, Madsbad, Perrild, Kristensen, & Axelsen, 2001) are commonly used as once-daily or twice-daily respectively injections as background insulin therapy. These insulin analogues have largely replaced the more traditional therapies of Isophane (Protaphane®, Humulin NPH®) (intermediate-acting insulin) and Lente (Ultralente®, Humulin L®) and Ultratard® (long-acting insulin). Glargine and Detemir provide a prolonged and reasonably consistent level of insulin which more accurately mimics insulin secretion in people without DM (Garber et al., 2012) unlike the traditional types of longer acting insulin. The onset of action of intermediate-acting insulin is around 90 minutes after injection, with the peak action at 4 to 12 hours and duration of 24 hours. The onset of action for long-acting insulin is around 4 hours, followed by a broad peak of action that lasts for 8 to 16 hours with a duration ranging from 20 to 36 hours.

Rapid-acting insulin

The preferred option for mealtime insulin in adults is one of the rapid-acting analogues: Insulin Aspart (NovoRapid®) or Insulin Lispro (Humalog®) or Insulin Glulisine (Apidra®). All have rapid onset of action (10–20 minutes) and short duration (3–5 hours) thus mimicking natural secretion of insulin following meals. Rapid-acting insulin is administered before meals and large snacks of more than 15 grams carbohydrate (equivalent to one slice of sandwich-thickness bread). It is ideal for adults with type 1 DM to have flexible insulin doses depending on their carbohydrate intake. Therefore it is important that management regimens for people with type 1 DM allow for a flexible lifestyle and that they have the opportunity to attend specific educational programs to provide them with the skills and knowledge required to assume a self-care role. Education programs such as DAFNE (Dose Adjustment For Normal Eating) (McIntyre, 2006) have been designed specifically for people with type 1 DM. A detailed description of the characteristics of various types of insulin can be found in pharmacology sources of evidence.

Continuous subcutaneous infusion of insulin (CSII)

The advent of portable and reliable subcutaneous infusion pumps has revolutionised the management of type 1 DM. Insulin pumps reduce the need for multiple daily injections and allows for better glucose control as the therapy is adjusted frequently. One drawback of using CSII is that equipment failure, including blockage or disconnection of the tube, can result in a rapid elevation of BGL. The pumps and the necessary consumables are expensive and not always covered by private health insurance, although consumables are available through the government-subsidised National Diabetes Support Scheme. Cost does prevent some people using pump therapy. Successful use of a pump is dependent upon frequent testing of BGL using Self-Blood Glucose Monitoring (SBGM) technique and the person's ability to accurately count carbohydrate intake (NICE, 2011).

Either rapid- or short-acting insulin is used in the insulin pumps. There are two specific modes of administration:

1 basal rate, meaning the continuous rate of insulin infused as a background dose
2 bolus rate, meaning the mealtime dose of insulin given as a bolus to cover the carbohydrate intake.

Specific education programs are required to enable people to use CSII effectively and safely and assistance should be available when required (NICE, 2011).

Type 2 diabetes

Unlike people with type 1 DM, people with type 2 DM do not require exogenous insulin to sustain life. Dietary modification and increased exercise is the first approach to management of people with type 2 DM particularly those who are overweight and with a BGL just above the normal range. Nevertheless, over the past decade the medication management of type 2 has changed significantly. Insulin is now commonly used when hyperglycaemia persists and the person is taking maximum doses of oral medications and new categories of oral medication have been introduced (American Diabetes Association, 2012; Colagiuri et al., 2009; Kamp, 2007).

Insulin-sensitising drugs

These medications lower BGL by sensitising the muscle and liver cells to insulin, which may improve the insulin resistance present in type 2 DM and increasing the uptake of glucose by cells (Kamp, 2007). Insulin-sensitising drugs have the advantage of lowering BGL without placing the person at risk of hypoglycaemia and are effective for people who are overweight or obese. Commonly used medications are Biguanide (Metformin®) or a thiazolidinedione. Recent research in the United Kingdom demonstrated that the use of Metformin® can significantly reduce the incidence of both micro-vascular and macro-vascular complications, although it can also cause gastrointestinal upset such as nausea, abdominal pain and diarrhoea. These medications are not suitable for all people and they should be introduced with caution due to their side effects (see chart below).

Insulin-stimulating drugs

Sulfonylurea derivatives are a class of antidiabetic drugs that are used in the management of type 2 DM. There are short-acting (e. g. tolbutamide) and long-acting (e. g. glimepiride) forms of these drugs and they act by increasing insulin release from the beta cells in the pancreas. A side effect of this mode of action is the potential for hypoglycaemia (low blood glucose), therefore the introduction of these drugs may be staged to assess dose response. Therapeutic dose adjustment is usually guided by SBGM results. Sulfonylureas are often used in combination with the insulin-sensitising drugs in order to address the major features of type 2: reduced insulin production and insulin resistance at the cell. The common forms of oral medication are shown in Table 26.2 (MIMS Australia Pty Ltd, 2012).

Drugs that focus on the incretin system

The oral dipeptidyl peptidase 4 (DPP4) inhibitors enhance circulating concentrations of glucagon-like peptide-1 (GLP1) and glucose dependent insulinotropic polypeptide (GIP) (Richter, Bandeira-Echtler, Bergerhoff, & Lerch, 2008). This causes an increase in glucose-dependent insulin secretion and a reduction in glucagon secretion. There is little risk of hypoglycaemia when using these medications alone or in combination with Metformin. A benefit of this class of drug is that they are reported to be weight neutral (Inzucchi et al., 2012). Injectable GLP1-receptor agonists mimic endogenous GLP1 therefore stimulating the pancreatic beta cells to produce insulin in a glucose-dependent manner; also appetite

TABLE 26.2

Oral agents for management of diabetes

DRUG	BRAND NAME	TABLET SIZE (mg)	MAX DAILY DOSE	ROUTE OF DISPOSAL	DURATION OF ACTION (hours)	MODE OF ACTION	CONTRAINDICATIONS	ADVERSE EFFECTS
Sulphonylureas								
Glibenclamide	Daonil Semi-Daonil Glimel	5, 2.5	20	Liver	10–15	Potentiate stimulated insulin release from pancreatic beta-cells Influence peripheral uptake of glucose	DKA, Type 1 DM, pregnancy, hypersensitivity to sulphonylureas, stress	Hypoglycaemia, GIT upset, skin reactions, LFT disturbance
Gliclazide	Diamicron	80	320	Kidney, Liver	12–15			
	Diamicron MR	30	120					
	Glyade	40	320					
	NIDEM	40	320					
Glimepiride	Amaryl	1, 2, 4	4	Kidney	Up to 24			
Glipizide	Minidiab Melizide	5	40	Kidney, Liver	Up to 24			
Thiazolidinediones								
Pioglitazone	Actos	15, 30, 45	45	Liver	1–8	Reduces insulin resistance Enhances insulin sensitivity	Pre-existing liver disease, HF, pregnancy, anaemia	Oedema, decrease Hb, hypercholesterolaemia
Biguanides								
Metformin	Diabex Diaformin Glucophage Glucomet NovoMet Glucohexal	500, 850, 1000	3000 [doses above 2000 are rarely used]	Kidney	5–6	Increases glucose uptake in skeletal muscle and fat Decreases appetite and GI absorption of glucose	DKA, serious renal impairment, chronic liver disease, history of lactic acidosis, PE, pregnancy	Nausea, GI discomfort, diarrhoea, macrocytic anaemia, lactic acidosis

Glucosidase inhibitor								
Acarbose	Glucobay	50, 100	600	Kidney	Up to 24	Delays CHO digestion	Pregnancy, lactation, hypersensitivity, renal impairment, bowel disease Not to be used in patients < 18 years	Flatulence, diarrhoea, nausea, skin reactions, ileus, hepatitis
Dipeptidyl peptidase-4 (DPP4) Inhibitors								
Sitagliptin Vildagliptin Saxagliptin Linagliptin	Januvia Galvus Onglyza Trajenta	25, 50, 100 50 5 5	100 100 5 5	Kidney Bile Salts GIT	Up to 24	Inhibits DPP-4 activity, increasing postprandial active incretin [GLP-1, GIP] concentrations, causing increase in glucose-dependent insulin secretion	Pregnancy, lactation, hypersensitivity, hepatic impairment Not to be use in patients < 18 years Caution in renal impairment *May be used in renal impairment*	Urticaria/angio-oedema, dizziness, headache, pancreatitis
New type of glucose-lowering injection therapy								
Glucagon-Like Peptide-1 (GLP-1) receptor agonists								
Exenatide	Byetta	5 mcg, 10 mcg	20 mcg	Kidney	Up to 12 hours	Activates GLP-1 receptors increasing glucose-dependent insulin secretion, slows gastric empting and increases satiety	Pregnancy, lactation, hypersensitivity, severe gastrointestinal disease, hepatic impairment Not to be use in patients < 18 years Caution in renal impairment	Nausea, GIT disturbances, urticaria/angio-oedema, acute renal failure, pancreatitis

is decreased as gastric emptying is slowed. It has been noted that the major advantage of this class of drug is modest weight reduction in most cases; however the side effects of nausea and vomiting may limit the tolerability of use.

Not all patients are suited to these therapies. Please note the precautions and potential side-effects listed in the table below (Inzucchi et al., 2012).

INSULIN THERAPY

Insulin therapy may be introduced when oral therapy is not effective or when patients have contraindications for glucose-lowering oral medications. It is important to note that the introduction of insulin therapy as a management strategy for a patient with type 2 DM does not change the diagnosis. People with type 2 DM who inject insulin are referred to as 'insulin requiring' and people with type 1 DM are 'insulin dependent'. Insulin therapy may be introduced in combination with tablets or as a replacement therapy depending on the patient's circumstances. Often less intense insulin regimens are used and the role for pre-mixed insulin preparations is more common in the management of type 2 DM. Insulin therapy is used in combination with Metformin®, a sulfonylurea or both. Goals for glucose control are individualised and may be more relaxed in older patients.

There is no consensus on when to prescribe insulin for people with type 2 DM, although-$HbA1_c$ level of more than 10% on more than one occasion is regarded by clinicians as an appropriate time to commence insulin. Frequently a small dose of insulin is required to start as the natural production of insulin declines, with the dose being increased as time passes. Introducing insulin reduces an individual's resistance to the insulin produced by their pancreas which allows their insulin to work more effectively. People with type 2 DM frequently start on one injection of long-acting insulin per day with short-acting insulin being added before meals if the BGL is not reduced.

Insulin is generally prescribed at either pre-supper or at bedtime. In clinical practice, insulin start doses are usually weight-related. Whilst it is true that insulin-requiring patients generally require large doses of insulin to achieve good glucose control (up to 2.0 units per kg per day), starting doses are usually much smaller and may be as low as 0.1 unit per kilogram per day. For example, a 100-kg person may be prescribed 10 units of long-acting insulin at bedtime in addition to oral medications. Insulin doses in type 2 DM are adjusted according to the person's specific response.

If insulin therapy is introduced because there are contraindications to tablet therapy, twice-daily doses of premixed insulin are often prescribed. The choice of premixed insulin is dependent on the individual's blood glucose profile. Start doses are usually estimated as 0.5 units per kilogram per day, with the total daily dose divided with 60% injected at breakfast and 40% injected at the evening meal. Therapeutic adjustment of insulin is dependent on the individual's health status and may be as frequent as daily for those patients who are acutely ill, although it is more common for weekly adjustments of doses for patients who are in the ambulatory or community setting.

Dietary interventions

Type 1 diabetes

The development of type 1 DM is not associated with obesity or a sedentary life style; however that is not understood by many people, including health professionals. As a result it is not unusual for children with type 1 diabetes and their parents to be criticised for contributing to development of type 1 DM. Nurses need to understand the differences between the two conditions and educate the community when they are aware of inaccurate perceptions.

While type 1 DM is not associated with weight gain, it is particularly important that people with that form of DM consider the type and quantity of carbohydrate they eat and the timing of meals relative to the administration of insulin to achieve optimal glycaemic control. This group is at particular risk of hyperglycaemia leading to DKA and hypoglycaemia leading to loss of consciousness (addressed later in this chapter under Acute Complications). Dietary counselling and education will assist people with type 1 DM to prevent those acute complications and also assist to slow the development and progression of both micro- and macrovascular complications which are invariably present to some degree in people who have had type 1 DM for more than 5 years (The Diabetes Control and Complications Trial Research Group, 1993).

Type 2 diabetes

Obesity is increasing in all developed countries and lifestyle modification, usually geared to weight management using both diet and exercise, is the major tool to achieve weight loss in those people who are overweight and obese. Researchers have unequivocally demonstrated that type 2 DM can be prevented, or at least delayed, by appropriate and timely lifestyle modification (Moore et al., 2007).

Nutritional management and education are the cornerstones of DM care (Dietitians Association of Australia New South Wales Branch Diabetes Interest Group, 2006). All people with type 2 DM (and when possible those with IGT) should have specialist assessment and education from a dietitian. Basic principles of regular meals, with emphasis on low fat, high fibre and controlled carbohydrate intake, are generally followed. The introduction of regular physical activity to achieve weight loss is essential; however recent studies have noted that resistance training provides the most overall benefit in the management of type 2 DM (Colagiuri et al., 2009).

The significance of dietary modification and weight loss in people who are at risk or have been diagnosed with type 2 DM cannot be over-emphasised. Obesity is the strongest known risk factor for type 2 DM and is associated with disturbances of carbohydrate, fat (dyslipidaemia) and protein metabolism in the community (Hossain, Kawar, & El Nahas, 2007). The combination of dietary advice and exercise has been demonstrated to achieve a significant reduction of glycated haemoglobin within 6 months of commencing the program (Moore et al., 2007).

Dietary advice for people with DM follows the healthy eating guidelines recommended for all people based on the food pyramid: high unrefined carbohydrate, some protein and low fat. For people with DM, the recommended diet is 25 to 30% of energy from fat and around 50% of the total energy from unrefined carbohydrate (Moore et al., 2007). These guidelines are consistent with the guidelines from the National Heart Foundation (National Vascular Disease Prevention Alliance, 2009).

In recent years the significance of the gylcaemic index (GI) of foods has attracted increasing attention from researchers and clinicians. The GI is the measure of the effect of different carbohydrate foods on BGLs. Foods with high GI are quickly digested and absorbed into the bloodstream causing the BGL to rise rapidly and stimulating a corresponding release of insulin (Brand-Miller, Hayne, Petocz, & Colagiuri, 2003; Gilbertson et al., 2001). Foods with low GI are digested and absorbed slowly causing a slow rise in the BGL and a slower and reduced release of insulin. Low GI foods include legumes and dairy products, whereas potatoes, rice and white bread have a high GI. The hormone insulin has a growth factor-like effect and high levels are associated with weight gain. The current line of thinking is that a steady release of glucose into the blood may have an insulin-sparing effect which, in conjunction with other interventions, contributes to optimal gylcaemic control for people with diabetes (Barclay et al., 2008).

Exercise

While regular exercise is not an intervention per se for the management of type 1 DM, regular exercise is recommended for health and wellbeing in all people. As shown above, exercise, particularly when combined with healthy eating, has a significant role in the prevention and progression of type 2 DM (Moore et al., 2007) and is a fundamental defence against type 2 and obesity (Colagiuri et al., 2009).

However, as all types of exercise require a readily available source of energy, adjustments in the patient's overall management strategy is required. People with type 1 DM need to take particular precautions before, during and after exercise. Prior to exercise people with type 1 need to check their BGL and if necessary eat some rapidly digested carbohydrate.

Exercise increases the sensitivity of muscle cells to insulin, which is one reason it is encouraged in people with type 2 DM, particularly those with insulin resistance and hyperinsulinaemia. Exercise improves insulin action and has a beneficial effect on cardiac risk factors (Chipkin, Klugh, & Chasan-Taber, 2001; Thomas, Elliott, & Naughton, 2007). Exercise assists the circulating insulin to enter the muscle where it acts to enable glucose to move from the blood into muscle. In people with type 1 DM the shift of glucose from the blood can result in hypoglycaemia. If exercise is to be sustained, for example in a game of football or tennis, the person may need to take additional carbohydrate during exercise. Exercise reduces insulin requirements in the hours after physical activity, therefore the person with type 1 DM should continue to monitor their BGL following exercise.

If there is too little insulin circulating at the time of exercise the body will convert fat into ketone bodies to provide energy to the cells, despite the elevated circulating glucose, resulting in ketosis. Exercise also stimulates the release of glucose from the liver, which can result in hyperglycaemia. Therefore, people with hyperglycaemia are advised not to exercise until the cause is determined and treatment initiated. Education in self-management must include guidelines for dietary or insulin adjustment prior to, during and following exercise to decrease the risk of hypoglycaemia and hyperglycaemia with ketosis (Colagiuri et al., 2009).

Many people with DM may find establishing an exercise program including resistance training challenging. The nurse should advise people to commence with gentle exercise such as a walking program or participation in gentle exercise classes and encourage the person to progress on to more strenuous forms of exercise as fitness improves. Prior to commencing an exercise program, the person with type 2 DM should discuss the planned exercise with his/her doctor. Foot care and appropriate types of shoes, cardiovascular function and self-monitoring should be discussed and education provided if necessary.

We have provided a brief background to the significance of healthy eating and appropriate exercise in the management of DM. Information describing specific nutrition and exercise interventions can be accessed elsewhere.

COMPLICATIONS OF DIABETES

Is this section we briefly outline DM-related complications. The care of people with complications requires a comprehensive management plan that is beyond the scope of this chapter, and we suggest that the reader refers to an appropriate reference (American Diabetes Association, 2012).

Acute complications

Hypoglycaemia

Hypoglycaemia (also referred to as 'a hypo') occurs when the person has taken insulin or one of the sulfonylurea drugs and has eaten insufficient carbohydrate causing the BGL to fall to below 4.0 mmol/L in adults. Other common causes of hypoglycaemia include excessive exercise without additional carbohydrate and rapid weight loss by people with type 2 without a reduction of medication. Over-medication is a less common cause, but may result from malfunctioning pen injecting devices, drawing up a larger dose because of poor eyesight or repeat doses of tablets. Children may exhibit symptoms of hypoglycaemia at higher BGLs than adults.

Hypoglycaemia is very common among people with type 1 DM, and those who are poorly controlled may experience episodes of hypoglycaemia most days. People with type 2 DM who inject insulin or take medications that stimulate insulin release are also at risk of hypoglycaemia although the episodes are usually less frequent than among people with type 1. Hypoglycaemic episodes, or 'hypos', are a frightening and embarrassing experience for people who experience them. Following a hypo, it is common for the person to experience severe headache, and waking in the morning with a headache may be a sign of a hypo during the night.

There are two major groups of signs and symptoms of hypoglycaemia:

1 sympathetic: weakness, sweating, tachycardia, palpitations, tremor, nervousness, irritability, tingling of the mouth and fingers and hunger
2 neuroglucopenic: headache, shivering, visual disturbances, mental dullness, confusion, amnesia, seizures and coma.

Hypoglycaemia may be managed quickly with little assistance if the person is able to recognise the symptoms and has a ready source of glucose available with a high (GI), such as glucose tablets, a third of a glass of regular soft drink or 5 to 7 jelly beans. This initial treatment is usually followed by one 15 g carbohydrate exchange of lower GI food, such as one slice of bread or two biscuits. However, if the person requires assistance, it is recommended that medical assistance is summoned, usually by telephoning for an ambulance. It is recommended that all patients with type 1 DM have a family member or friend who is able and willing to administer a glucagon injection. Glucagon is a hormone, which is secreted from the alpha cells of the pancreas. Its action is the opposite to insulin: glucose is released from the liver thus reversing the hypoglycaemia (Harmel & Mathur, 2004).

Long-term complications

The avoidance of both short- and long-term complications is one of the goals of the management of DM. Long-term complications of DM are caused by the disturbance in metabolism triggered by the absolute or relative lack of insulin over a long duration. DM is a leading cause of renal failure (nephropathy), blindness (retinopathy), coronary vascular disease and amputation of lower limbs (neuropathy). Some health professionals are reluctant to discuss the complications, particularly at the time of diagnosis. Nurses need to be familiar with the complications and have sufficient knowledge to discuss them with people with diabetes and their families.

Long-term complications may be categorised in three major groups:

1 micro-vascular (small vessel disease) — this category includes retinopathy and nephropathy
2 macro-vascular (large vessel disease) — this category includes coronary artery disease, peripheral vascular disease and cerebral vascular disease
3 neuropathy (both autonomic and peripheral nervous systems).

The specific pathophysiology for the formation of diabetic complications is not clear. However, chronically elevated BGLs appear to be a major component for the development

TABLE 26.3
Screening for long-term complications

TEST TO BE CONDUCTED	TIMING/FREQUENCY
HbA_{1c} (average BGL for last 2–3 months)	3 monthly
Review of SBGM	3 monthly (compare to HbA_{1c})
Wt/Ht (BMI)	3 monthly
Blood pressure	3 monthly
Blood lipid profile	6 monthly
Feet examination	6 monthly
Microalbuminuria	Annually
Eye examination	Annually
Self-management skills	Annually
Healthy eating plan	Annually

of these complications (Stratton et al., 2000; The Diabetes Control and Complications Trial Research Group, 1993; The United Kingdom Prospective Study 33, 1996). Abnormalities in the connective tissues in blood vessels are associated with elevated levels of complex compounds known as advanced glycosylation end-products (AGEs). These products may well be the key to the formation of both micro- and macrovascular complications (McDermott, 2002). Neuropathic complications, however, appear to be more closely associated with the demyelination and axonal damage possibly due to the accumulation of sorbitol in the nerve structures (McDermott, 2002).

The landmark diabetes trials (The Diabetes Control and Complications Trial Research Group, 1993; The United Kingdom Prospective Study 33, 1996) noted the relationship between glucose control and reduced risk of development of complications. Results of both trials stressed the importance of early diagnosis and treatment of all complications and associated conditions such as hypertension and mixed dyslipidaemia.

Whilst screening for long-term complications is strongly recommended (American Diabetes Association, 2012), the challenge may be persuading people with DM to attend for various tests which are often time-consuming, therefore a focus on secondary health promotion is needed. An explanation of the reasons for testing is essential. As wellness is the goal for management of all chronic diseases, the regimen of testing may be referred to as a 'wellness program' or 'cycle of care'. The recommended annual cycle of screening for complications is presented in Table 26.3.

SELF-MANAGEMENT

Patient education

Patient education is recognised as an essential component of diabetes management (Colagiuri et al., 2009; Corser, Holmes-Rovner, Lein, & Gossain, 2007) and is best provided by a multidisciplinary team comprising practitioners with specialist knowledge and skills in diabetes care, GPs and including the person with diabetes and their supporters/carer(s). Medical practitioners, nurses, dietitians, podiatrists and psychologists (when available) should collaborate to ensure the best outcomes for people with DM. Research in the fields of psychology, human behaviour, social learning theory and health education has improved our understanding of the problems that underlie relapse from self-care regimens in chronic disease (Colagiuri et al., 2009; Corser et al., 2007) and underpin the formal education programs for people with DM.

Over recent years the emphasis of, and approaches to, DM patient education have changed, due in part to an increased understanding of the complex relationship between adherence to treatment and glycaemic control (Seley & Weinger, 2007; The Diabetes Control and Complications Trial Research Group, 1993; The United Kingdom Prospective Study 33, 1996). People with DM and their support people are required to make daily decisions in order to balance diet, physical activity and medication to achieve their optimum level of control (Colagiuri et al., 2009).

People with DM are required to comprehend and act on content covering an extensive list of topics including the carbohydrate content of various foods and menu design, the action of oral agents and insulin, precautions related to exercise, managing DM during concomitant illness and screening for complications, signs of onset of complications and SBGM. Education sessions are most effective when they focus on developing skills that enable the person to proactively adjust their treatment to account for variations in their day-to-day routines and to identify potential causes of hypo- and hyperglycaemia.

In tandem with the changing emphasis of patient education, value outcomes have also changed (Bradshaw, Richardson, & Kulkarni, 2007; Bradshaw et al., 2007). Adherence to treatments is no longer the only outcome measured. Teaching is no longer limited to a checklist of do's and don'ts on the assumption that information equates with understanding, awareness and confidence in people's abilities to make the necessary adjustments in their lives (Colagiuri et al., 2009).

Nurses need to be familiar with the information that is provided to people and to provide a supporting and reinforcing role to assist people to make the necessary lifestyle changes. The challenge for nurses is to translate a treatment regimen into a plan of care that a person with DM and their support people can follow. While the role and functions of specialist diabetes educators have been described (Seley & Weinger, 2007) as well as standards of practice developed as a basis for professional accreditation and service provision (American Association of Diabetes Educators, 2007; Australian Diabetes Educators Association, 2003), nurses working in all clinical settings will be required to provide care and, in the absence of specialist practitioners, provide education and ongoing follow up to people with DM. The professional associations have developed resources that assist health professionals to provide care to people with DM. You will find useful resources developed by the Australian Diabetes Educators Association (ADEA) on the association's website (http://www.adea.com.au).

Self-blood glucose monitoring

Self-blood glucose monitoring (SBGM) is an important adjunct to the management of people with DM. Regular tests using a home blood glucose monitor (HBGM) assist the person with DM and their health professionals to maintain the balance between medications, diet and exercise on a day-to-day basis and identify trends over time. People who inject insulin are particularly advised to perform regular monitoring and record results which are used to guide insulin doses (ADEA, 2010; Farmer et al., 2007). While the importance of SBGM in management of people who are not taking insulin therapy has recently come in to question (Farmer et al., 2007), most people with DM benefit from regular surveillance.

ADEA's *Position Statement: Use of Blood Glucose Meters* (ADEA, 2010) recommends that people using insulin therapy be encouraged to perform SBGM. The ADEA position

CASE STUDY 26.1 Issues for dietary management in culturally diverse groups

Mr A is a 78-year-old man admitted to the stroke unit with provisional diagnosis of TIAs or syncope. He has lived in Australia since 1995 but speaks only limited English. He was accompanied by his son. The medical history was taken in the emergency department. Clinical observations noted: radial pulse rate 125 bpm irregular; blood pressure (BP) 145/62; respiratory rate 28 bpm. Results of blood analysed for urea, electrolytes, creatinine (UECs) were within normal limits (plasma glucose was not ordered). Haematological profile was described as unremarkable. An electrocardiograph (ECG) identified acute inferior changes with ST-segment elevation.

A healthcare interpreter speaking Arabic was booked for the next day, when a full nursing assessment was conducted. During this assessment Mr A stated that he had had diabetes in 2001 but after taking insulin injections for a couple of months, he was started on tablets but 'they ran out a few years ago'. Other medical history included essential hypertension and intermittent central chest pain associated with exercise for several months. Nursing staff noted his ECG and troponin levels confirm AMI complicated by pulmonary oedema. Also random capillary blood glucose estimation was attended with the post breakfast result of 13.1 mmol/L. No formal measurements of blood glucose or HbA_{1c} had been ordered on admission due to the absence of history of DM being noted by ED medical staff. Mr A lives with his extended family and his daughter-in-law is his main carer.

The nursing staff notified the medical team and suggested investigations of formal blood glucose and HbA_{1c}, in addition to ward-based capillary blood glucose levels pre-meals. A 'diabetic diet' was also ordered. Referrals were made to the diabetes educator, dietitian and cardiac rehabilitation nurse. The discharge planner was notified of admission as Mr A may require support post discharge.

Mr A's general practitioner was contacted by the medical staff and a comprehensive list of prescribed medications was provided. The Arabic-speaking registrar discussed the prescribed medication list with Mr A. It was discovered that he was not taking any of the prescribed medications as he stated that there were just too many. The medical staff prescribed an ACE inhibiter for BP, Diamicron MR for diabetes and aspirin as an anticoagulant.

The following is a chart of the ward-based capillary BGL:

BEFORE BREAKFAST	BEFORE LUNCH	BEFORE DINNER	BEFORE BED
6.1	12.8	3.4	16.7
7.8	8.1	19.8	27.1
7.0	16.8	2.3	6.1
8.7			

It was noted by the nursing staff that Mr A had been eating the food that the family had been bringing from home in addition to the food provided by the hospital. Mr A's carbohydrate intake could be twice that recommended by the dietitian. As a result his BGL was variable. The family told the nursing staff that it was food from home, and they thought that their father would prefer the food from home as he doesn't like 'Aussie food' and 'anyway we always bring food when people are ill'. Mr A was bored

CASE STUDY 26.1 Issues for dietary management in culturally diverse groups — cont'd

and hungry in hospital so he ate the food provided by both the hospital and his family. Following a family discussion Mr A decided to only eat the food from home and the family agreed to bring all his meals from home. His daughter needed to discuss Mr A's dietary requirements with the dietitian. Mr A's blood glucose levels became more stable when the diet was modified, however the medical staff prescribed Diamicron MR 120 mg and a single dose of Glargine 10 units at 21:00 hrs.

The diabetes educator conducted family education sessions with the assistance of the Arabic-speaking healthcare interpreter. These sessions addressed self-management in diabetes. Topics included: what is diabetes; importance of controlling blood glucose levels for short- and long-term health; self blood glucose monitoring; and the role of Diamicron MR and Glargine insulin as therapy. A clear explanation that there was no cure for diabetes was emphasised. Techniques for self-injection using a Solostar device, basic principles regarding storage and supply of insulin, injection site selection and rotation and needle disposal were also explained.

The dietitian performed a full nutritional assessment including preference in diet. Basic principles of the diet recommended for diabetes management including GI were explained, with particular emphasis on size of meal, avoiding missing meals and only having one large meal each day. In Arabic culture it is usual for families to eat a large evening meal and many family members will not eat either breakfast or lunch. Mr A likes both Turkish-style coffee [highly sweetened with sugar] and Lebanese sweet pastries. Information about how these goods can be included in the diabetic diet, when eaten occasionally and in small servings, has also been included in the education sessions.

Post discharge from the ward Mr A has been attending his local diabetes centre for ongoing management and further education. He feels well and is now taking his prescribed medications regularly and his blood glucose control is classified as acceptable.

statement recommends that all people with diabetes using insulin therapy be encouraged to perform blood glucose monitoring. The testing regimen needs to be developed specifically for the individual, therefore the support of appropriately trained health professionals is recommended. Factors such as age, culture, dexterity and physical and intellectual capabilities, level of control required, current medication regimen and motivation are taken into account by the health professional. People testing their blood for glucose also need to receive comprehensive education because effective SBGM requires more than an accurate technique. Effective self-management also requires the individual to understand and interpret their blood glucose levels in order to be able to apply the results as a part of their self-management (ADEA, 2010).

CONCLUSION

DM, particularly type 2, affects the lives of many Australians. Type 1 and type 2 DM cause significant disability and premature death and the incidence is increasing at a rate that is

Reflective questions

1 How would you respond to the statement 'I used to have diabetes but now I lost some weight and follow the diet given to me by the dietitian and now I am cured'?

2 Although John is only 5 years old, he is very familiar with the regimen he must follow to manage his diabetes. His mother does not understand why he ate a bag of lollies when he knows that sugar raises his blood glucose levels and makes him very sick. How would you counsel her?

3 Mr Jones is prescribed insulin as part of his treatment for type 2 diabetes. He has had three episodes of hypoglycaemia this week when he usually has one or two episodes each month. What investigations should the nurse perform?

referred to as 'an epidemic' (Dunstan et al., 2002). DM is one of the health priorities identified by the Commonwealth Government of Australia.

Management of DM is increasingly complex, reflecting advances in technology and approaches to management of all chronic disorders. While the management of DM has developed to be an area of speciality practice, and professional sub-groups have been established to support nurses (Australian Diabetes Educator's Association), medical practitioners (Australian Diabetes Society) and dietitians (Dietitians Association of Australia), nurses working in all clinical settings will be caring for large numbers of people with diabetes.

The management of diabetes involves a combination of medication, exercise and diet, each individualised to a person's needs and health goals. Some people are required to adopt substantial lifestyle change and self-discipline to achieve their optimum BGL. Changing long-held practices, attitudes and priorities is difficult for people; however once diagnosed with diabetes all activities need to be planned around the treatment. When a person is diagnosed with diabetes, particularly type 1, the opportunity for much of the spontaneity we take for granted is lost.

The role of the nurse in the management of DM is considerably more complex than teaching people how to test blood glucose and inject insulin. As is the case in the management of other chronic disorders that require the person to change their lifestyle, nurses frequently adopt the roles of educator, coach and motivator. It is difficult to put yourself in the shoes of another and there is a tendency for some clinicians to focus on the signs and overlook the underlying cause. For example, the reason a person with type 1 DM presents with a life-threatening episode of DKA could be as diverse as a malfunctioning insulin pen device through to an underlying psychiatric issue. The nature of nursing care enables us to talk with people and, in the process of doing that, we may identify the clues.

My purpose in writing this chapter was to provide an overview of DM and introduce the reader to the principles and goals of management. DM is a complex disorder. However, the management is well described in various textbooks and journal articles. We recommend that readers seek detailed information when they are caring for a person with DM to assist the team of health professionals and the person to work together to achieve the best outcomes.

Recommended reading

Deakin, T. A., McShane, C. E., Cade, J. E., et al. (2005). Group-based training for self-management strategies in people with type 2 diabetes mellitus. *Cochrane Database of Systematic Reviews*, Issue 2. Art. No: CD003417. doi: 10.1002/14651858.CD003417.pub2

Renders, C. M., Valk, G. D., Griffin, S. J., et al. (2009). Interventions to improve the management of diabetes mellitus in primary care, outpatient and community settings. *Cochrane Database of Systematic Reviews*, Issue 4. Art No: CD001481. doi: 10.1002/14651858.CD001481

Malanda, U. L.,Welschen, L. M. C., Riphagen, I. I., et al. (2012). Self-monitoring of blood glucose in patients with type 2 diabetes mellitus who are not using insulin. *Cochrane Database of Systematic Reviews*, Issue 1. Art No: CD005060. doi: 10.1002/14651858.CD005060.pub3

Misso, M. L., Egberts, K. J., Page, M., et al. (2010). Continuous subcutaneous insulin infusion (CSII) versus multiple insulin injections for type 1 diabetes mellitus. *Cochrane Database of Systematic Reviews*, Issue 1. Art No: CD005103. doi: 10.1002/14651858.CD005103.pub2

Thomas, D., Elliott, E. J., & Naughton, G. A. (2009). Exercise for type 2 diabetes mellitus. *Cochrane Database of Systematic Reviews*, Issue 3. Art No: CD002968. doi: 10.1002/14651858.CD002968 .pub2

Useful website

Australian Diabetes Educators Association: http://www.adea.com.au

References

Aguilar-Salinas, C., Rojas, R., Gonzalez-Villalpando, C., et al. (2006). Design and Validation of a Population-Based Definition of the Metabolic Sydndrome. *Diabetes Care*, *29*(11), 2420–2426.

Alberti, K. G. M. M., Zimmet, P., Shaw, J., et al. (2004). Type 2 Diabetes in the Young: The Evolving Epidemic. *Diabetes Care*, *27*(7), 1798–1811.

American Association of Diabetes Educators. (2007). National Standards for Diabetes Self-Management Education. *Diabetes Care*, *30*, 1630–1637.

American Diabetes Association. (2007). Diagnosis and Classification of Diabetes Mellitus. *Diabetes Care*, *30*(Suppl. 1), S42–S47.

American Diabetes Association. (2012). Standards of Medical Care in Diabetes — 2012. *Diabetes Care*, *35*(Suppl. 1), S11–S63.

Australian Diabetes Educators Association. (2010). *Position Statement. Use of Blood Glucose Meters.* Canberra: Australian Diabetes Educators Association.

Australian Bureau of Statistics. (May 2012). *Year Book Australia, 2012.* Canberra: Author.

Australian Diabetes Educators Association. (2003). *National Standards of Practice for Diabetes Educators.* Canberra: Australian Diabetes Educators Association.

Australian Institute of Health and Welfare. (2002). *Diabetes: Australian facts 2002* (AIHW Cat. No. CVD 20 (Diabetes Series No 3)). Canberra: AIHW.

Australian Institute of Health and Welfare. (2011). *Diabetes prevalence in Australia: detailed estimates for 2007–2008.* Canberra: AIHW.

Barclay, A., Petocz, P., McMillan-Price, J., et al. (2008). Glycemic index, glycemic load, and chronic disease risk — a meta-analysis of observational studies. *American Journal of Clinical Nutrition*, *87*(3), 627–637.

Bonadonna, R., Cucinotta, D., Fedele, D., et al., The Metascreen Writing Committee. (2006). The Metabolic Syndrome Is a Risk Indicator of Macrovascular and Macrovascular Complications in Diabetes. *Diabetes Care*, *29*(12), 2701–2707.

Bradshaw, B., Richardson, G., & Kulkarni, K. (2007). Thriving with Diabetes. An Introduction to the Resiliency Approach for Diabetes Educators. *The Diabetes Educator*, *33*(4), 643–649.

Bradshaw, B., Richardson, G., Kumpfer, K., et al. (2007). Determining the Efficacy of a Resiliency Training Approach in Adults with Type 2 Diabetes. *The Diabetes Educator*, *33*(4), 650–659.

Brand-Miller, J., Hayne, S., Petocz, P., et al. (2003). Low-Glycemic Index Diets in the Management of Diabetes. A meta-analysis of randomized controlled trials. *Diabetes Care*, *26*(8), 2261–2267.

Chipkin, S., Klugh, S., & Chasan-Taber, L. (2001). Exercise and diabetes. *Cardiology Clinics, 19*(3), 489–505.

Colagiuri, R., Girgis, S., Eigenmann, C., et al. (2009). *National Evidence Based Guideline for Patient Education in type 2 Diabetes.* Canberra: Diabetes Australia and the NHMRC.

Corser, W., Holmes-Rovner, M., Lein, C., et al. (2007). A Shared Decision-Making Primary Care Intervention for Type 2 Diabetes. *The Diabetes Educator, 33*(4), 700–708.

Craig, M. E., Twigg, S. M., Donaghue, K. C., et al. (2011). For the Australian Type 1 Diabetes Guidelines Expert Advisory Group. *National evidence-based clinical careguidelines for type 1 diabetes in children, adolescents and adults.* Canberra: Australian Government Department of Health and Ageing.

De Fronzo, R., Ferrannini, E., Keen, H., et al. (2004). *International Textbook of Diabetes Mellitus* (*Vol. 1*). Chichester: John Wiley & Sons.

Dietitians Association of Australia New South Wales Branch Diabetes Interest Group. (2006). *Evidence Based Practice Guidelines for the Nutritional Management of Type 2 Diabetes Mellitus for Adults.* Sydney: Author.

Dunstan, D., Zimmet, P., Welbourne, T., et al. (2002). The Rising Prevalence of Diabetes and Impaired Glucose Tolerance. *Diabetes Care, 25*(5), 829–834.

Fajans, S., & Bell, G. (2011). MODY: history, genetics, pathophysiology, and clinical decision making. *Diabetes Care, 34,* 1878–1884.

Farmer, A., Wade, A., Goyder, E., et al. (2007). Impact of self-monitoring of blood glucose in the management of patients with non-insulin treated diabetes: open parallel group randomized trial. *British Medical Journal, 335*(7611), 132–139.

Garber, A. J., King, A. B., Prato, S. D., et al. (2012). Insulin degludec, an ultra-longacting basal insulin, versus insulin glargine in basal-bolus treatment with mealtime insulin aspart in type 2 diabetes (BEGIN Basal-Bolus Type 2): a phase 3, randomised, open-label, treat-to-target non-inferiority trial. *The Lancet, 379*(9825), 1498–1507.

Gilbertson, H., Brand-Miller, J., Thorburn, A., et al. (2001). The Effect of Flexible Low Glycemic Index Dietary Advice Versus Measured Carbohydrate Exchange Diets on Glycemic Control in Children With Type 1 Diabetes. *Diabetes Care, 24*(7), 1137–1143.

Harmel, A., & Mathur, R. (2004). *Diabetes Mellitus Diagnosis and Treatment* (5th ed.). Philadelphia: Saunders.

Hermansen, K., Madsbad, S., Perrild, H., et al. (2001). Comparison of the Soluble Basal Insulin Analog Insulin Detemir With NPH Insulin. *Diabetes Care, 24*(2), 296–301.

Hossain, P., Kawar, B., & El Nahas, M. (2007). Obesity and Diabetes in the Developing World — A Growing Challenge. *The New England Journal of Medicine, 356*(3), 213–216.

Inzucchi, S., Berngenstal, R., Buse, J., et al. (2012). Management of Hyperglycemia in Type 2 Diabetes: A Patient-Centered Approach. Position Statement of the American Diabetes Association (ADA) and the European Association for the Study of Diabetes (EASD). *Diabetes Care, 35*(Suppl. 1), S11–S63.

Kamp, M. (2007). Oral Medications and Type 2 diabetes. *Diabetes Management Journal, 19,* 28–29.

Karvonen, M., Viik-Kajander, M., Libman, I., et al. (2000). Incidence of Childhood Type 1 Diabetes Worldwide. *Diabetes Care, 23*(10), 1516–1526.

Katzmarzyk, P., Church, T., Janssen, I., et al. (2005). Metabolic Syndrome, Obesity, and Mortality. *Diabetes Care, 28,* 391–397.

Lee, A., Hiscock, R., Wein, P., et al. (2007). Gestational Diabetes Mellitus: Clinical Predictors and Long-Term Risk of Developing Type 2 Diabetes. *Diabetes Care, 30*(4), 878–883.

McDermott, M. (2002). *Endocrine Secrets.* Philadelphia: Hanley & Belfus.

McElduff, A., & Yue, D. (2007). Inhaled insulin: where are we and where might we go? *The Medical Journal of Australia, 186*(8), 390–391.

McIntyre, H. D. (2006). DAFNE (Dose Adjustment For Normal Eating): structured education in insulin replacement therapy for type 1 diabetes. *Medical Journal of Australia, 108*(7), 317–318.

MIMS Australia Pty Ltd. (2012). MIMS Australian Decision Support. Retrieved October 21, 2012, from UBM Medica Australia Pty Ltd http://www. mims.com.au/

Moore, H., Summerbell, C., Hooper, L., et al. (2007). Dietary advice for treatment of type 2 diabetes mellitus in adults (Review). *Cochrane Library* CD004097.

National Institute for Health and Clinical Excellence (NICE). (2011, revised). Continuous subcutaneous insulin infusion for the treatment of diabetes mellitus. Review of technology appraisal guidance 57. *Technology appraisal guidance 151*. London (UK): Author.

National Vascular Disease Prevention Alliance. (2009). *Guidelines for the assessment of absolute cardiovascular disease risk*. Canberra: National Health and Medical Rsearch Council.

Ratner, R., Hirsch, I., Neifing, J., et al. (2000). Less Hypoglycaemia with Insulin Glargine in Intensive Insulin Therapy for Type 1 Diabetes. *Diabetes Care, 23*(5), 639–643.

Rewers, M., Zaccaro, D., D'Agostino, R., et al. (2004). Insulin Sensitivity, Insulinemia, and Coronary Artery Disease. *Diabetes Care, 27*(3), 781–787.

Richter, B., Bandeira-Echtler, E., Bergerhoff, K., et al. (2008). Dipeptidyl peptidase-4 (DPP-4) inhibitors for type 2 diabetes mellitus. *Cochrane Database Systematic Reviews 2008*.

Riddle, M., & Karl, D. (2012). Individualizing Targets and Tactics for High-Risk Patients With Type 2 Diabetes. Practical lessons from ACCORD and other cardiovascular trials. *Diabetes Care, 35*, 2100–2107.

Rosenstock, J., Cappelleri, J., Bolinder, B., et al. (2004). Patient Satisfaction and Glycaemic Control After 1 Year With Inhaled Insulin (Exubera) in Patients With Type 1 or Type 2 Diabetes. *Diabetes Care, 27*(6), 1318–1323.

Rosenstock, J., Lorber, D. L., Gnudi, L., et al. (2010). Prandial inhaled insulin plus basal insulin glargine versus twice daily biaspart insulin for type 2 diabetes: a multicentre randomised trial. *The Lancet, 375*(9733), 2244–2253.

Seley, J., & Weinger, K. (2007). The State of the Science on Nursing Best Practices for Diabetes Self-Management. *The Diabetes Educator, 33*(4), 616–626.

Skyler, J., Cefalu, W., Kourides, I., et al. (2004). Efficacy of inhaled human insulin in type 1 diabetes mellitus: a randomised proof-of-concept study. *The Lancet, 357*(9253), 331–335.

Stratton, I., Adler, A., Andrew, H., et al. (2000). Association of glycaemia and macrovascular and microvascular complications of type 2 diabetes (UKPDS 35): prospective observational study. *British Medical Journal, 321*, 405–412.

The Diabetes Control and Complications Trial Research Group. (1993). The Effect of Intensive Treatment of Diabetes on the Development and Progression of Long-term Complications in Insulin-Dependent Diabetes Mellitus. *The New England Journal of Medicine, 329*(14), 977–986.

The Diabetes Prevention Trial — Type 1 Study Group. (2005). Effects of Oral Insulin in Relatives of Patients With Type 1 Diabetes. *Diabetes Care, 28*(5), 1068–1076.

The United Kingdom Prospective Study 33. (1996). Intensive blood glucose control with sulphonylureas or insulin compared with conventional treatment and the risk of complications in patients with Type 2 Diabetes. *The Lancet, 352*, 837–853.

Thomas, D., Elliott, E., & Naughton, G. (2007). Exercise for type 2 diabetes mellitus. Retrieved July 20, 2007, from http://www.thecochranelibrary.com

Wang, F., Carabino, J., & Vergara, C. (2003). Insulin glargine: a systematic review of a long-acting insulin analogue. *Clinical Therepautics, 25*(6), 1541–1577.

World Health Organization. (1999). *Definition, Diagnosis and Classification of Diabetes Mellitus and its Complications*. Geneva: World Health Organization Department of Noncommunicable Disease Surveillance.

CHAPTER 27

Stephen Neville
Mark Henrickson

HIV/AIDS

Learning objectives

When you have completed this chapter you will be able to:

- understand the history, presentation and the contemporary management of people living with HIV/AIDS
- restate health-promoting measures to reduce the transmission of HIV infection and to encourage risk reduction in people living with HIV
- be aware of the social and professional stigma associated with living and working with HIV/AIDS
- examine your own attitudes towards people living with HIV/AIDS
- be able to provide an appropriate basic health service to people with HIV/AIDS.

Key words

HIV prevention, HIV testing, HIV transmission, opportunistic diseases, stigma

INTRODUCTION

There have been few modern diseases that have captured the public imagination in so short a period of time as human immunodeficiency virus (HIV) and its fulminate expression, acquired immune deficiency syndrome (AIDS). The way the disease appeared to emerge so suddenly in the developed world in the late 1970s — the severity of the symptoms; its disfiguring, wasting and painful impact on people diagnosed with the condition;

and the inevitably fatal nature of the diagnosis — gave rise to a climate of fear. Yet we have discovered more about HIV/AIDS in a shorter period of time than any disease in history. HIV/AIDS has today become a chronic, manageable condition, although still life-threatening.

Rather than attempting to provide a definitive and exhaustive overview of this complex disease, three case studies will focus on some key issues associated with living with HIV in Australasia. The chapter begins with an overview of HIV/AIDS and provides a context for the development of your knowledge and understanding about the disease and its prevention. Case Study 27.1 is about an older homosexual man living with HIV who has been admitted to hospital for treatment and stabilisation before being discharged home. Case Study 27.2 is about a transgendered sex worker who is a regular street drug user. Case Study 27.3 is about a young married African migrant woman with two young children. Each of these cases represents the types of people living with HIV/AIDS who you may come across in healthcare settings when working as a nurse in Australasia.

BACKGROUND

There is compelling evidence that the viral ancestor of HIV existed in humans from the early decades of the twentieth century. It probably crossed into a very small pool of humans in south central Africa who were hunting species of monkeys infected with a related virus (Pepin, 2011). Once a viral reservoir was created in the human population largely due to post-colonial healthcare practices and sex workers (Pepin, 2011), what we now know as HIV appears to have travelled along major transportation routes throughout Africa, and from these networks to airports in major cities around the world, where it took hold in vulnerable populations. In many ways HIV may be the first disease of modern transportation, and has served as a brutal reminder of how quickly infectious diseases can spread around an unprepared world.

Since 1984 AIDS has been understood to be caused by HIV, although even at the time of writing there are some researchers and politicians who continue to deny the role of HIV in AIDS. Since HIV disease is much more common and comprehensive than AIDS we will mostly use the term 'HIV' in this chapter from now on. HIV has been associated from its earliest days with stigmatised communities and, tragically, in many countries and regions much of that stigma has remained (Sullivan & Wolitski, 2008). In the early days of the epidemic, populations that were most affected in developed nations — men who had sex with other men; injecting drug users; the poor; African migrants and refugees; and other communities of colour — were socially and politically marginalised. Children and people who were infected through infected blood products were referred to as 'innocent victims', implying that others were somehow 'guilty'. This contributed to the marginalisation of large groups of people living with HIV. Some religious and political leaders even spoke of AIDS as 'God's punishment'.

When an individual is infected with HIV, they must deal not only with the medical aspects of the condition, but also with the social dimensions. Gay men, for instance, may have to endure homophobic (irrational fear of gay people) reactions, resulting in isolation from their families and friends (Henrickson & Neville, 2012); one African migrant referred to herself as 'standing in the fire' — that is, as already dead to her family (Fouché et al., 2011). Consequently, HIV is as much a social diagnosis as it is a medical diagnosis. For some bisexual or gay men, a diagnosis with HIV may be the first time their families have had any idea about their son's or husband's or father's sexual behaviours or identity.

STATISTICS, TRANSMISSION AND PREVENTION

Statistics

By the end of 2010, UNAIDS estimated that there were approximately 34 million people worldwide living with HIV (UNAIDS, 2011). In Australia, as of 30 June 2011, an estimated 31 060 people were reported to be living with HIV (National Centre in HIV Epidemiology and Clinical Research, 2010). Figures for 2010 in New Zealand are much lower, with an estimated total number of 3474 people ever having being diagnosed with HIV (Fouché et al., 2011). It is important to remember that while overall population prevalence may be low, different groups within a population may have relatively high prevalence and that within some groups there may be high rates of unidentified infection (Saxton et al., 2012).

Transmission

HIV is an unstable and fragile virus that can only be transmitted through direct human-to-human contact. Its transmission is via infected blood, semen, vaginal secretions or breast milk (Stolley & Glass, 2009). HIV cannot be transmitted through kissing or hugging, insect bites or other casual, household or ordinary workplace contact. Sexual intercourse, whether anal or vaginal, is the most common method of transmitting the virus (Lewis et al., 2011). Recent studies have found that circumcising men can reduce the rates of HIV infection, particularly in heterosexual populations (Westercamp et al., 2012).

HIV can be transmitted through exposure to contaminated blood products or the use of contaminated syringes, needles and other street drug paraphernalia. Even microscopic amounts of blood left in drug-use equipment can transmit HIV if they are not thoroughly disinfected. Therefore, people who choose to inject drugs such as opiates (including heroin and morphine), amphetamine-type stimulants, so-called 'party drugs' and steroids (used by some body-builders and transgendered persons) must never share any of their injecting equipment with anyone else. Syringe exchange schemes encourage safer drug use behaviours (Turner et al., 2011). Both New Zealand (see www.needle.co.nz) and Australia have expanded needle access for drug users. In addition, medically supervised injecting centres provide an opportunity to educate injecting drug users about reducing their risk of HIV if they are going to continue to inject drugs (DeBeck et al., 2011).

Injecting street drugs is also strongly associated with unsafe sexual practices (Goldenberg et al., 2012), because not only may people begin to exchange sex for drugs when the money runs out, but their judgment about what is safe may be impaired. The relationship between substance use and sexual risk taking is strongly supported in the literature. Goldenberg et al.'s (2012) study found sex workers who injected illicit drugs were more likely to be depressed and as a consequence have sex without using a condom.

Tattooing and cultural rituals such as tatau and moko may involve exposure to infected blood; practitioners and clients must be sure that they are both well protected from infection. Appropriate sterilisation of all equipment and the use of gloves and other personal protective equipment must be routine, even in these very traditional cultural activities. There is also a small risk to people receiving blood and blood products. However, in developed nations the routine screening of blood donors and blood products has made the risk for HIV transmission in this way negligible (Australian Red Cross Blood Service, 2012).

Needlestick injuries can also result in transmission of the virus, as can splash exposures of infected products on skin with an open lesion or into the eye (Lewis et al., 2011). All healthcare organisations have prevention and post-exposure protocols, and all healthcare workers should be familiar with them. The standard guidelines for preventing healthcare associated infections can be found in the recommended text by Durham and Lashley (2010, p. 159).

Perinatal transmission of the HIV virus from mother to infant can occur prenatally, at the time of delivery or through breastfeeding. People who live in the same home as a person with HIV and/or visitors will need good information on how the virus is and is not transmitted; the website of the Centre for Disease Control and Prevention has good basic prevention information (www.cdc.gov/hiv/resources/factsheets/transmission.htm).

Prevention

People who choose to be sexually active can prevent infection with HIV or any of the other blood-borne, sexually transmitted diseases by putting a latex barrier between themselves and the virus. This means correctly using a fresh latex condom, together with a water-based lubricant, for penetrative sexual activity every time.

Risk-reduction messages can vary from one country to another, based on local circumstances, cultural norms and politics. For instance, in New Zealand the New Zealand AIDS Foundation advocates the use of a condom and lubricant for every sexual encounter in all situations where men have sex with men. However, in Australia, as well as other parts of the world, the health education message promoting the use of a condom every time is applied only in certain situations (Neville & Adams, 2009); for example, if a person is HIV-positive or is having sexual encounters with multiple partners. Some studies have found, however, that people in relationships are likely to ignore safer sex guidelines and utilise monogamy as a way to manage the risk of being exposed to HIV (Adams & Neville, 2009); this puts both partners at risk. In some cultural groups, however, if a woman asks her male partner to use a condom, the request may be interpreted that the woman does not trust her partner, or that the woman herself is involved in other sexual relationships; this interpretation can even lead to partner violence (Hendriksen et al., 2007).

Every opportunity should be taken by nurses to reinforce safer sex and harm reduction messages about drug use so that patients are not put at risk because of their behaviour, and that they do not put themselves at increased risk for infection or re-infection from others. Great care must be taken, however, not to scold, judge or frighten clients who have difficulty adhering to treatments, safer sex or drug use guidelines or medical appointments. There is no evidence anywhere to suggest that such approaches work (Stevens & Hildebrandt, 2009). It is much more efficient to spend some extra time listening to a patient and collaborate with them to plan their own solutions than it is to risk losing them altogether. A woman who is trading sex for drugs or for money to feed her child is not going to change her entire life simply because she has begun a new medication; HIV is probably quite a low priority for her, coming somewhere after housing, food, utility bills, clothing, transportation or mobile phone chargers. Only by carefully building a trusting relationship will the nurse encourage the person with HIV to make their health more of a priority.

One of the emerging issues in nursing is HIV discrimination in the workplace. Recent research has found that nurses with HIV experience stigma, violations of their privacy, workplace gossip and employment discrimination (Fouché et al., 2011). There is no reason that people with HIV cannot work as nurses; standard precautions protect nurses, patients and colleagues. As long as nurses are not having unprotected sex with their colleagues or sharing non-sterile injection equipment with them, there is no workplace risk for acquiring HIV from a colleague. Workplace stigma and discrimination is both unnecessary and illegal. Good information, mutual respect and an overall positive environment will prevent unnecessary difficulties in the healthcare workplace.

BOX 27.1
How to use a male condom

Make sure the condom package is not broken or punctured. Check the 'use-by date' on the condom package to ensure that the condom has not passed its use-by date. Do not open it with any sharp object, or with your teeth. Do not use oil-based lubricants such as baby oil, petroleum jellies or moisturisers with the condom because they can degrade the latex. Do use purpose-formulated water-based lubricants.

1. When you remove the condom, ensure that it is not brittle, dried out or damaged in any way. Note which way the condom is rolled; if you start to put the condom on the penis and notice that the condom is backwards, do not simply turn it over; discard it and get a fresh one.
2. Place the condom at the end of the hard penis (if the penis is uncircumcised, pull back the foreskin first). Then pinch the tip of the condom to squeeze out the air and unroll the condom until it reaches the base of the penis. A drop of lubricant inside the condom can increase sensitivity, but too much lubricant may cause it to slip off.
3. Make sure the condom is secure and unbroken, and that there is room for the ejaculate (come) at the tip. Insert the penis into your partner.
4. After you have ejaculated (come), while the penis is still hard hold the condom at the base so it does not slip off as you withdraw. Remove the condom, being careful not to spill the fluid inside. Discard the condom.

Remember, with condoms, practice makes perfect. You can always ask your partner for help.

Testing for HIV

Testing for HIV has become much simpler over the past two decades. The 'HIV test' is actually a test for antibodies to HIV. Testing is usually done with blood, although tests using oral mucosa and so-called rapid tests using finger sticks are available in some regions. A negative test simply means that the analysis was unable to detect antibodies to HIV; a repeat test in 3 months is recommended for individuals at high risk for infection, and particularly when the last possible exposure was less than 12 weeks prior to the test.

HIV testing should always be linked to supportive risk-reduction education to help an individual reduce their risk of exposure to HIV, or to prevent transmitting HIV to someone else if they are already infected. For HIV-positive people it is not possible to determine who infected them simply through taking a HIV test.

PROGRESSION AND TREATMENT

Progression

HIV is a progressive condition with a predictable trajectory. Different clinical features appear, depending on the stage of disease. One marker of immune system functioning is CD4 cells. Since HIV attacks the immune system, a decrease in the number of functional CD4 cells can be used as a marker for the progression of the disease. Stages of HIV can be classified as:

- acute HIV infection (at the time of infection)
- early infection (CD4 >500/microL of blood)

- early symptomatic disease (CD4 between 200 and 499/microL)
- a diagnosis of AIDS (CD4 < 200/microL).

Acute HIV infection is also called 'acute retroviral syndrome' or a 'seroconversion illness'. After exposure to the HIV virus it may take between three and 12 weeks for seroconversion to occur (Lewis et al., 2011). People may present to health practitioners with flu-like viral symptoms and lymphadenopathy, or may be clinically asymptomatic and may only be diagnosed after formal HIV testing.

The early infection stage may last from several months to up to 10 years or more. During this time the person is infectious, but may be clinically asymptomatic, or only experience mild symptoms, which health professionals may put down to being viral in nature (Klebert, 2010). However, because the virus continues to replicate during this period, without treatment the body's immune system can become increasingly impaired. This may cause early symptoms associated with being HIV-positive. Some examples of early symptoms include:

- persistent high temperatures
- night sweats
- diarrhoea
- fatigue
- headaches
- localised infections (e.g. oral or vaginal thrush)
- persistent and frequently generalised lymphadenopathy.

The transition from being HIV-positive to having a diagnosis of AIDS is marked by the presence of opportunistic infections and/or a CD4 count <200/microL. A diagnosis of AIDS marks the transition to the final stage of the disease. The Centers for Disease Control in the United States have developed a useful set of diagnostic criteria that supports a diagnosis of AIDS (see www.cdc.gov/mmwr/preview/mmwrhtml/00018871.htm).

TREATMENTS

In developed nations, the treatment and management of HIV is a relatively fast-moving environment, and new therapies, new drugs and new combinations of drugs are becoming available frequently. For a current and comprehensive list of drugs available for treatment and management of HIV disease see the website of the New Zealand AIDS Foundation (www.nzaf.org.nz/positive-people/living-with-hiv/current-treatments).

Since the more HIV there is in the body ('viral load') the more damage the virus can do, the management of HIV infection is focused around preventing HIV from replicating itself. Because of the way it replicates, HIV is known as a 'retrovirus'; and the group of drugs that interfere with the replication process at various stages are called 'antiretrovirals' (ARVs; sometimes these are called 'highly active antiretroviral therapies', or HAART). The major classes of antiretroviral agents include the oldest class of such drugs, the nucleoside/nucleotide reverse transcriptase inhibitors (Stolley & Glass, 2009). The non-nucleoside reverse transcriptase inhibitors were the next class of drugs to be developed. Protease inhibitors and the fusion inhibitors were the next class of drugs to be developed and have been made available most recently. Combinations of antiretrovirals are usually used because HIV is very mutable, and can develop resistance to one or more of these drugs. Antiretrovirals must be taken exactly as prescribed, and care must be taken to follow instructions related to food intake (and the kinds of food), liquids and sleep habits, as diet can affect the way the body processes these drugs. These drugs can often have significant side-effects, including psychotropic effects such as vivid dreams. Patients should be encouraged to be highly adherent to prescribed medication regimens, as individuals can develop resistance to medications in a relatively short period of time if they miss doses, or take unplanned 'drug holidays'.

Strategies to support adherence to medication can include planning dosing around mealtimes, sleep routines or other regularly scheduled activities such as regular television or radio programs. Cues such as pillboxes or mobile phones with alarms, text message reminders and enlisting the support of partners or friends may also help adherence. If the person with HIV continues to use non-prescribed drugs, street drugs or alcohol regularly these may interfere with their medication routine and their awareness of time and mealtimes. If the person is having particular difficulty managing the side-effects of a drug, which can be quite dramatic (e.g. a condition called lipodystrophy is the result of a redistribution of body fat, which can be very disfiguring), this should be brought to the attention of the doctor or nurse so that these side-effects can be medically managed, or alternative therapies considered.

In Case Study 27.1, as part of the nursing assessment, the key nursing issues are identified, as well as interventions to address these issues.

CASE STUDY 27.1

Eric is a 68-year-old retired Caucasian male who has lived with a diagnosis of HIV for the last 15 years. He has no other significant health issues other than those related to his HIV status. Eric identifies as gay, has not been in a sexual relationship since his diagnosis and does not have good support networks from either family or friends. He lives alone with his pet budgie called 'Archie' and has one friend, Charles, who lives close by. Eric tells you that his long-term partner died of AIDS 10 years ago and over the years he has witnessed not only his partner but a large number of his close friends die from the disease. He has little savings and is reliant on a government-funded benefit for income. Eric was admitted to hospital with flu-like symptoms, weight loss, dehydration, oral candidiasis, fatigue and decreased mobility. He is diagnosed with psittacosis (also called 'bird flu'), a bacterial infection caused by *Chlamydia psittaci*, an organism transmitted from birds to humans.

The psittacosis has responded well to antibiotic treatment and Eric is now being prepared to be discharged home. His hospital stay has coincided with your placement in the medical unit. The nurses you have been preceptored with have mainly been responsible for his care. Consequently in conjunction with the registered nurses, you have been involved in the provision of nursing care to Eric and have a good understanding of issues that he faces as he struggles to adjust to living with this chronic and now debilitating illness.

Fatigue

A key issue is Eric's fatigue, related to dehydration, malnutrition and the residual effects of having psittacosis. Constant tiredness is one of the common complaints associated with HIV particularly in older adults and it is known to cause anxiety, depression and sleep disturbance which ultimately negatively impacts on quality of life (Lerdal et al., 2011). The nurse will need to work with Eric to identify the factors contributing to fatigue, plan activities and provide him with assistive devices. This is especially important considering he lives alone. For example:

- provide a shower stool and other occupational therapy aids
- develop a daily plan that includes regular rest periods
- include the involvement of an occupational therapist.

Feeling constantly tired also affects Eric's ability to mobilise.

Activity intolerance

Another key issue is activity intolerance related to muscle atrophy, fatigue, peripheral neuropathy, decreased nutritional intake and the side-effects of HIV-related medications. Peripheral neuropathy is an issue that specifically affects people with HIV, manifesting as either acute or chronic pain, and contributes to problems associated with maintaining activity levels (Black & Hawks, 2009). It is important in Eric's case to:

- administer pain medications as prescribed and monitor the effects
- ensure a physiotherapist is involved in Eric's care
- encourage the use of non-pharmacological treatments for pain, for example the use of a transcutaneous electrical nerve stimulation (TENS) machine
- assess footwear to ensure it is comfortable and appropriate for exercise
- work with Eric to develop an exercise program that he enjoys and will increase his physical activity levels and endurance, and maintain lean muscle mass.

Weight loss and malnutrition also limit Eric's ability to maintain lean muscle mass and remain active.

Weight loss

Eric's weight loss is related to a sore mouth as a result of having chronic oral candidiasis dehydration and decreased nutritional intake. Weight loss remains a common consequence of HIV infection. Factors that contribute to weight loss include low food intake (due to side-effects of drugs, opportunistic infections in the mouth making eating painful and digestive tract infections), poor nutrient absorption (due to HIV-related infections and the presence of diarrhoea) and altered metabolism (due to fever) (Thompson et al., 2012). One of the reasons for Eric's admission was that he had contracted psittacosis and presented with oral thrush. Oral thrush has been shown to contribute to weight loss (Gallant, 2009). People with HIV therefore need more calories just to maintain their body weight. In Eric's case the nurse should:

- encourage small frequent meals that are highly nutritious and appetising
- if oral thrush remains, advise Eric to avoid spicy and acidic foods (such as citrus and fruit juices), replacing with non-irritating foods (such as eggs, cream soups)
- encourage an adequate fluid intake and intake of foods high in potassium (such as bananas) especially if Eric experiences episodes of diarrhoea
- encourage Eric to weigh himself weekly, document his weight and inform his health practitioner of any significant changes
- ensure a dietitian works with Eric to assist with the establishment of appropriate nutritional principles to delay the progression of the disease and have a positive impact on his quality of life.

Coping with loss

A major issue for Eric is coping with loss related to reduced quality of life, the loss of his partner 10 years ago and having no family. As already identified, a diagnosis of HIV has transformed from one of terminal illness to one of chronic illness. In the 1980s people who had HIV might have asked the question, 'How am I going to live what little life I have left?'. This may have been the case for Eric's partner. However, Eric is faced with the question, 'Who am I to outlive my lover?'. Eric's partner was also his major source of social and emotional support. He watched the man he loved die and had to deal with the inevitable feelings of bereavement and grief. Eric's personal turmoil leaves him vulnerable to what Machado (2012) identifies as social isolation, loneliness, depression, suicide ideation, substance abuse and non-adherence to prescribed treatment regimens. In addition, Eric is going to have to find his pet bird, Archie, a new home. This is extremely distressing for Eric as Archie is a major source of social support. Consequently the nurse should:

- reinforce the importance of consistently taking his medications and attending his appointments with his healthcare provider
- ensure the involvement of a social worker who works in the area of HIV to assess his psychosocial status and help provide links to the appropriate community services
- encourage participation in HIV support groups and contact with his local HIV organisation
- encourage involvement in other community organisations where Eric may be able to meet new people and expand his social network
- with Eric's permission, include his friend Charles in the discharge planning meetings
- work with Eric to find a suitable home for Archie and provide education to ensure he is not at risk of contracting psittacosis again
- offer appropriate referral to counselling, psychotherapy or other support workers.

As can be seen from Case Study 27.1 many of the issues associated with HIV are interrelated. For example, weight loss and dehydration contribute to Eric's fatigue, which concomitantly decreases mobility, leading to muscle atrophy and further weight loss. All these physiological disturbances affect his quality of life, an important concept for nurses to consider when working with people who have a chronic illness.

CASE STUDY 27.2

Fa'atasi is a 23-year-old fa'afafine who now lives in Auckland. A fa'afafine is a Samoan cultural term for someone who was born a biological male, who embodies both male and female characteristics, but takes on the cultural role of a woman, and presents publicly and socially as a woman. Fa'atasi is unemployed, although she has worked casually as street sex worker. She tested positive for HIV 4 years ago. She does not have a regular doctor, but sometimes turns up at the sexual health clinic when she suspects she may have an STI or is otherwise not feeling well. Fa'atasi uses cannabis, alcohol and amphetamine-type stimulants (ATS) when she is engaged in sex work. She has a strong support community within the Pacifica transgendered community.

In Case Study 27.2, as part of the nursing assessment the key nursing issues are identified, as well as interventions to address these issues.

Sexually transmitted infections

Fa'atasi's repeated diagnosis with sexually transmitted infections is concerning because it means that she is not practising safer sex. Particularly concerning is the emergence of drug resistant gonorrheae in Australasia and globally (Bratt et al., 2009). Nursing interventions will include safe sex education and reinforcement of risk reduction plans already in place. It is important not simply to lecture Fa'atasi on safer sex or sex work, because she will have heard them before. Rather it will be more productive to help her identify ways that she can take responsibility for reducing her own risks of STIs, and reducing her risks of transmitting STIs and HIV to others. Using aiga (family) as a model, and perhaps drawing on her own spiritual or religious beliefs, Fa'atasi can be assisted to develop a plan to reduce her sexual risk even when she is engaged in sex work. Sex work can be very risky, so it is also important to ensure that Fa'atasi has a safety plan while on the streets and that she is aware of the resources available to her. Assessment for violence or rape may be necessary, as many street sex workers are victims of both. Her relationships with clinic staff and with her Pacifica community are strengths.

Substance use

Fa'atasi's substance use, particularly ATS, puts her and other users who may share her drug using equipment at greatly increased risk of all blood-borne pathogens, including reinfection with HIV. Equally importantly, people who use ATS may make decisions about sexual activity which may increase their risk of disease transmission. The nurse will reinforce the importance of education on reducing the harms of substance use and consider a referral to a substance use treatment program.

Medical appointments

Fa'atasi does not have regular medical appointments to monitor her HIV. While HIV does not appear to be the major presenting issue at the moment, it is important that she is monitored regularly in order to prevent opportunistic infections and to assess whether antiretroviral medication may be appropriate. In collaboration with Fa'atasi and the clinical team, the nurse will develop strategies to support her adherence to medical appointments, such as introducing her to the medical team, ensuring that she has access to transportation, encouraging her to bring a support person to appointments or ensuring that appointments are available at convenient times of the day. Incentives could be offered, such as meals or social events. The clinic staff must also be prepared for Fa'atasi by ensuring that all staff treat her respectfully from the moment she walks in the door. Respectful treatment can include things like ensuring that staff use female pronouns and learn respectful greetings in Samoan, or allowing her to use the female toilet.

There may be other significant social issues in Fa'atasi's life that should be considered and assessed. Working casually as a sex worker suggests that her financial resources are fragile, which may put her housing, food and other essentials at risk. Her legal residency status may need to be clarified, and she may have outstanding legal issues which will need to be addressed. Other issues that may need to be explored include income and/or employment alternatives to sex work; access to medications; and social and family supports. A referral to a social worker or case manager should be considered to assess these issues.

In Case Study 27.3, as part of the nursing assessment the following key nursing issues are identified, as well as interventions to address these problems.

CASE STUDY 27.3

Ruth is a 29-year-old migrant to New Zealand from Somalia. She has been married for 8 years and has two children, ages 3 and 7. Ruth and her husband are both Muslim. Ruth's husband came to New Zealand 5 years ago, almost 1 year before Ruth, in order to begin his new job and establish a home for Ruth and the children. During that time Ruth had a brief affair with another man in Somalia. Ruth works evenings as a care worker in a nursing home. About a year ago Ruth and her husband underwent routine health screening for her permanent residency visa. Ruth was told that she was HIV positive. She was also PPD+. Ruth's husband is HIV negative. They have no other family in New Zealand. Ruth sees her doctor, who has treated her for vaginal candidiasis and is prophylaxing her for tuberculosis.

Ruth has told no one except her husband about her HIV status. She tries to avoid other African migrants because she 'feels dirty inside her', and thinks that if anyone sees her they will know about her. She is keenly aware of how small immigrant African communities are, and knows how much everyone gossips. She feels overwhelmed by her diagnosis and is sure that she will die, because everyone she knew with AIDS in Somalia has died. She is deeply religious, however, and believes her disease is punishment for her brief affair. Nevertheless, she feels hurt and angry with her husband because she feels he does not understand her, although she understands his sense of anger and betrayal. She presents with fever, nausea and vomiting, headache and fatigue. She missed her last menstrual period.

Medical presentation

Ruth needs to be assessed for progression of her HIV disease, including opportunistic diseases such as cryptococcal meningitis. The doctor may repeat her CD4 and viral load testing to determine the current state of her immune system. The nurse will provide or review education about HIV and HIV treatments and opportunistic infections.

Pregnancy testing

Ruth has missed her period. It is possible that a pregnant mother can transmit HIV to her baby either during gestation or during the birth process. This is often called 'vertical' transmission. Although the risks of vertical transmission have been greatly reduced today with antiretroviral therapies, women with HIV should carefully consider the risks to themselves and to their babies before they become pregnant. Many countries now routinely test for HIV including '… the use of rapid HIV tests at delivery for women of unknown HIV status, and the use of antiretroviral therapy by HIV-infected women during pregnancy and by infants after birth' (Stolley & Glass, 2009, p. 194). Ruth should be advised of these concerns and risks.

Partner education

Ruth's husband needs to be educated about HIV disease and risk reduction; and probably re-testing would be recommended for him if he has been sexually active with Ruth without a condom.

Testing of children

Although this case does not provide information about the children, the birth of at least one of them fell after the time when Ruth may have been infected with HIV. Therefore assessing these children for HIV infection is important. We have not included a section on paediatric HIV disease in this chapter, as it is quite a different disease presentation and merits attention all on its own.

Social factors

In addition to these issues, it is apparent that there are a number of other social factors that are contributing to Ruth's current health and mental health status. These include:

- her apparent social isolation
- her perception of her disease, which will relate to her motivation to care for herself
- her relationship with her husband
- her legal and immigration status, which may affect her treatment options and her ability to stay in the country
- permanency planning for the children, should her health deteriorate rapidly.

INTERVENTIONS

Since HIV is a syndrome that may affect many body systems, people may present with a number of possible symptoms, conditions and opportunistic infections, each of which requires careful assessment, planning (include the person, their family and significant others) and intervention. This section will expand the above discussion on treatment of HIV to include:

- an overview of opportunistic diseases
- collaboration with other allied health professionals.

As you read the material presented in the following sections think about how some of these interventions have affected, or could affect, Eric, Fa'atasi and Ruth.

Opportunistic infections

One of the ways HIV damages the body is by impairing the immune system that would normally protect the body against an array of pathogens. These are commonly referred to as opportunistic infections, which in a person who doesn't have HIV pose no problems but in someone with HIV are problematic. These opportunistic infections can involve every body system. Both Eric and Ruth present with opportunistic infections; Eric with *Chlamydia psittaci* (bacterial) and oral candidiasis (fungal) and Ruth with vaginal candidiasis (fungal). Ruth is also taking antibiotics prophylactically to help prevent her getting mycobacterium tuberculosis (bacterial), another opportunistic infection. Lewis et al. (2011) identify the following opportunistic infections that may occur in people with HIV in addition to those presented above:

- *Chlamydia psittaci* (bacterial)
- cryptococcosis (fungal)
- histoplasmosis (fungal)
- toxoplasmosis (protozoal)
- cryptosporidium organisms (protozoal)
- cytomegalovirus (viral)
- herpes simplex types 1 and 2 (virus)
- Kaposi's sarcoma (cancer).

All nurses need to have an extensive knowledge and understanding of the array of opportunistic infections that commonly present themselves in people who have HIV. Doing so will ensure that they are in a position to monitor, report and appropriately intervene in a timely manner. The early recognition of changes to a person's health status benefits the person and their family or significant other from further distress and hospitalisation. Healthcare occurs in an environment where health resources are scarce, fiscal restraint on healthcare delivery is a reality and hospitalisation is expensive (Jones, 2011). Consequently the early detection and treatment of health issues in people living with lifelong conditions like HIV/AIDS to prevent hospital admissions is one way of ensuring the health dollar goes further.

Collaboration with allied health professionals

As can be seen in the case studies, HIV impacts on all aspects of an individual's life. It is therefore important to take the broadest possible view of the disease process and involve allied health professionals as necessary — and it is almost always necessary. Many clients may present with, for instance, mental health issues, gender or sexual identity issues or substance misuse or dependency; in such cases, psychologists, psychiatrists, social workers, counsellors or substance misuse professionals may be helpful. If a person is having legal, financial, immigration, employment, housing, relationship or childcare problems, those concerns may distract them from taking care of themselves, and may affect access to or adherence to treatments; a referral to a social services worker will be in order. Other allied health professionals that have been or may in the future be recommended to contribute to Eric's, Fa'atasi's and Ruth's care include physiotherapists, occupational therapists, dietitians, podiatrists and pharmacists.

Much of nursing and medicine's work with people who live with HIV focuses on the psycho-physical aspects of the disease, keeping people alive as well as free from the harmful effects of HIV-related opportunistic infections. Many people with HIV use complementary and alternative medicine (CAM) in combination with biomedical (or 'allopathic') therapies to manage the effects of their chronic illness. For example, those who report chronic or unmanageable pain may find benefit from massage or acupuncture. In addition, some people with HIV may be either socially isolated or live with family or partners who may be afraid to touch them; therefore massage may provide the only opportunity for these people to be touched in a non-clinical or non-painful way. While there are many CAM therapies available, below is a list of some of those identified by Raper (2010) as being more commonly used. As you read through these, identify those that might be useful to encourage Eric, Fa'atasi and Ruth to consider:

- acupuncture
- herbal medicine
- manipulative and body-based therapies
- homeopathy
- meditation
- chiropractic
- the use of oil or incense
- reflexology
- massage
- meditation.

In summary, care for people with HIV must be understood as a team effort, with every person contributing their expertise.

Family and carers

The role of families and carers in HIV disease management is complex because many people with HIV are socially isolated either by choice or because they have been rejected by their families. In addition, families and carers themselves may be subject to stigma from their communities (Fouché et al., 2011). Fortunately, there are a number of HIV service organisations located throughout Australasia that can provide support to individuals living with HIV and their families (see the resources listed in the recommended reading and useful website sections at the end of this chapter). It is also important to recognise that there are many different constellations of families. As reflected in the case studies, people with HIV may have same- or opposite-sex partners; they may have children or parents, or grandparents; they may have people who are very close friends who accompany them to medical appointments and who help out at home. All these people will bring their own understandings of disease and wellness, confusion and clarity, despair and hope.

The most important thing that people both infected and affected by HIV need is information. They need to know that their healthcare providers will provide care and information and not judgment. There is a social stigma attached to having HIV that permeates society, negatively affecting quality of life and manifesting as affective symptoms of depression that can progress to suicide ideation (Machado, 2012). The people represented in the case studies are all susceptible to negative social attitudes related to their HIV status and their sexual orientation (Eric and Fa'atasi), for being a sex worker as well as using drugs (Fa'atasi) and for being a member of an ethnic minority (Ruth).

Frequently nurses are the first point of contact for people living with chronic illnesses such as HIV and spend more time with this group of people when compared with other health professional groups. It is therefore vital that nurses develop therapeutic relationships with people living with HIV, their families and significant others that are non-judgmental and accepting. The development of a supportive relationship based on these principles is more likely to positively influence health and wellbeing, including the adherence to treatment regimens (Neville & Henrickson, 2009).

As demonstrated in the case studies, nurses need to have a sound understanding of the principles of chronic illness such as HIV so they can reassure and support the family in the following ways:

- explaining that there will be good days and bad days as part of the illness experience
- providing education about the often complicated regimen of medications and the potential side effects of these medications
- reinforcing the importance of adhering to drug and treatment regimens — this is especially important in HIV/AIDS as lack of adherence can lead to drug resistance
- making sure the family understand the disease trajectory so they can monitor and provide a useful source of information to the health professionals they come in contact with
- reinforcing that people respond differently to challenges associated with living with HIV; for example, some people become profoundly depressed, some may even be affected by primary HIV and secondary infections of the brain itself, which result in mood changes and thought disorders, affecting the individual's ability to self-care; some people, however, may find new meaning and purpose, or a renewed sense of spirituality in their lives
- encouraging families and carers to be mindful of the stressful and even exhausting nature of supporting someone living with HIV and advising them about who to

Reflective questions

1. How can nurses ensure that people with HIV are provided with optimal care when engaging with health service organisations?
2. What areas of knowledge do you need to add to your skills in order to provide an appropriate health service for people living with HIV?
3. As a nurse what role do you have in preventing the spread of HIV?

call for help, respite care, advocacy or professional assistance when required — they should be encouraged to keep a directory of emergency phone numbers and phone numbers for community support agencies in an accessible location

- ensuring that families know that spiritual support is available for them and the person with HIV and where to access this support. The local AIDS service organisation will be an invaluable resource.

The provision of healthcare is highly political and nurses engage with the socio-political context of healthcare provision and the impact it has on consumers of healthcare services (Neville & Henrickson, 2009). Consequently, HIV can be seen as a political diagnosis; the lives of people living with an HIV-related illness are directly affected by government or private sector decisions and policies about, for example, what medications will be available (and at what cost), what services will be funded and which clinical trials they may have access to. Nurses need to be able to support and prepare families and caregivers to face the various political challenges that impact on the health and wellbeing of their family member living with HIV.

CONCLUSION

HIV shares many of the attributes associated with other chronic illnesses, including tiredness, a decrease in quality of life, an inability to independently undertake activities of daily living and being dependent on others. People living with a chronic illness, no matter what disease it is, are likely to have contact with healthcare, government and social service organisations. Most importantly, they will all come in contact with nurses at some stage of their illness experience. Nurses working in any area where they are likely to come in contact with people living with HIV need to have appropriate knowledge and skills in order to provide a quality and holistic healthcare experience for this group of people.

Recommended reading

Durham, J., & Lashley, F. (Eds.) (2010). *The person with HIV/AIDS. Nursing perspectives* (4th ed.). New York: Springer Publishing Company.

Gallant, J. (2009). *100 questions & answers about HIV and AIDS*. Boston: Jones and Bartlett Publishers.

Useful websites

Centers for Disease Control in the United States. www.cdc.gov/mmwr/preview/mmwrhtml/00018871.htm

Center for Disease Control and Prevention. www.cdc.gov/hiv/resources/factsheets/transmission.htm

The Australian Research Centre in Sex, Health and Society. www.hivpolicy.org/biogs/HPE0160b.htm

The New Zealand AIDS Foundation. www.NZAF.org.nz

The World Health Organization. www.who.int/en/

References

Adams, J., & Neville, S. (2009). Men who have sex with men account for nonuse of condoms. *Qualitative Health Research, 19*(12), 1669–1677.

Australian Red Cross Blood Service. (2012). Safety and testing. Retrieved July 12, 2012, from http://www.donateblood.com.au/page.aspx?IDDataTreeMenu=41&parent=30

Black, J., & Hawks, J. (Eds.) (2009). *Medical-surgical nursing. Clinical management for positive outcomes* (8th ed.). St Louis: Elsevier Saunders.

Bratt, G., Edlund, M., Cullberg, M., et al. (2009). Sexually transmitted infections (STI) in men who have sex with men (MSM). *The Open Infectious Diseases Journal, 3*, 118–127.

DeBeck, K., Kerr, T., Bird, L., et al. (2011). Injection drug use cessation and use of North America's first medically supervised safer injecting facility. *Drug and Alcohol Dependence, 113*, 172–176.

Durham, J., & Lashley, F. (Eds.) (2010). *The person with HIV/AIDS. Nursing perspectives* (4th ed.). New York: Springer Publishing Company.

Fouché, C., Henrickson, M., Poindexter, C., et al. (2011). *Standing in the fire: Experiences of HIV positive Black African migrants and refugees living in New Zealand.* Auckland: University of Auckland. Retrieved May 22, 2013, from http://www.education.auckland.ac.nz/webdav/site/education/shared/about/schools/chsswk/docs/HIV%20BAM_Research%20Report_%20August2011-web.pdf

Gallant, J. (2009). *100 questions & answers about HIV and AIDS.* Boston: Jones and Bartlett Publishers.

Goldenberg, S., Rangel, G., Vera, A., et al. (2012). Exploring the impact of underage sex work among female sex workers in two Mexico-US border cities. *AIDS and Behavior, 16*, 969–981.

Hendriksen, E., Pettifor, A., Lee, S., et al. (2007). Predictors of condom use among young adults in South Africa: The reproductive health and HIV Research Unit National Youth Survey. *American Journal of Public Health, 97*(7), 1241–1248.

Henrickson, M., & Neville, S. (2012). Identity satisfaction over the lifecourse in sexual minorities. *Journal of Gay & Lesbian Social Services, 24*(1), 80–95.

Jones, R. (2011). Hospital admission rates for COPD: The inverse care law is alive and well. *Thorax, 66*, 185–186.

Klebert, M. (2010). Managing symptoms in HIV disease. In J. Durham & F. Lashley (Eds.), *The person with HIV/AIDS. Nursing perspectives* (4th ed., pp. 293–320). New York: Springer Publishing Company.

Lerdal, A., Gay, C., Aouizerat, B., et al. (2011). Patterns of morning and evening fatigue among adults with HIV/AIDS. *Journal of Clinical Nursing, 20*, 2204–2216.

Lewis, S., Dirksen, S., Heitkemper, M., et al. (Eds.), (2011). *Medical-surgical nursing: Assessment and management of clinical problems* (8th ed.). St Louis: Elsevier.

Machado, S. (2012). Existential dimensions of surviving HIV: The experience of gay long-term survivors. *Journal of Humanistic Psychology, 52*(1), 6–29.

National Centre in HIV Epidemiology and Clinical Research. Australian HIV Surveillance Report, Vol 26, No 1, January 2010.

Neville, S., & Adams, J. (2009). Condom use in men who have sex with men: A literature review. *Contemporary Nurse, 33*(2), 130–139.

Neville, S., & Henrickson, M. (2009). The constitution of 'lavender families': A LGB perspective. *Journal of Clinical Nursing, 18*(6), 849–856.

Pepin, J. (2011). *The origins of AIDS*. Cambridge, UK: Cambridge University Press.

Raper, J. (2010). The medical management of HIV disease. In J. Durham & F. Lashley (Eds.), *The person with HIV/AIDS. Nursing perspectives* (4th ed., pp. 221–292). New York: Springer Publishing Company.

Saxton, P., Dickson, N., McAllister, S., et al. (2012). HIV prevalence among men who have sex with men in New Zealand 1985–2009: 25 years of public health monitoring. *International Journal of STD & AIDS, 23*, 274–279.

Stevens, P., & Hildebrandt, E. (2009). Pill taking from the perspective of HIV-infected women who are vulnerable to antiretroviral treatment failure. *Qualitative Health Research, 19*, 593–604.

Stolley, K., & Glass, J. (2009). *HIV/AIDS. Health and medical issues today*. Santa Barbara, California: Greenwood Press.

Sullivan, P., & Wolitski, R. (2008). HIV infection among gay and bisexual men. In R. Wolitski, R. Stall & R. Valdiserri (Eds.), *Unequal opportunity. Health disparities affecting gay and bisexual men in the United States* (pp. 220–247). New York: Oxford University Press.

Thompson, T., Lee, M., Clarke, T., et al. (2012). Prevalence of gastrointestinal symptoms among ambulatory HIV patients and a control population. *Annals of Gastroenterology, 25*, 1–6.

Turner, K., Hutchinson, S., Vickerman, P., et al. (2011). The impact of needle and syringe provision and opiate substitution therapy on the incidence of hepatitis C virus in injecting drug users: pooling of UK evidence. *Addiction, 106*(11), 1978–1988.

UNAIDS. (2011). *How to get zero. Faster. Smarter. Better. UNAIDS world AIDS day report 2011.* Geneva: United Nations.

Westercamp, M., Kawango, E., Jeckaniah, N., et al. (2012). Circumcision preference among women and uncircumcised men prior to scale-up of male circumcision for HIV prevention in Kisumu, Kenya. *AIDS Care: Psychological and Socio-medical Aspects of AIDS/HIV, 24*(2), 157–166.

CHAPTER 28

Patsy Yates

Cancer

Learning objectives

When you have completed this chapter you will be able to:

- appreciate the trajectory of cancer as a chronic disease and its implications for the physical and psychosocial wellbeing of people affected by cancer
- identify key principles for reducing the risk and identifying cancer early
- discuss factors influencing quality of life for people affected by cancer across the disease trajectory
- describe the information and support needs for people affected by cancer
- identify interventions to enhance quality of life for people at all stages of the cancer trajectory.

Key words

cancer, treatment effects, quality of life, survivorship, supportive care

INTRODUCTION

Cancer is a chronic and complex set of diseases. On average, one in two Australians will develop cancer and one in five will die from it before the age of 85 (Australian Institute of Health and Welfare and Australasian Association of Cancer Registries [AIHW & AACR], 2010). While cancer continues to be one of the most common causes of death amongst adult Australians and New Zealanders, considerable progress has been made in controlling this disease in recent years. The 5-year relative survival rate in Australia is around 61% (up from 47% for those diagnosed in the period from 1982–1986) (AIHW & AACR, 2010). In

New Zealand, 5-year relative survival rates are similarly increasing, currently at 63% (Ministry of Health, 2012). This progress means that there are an estimated 775 000 Australians alive today who have a history of cancer (AIHW, 2012). Such scientific advances mean that cancer today is considered a chronic disease.

Cancer is a set of diseases which have a natural history and course of progression, treatments and outcomes in the short and long term which vary markedly. This means that the experiences and needs of people at risk or affected by cancer will vary considerably. While it is a disease that does not have a series of well-marked events, critical points at which health professionals may intervene to improve cancer outcomes can be identified. For well communities these critical points include opportunities for reducing the risk of cancer and detecting the cancer early. For those with a diagnosis of cancer, critical points include opportunities for ensuring the best possible treatment and support during and after treatment and providing best care at end of life for those whose disease progresses (National Health Priority Action Council [NHPAC], 2006).

Responding effectively to meet the needs of the person affected by cancer at these critical intervention points requires an appreciation of cancer as a chronic disease, and the factors which may influence an individual's experiences and responses at key phases along this journey.

REDUCING RISK AND DETECTING CANCER EARLY

Behaviours which contribute to the development of the cancer

The cellular changes that characterise cancer are initiated by various degrees of interaction between endogenous biological and exogenous carcinogenic factors, including tobacco, alcohol, occupational exposure, environmental pollution, food contaminants, medicinal drugs, radiation, chronic infections, diet and nutrition, immunosuppression, genetic susceptibility and reproductive factors and hormones (International Agency for Cancer Control [IARC], 2008). Modifiable behavioural factors can thus play an important role in the development of cancer. The prevention of cancer, especially when integrated with the prevention of chronic diseases and other related problems, offers the greatest public health potential and the most cost-effective long-term method of cancer control (IARC, 2008).

Evidence to support the implementation of strategies to prevent cancer is growing. The World Health Organization (WHO) claims that we now have sufficient knowledge to prevent around 40% of all cancers (WHO, 2007), with evidence to support the effectiveness of interventions to address modifiable behavioural risk factors in areas including: tobacco control; exposure to ultraviolet radiation; diet; physical activity; overweight and obesity; and alcohol. The Cancer Council Australia (TCCA) has defined evidence-based policy targets for cancer prevention and recommended actions for health and community organisations and individual health professionals to achieve their proposed targets (TCCA, 2007). A summary of these recommended actions is presented in Box 28.1.

Participation in cancer screening programs

For the majority of cancers, outcomes are dramatically improved when the cancer is detected early. Promoting participation in early detection programs is a critical concern for health professionals in all areas of practice. In the context of cancer, early detection can be achieved through population screening programs (such as screening mammography, cervical cancer screening or faecal occult blood testing), opportunistic screening (such as through informal health checks) and diagnostic screening (that is, when a person

BOX 28.1
Cancer prevention aims: The Cancer Council Australia

Tobacco:

prevent the uptake of smoking

encourage and assist as many smokers as possible to quit as soon as possible

eliminate harmful exposure to tobacco smoke for non-smokers

where feasible, reduce the harm associated with continuing use of, and dependence on, tobacco and nicotine.

Ultraviolet radiation:

change the attitudes, knowledge and skills of individuals, particularly young people, about skin cancer and sun protection

develop strategies for the early detection and effective diagnosis of skin cancer

achieve health settings, organisations, products, policies and practices that promote sun protection

strengthen the community's capacity for coordinated action on skin cancer prevention

inform the design, implementation and evaluation of skin cancer prevention strategies.

Nutrition:

consume nutritionally adequate and varied diets based primarily on foods of plant origin such as vegetables, fruit, pulses and wholegrain cereals, as well as lean meats, fish and low fat dairy products

ensure children have a nutritionally adequate and varied diet along similar lines with appropriate moderation to suit different age groups

maintain a healthy body weight through a balance of food intake and physical activity.

Physical activity:

maintain a least a minimum level of physical activity: for adults at least 30 minutes of moderate-intensity activity on most days of the week; for children and adolescents at least 60 minutes

participate in physical activity of longer duration and higher intensity, to further reduce colon cancer risk, where possible across the lifespan

maintain a health body weight through a balance of food intake and physical activity.

Overweight and obesity:

maintain a health body weight throughout life by means of a balance of food intake and physical activity

consume nutritionally adequate and varied diets based primarily on foods of plant origin such as vegetables, fruit, pulses and wholegrain cereals, as well as lean meats, fish and low fat dairy products

adopt a physically active lifestyle

ensure children have a nutritionally adequate and varied diet and adopt an active lifestyle appropriate to different age groups.

Alcohol:

increase awareness of the link between alcohol consumption and cancer risk among health authorities, health professionals and the community

encourage efforts to reduce alcohol consumption.

Source: The Cancer Council Australia (2007).

presents with symptoms for investigation). While familial cancers that are caused by inherited genetic mutations account for only around 5–10% of cancers, the growth in understanding of many of the genes responsible for heritable mutations is also raising a range of issues in relation to cancer screening (National Health and Medical Research Council, 1999).

Despite the importance of early detection, rates of participation in screening programs vary between different social demographic groups. For example, women from a non-English-speaking background and Aboriginal and Torres Strait Islander women have lower participation rates in mammographic screening programs (Breast Screen Australia, 2009). Understanding barriers to cancer screening enables health professionals to implement targeted intervention strategies to promote participation. For example, barriers to cancer screening that are potentially amenable to intervention include financial concerns, concern about radiation, embarrassment, poor access, anxiety about test results, inconvenience, forgetting or procrastination and discomfort associated with the screening test (TCCA, 2007). The *National service improvement framework for cancer* (NHPAC, 2006) has defined principles which should underpin optimal services in relation to cancer screening. These principles are described in Box 28.2. They provide a framework for health professionals to

BOX 28.2
National service improvement framework for cancer: Optimal services: Finding cancer early

People will have access to high quality population screening programs.

People will have information about population screening programs for cancer including:

- the purpose of the screening, its benefits, downsides and limitations and differences between cancers
- which cancers can be detected early
- information to assist in their decision about whether to participate in population screening programs
- information appropriate for people from disadvantaged groups, especially Aboriginal and Torres Strait Islander people and people from culturally and linguistically diverse backgrounds.

Cost effective population screening programs will be readily accessible to all Australians and their participation will be facilitated by:

- people will not be prevented from participating by cost or access barriers
- Aboriginal and Torres Strait Islander people and people from culturally and linguistically diverse backgrounds will have access to services appropriate to their needs, and targeted to special barriers to participation
- health professionals will provide advice about participation in population screening programs to eligible people
- information about reasons for screening and screening intervals will be provided to all participants, and reminders sent when screening is due.

Source: National Health Priority Action Council (2006).

consider areas in which they may intervene to ensure optimal outcomes from cancer screening at the population and individual level.

ENSURING BEST POSSIBLE TREATMENT AND SUPPORT DURING AND AFTER ACTIVE TREATMENT

Issues of quality of life in relation to cancer

The cancer disease process and contemporary cancer treatments present many challenges to an individual's quality of life. Cancer is a multi-system disease, and its treatments are typically multi-modal, including surgery, chemotherapy, radiotherapy, biotherapy and/or hormone therapy. Cancer treatment programs also tend to be long term, often requiring several administrations or doses delivered over a period of many months. Each of these treatments is associated with a range of short-term and longer-term effects on an individual's quality of life.

The presence and severity of the effects will vary from individual to individual, although the factors underlying these differences are not completely understood. Quality of life concerns for the person affected by cancer thus include many physical, psychosocial and practical issues and, for some, end of life concerns. Box 28.3 provides a summary of the key quality of life concerns that may be experienced by people affected by cancer, many of which persist during and after treatment for cancer.

With improvements in cancer treatment, survival from cancer has been extended. A growing body of research has highlighted that cancer survivors have a unique set of health and support needs. For the majority of people diagnosed with cancer, the disease and its effects thus become chronic in nature. The specific risk for recurrence or late effects experienced by an individual who has undergone treatment for cancer will usually depend on the specific site, histology of their disease, the treatments they received, when those treatments were delivered (since regimens and techniques change over time), the length of time that has elapsed since those exposures and underlying risk factors independent of their cancer or its treatment (Institute of Medicine [IOM], 2006). Moreover, as cancer is largely a disease of the elderly, determining the late effects of the cancer disease and treatment process from unrelated co-morbid conditions can be difficult (IOM, 2006). While there is considerable heterogeneity in post-treatment experiences for people with cancer, a number of common quality of life concerns have been identified for cancer survivors. These are summarised in Box 28.4.

Cancer is a life threatening disease. Unfortunately, despite developments in cancer treatments, nearly 40% of those diagnosed with cancer will ultimately die from their disease. For those who have disease recurrence, or for those whose disease is progressing, some important and unique quality of life concerns arise during end-of-life care. Some of these concerns are presented in Box 28.5.

Our review of quality of life concerns for people affected by cancer as a chronic disease highlights the significant impact of this disease on day-to-day living, both during and following the treatment process. Indeed, many people asked about their experience of cancer can describe numerous examples of how the problems resulting from cancer or its treatment affect their daily activities in the short and longer term. Nurses are well placed to respond to these concerns, by assessment of the factors contributing to these problems, and applying evidence-based interventions relevant to the individual's needs.

BOX 28.3
Summary of the major issues faced by people with cancer

EMOTIONAL AND SOCIAL ISSUES

Psychological issues:

body image
sexuality
interpersonal problems
new relationships post diagnosis
stress and adjustment reactions/severe emotional distress
anxiety, depression, PTSD.

Practical issues:

costs
reconstructive surgery
lymphoedema
travel and accommodation
other support needs
loss of income
difficulties with business dealings
legal issues related to advanced disease.

SURVIVAL ISSUES

Physical issues:

nausea and vomiting
pain
fatigue
fertility
lymphoedema
disfigurement
odour
incontinence
bowel dysfunction
cognitive problems
communication difficulties
malnutrition
respiratory symptoms.

End of life concerns.

Source: National Breast Cancer Centre and National Cancer Control Initiative (2003).
In February 2008, National Breast Cancer Centre (NBCC), incorporation the Ovarian Cancer Program, changed its name to National Breast and Ovarian Cancer Centre (NBOCC). On 30 June 2011, NBOCC amalgamated with Cancer Australia, to form a single national agency, Cancer Australia.

NURSING RESPONSES TO KEY QUALITY OF LIFE CONCERNS FOR PEOPLE AFFECTED BY CANCER

Altered mobility and fatigue — relationship to activities of daily living

Many people undergoing cancer treatment identify fatigue as a frequent and significant treatment side effect and that this is a symptom that persists long after treatment ends (Goedendorp et al., 2012). Fatigue is an almost universal symptom reported across diagnostic and treatment categories at all phases of the lifespan, being as high as 90–100% for people with advanced disease. Qualitative studies have identified that people describe cancer-related fatigue as making them feel angry, frustrated and depressed, as it prevents them from doing some of the most basic day-to-day activities and has major impacts on

BOX 28.4
Quality of life concerns for cancer survivors

Physical issues:

- fatigue
- reduced function
- dysphagia, heartburn, altered taste and smell, problems with saliva
- physical sequelae (stoma, scars, disfigurement)
- lymphoedema
- pain.

Sexual issues:

- sexual difficulties
- vaginal dryness, stenosis.

Emotional issues

- fear, anxiety, distress
- reflection on values, sense of identity
- relationship concerns
- sense of guilt
- concerns about recurrence
- concerns about family.

Social concerns:

- changes to relationships
- employment concerns
- financial concerns.

Source: National Breast Cancer Centre and National Cancer Control Initiative (2003).
In February 2008, National Breast Cancer Centre (NBCC), incorporation the Ovarian Cancer Program, changed its name to National Breast and Ovarian Cancer Centre (NBOCC). On 30 June 2011, NBOCC amalgamated with Cancer Australia, to form a single national agency, Cancer Australia.

BOX 28.5
Quality of life concerns at end of life

- Symptoms, including nausea, pain, dyspnoea, fatigue, anorexia, vomiting, constipation, abdominal bloating, lymphoedema.
- Decreased ability to perform activities of daily living and self-care.
- Grief, anxiety, depression, adjustment problems.
- Disrupted social relationships, concerns about family.
- Existential and spiritual distress.

Source: National Breast Cancer Centre and National Cancer Control Initiative (2003).
In February 2008, National Breast Cancer Centre (NBCC), incorporation the Ovarian Cancer Program, changed its name to National Breast and Ovarian Cancer Centre (NBOCC). On 30 June 2011, NBOCC amalgamated with Cancer Australia, to form a single national agency, Cancer Australia.

BOX 28.6
Treatable factors contributing to fatigue

Medication side effects
Pain
Emotional distress
- Depression
- Anxiety

Anaemia
Sleep disturbance
Nutritional disturbances
- Weight/caloric intake changes
- Fluid electrolyte imbalance

Decreased functional status
- Decreased activity
- Decreased physical fitness

Comorbidities
- Alcohol/substance abuse
- Cardiac dysfunction
- Endocrine dysfunction
- Gastrointestinal dysfunction
- Hepatic dysfunction
- Infection
- Neurological dysfunction
- Pulmonary dysfunction
- Renal dysfunction

Source: Ann M. Berger et al., NCCN Clinical Practice Guidelines in Oncology (NCCN Guidelines®) Cancer related fatigue V1.2013 (c) 2013 National Comprehensive Cancer Network, Inc. Available at NCCN.org. Accessed October 28th, 2012.

social lives (Scott, Lasch, Barsevick, & Piault-Louis, 2011). In contrast to healthy individuals, people with cancer have fatigue that is more persistent and distressing (Goedendorp et al., 2012). The exact mechanisms of cancer-related fatigue are not well understood, but may involve pro-inflammatory cytokines, circadian rhythm de-synchronisation or skeletal muscle deregulation (NCCN®, 2013). Box 28.6 presents a summary of the factors which may contribute to fatigue in people affected by cancer, highlighting the multidimensional nature of this problem.

Assessment of the factors contributing to an individual's fatigue is integral to effectively managing this problem. Recent research has highlighted a number of interventions that nurses can use to manage cancer-related fatigue, during treatment and in the post-treatment phase. These interventions include:

- patient/family education and counselling; for example, information about patterns of fatigue
- general strategies; for example, energy conservation, distraction

- non-pharmacological strategies; for example, activity enhancement; psychological interventions (stress management, relaxation); attention-restoring therapy; nutrition consultation; sleep therapy; family interaction (NCCN, 2013).

People with cancer may also experience altered mobility and function as a result of their disease or its treatment. This can be due to the impact of a primary cancer on corticospinal and corticobulbar tracts (e.g. with some brain tumours) or the secondary effects of metastatic disease (e.g. spinal cord compression or other obstructions) (Pearce, 2005). It may also be due to the impact of treatments (e.g. restrictions due to surgery, or alterations from the neurotoxic effects of cancer treatments that result in peripheral neuropathies). Other disease- and treatment-related symptoms, such as pain or fatigue, may also result in impaired mobility. Strategies for optimising function for the person affected by cancer will thus be influenced by the specific factors causing the impaired function. There is increasing evidence, however, that exercise has a number of physical and psychological benefits for people both during and following cancer treatment (Mishra et al., 2012). Available reviews indicate that exercise interventions during adjuvant treatment for breast cancer can be regarded as a supportive self-care intervention which results in improved physical fitness and the capacity for performing activities of daily life (Markes, Brockow, & Resch, 2007). There is limited research investigating the role of rehabilitative interventions to improve function in the longer term following completion of cancer treatment.

Body image — impact for the person and their family carers

Living with cancer may affect *personal* self-concept (facts about the self or a person's self-opinion); *social* self-concept (perceptions of how one is regarded by others); and self-ideals (perceptions of oneself with respect to how one would like to be) (National Breast Cancer Centre and National Cancer Control Initiative [NBCC & NCCI], 2005, p. 16). That is, a diagnosis of cancer can threaten one's confidence in their body, and raise existential challenges which alter the way we think about our place in the social world. Moreover, cancer treatments can produce various temporary changes (e.g. hair loss, weight loss, weight gain and alterations in the appearance of the skin) and permanent alterations (e.g. minor scarring, loss of a body part or loss of bodily and sexual function) in a patient's physical appearance (NBCC & NCCI, 2005).

These types of bodily changes have been identified as being of concern for patients with many different types of cancers, including breast, prostate, gynaecological, head and neck, laryngeal and skin cancers (NBCC & NCCI, 2005). As many as 52% of people diagnosed with cancer identify that having support to deal with changes in their body is important (Soothill et al., 2001). These concerns about body image can last long after completion of cancer treatment. One study identified that 16–54% of women post-treatment reported dislike for a given body image item (e.g. 'My body is sexually unappealing'; 'I dislike my physique'; 'I am physically unattractive'), and 11%–34% of men reported dislike for the same items (DeFrank, Mehta, Stein, & Baker, 2007).

It is important for nurses to explore whether the patient has significant concerns about the impact of treatments on their body or sense of self. Possible questions to prompt discussions about these concerns include (NBCC & NCCI, 2005, p. 87):

> We don't often talk about it, but cancer certainly changes how we feel about ourselves. Many people tell me that they do have concerns about how they will look, and how they will feel about themselves after treatment. Is this something that you feel you could discuss with me?

A range of practical prosthetic or rehabilitative devices or procedures may be suitable for some people affected by cancer. For example, reconstructive surgery for breast cancer can be offered to improve a woman's body image. Other supportive and educative interventions that may assist include programs such as the *Look Good … Feel Better* program. The purpose of the program, which is widely available through Cancer Councils and specialist cancer settings, is to help people manage the appearance-related side effects of chemotherapy and radiotherapy, thereby helping to restore appearance and self image.

FAMILY AND CARERS OF PEOPLE AFFECTED BY CANCER

Cancer is a disease experienced by the whole family. Studies suggest that couples react to cancer as an 'emotional system' as the distress experienced by the person with cancer is closely linked with the emotional wellbeing of the family (Northouse, 2012). Family members can also play an important role as caregivers, providing physical, practical and emotional support to meet the diverse needs of their relative. The needs and concerns of families are therefore considerable across all phases of the cancer journey. Studies suggest that common needs of caregivers during treatment can be: having questions answered; being assured best treatment is being provided; knowing the outcomes of illness; having explanations given in terms that are understandable; and being informed of changes in their relative's condition (Nikoletti, Kristjanson, Tataryn, McPhee, & Burt, 2003). During this time, families also often have to adjust to different roles and deal with strains associated with changes to social functioning and interpersonal relationships.

Studies have also reported that the majority of partners of people affected by cancer report at least one supportive care need 1–11 years post diagnosis, indicating the ongoing impact of cancer (Hodgkinson et al., 2007). Approximately half of partners surveyed reported at least one unmet need, most frequently in the domains of relationships, information and partner impact. The most frequently endorsed unmet needs by partners were 'help to reduce stress in their partner's life', 'accessible hospital parking' and 'local health care services' (Hodgkinson et al., 2007).

The needs of family members at the end of life become of particular importance, as family caregivers often take on substantial caregiving roles while at the same time having to deal with the distress associated with losing a loved one. Some unique family-related challenges for health professionals when caring for families at end of life include high symptom distress, strained family relationships, feelings of abandonment, competing outside demands (e.g. work), lack of financial and community support and poor self-care (exercise, diet) (Northouse, 2012).

A range of interventions can be applied to support family caregivers throughout the cancer journey. These interventions need to be based on a comprehensive assessment of family needs and fall into four categories: providing information; providing psychological support; providing physical support; and mobilising resources (Ferrall, 2006). Such supportive interventions can be delivered through family conferences, skills training, problem solving, caregiver training and information resources. Enabling access to additional support services such as respite, home modification or community support groups to deal with the longer-term impact of cancer as a chronic disease may also be helpful (Ferrall, 2006).

EDUCATION AND SUPPORT FOR THE PERSON AND FAMILY AFFECTED BY CANCER

The emotional and support needs of people affected by cancer are wide-ranging and profound. These psychosocial needs are significant, and frequently go undetected and unmet

(NBCC & NCCI, 2005). Screening all patients for supportive care needs is an essential component of nursing practice in all settings. For example, the Supportive Care Screening Tool developed by Peter MacCallum Cancer Centre (http://supportivecancercarevictoria.org/Resources/rDOCs/Screening_Tools_Summary.pdf) comprises a checklist covering aspects of the individual's health and wellbeing to enable identification of needs. These areas include:

- communication and understanding
- physical health
- emotional health
- activities of daily living
- support and coping
- use of support services
- information requirements.

Once needs have been identified, responses that are targeted and tailored to an individual's needs are required. A tiered model of care has been suggested as a stepped care approach that aims to match the patient's or family member's level of distress and expressed need to an appropriate level of psychosocial intervention (Steginga, Hutchinson, Turner, & Dunn, 2006). Components in this tiered model include:

- universal care: information, brief emotional and practical support (e.g. healthcare team, Cancer Helpline)
- supportive care: emotional, practical, spiritual care, psycho-education, values-based decision support, peer support (e.g. social worker, peers, chaplain, Cancer Helpline)
- extended care: counselling, time-limited therapy, skills training (e.g. psychologist, social work, tele-based cancer counselling service)
- specialist care: specialised therapy for depression, anxiety, relationship problems (e.g. psychologist, psychiatrist, tele-based cancer counselling service)
- acute care: intensive or comprehensive therapy for acute and complex problems (e.g. mental health team, psychiatrist).

According to this model, services are provided according to the level of need. Importantly, as a minimum, all persons require access to the components of universal care, including information and brief emotional and social support. Such informational and supportive interventions are fundamental elements of nursing care for people affected by cancer at all stages of the journey.

Specifically, education for the person and family affected by cancer involves a series of structured or non-structured experiences designed to help the person and their family to develop knowledge and self-care abilities needed to manage the impact of cancer and its treatments on their wellbeing. For the nurse seeking to design an effective educational intervention for people with cancer, there appears an overwhelming number of considerations to be taken into account. For example, issues to be considered may include what type/s of educational process should be employed, what the focus (content, topics) of the educational intervention should be and what is the ideal context and most appropriate methods for delivering an intervention. Current evidence suggests that a multi-faceted approach, in which information is provided by healthcare professionals using a variety of media, may best satisfy most people, and that it is important to elicit and respond to the individual's own concerns and information needs (NBCC & NCCI, 2005). Issues related to the accessibility of an intervention to various groups, the responsiveness of an intervention to diverse contexts and needs as well as the efficiency with which interventions can be delivered are also important considerations for healthcare providers.

One model to guide nurses is the TEC model (tailored education and coaching). The TEC model is a brief, patient-centred model that is underpinned by social cognitive theory. The components of the TEC model include:

- assessment of current knowledge, attitudes and preferences (values)
- correction of misconceptions about the disease, treatment and/or side effects
- teaching of relevant concepts — this could include self-management skills, as well as increasing confidence when communicating with the health team
- planning which includes identifying goals, matching strategies to goals
- rehearsal using role play exercises
- portrayal of learned skills (Glasgow, Davis, Funnell, & Beck, 2003).

CONCLUSION

A diagnosis of cancer is an enormously distressing and disruptive experience for the person diagnosed and their family. As a multi-system disease, which typically requires multiple systemic treatments over long periods of time, cancer is today a chronic disease. There are many points throughout the cancer journey where nurses can intervene to improve a person's quality of life. In particular, nurses are well placed to provide information and supportive care to help promote a person's health and wellbeing and enhance the person's ability to prevent and manage disease- and treatment-related effects in the short and longer term. Cancer is a chronic disease which can have long lasting impacts for the person and their family. Applying best available evidence to manage these impacts has the potential to significantly reduce mortality and morbidity from the disease.

CASE STUDY 28.1

Mrs Jones is a 58-year-old woman with three children and two grandchildren who has just undergone routine screening mammography in the nearby breast screen service. Mrs Jones is accompanied by her husband as she returns to her GP for discussion of the results. Mrs Jones' GP explains that the mammography indicates she has evidence of breast cancer, and she will need to be referred to the breast clinic at the local hospital for follow-up. Mrs Jones and her husband are extremely distressed and shocked. While Mrs Jones is slightly overweight, she does not understand how she could have developed this cancer. She explains that she has not attended the routine screening mammography when she received reminder letters in recent years because she has been too busy with her new grandchildren and work commitments. Mrs Jones is anxious to find out more information about what is likely to happen, and searches the internet to find information to answer her questions. The practice nurse at the GP clinic spends some time talking with Mr and Mrs Jones about the planned visit to the breast clinic, and assists them to make an appointment at the centre. The nurse ensures all appropriate clinical information and diagnostic tests are forwarded to the clinic as part of the referral.

CASE STUDY 28.1 — cont'd

Mrs Jones is referred to a multidisciplinary team at the cancer centre for treatment planning. Following breast conserving surgery for early stage breast cancer, she undergoes a course of adjuvant chemotherapy and radiotherapy. Her treatment goes well; however, she experiences a range of side effects including oral mucositis, persistent nausea and fatigue. The nurses in the treatment centre teach Mrs Jones and her husband how to prevent and treat her side effects. They provide a range of written resources so that they can manage at home, including information about what signs or symptoms should prompt Mrs Jones to return to her doctor or call the clinic for advice between treatments.

During the treatment program, Mr Jones also tells the nurse he is having trouble coping with his wife's diagnosis. He feels helpless, not knowing what he can do to help her. He also worries about their future and if the cancer will return. The nurses refer Mr Jones to information resources provided by the local cancer council and teach him some techniques to help him relax. Mr Jones also tells the nurse that he has convinced his wife to visit a naturopath to see if they can do anything to help her beat her cancer. The nurse provides information to Mr Jones from the local cancer council about the use of complementary and alternative medicines in cancer. The nurses encourage Mr and Mrs Jones to discuss any decisions with them and with the doctor.

Mrs Jones completes her treatment and talks with nurses about diet and exercise recommendations that would help her to maintain her health into the future. She says she has read lots of information on the internet, but is not sure what sources of information she should access to ensure it is reputable. She is also keen to establish an exercise program that fits with her busy schedule, including work and looking after her grandchildren.

Twelve months after completing her treatment, Mrs Jones is returning for another routine check-up. She says the fatigue is still a problem, and still worries a lot about her cancer returning, and that these visits for check-ups are especially hard for her husband. She says her life is now very different as a result of her cancer. She is maintaining a regular exercise program and has lost a few kilos to be at a healthy weight. Mrs Jones admits her relationship with her husband has changed, as he seems to want to 'wrap her in cotton wool'. She also says it has been helpful to access a local support group, as she finds it helpful to be able to talk about what is worrying her and her fears about the future with others who are going through the same experience.

Reflective questions

1 What are likely to be some of the major physical, psychological and social concerns of a person during and following treatment for cancer? How might these needs change for a person whose cancer recurs, and whose illness progresses?

2 How would you respond to questions from a person with cancer about what they can do to optimise their health during and following treatment for cancer? What community and information resources are available in your region to assist the person affected by cancer?

3 What are some of the key features of an effective education program for people with cancer?

Recommended readings

Brown, C. (Ed.) (2009). Guide to Oncology Symptom Management. Pittsburgh, PA: Oncology Nursing Society.

Fitch, M. I. (2006). Programmatic approaches to psychosocial support. In R. M. Carroll-Johnson, L. M. Gorman & N. J. Bush (Eds.), *Psychosocial nursing care along the cancer continuum* (2nd ed., pp. 419–438). Pittsburgh, PA: Oncology Nursing Society.

Institutes of Medicine. (2006). *Implementing Cancer Survivorship Care Planning*. Washington: Author.

National Breast Cancer Centre and National Cancer Control Initiative [NBCC & NCCI]. (2005). *Clinical guidelines for the psychosocial care of adults with cancer*. Canberra: National Health and Medical Research Council.

Olver, I. (Ed.) (2011). *The MASCC Textbook of Cancer Supportive Care and Survivorship*. New York: Springer.

References

Ann, M. Berger, et al. *NCCN Clinical Practice Guidelines in Oncology (NCCN Guidelines®) Cancer related fatigue V1.2013 (c) 2013*. National Comprehensive Cancer Network, Inc. Available at NCCN.org. Accessed October 28th, 2012.

Australian Institute of Health and Welfare and Australasian Association of Cancer Registries [AIHW & AACR]. (2010). *Cancer in Australia: An overview, 2010*. Canberra: Author.

Australian Institute of Health and Welfare [AIHW]. (2012). *Cancer survival and prevalence in Australia: period estimates from 1982 to 2010. Cancer Series no. 69. Cat. no. CAN 65*. Canberra: AIHW.

Breast Screen Australia. (2009). *Breast Screen Australia Evaluation: Final Evaluation Report, Commonwealth of Australia*. Canberra: Commonwealth of Australia.

DeFrank, J., Mehta, C., Stein, K., et al. (2007). Body image dissatisfaction in cancer survivors. *Oncology Nursing Forum*, *34*(3), 625–632.

Ferrall, S. (2006). Caring for the family caregiver. In R. Carroll-Johnson, L. Gorman & N. Bush (Eds.), *Psychosocial nursing care along the cancer continuum* (pp. 603–610). Pittsburgh: Oncology Nursing Society.

Glasgow, R., Davis, C., Funnell, M., et al. (2003). Implementing practical interventions to support chronic illness self-management. *Joint Commission Journal on Quality and Safety*, *29*(11), 563–574.

Goedendorp, M., Andrykowski, M., Donovan, K., et al. (2012). Prolonged impact of chemotherapy on fatigue in breast cancer survivors: a longitudinal comparison with radiotherapy-treated breast cancer survivors and noncancer controls. *Cancer*, *118*(15), 3833–3841.

Hodgkinson, K., Butow, P., Hobbs, K., et al. (2007). Assessing unmet supportive care needs in partners of cancer survivors: The development and evaluation of the Cancer Survivors' Partners Unmet Needs measure. *Psychooncology*, *16*, 805–813.

Institutes of Medicine. (2006). *Implementing Cancer Survivorship Care Planning*. Washington: Author.

International Agency for Cancer Research. (2008). *World Cancer Report*. Lyon: IARC Press.

Markes, M., Brockow, T., & Resch, K. (2007). Exercise for women receiving adjuvant therapy for breast cancer. *Cochrane Database of Systematic Reviews*, Issue 4. Art No: CD005001. doi: 10.1002/14651858.CD005001.pub2

Ministry of Health. (2012). *Cancer Patient Survival Change Over Time Update: Covering the Period 1994 to 2009*. Wellington: Ministry of Health.

Mishra, S., Scherer, R., Snyder, C., et al. (2012). Exercise interventions on health-related quality of life for people with cancer during active treatment. *Cochrane Database of Systematic Reviews*, Issue 8. Art No: CD008465. doi: 10.1002/14651858.CD008465.pub2

National Breast Cancer Centre and National Cancer Control Initiative. (2003). *Clinical practice guidelines for the psychosocial care of adults with cancer*. Camperdown, NSW: National Breast Cancer Centre.

National Health and Medical Research Council. (1999). *Clinical practice guidelines. Familial aspects of cancer: A guide to clinical practice*. Canberra: Author.

National Health Priority Action Council (NHPAC). (2006). *National Service Improvement Framework for Cancer*. Canberra: Australian Government Department of Health and Ageing.

Nikoletti, S., Kristjanson, L., Tataryn, D., et al. (2003). Information needs and coping styles of primary family caregivers of women following breast cancer surgery. *Oncology Nursing Forum*, *30*(6), 987–996.

Northouse, L. (2012). The impact of caregiving on the psychological well-being of family caregivers and cancer patients. *Seminars in Oncology Nursing*, *28*(4), 236.

Pearce, J. (2005). Alterations in mobility, skin integrity, and neurological status. In J. Itano & K. Taoko (Eds.), *Core curriculum for oncology nursing* (3rd ed.). Philadelphia: W. B. Saunders.

Scott, J., Lasch, K., Barsevick, A., et al. (2011). Patients' experiences with cancer-related fatigue: A review and synthesis of qualitative research. *Oncology Nursing Forum*, *38*(3), E191–E203.

Steginga, S., Hutchinson, S., Turner, J., et al. (2006). Translating psychosocial care: Guidelines into action. *Cancer Forum*, *31*(1), 28–31.

Soothill, K., Morris, S. M., Harman, J., et al. (2001). The significant unmet needs of cancer patients: Probing psychosocial concerns. *Supportive Care in Cancer*, *9*, 597–605.

The Cancer Council Australia. (2007). *National Cancer Prevention Policy 2007–09*. NSW: Author.

World Health Organization. (2007). *Cancer Control: Knowledge into Action. WHO Guide for Effective Programs. Prevention.* Retrieved November 12, 2012, http://whqlibdoc.who.int/publications/2007/9241547111_eng.pdf

INDEX

Page numbers followed by 'f' indicate figures, 't' indicate tables, and 'b' indicate boxes.

K

L

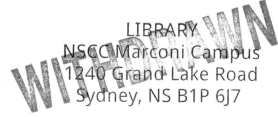